Cardiovascular Physiology

CARDIOVASCULAR PHYSIOLOGY

William R. Milnor, M.D.
PROFESSOR OF PHYSIOLOGY
THE JOHNS HOPKINS UNIVERSITY
SCHOOL OF MEDICINE

New York   Oxford
OXFORD UNIVERSITY PRESS
1990

Oxford University Press

Oxford   New York   Toronto
Delhi   Bombay   Calcutta   Madras   Karachi
Petaling Jaya   Singapore   Hong Kong   Tokyo
Nairobi   Dar es Salaam   Cape Town
Melbourne   Auckland
and associated companies in
Berlin   Ibadan

Copyright © 1990 by Oxford University Press, Inc.

Published by Oxford University Press, Inc.,
200 Madison Avenue, New York, New York 10016
Oxford is a registered trademark of Oxford University Press

Library of Congress Cataloging-in-Publication Data
Milnor, William R.
Cardiovascular physiology / William R. Milnor.
p.   cm. Includes bibliographical references.
ISBN 0-19-505884-4
1. Cardiovascular system—Physiology.   I. Title.
[DNLM: 1. Cardiovascular System—physiology.
WG 102 M659c]   QP102.M55   1990   612.1—dc20   DNLM/DLC
for Library of Congress   89-23002

9 8 7 6 5 4 3 2 1
Printed in the United States of America
on acid-free paper

To
Kathy
Bill
and R.J.

PREFACE

Cardiovascular physiology has expanded to such an extent that most of us must be content to cultivate only a small segment of it, yet we cannot do without some broad sense of the field as a whole. The present work is an attempt to address that need by surveying the subject in a comprehensive although by no means exhaustive manner.

This book has two purposes. It is intended to serve as an introduction to the subject for the beginning medical or graduate student, and at the same time to be of value as a reference work for advanced readers. More information is provided than is usually covered in a first-year course, but I have found that students welcome the chance to explore in some depth the topics that arouse their interest. Readers approaching the subject for the first time will want to become acquainted in a general way with the subject matter of each chapter, but they should feel no compulsion to study every detail in every section. A list of sections suitable for an introductory course follows the Table of Contents.

For those who are already familiar with the elements of cardiovascular physiology, I have tried to provide more detailed information and to point the way to the scientific literature by citing selected reviews and research papers. My goal has been a volume that meets the needs of students at all levels, including cardiologists and investigators in other fields, a work of reference that is intermediate between the most elementary textbooks and definitive works like the *Handbook of Physiology* series published by the American Physiological Society.

The references include older papers as well as recent publications. Physiology is not a new science, and on some matters the original reports are still the best source of information. The subject is one with a long history and a promising future, in which the fundamental mechanisms of physiological regulation are slowly being uncovered. Indeed, the fascination of physiology today lies in the resonance between earlier observations and modern cell physiology—the explanation of well-known biological phenomena by new discoveries at the molecular level. Access to microcosmic events has greatly advanced the understanding of intact, living organisms, the goal to which the physiologist is committed. Many important questions remain unanswered, however, as I have indicated throughout this volume.

In writing this survey I have been keenly aware of the debt owed to my teachers and associates, which I acknowledge with gratitude. The late Dr. Philip Bard, my first teacher in physiology, was a scientist whose breadth of mind and fascination with living things communicated themselves to everyone around him. The colleagues with whom I have shared the excitement of research since then are too numerous to list, but each of them has contributed to my education and to happy recollections of our work together. As every teacher knows, my students have also been a constant source of stimulation, and my thanks go to them for keeping me on my toes.

Finally, I welcome the opportunity to express my appreciation to the organizations that have supported my research work: the National Institutes of Health, the National Science Foundation, the American Heart Association and its Maryland affiliate, and the Howell-Cannon Fund.

Baltimore   W.R.M.
June 1989

CONTENTS

Sections Recommended for an Introductory Course in Cardiovascular Physiology, xiii

1. The Circulatory System, 3
Structure and Function, 3
Blood Pressure and Blood Flow, 17
Control and Regulation of the System, 20
Cellular Receptors, 21

2. Normal State of the Circulation, 29
Definitions of Normality, 30
Cardiac Output, 31
Dimensions of the System, 39
Pulsations of Pressure, 43
Pulsatile Blood Flow, 49
Effects of Age, 52
The Influence of Body Size, 54

3. Properties of Cardiac Cells, 62
Morphology, 62
Cell Receptors, 69
Excitation of the Heart, 70
Transmembrane Potentials, 76

Mechanisms of Conduction, 88
Myocardial Contraction, 90
Cardioactive Agents, 102

4. **The Heart as a Pump,** 111
    Events of the Cardiac Cycle, 111
    Determinants of Ventricular Function, 116
    Cardiac Output and Work, 127
    Interaction Between Heart and Circulation, 131
    Cardiac Failure, 135

5. **Electrical Activity of the Heart,** 140
    The Cardiac Electrical Field, 140
    Electrocardiography, 143
    Disturbances of Conduction, 153
    Disturbances of Rate and Rhythm, 155

6. **Principles of Hemodynamics,** 171
    Steady Flow, 172
    Vascular Distensibility, 184
    Pulsatile Pressure and Flow, 198
    Branching Systems, 212
    Circular Systems, 214
    Hemodynamic Effects of Vasomotor Activity, 215

7. **The Cardiovascular Control System,** 219
    Central Nervous System, 220
    Cardiovascular Sensors, 225
    Extrinsic Sources of Afferent Signals, 243

8. **Autonomic and Peripheral Control Mechanisms,** 249
    Autonomic Nervous System, 249
    Endocrine Control, 267
    Paracrine Control, 271
    Integrated Reactions to Stress, 277

9. **Vascular Smooth Muscle and Its Regulation**, 290

Structure and Function, 291
Vascular Heterogeneity, 297
Neural Excitation, 299
Other Modes of Excitation, 301
Depolarization, 309
Excitation–Contraction Coupling, 312
Mechanical Behavior, 314

10. **Capillary and Lymphatic Systems**, 327

Architecture, 328
Hemodynamics, 333
Flux Through the Capillary Wall, 336
Lymphatic System, 351

11. **Pulmonary Circulation**, 357

Fetal and Neonatal Circulations, 358
Vascular Structure, 360
Pulmonary Hemodynamics, 362
Control and Regulation, 375
Extravascular Forces and the Pulmonary Circulation, 379
Vascular Endothelium, 382

12. **Regional Circulations**, 387

Autoregulation, 388
Cerebral Circulation, 392
Coronary Circulation, 400
Circulation to the Skin, 407
Splanchnic Circulation, 411
Renal Circulation, 416
Skeletal Muscle, 422

13. **The Circulating Fluid: Blood**, 429

Cellular Elements, 430
Physical Properties of Blood, 431
Blood Volume, 436
Regional Volumes, 443
Redistribution of Blood Volume, 445

14. Methods of Measurement, 454

Instrumentation, 455
Pressure and Force, 457
Cardiac Output, 460
Regional Blood Flows, 467
Pulsatile Blood Flow, 470
Imaging Methods, 475
Computers, 477

Index, 483

SECTIONS RECOMMENDED FOR AN INTRODUCTORY COURSE IN CARDIOVASCULAR PHYSIOLOGY

1. Introduction, 3–15, 17–18, 21–23
2. The normal state; cardiac output, 29, 31–37
   Blood pressure and blood flow, 33, 44–51
3. Myocardial cells; innervation, receptors, 62–70
   Excitation, membrane potentials, 71–76, 83–88, 91–98
4. The cardiac cycle; ventricular function, 111–115
   Control and regulation of the heart, 116–127
5. Electrical activity of the heart, 140–141
6. Principles of hemodynamics, 171–180, 200–203
   Reflected waves in the aorta, 212–214
7. Cardiovascular regulation; baroreceptors, 225–232
   Chemoreceptors, 239–242
8. Autonomic nervous control, 249–263
   Endocrine mechanisms, 267–271
   Responses to exercise, 282–284
9. Properties of vascular smooth muscle, 290–296, 298, 312–315
10. Capillary structure and dynamics, 327–334
    Flux through capillary wall, 336–339
    Lymphatic system, 351–354
11. Pulmonary circulation, fetal and adult, 357–360, 362–369
    Pulmonary vascular control and regulation, 376–379
12. Autoregulation, 388–390
13. Properties and constituents of blood, 429–434
    Blood volume, 436–438

Cardiovascular Physiology

Physiologists and physicians must always consider organisms as a whole and in detail at one and the same time, without ever losing sight of the special conditions of all the particular phenomena that constitute the individual. Yet particular facts are never scientific: only generalizations can establish science. Here we must avoid a double stumbling-block; for if excess of detail is antiscientific, excessive generalization creates an ideal science no longer connected with reality.

Claude Bernard, *Introduction a l'étude*
de la médecine expérimentale, 1865

1

THE CIRCULATORY SYSTEM

To begin with a general view of the subject that will be examined more closely later, this chapter presents the salient features of cardiovascular physiology in broad outline. In the course of this preliminary survey, three topics are considered in some detail because they are relevant to virtually all subsequent chapters: the manifold functions of the endothelial cells that line all blood vessels, the role of cell membrane receptors as regulatory agents, and the rationale for using intricate models of the circulation as tools in research.

Structure and Function

The heart and blood vessels are essentially a transportation system that supplies all the cells of the body, delivering essential materials and carrying away the waste products of metabolism. Using blood as the vehicle, the system carries nutrients, oxygen, carbon dioxide, hormones, and many other substances required for proper function of the organism. Fats and carbohydrates are moved from storage depots to regions where they are utilized, leukocytes and immune antibodies are delivered to sites where they are needed, and circulating materials involved in blood coagulation guard the integrity of the vessels.

The circulatory system consists of the heart, arteries, capillaries, and veins, each with a distinctive architecture and function. The arteries carry blood from the heart to the periphery, branching in a more or less orderly fashion until they reach capillary beds. Capillaries are thin-walled tubes, 5 to 10 μm in diameter, made up of a single layer of endothelial cells. They form a diffuse, freely anastomosing network, varying somewhat in pattern in different

3

organs but always in close proximity to the cells they serve. Blood flows from capillaries into microscopic veins, and subsequently into a venous system that mirrors the design of the arterial tree, with the veins coming together in fewer vessels of increasing diameter as they approach the heart. Blood travels through two such systems in succession. The left side of the heart pumps blood into the aorta and *systemic circulation,* whence it returns through the veins to the right heart. The right ventricle then propels the blood into the pulmonary artery and the *pulmonic circulation,* where exchange between blood and respiratory gases occurs.

The bloodstream thus moves in a circle, from the heart to the periphery and back again, a fact that escaped recognition for centuries. Credit for discovering the circulatory nature of the process belongs to William Harvey (1578–1657), who published his conclusion in a work[7] that is a landmark in experimental biology. Earlier observers had encountered signs of the circular motion of blood, but the fragments of evidence were ignored because they conflicted with the writings of Galen in the second century. Harvey not only rejected such uncritical acceptance of ancient authority but also buttressed his arguments with carefully detailed accounts of his experiments, establishing clearly the principle that

> blood is pushed by the beat of the left ventricle and distributed through the arteries to the whole body, and back through the veins to the vena cava, and then returned to the right auricle, just as it is sent to the lungs through the pulmonary artery from the right ventricle and returned from the lungs through the pulmonary veins to the left ventricle. . . .[7]

Transfers between blood and tissues take place through the capillary wall, but indirectly through the medium of the *extracellular fluid* that bathes all cells. Claude Bernard[1] named this pervasive extravascular and extracellular fluid the *milieu interieur,* an internal environment kept constant by a host of regulatory mechanisms. The relatively constant chemical composition of this compartment, communicating on the one hand with the bloodstream and on the other hand with the cells of each organ, makes survival possible in a wide range of external environments.

Heart

The mammalian heart is, in effect, two conjoined pumps, one sending blood through the lungs and the other to the rest of the body. Its complicated architecture is an evolutionary development that is retraced in the embryo. In the lowest forms that possess an analogous structure, the heart is a simple muscular tube, and its contraction propels blood rather inefficiently through a single circulation. Higher on the evolutionary scale, two distinct regions appear in this tube, separated by a valve. Blood enters first a thin-walled, muscular sac (atrium) and then a thick-walled, muscular chamber (ventricle). The atrium provides a storage site for blood returning from the circulation while the ventricle is contracting. Atrial contraction occurs just before the next ventricular contraction and thus helps to fill the thicker chamber.

A later and more significant evolutionary development is the extension of septi into the atrium and ventricle. These partitions become complete in birds and mammals, creating the four-chambered heart. The blood leaving the lungs, high in oxygen and low in carbon dioxide, is now delivered by the left heart directly to the organs of the body, uncontaminated by systemic venous blood. The blood draining from the organs into the veins travels to the right heart and thus to the lungs, where the oxygen is replenished and the carbon dioxide produced by metabolism is discharged. Valves between each atrium and ventricle and at the ventricular exits prevent retrograde movement of blood, so that the rhythmic contractions of the heart propel blood forward in a highly effective manner. The flow pathway now leads from the systemic veins into the right atrium, right ventricle, pulmonary artery, pulmonary vessels, pulmonary veins, left atrium, left ventricle, aorta, and so into the systemic vessels.

The two ventricles contract simultaneously, and the left ventricle ejects the same amount of blood as the right with each hearbeat, apart from trivial differences that average out in a few beats. More energy and higher pressure are required to move blood through the systemic circulation than through pulmonary vessels, and the muscular wall of the left ventricle is much thicker than that of the right. The stimulus for muscle contraction is generated by the *pacemaker,* a group of cells in the right atrial wall, and excitation spreads in an orderly sequence through the atria and ventricles. A specialized conducting system conveys the excitatory impulse across the atrioventricular boundary and over the inner surface of both ventricles. The spread of excitation takes less than 0.1 sec in the human heart, but its sequence ensures efficient ejection of blood by the resulting mechanical contraction. The contractile process is one in which the muscle fibers generate force and tend to shorten, raising pressure in the ventricles and ejecting blood into the aorta and pulmonary artery. The period of active contraction (*systole*) is followed by an interval in which muscle relaxes and the ventricle fills again before the next beat (*diastole*). The pressures generated in the heart chambers cause the four cardiac valves to open and close at appropriate times. This intricate sequence, referred to as the *events of the cardiac cycle,* is reviewed in Chapter 4.

Blood vessels

Arteries

Blood ejected from the left and right ventricles enters the aorta and main pulmonary artery, respectively, and the subsequent branching of these primary vessels is tree-like. Major branches leave the aorta at points dictated by the position of the organs they supply. In the pulmonary system the branching pattern is more regular, and each branch is shorter. Bifurcation into two more or less similar branches is common in both circulations, but many other types of division also occur. The result is an arborization into more and more vessels of smaller and smaller diameter. The sequence of vessels and their relative dimensions in the canine mesenteric vascular bed are listed in Table 1.1, although the values given are only rough approximations. The overall pattern in most other regions is similar.

Although the caliber of the arteries becomes smaller at each point of division, the total cross section of the branches usually increases (Chapter 2). In simple bifurcation, the ratio of the total cross section of the two branches to that of the parent vessel oridinarily ranges from 1.2 to 1.7. Subdivisions do not occur with perfect geometric regularity, however. At some points, a single small lateral branch may arise from a large vessel; at others, one small artery may divide into many branches. Overall, the total cross section of the arterial tree continually expands toward the periphery, increasing 100-fold between the aorta and terminal arterioles, and to an even greater extent in the capillary bed. Because the same volume of blood passes through each transverse section across the systemic vascular bed per unit time, the velocity of the blood falls progressively from an average of about 18 cm/sec in the aorta to less than 0.2 cm/sec in the terminal arterioles. The process is reversed in the veins, and blood accelerates as the venous total cross section diminishes.

The thickness of the arterial wall is approximately 10% of the vessel radius in the primary and secondary aortic branches, but the ratio of the wall to the lumen increases in the distal arterial tree (Figure 1.1). The walls of the arteries and veins contain a mixture of tissues. The *intima* consists of a single layer of endothelial cells that line the vessel. The outermost layer, or *adventitia,* is mainly connective tissue that merges with surrounding structures. The relatively wide region between these two layers, the *media,* contains elastin, collagen, and smooth muscle, all embedded in an amorphous mucupolysaccharide *ground substance.* All of these components have viscoelastic properties, elastin being relatively extensible and collagen very stiff (Chapter 6). The elasticity of the vascular smooth muscle varies with contractile activity, and contraction or relaxation of the muscle cells is the mechanism by which small vessels are constructed or dilated. The arteries and veins are also elastic structures, and

Table 1.1. Dimensions of Canine Mesenteric Vascular Bed[a]

VESSEL	TOTAL NUMBER	RADIUS (CM)	TOTAL CROSS-SECTION (CM²)	LENGTH (CM)	MEAN VELOCITY (CM/SEC)	PRESSURE DROP (MM HG)	VOLUME (% OF TOTAL)
Mesenteric artery	1	0.15	0.07	6.00	16.80	0.8	2.5
Main branches	15	0.05	0.12	4.50	10.10	3.2	3.2
End branches	45	0.03	0.13	3.91	9.30	7.4	3.0
Arterial bed							
Intestinal branches	1,899	0.0068	0.28	1.42	5.80	23.5	2.3
Last branches	26,640	0.0025	0.52	0.11	2.10	7.2	0.3
Branches to villi	328,500	0.00155	2.48	0.15	0.48	5.4	2.2
Arteries of villi	1,051,000	0.00122	4.91	0.20	0.28	8.1	5.9
Capillaries of villi	47,300,000	0.00040	23.78	0.04	0.05	2.4	5.7
						58.0	25.1
Veins at base of villi	2,102,400	0.00132	11.51	0.10	0.10	1.0	6.9
Presubmucosal veins	131,400	0.00375	5.80	0.10	0.20	0.3	3.5
Submucosal veins	18,000	0.0064	2.32	0.15	0.51	0.4	2.1
Short intestinal veins	28,800	0.0032	0.93	1.10	1.30	2.5	6.1
Intestinal veins	1,899	0.0138	1.14	1.42	1.40	1.4	9.6
Mesenteric veins							
Last branches	45	0.075	0.79	3.91	1.50	0.2	18.4
Middle branches	15	0.12	0.67	4.50	1.70	0.1	18.2
Main vein	1	0.3	0.28	6.00	4.20	0.1	10.1
						6.0	74.9

[a]From data of Schleier.[23]

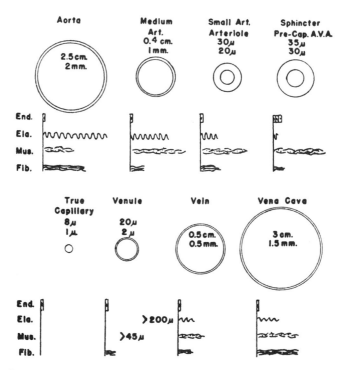

Figure 1.1. Size, wall thickness, and relative amounts of the four major components of human blood vessels. Diameter is indicated below name of vessel, and wall thickness below that. (Reproduced from Burton,[16] with permission of the American Physiological Society)

their diameter is affected by blood pressure. The normal pulsations of pressure expand the diameter of large arteries with each heartbeat.

The aorta and pulmonary artery, together with their major branches, contain relatively large amounts of elastin and are sometimes called *elastic* arteries. More distal branches, with prominent layers of smooth muscle (Figure 1.1), are labeled *muscular* arteries. These terms are widely used and make a valid point, but virtually all blood vessels are distensible, and all except capillaries contain some of each of the three major wall components—elastin, collagen, and muscle. The terms were originally adopted as a way of emphasizing the role of the ascending aorta and main pulmonary artery in transforming the discontinuous ejection of blood from the ventricles into a pulsatile but continuous flow in the peripheral arteries. Because of the elasticity of these major arterial trunks and their proximity to the ventricles, they are distended by each ejection. At the end of ventricular contraction, when the aortic and pulmonic valves have closed, the energy stored elastically in the walls of these arteries provides pressure to move the blood forward during diastole. The systolic distention is not large, perhaps 6% of the diameter in the ascending aorta and 2% in the abdominal aorta, but it suffices to maintain flow in the periphery when the ventricles are at rest.

The architecture and dimensions of the arterial tree are major factors in determining the amount of energy needed to move blood through the system. Most of the energy is expended in overcoming a kind of friction between the blood, a viscous substance, and the lining of the vessel (Chapter 6). The smaller the diameter of a vessel and the greater its length, the greater the energy needed to push a given fluid volume through it per unit time. The physical properties of a vascular bed thus oppose the flow of blood, in a sense, and this opposition is expressed in a parameter called the *vascular resistance* (Chapter 6). One manifestation of resistance is the continuous decrease in blood pressure throughout the length of the vascular system. The ventricle supplies the initial driving pressure, and the subsequent changes can be represented by a *pressure profile* like that in Figure 1.2.

When the blood has traversed the systemic veins and reached the right ventricle, that chamber provides the force to drive it through the pulmonary

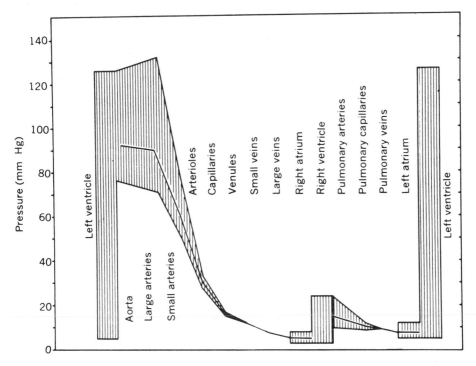

Figure 1.2. Typical blood pressures in human cardiovascular system. *Solid line* indicates mean pressure; *shaded area* the pulsations from systole to diastole.

circuit, again with a progressive decrement in pressure throughout the bed. Although the right heart pumps the same volume per minute as the left heart, pulmonary vascular resistance is lower than systemic resistance, and the pressures are consequently lower in the pulmonary vessels. The difference in resistance arises from the relatively short length of the vessels in the lung, the large number of parallel channels in the pulmonary microcirculation, and the greater degree of normal arteriolar constriction in the systemic bed.

The greatest drop in pressure occurs in the smallest vessels, those with diameters less than 0.5 mm. Control of blood flow to each region resides in this terminal part of the arterial tree, especially in arterioles with a diameter less than 0.2 mm, because very small changes in caliber can produce large changes in vascular resistance (Chapter 6). Contraction of smooth muscle in the vascular wall tends to decrease the diameter of the vessel, and relaxation of the muscle tends to increase it. Inasmuch as vessel diameter is a major factor in determining pressure–flow relationships, vascular smooth muscle provides a mechanism for control and regulation of blood pressure and flow in all parts of the body.

Large arteries like the aorta, pulmonary artery, and their major branches also contain smooth muscle, but its contraction decreases the diameter of the vessels only slightly, and their resistance to flow is small in any case. The principal effect of muscle activity in these arteries is on the elasticity of the vascular wall, which influences the transmission of pulse waves through the system (Chapter 6). The metabolic needs of the tissues in the wall of a large artery are supplied in part by *vasa vasorum,* tiny vessels that originate from branches of the artery itself and return to penetrate the wall. Endothelial cells are exposed to direct diffusion of substances from the adjacent bloodstream.

The arterial tree is thus not a mere passive conduit, but a system with properties that change appropriately from origin to termination in capillary beds. The largest arteries distend to accommodate part of the ventricular output during systole and recoil to move it forward in diastole. Arterioles control local hemodynamic conditions, regulating blood flow to each region.

Microcirculation

Arterioles, capillaries, and venules are often spoken of as the *microcirculation.* The capillary bed is made up of endothelial tubes 5 to 10 μm in diameter, their walls consisting of a single layer of endothelial cells. These tubes form a network quite unlike the tree-like branching pattern of the arteries, and many alternate pathways through this complex meshwork are possible (Figure 10.1). No one segment extends far before sending off lateral channels that anastomose with adjoining segments. Blood enters the capillaries through terminal arterioles, which contain smooth muscle and are 10 to 20 μm in diameter at their junction with the capillary bed, and leaves through venules that are more numerous, slightly larger, and endowed with less smooth muscle. At some points, muscular *arteriovenous anastomoses* connect terminal arterioles directly to venules, bypassing the true capillaries.

Capillary beds are the delivery points served by the arterial and venous transportation systems. Oxygen, nutrients, hormones, and many drugs reach the cells of the body by passing through the capillary wall into the extracellular spaces of the peripheral tissues. Conversely, waste products enter the bloodstream and are carried to the lungs, liver, or other organs for disposal. Architecture and flow dynamics in the capillaries are ideally suited to such exchange, presenting an enormous membrane surface to relatively slow-moving blood. The best estimates in man suggest a capillary surface area of perhaps 60 m^2 in systemic capillaries and 40 m^2 in pulmonary capillaries. Exchange rates across the capillary wall are determined by its inherent permeability and the physicochemical forces acting on it (Chapter 10).

Observations *in vivo* show that the capillary segments in a microscopic field tend to be either fully open or fully closed. Although they lack an inherent contractile mechanism, they are held open or allowed to collapse by the level of intracapillary pressure, which is controlled by the arterioles upstream and the venules downstream. The smooth muscle of these precapillary and postcapillary vessels is innervated, and also responds to direct contact with certain vasoactive substances.[12] The capillaries themselves are not supplied with nerve fibers. The histological density of capillaries varies from one organ to another, and they are rarely all open at the same time in any region. The fraction open in inactive skeletal muscle, for example, has been estimated at 1%. The elaborate pattern of capillary beds, posed between the arterioles and venules that exert hemodynamic control, makes the system one that can be regulated over a wide range to meet physiological demands.

Veins

The veins constitute a second vascular tree, beginning with venules and converging to form larger and larger trunks. Their walls are thinner than those of arteries of comparable diameter and contain less smooth muscle. As a rule, veins are more numerous than arteries at each level of the circulation. The smooth muscle of the venules, like that of the arterioles, is subject to stimulation by the nervous system and by chemical agents, providing a controllable postcapillary resistance. The resistance of venules is smaller than that of arterioles, but these pre- and postcapillary vessels together form the mechanism for regulating capillary pressure and flow (Chapter 10).

The large veins offer little resistance to blood flow, but activation of their smooth muscle has profound hemodynamic consequences. Roughly two-thirds of the total blood volume resides in veins (Table 1.2), so a relatively small decrease in their diameter can displace a significant amount of blood into other

Table 1.2. Estimated Distribution of Blood in the Vascular System of an Adult Human

REGION	VOLUME		
	MILLILITERS	PERCENT OF TOTAL	
Heart (diastole)	360	6.4	(6%)
Pulmonary			
Arteries	130 ⎫	2.3 ⎫	
Capillaries	150 ⎬ 440	2.7 ⎬	(8%)
Veins	160 ⎭	2.9 ⎭	
Systemic			
Aorta, large arteries	300 ⎫	5.4 ⎫	
Small arteries	500 ⎪	8.9 ⎪	
Capillaries	300 ⎬ 4800	5.4 ⎬	(86%)
Small veins	2700 ⎪	48.1 ⎪	
Large veins	1000 ⎭	17.9 ⎭	
	5600	100.0	

parts of the circulation (Chapter 13). For this reason, veins are referred to as *capacitance vessels,* in contrast to the arteriolar and venular *resistance vessels,* and the venous system functions as an adjustable *blood reservoir.*[20] The distensibility of veins makes it possible for small changes in pressure to alter their volume appreciably. Unlike the major arteries, which tend to retain a cylindrical shape and an open lumen even when distending pressure is absent, the thin-walled, large veins can collapse at low pressures. The external jugular vein in humans, for example, is almost completely collapsed in the erect posture. Veins in the skin play a part in regulating the temperature of the body, as well as serving the usual circulatory function (Chapter 12).

A distinctive structural feature of large veins in the extremities is the presence of valves that prevent retrograde flow. These valves recur at more or less regular intervals along the vessel and preserve the forward motion of blood toward the heart. They also interrupt the vertical columns of blood that would otherwise produce large hydrostatic pressures in the veins of the lower extremities in humans standing erect. Contractions of the skeletal muscles that surround deep vessels of the extremities compress the veins, and the valves allow such compression to move blood forward but prevent backward flow. This phenomenon, called *muscle pumping,* helps to return blood to the heart and contributes significantly to the circulatory process during exercise. Valves can be demonstrated in superficial veins of humans without dissection, a fact used by William Harvey in proving that venous blood moves in only one direction, toward the heart (Figure 1.3). His description is still worth noting as an example of scientific inference from a very simple experiment:

> The valves are present solely that blood may not advance from the center of the body into the periphery through the veins, but rather from the extremities to the center. . . . This fact may be more clearly shown by tying off an arm of a subject as if for blood letting [*AA*, Figure 1.3]. There will appear at intervals . . . knots or swellings [*B* to *F*] not only where there is branching but also where there is none. These are caused by the valves. If you will clear the blood away from a nodule or valve by pressing a finger below it [*H*], you will see that nothing can flow back, being entirely prevented by the valve. . . . If you press downward against valve O, you will note that nothing can be forced through it. From many such experiments it is evident that the function of the valves in the veins is the same as that of the three sigmoid valves placed at the opening of the aorta and pulmonary artery—to prevent, when they are closed, the reflux of blood passing over them.[7]

This demonstration was only one of many pieces of evidence that led Harvey to conclude that blood moves in a circle, from the heart to the periphery and back again by a different route. Like all great discoveries, this one changed our thinking so fundamentally that it is now difficult to imagine how anyone could have believed otherwise.[6]

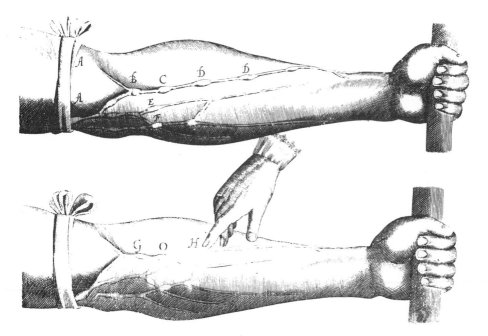

Figure 1.3. From William Harvey's presentation of experiments on valves and blood flow in superficial veins[7] (see text).

Blood

The volume and physical properties of the fluid that fills the cardiovascular system play a central role in physiology. The total blood volume in man is normally 60 to 80 ml per kilogram of body weight, or about 5 liters in an average adult male (Chapter 13). About half of this volume is fluid, and the other half consists of blood cells, chiefly erythrocytes. The heart and blood vessels resemble a closed elastic container filled with blood (assuming a steady state of exchange in the capillaries). This compartment has been filled under pressure, so to speak, so that it is slightly distended. When the heart ceases to beat, arterial pressure falls and venous pressure rises until an equilibrium is reached throughout the system. This equilibrium, which occurs in a few minutes, is called the *mean circulatory filling pressure (MCFP)* and represents the relationship between vascular elastic capacity and blood volume (Chapter 6).

The equilibrium pressure can be measured in experimental animals by imposing transient cardiac arrest or fibrillation for a few minutes; it is normally about 9 mm Hg. The intravascular pressures observed *in vivo* are, consequently, the sum of the MCFP and the driving force generated by the ventricles. As might be expected, stimuli that cause venoconstriction elevate the MCFP. The distensibility of the vascular system is thus one of the factors that determine blood pressure. The volume of blood in each part of the circulation depends on the local pressures and vessel elasticity, and a kind of dynamic equilibrium is maintained. Table 1.2 summarizes the normal distribution of volume among the various segments of the system in humans.

One of the important attributes of blood is its *viscosity,* a physical property defined by Newton as "a lack of slipperiness between the layers of a fluid." Blood viscosity is a key variable in the relation between pressure and flow in the vascular system, because the viscosity of a fluid is a major factor in determining the energy required to move it through a tube (Chapter 6). Blood is a suspension, not a pure fluid, and its viscosity varies with the concentration of cells and plasma proteins.

The ratio of the red cell volume to the total volume in a blood sample is called the *hematocrit,* a name taken from the centrifugation tube used to measure it. The hematocrit of the overall blood volume in man is about 0.40, and that of venous blood samples averages 0.45. Regional hematocrits differ widely, amounting to as much 0.80 in the spleen and bone marrow and as little as 0.20 in some parts of the kidney (Chapter 13). These values represent the ratios in one region at any instant. The surprising variations indicate that blood cells and plasma travel at different velocities and, to some extent, through different pathways. Such discrepancies are easy to imagine in the bone marrow, where red cells are manufactured and temporarily stored in out-of-the-way spaces, but they are more difficult to picture elsewhere. The cause of the nonuniformity is debatable, and several theories have been proposed. One hypothesis emphasizes the tendency of red cells to concentrate in relatively rapid axial streams in arteries, allowing more plasma than cells to leave the vessel at branch points *(plasma skimming)*. Another hypothesis makes the structure of local microcirculations responsible, assuming that certain channels favor the passage of either red cells or plasma. Some capillaries have a lumen smaller than the diameter of a red cell, for example, and erythrocytes are temporarily deformed in squeezing through them.

Lymphatic system

Another vascular system exists in parallel with the blood vessels, namely, a network of *lymphatic channels* (Chapter 10). These vessels originate in extracellular spaces as microscopic, thin-walled tubes that resemble blood capillaries except for being closed at one end. These *lymph capillaries* lead to larger channels, which converge into progressively wider conduits and eventually drain into large veins near the heart. The lymphatic system is filled with *lymph,* a fluid containing solutes that diffuse from the interstitial space and leukocytes. Lymphatic flow is directed toward the heart by one-way valves in many of the larger channels, but the only motive force is external compression by the activity of skeletal muscles. The flow pathway leads through numerous lymph glands.

Endothelium

The endothelial cell lining of the blood vessels has come to be recognized as a virtual organ system in itself.[11] The permeability of this lining is one route of communication between blood and vascular smooth muscle (Chapter 10), but at least five other important physiological functions are served by endothelial cells:

1. *Release of endothelium-derived relaxing factor (EDRF):* Stimulation of cells of the vascular endothelium causes them to release nitric oxide,[21] and perhaps other substances, that relax smooth muscle in the wall of the vessel. This relaxation is mediated by muscarinic cholinergic receptors of the endothelial cell and accounts for the vasodilatation produced by acetylcholine. Similar endothelium-dependent relaxation can be produced by a number of other endogenous vasoactive substances (Chapter 8). Beta-adrenergic receptors and an adenylate cyclase system (see below) have also been identified in endothelial cells.[24]

2. *Clearance of specific vasoactive substances from the circulation:* Endothelial cells can take up certain materials from the bloodstream and metabolize them. Pulmonary arterioles and capillaries are the principal sites of this process, although the endothelium of other vessels performs the same function to a limited extent. Norepinephrine, 5-hydroxytryptamine, and bradykinin are cleared from the blood in a single passage through the pulmonary vascular bed, and angiotensin-I is completely converted to angiotensin-II (Chapter 11). The metabolic and relaxing functions of endothelium are both modulated by the partial pressure of oxygen; anoxia decreases the relaxant effect of acetylcholine, for example, and hyperoxia decreases the pulmonary endothelial conversion of angiotensin-I to angiotensin-II.

3. *Synthesis of prostaglandins:* Endothelial cells synthesize fatty acids called *prostaglandins,* which have a variety of physiological actions (Chapter 8). Some members of this chemical class stimulate smooth muscle contraction, whereas others inhibit it. Prostaglandins are synthesized from arachidonic acid within endothelial cells, and can be released through their luminal surface into the bloodstream or through the abluminal surface into interstitial spaces adjoining smooth muscle. Prostaglandins are not circulating regulators of vascular smooth muscle tone, because they are rapidly metabolized. The production of prostaglandins is enhanced by a number of biological substances, including histamine, and by the shearing force exerted on endothelium by the motion of blood (Chapter 6). Local concentrations of prostaglandins inhibit platelet aggregation in the blood.

4. *Antithrombogenic activity:* Blood clots rapidly when removed from the vascular system, and preservation of its fluid state *in vivo* depends largely on the endothelium. The luminal surface of endothelial cells is antithrombogenic because of the presence of heparin-like compounds and a net negative charge. The distribution of anionic and cationic sites on this surface is also the mechanism for selective transport of some molecules, including most plasma proteins, across the endothelial barrier.[4] Endothelial cells manufacture both coagulant and anticoagulant substances, the relative amounts mitigating fibrin formation and platelet aggregation under normal conditions.

5. *Regulation of mitosis and development of vascular smooth muscle:* Endothelial cells can produce substances that include both stimulators and inhibitors of muscle cell division.[3] This phenomenon has been studied principally in cultures, where it has been shown that endothelial and smooth muscle cells grown in the same bathing medium, but not in contact, produce substances that inhibit cell growth. In intact blood vessels, the removal of large areas of endothelium leads to the transformation of some smooth muscle cells into a kind of pseudoendothelium. These cells retain some of their contractile characteristics and morphology, but after some months they produce prostaglandin I_2–

like true endothelial cells (Chapter 8). Such observations suggest that the endothelium plays an essential role in the responses to vascular injury and possibly in the normal growth and development of blood vessels. Endothelial cells play some part in events associated with immune responses, as well as in vascular inflammation or injury, although under normal conditions the endothelium appears to be immunologically unreactive.

As if this extraordinary range of functions were not enough, recent observations raise the possibility that endothelial cells are mechanically active. Their cytoskeleton includes filaments of actin and other proteins that bear stress. Norepinephrine, epinephrine, and probably 5-hydroxytrypamine promote the assembly of these *stress fibers* in cultured endothelial cells, whereas histamine appears to disassemble them and cause the cells to contract.[25] Histamine is a substance that increases the permeability of capillaries in allergic reactions. It is tempting to suppose that it does so by ultramicroscopic contraction of endothelial cells, enlarging the clefts between them. Much more needs to be learned about the physical properties of endothelial cells, including the significance of stress fibers and electrostatic phenomena at the cell surface, which may well be of great importance to endothelial permeability in the microcirculation.

Blood Pressure and Blood Flow

Each contraction of the heart confers a finite amount of mechanical energy on the blood ejected into the aorta and pulmonary artery. The pressure and flow of blood in the vascular system arise from this energy, but they also depend on the physical properties of the vascular tree, namely, the dimensions of the vessels, the viscosity of blood, and the viscoelasticity of vascular walls. The body of knowledge concerned with the relationships among these variables in living animals is called *hemodynamics*. The relationships are defined by known physical laws of force, motion, and viscoelasticity, and equations can be written that express quite accurately the pressure and velocity of fluids moving through tubular models. Similar equations apply to the cardiovascular system and are used extensively in research and clinical medicine. Although the complex, asymmetrical structure of the heart and vascular tree makes it difficult to derive exact equations for the conditions *in vivo,* good approximations have been developed (Chapter 6).

The simplest quantitative treatments of hemodynamics consider only average pressures and flows, ignoring the peaks and valleys of the pulsations. Blood flow, for example, is often expressed as the *cardiac output,* the number of liters of blood pumped per minute by each ventricle, averaged over several heartbeats. The systolic and diastolic pressures measured in humans by the

routine clinical arm-cuff method not only provide those maximum and minimum values, which are an important aspect of the pulsations, but also permit
a rough estimate of mean pressure in large arteries. Mean blood flow is essentially the same at all cross sections of the arterial tree, the same in the total
population of peripheral arterioles as in the ascending aorta. Mean pressure,
however, falls continually from the ascending aorta to the terminus of the venae
cavae, an indication that the energy imparted to the blood by ventricular ejection is gradually dissipated as it travels through the vascular system. As we
have already seen, the decrement in pressure per unit length of the system, or
vascular resistance, is greatest in the microcirculation. The relative resistance
of each organ system determines the fraction of the cardiac output delivered to
it.

The pulsations of pressure and flow with each heartbeat have also been
analyzed theoretically and quantitatively (Chapter 6). In general, the amplitude
of these pulsations becomes smaller with the distance from the heart, diminishing to small but detectable levels in the capillary bed. This attenuation, like
that of mean pressure, is a function of the physical properties of the system.
These properties determine the ratio of pulsatile pressure to pulsatile flow,
which is expressed in a frequency-dependent parameter called *vascular impedance* (Chapter 6), the pulsatile analogue of resistance. In addition, pulse waves
are partially reflected back toward the heart at some points, affecting the overall pattern of pulsatile waveforms in the arterial tree. Cardiac performance can
be characterized by time-varying data on the pulsatile characteristics of intracardiac pressures, force in the ventricular wall, velocity of shortening of muscle
fibers, or external cardiac work (Chapter 4).

Although mathematical analysis of pulse waves in the circulation has been
employed mainly in research work, it is now becoming more common in clinical
settings, and many diagnostic laboratories handle such analysis routinely by
computers. Some of the results have broad practical implications. The waveforms of arterial pressure observed in various mammals, for example, can be
understood in terms of reflected wave effects, and the arterial pulse wave velocity in man may be one index of the risk of heart disease (Chapter 2).

Hemodynamic models of the circulation

The number of variables involved in cardiovascular function is so great,
and the regulation in living animals so efficient, that it is difficult to grasp the
quantitative relation of any single element in the system to all the others. For
example, constriction of the veins tends to raise arterial blood pressure by displacing blood from one compartment to the other, but to what extent can reflex
arteriolar dilatation counteract this effect? How much can the cardiac output

be raised by tachycardia alone, with no change in volume ejected per stroke, considering that time must be available between beats for ventricular filling?

Controlled experiments are one way of answering such questions, keeping all but a few relevant variables constant. This is the classical method of investigation, frequently applied in isolated vessels or organs. It is the foundation of most physiological knowledge and continues to be an essential procedure in research, but the designer of an experiment is always uneasily aware that the physiological events observed may be different from those in the living animal, where the regulatory systems are always at work. One development that has helped to avoid the limitations of this approach is the design of miniature transducers and noninvasive techniques that increase the number of variables that can be measured without interfering with normal function in live animals. A quite different path has been taken by investigators who study isolated cardiovascular cells under tightly controlled conditions, and the range between these two extremes, from intact organisms to single cells, represents the domain of current research.

Mathematical models are one way of fitting together experimental data from these diverse sources, offering tentative answers, at least, to questions about integrated function. Such models are most useful in research laboratories, but the principles are identical to those used in everyday reasoning, and formal models are resorted to only when the number of components and variables in a system makes it impossible to answer questions about it "off the cuff." The circular nature of the cardiovascular system puts a particular strain on cause-and-effect reasoning, inasmuch as conditions in each segment exist in a dynamic equilibrium with those elsewhere.

Many investigators have embodied their observations in sets of mathematical equations that constitute models of the heart and blood vessels. These constructs range in complexity from the *Windkessel* (Chapter 6), a model of a simple, distensible chamber emptying through a resistance, to formulae for the transmission of pulse waves through the arteries, borrowed from electrical engineering. Their purpose is not merely to imitate the input and output of a physiological system, but to represent its components and their known relationships as realistically as possible. Digital computers have made this task much simpler, not merely by easing the burdens of numerical analysis but also by giving the investigator freedom to express hypotheses in the most appropriate mathematical and logical forms.

The value of such models lies in their explicitness and predictive ability. The necessity of stating the conditions explicitly becomes clear as soon as one tries to express the behavior of a system in equations, and previously unrecognized assumptions often come to light. When a consistent, clearly defined model has been devised, predicting the consequences of changing one or more variables is straightforward. The result may be the discovery of relative insensitivity to changes in some properties and great sensitivity to changes in others *in the model*. At other times, a model may suggest the crucial importance of some variable that has not been experimentally measured. The one conclusion to be avoided is that we have thereby discovered something about living tissue, for that conclusion can be reached only by experiments on the tissue itself. Models, in other words, are primarily a means of generating new hypotheses, which can then be tested in the laboratory. Sometimes direct experimental confirmation is technically impossible at present, and the model prediction can only serve as a tentative theory until new methods are invented. The total volume of the venous system, for example, cannot be measured directly, and the accepted estimates (Tables 1.1 and 1.2) are derived from models based on data extrapolated from measurements of the dimensions of a few vessels.

Control and Regulation of the System

The cardiovascular system adapts itself to the needs of the organism, meeting any demands made by changes in external or internal conditions. The circulation can maintain normal blood pressures in the face of trauma and hemorrhage, for example. The pacemaker and conduction system of the heart, the striated muscle of the cardiac chambers, and the smooth muscle of blood vessels are the *effectors*, the structures that effect this adaptation, and each of these tissues responds to the commands of an elaborate control system. The command signals are generated in three different ways: by the central nervous system, by blood-borne agents, and by the local action of certain substances that are produced in the tissue concerned (Chapter 8).

The central nervous system receives information from many different sources, ranging from specific sensors in the arteries to emotion-laden visual images, and it integrates this information in ways still only partially understood. Appropriate signals are then sent out over a sequence of nerve pathways, ultimately causing a nerve terminal to release a *neurotransmitter*, a substance that stimulates or inhibits effector tissues. Norepinephrine and acetylcholine are the best-known transmitters in the cardiovascular system, but others have now been identified (Chapter 8). The nerves involved are mainly those of the *autonomic* division of the central nervous system, and they are distributed to the heart and to blood vessels in virtually all parts of the body.

The signals sent out by the brain are selective in the sense that they may be transmitted to some organs and not others, depending on the needs of the moment. The heart rate may be made to increase with little change in the vascular system, for example, or blood vessels may be made to dilate in skeletal muscle but not elsewhere. Many of these responses take the form of cardiovascular *reflexes,* in which the signals returned to the brain from a particular type of sensor evoke a characteristic set of output signals and responses. Such reflex responses are often modified in accordance with other data processed simultaneously by the central nervous system, however. The continuous function of central controls and peripheral sensors ensures that the system is regulated or, in other words, that the desired goal is achieved.

Although the autonomic nervous system is a major factor in the proper function of the circulation, other mechanisms are equally important. *Endocrine* secretions from the adrenal and other glands are carried by the bloodstream to act on the heart and vessels, and *paracrine* substances made by cells in many parts of the body stimulate adjacent cardiovascular tissues. Epinephrine from the adrenal medulla is perhaps the classical example of a blood-borne, or endocrine, agent. Purely local control of smooth muscle in small vessels is exerted by a long list of substances[12]—purine nucleotides, histamine, and the local partial pressures of oxygen and carbon dioxide, to name but a few (Chapter 9).

These control systems, acting in concert, give the organism a large repertoire of potential stimuli and responses, precise adjustments to meet challenges from the external environment or, for that matter, from pathological internal conditions. The final links are the interface between control system and effector cell and the behavior of the effector tissue. As is evident from the preceding discussion, all transmission of messages to cardiovascular effectors is chemical in nature, whether delivered by neural or other routes. In the great majority of cases, the receiving station for these control signals is a specific protein in the cell membrane, called a *receptor.*

Cellular Receptors

The discovery that specific receptors regulate the behavior of most cells is one of the major advances of modern biology. Information on this subject is expanding rapidly, and many reviews are available.[2,5,8] The receptors with which we are concerned here are discrete protein molecules inserted into the cell membrane. These entities should not be confused with the quite different vascular receptors, specialized nerve endings that are sensitive to stretch or chemical stimulation (Chapter 8). Clinical medicine and research have benefitted enormously from the growing understanding of receptor-mediated cardiovascular control. Drugs that act on certain receptors can provide controlled vasodilatation, vasoconstriction, or effects on the heart, for example, and many such compounds have found a place in medical therapy.

There are many different kinds of cell receptors, and each type binds to certain biologically active substances that are released by nerve fibers or other tissues, thus transmitting signals from one cell to others. The binding between transmitter and receptor is a very specific molecular matching; only the levo-rotatory optical isomers of norepinephrine and epinephrine bind to adrenergic receptors with high affinity, for instance. References to these catecholamines throughout this volume denote the physiologically active isomers unless otherwise qualified. The transmitter-bound receptor alters other parts of the membrane or the cell interior, in some cases by acting on ion channels and in others by activating or causing the synthesis of another substance, a *messenger* that initiates a series of intracellular events. This train of signals is referred to as the *coupling* of receptor to response. The chemical structure of some receptors is known, and in some instances the gene for the receptor has been cloned. Historically, the properties of receptors in a particular tissue were first determined by the functional responses to transmitters or drugs, and that approach is still an important source of information. Techniques developed more recently depend on the binding of radioisotopes or antibodies to the receptors, which is the basis of radioligand, autoradiographic, and histoimmunological methods.

Receptors are usually named after their physiological transmitter: *adrenergic* for those bound by adrenaline and noradrenaline (alternative names of epinephrine and norepinephrine, respectively), *cholinergic* for those bound by acetylcholine, and so on. In some cases these classes include two or more types, as illustrated by the alpha-adrenergic and beta-adrenergic receptors. Further subdivision into subtypes (e.g., alpha$_1$, alpha$_2$) is based on binding properties and responses to selective drugs (see below). Tissues vary widely in the types of receptors possessed by their cells and in the number per cell. For example, the concentration of alpha-adrenergic receptors (sometimes called *alpha-adrenoceptors*) is much higher in the brain than in vascular smooth muscle. The best-known cardiovascular receptors are the alpha-adrenergic,[2,5] beta-adrenergic,[13] and muscarinic cholinergic[10] species, but others are continuously being added to the list. The receptor-influenced cells of most interest in the present context are those of the heart (Chapter 3), vascular smooth muscle (Chapter 9), endothelium, and nerve terminals.

The characteristic cellular response to activation of a receptor depends on the nature of the cell, as well as the ligand and the kind of receptor. A specific receptor type may cause contraction in muscle but secretion in glandular cells. The response does not depend on the source of the ligand, being essentially the same whether the transmitter is neurally released, delivered by the bloodstream, or generated by nearby cells. The effect on the cell may be excitatory or inhibitory, and its magnitude is usually directly related to the number of transmitter-bound receptors, although often in a nonlinear way. When the binding of an agent to a receptor evokes a characteristic train of messengers and a cell response, that agent is referred to as an *agonist* for that receptor. Drugs that bind to a receptor but do not evoke the usual response are called *antagonists* because they can compete with agonists for binding sites.

Receptor numbers are not permanently fixed quantities. Individual receptors are continually withdrawn into the cell, degraded, and replaced by newly synthesized proteins. The rate and net result of such turnover are influenced by a number of factors, including agonist concentration. The number of alpha receptors per smooth muscle cell, for example, can be increased over a period of days by raising the level of norepinephrine or cyclic AMP to which the tissue is exposed.[17]

Messengers

The coupling of receptors to the final cell response is carried out by a complex chain of intracellular reactions. A long list of putative messengers is currently under study, and three in particular have been identified in cardiovascular tissues: Ca^{2+}, cyclic nucleotides, and certain products of phosphoinositide metabolism. Calcium plays a key role in the reactions of many cell types, and its importance in vascular smooth muscle and the myocardium is discussed elsewhere in this volume (Chapters 3 and 9). Activation of alpha-adrenergic receptors raises $[Ca^{2+}]_i$. Stimulation of beta-adrenergic receptors increases intracellular cyclic AMP, which in turn leads, in myocardial cells, to a rise in $[Ca^{2+}]_i$. Current research suggests that breakdown products of phosphoinositides are part of the messenger chain for alpha$_1$-adrenergic and muscarinic cholinergic receptors.

Cyclic nucleotides

Cyclic AMP (cyclic adenosine-3′,5′ monophosphate) appears in virtually all cell types and has been implicated in the regulation of a host of biological processes. It activates specific protein kinases, which phosphorylate and thereby alter the activity of certain proteins. Alpha$_2$-, but not alpha$_1$-adrenoceptors, use this messenger in some tissues. Degradation of cyclic AMP occurs by hydrolysis to 5′-AMP under the influence of cyclic nucleotide phosphodiesterase, and inhibition of that enzyme is presumably the basis for smooth muscle relaxation by some drugs.

Agonist-bound beta-adrenoceptors activate adenylate cyclase in the cell membrane, which produces cyclic AMP from adenosine triphosphate (ATP).[13] The ultimate effect of increased intracellular cyclic AMP varies in different tissues, apparently as a function of the particular protein kinase possessed by the cells. Beta-agonists *enhance* the contractility of myocardial cells, for example, but cause *relaxation* of vascular smooth muscle. In the case of cardiac muscle, beta-activation by catecholamines causes a rise in cyclic AMP that precedes contraction and an influx of Ca^{2+}, so the inotropic effect is presumably the result of increased $[Ca^{2+}]_i$ (Chapter 3).

The properties of the beta-adrenoceptors themselves seem to be the same in blood vessels as in the heart, implying that the contrast between their positive inotropic action in cardiac muscle and the negative inotropism in vascular smooth muscle is a matter of messengers distal to the elevation of cyclic AMP. The steps that translate an increase of intracellular cyclic AMP into smooth muscle relaxation remain open to question, although the two phenomena are quantitatively related. The most probable explanation is that phosphorylation by cyclic AMP lowers the affinity of the myosin light chain for the calcium–calmodulin complex (Chapter 9). Other theories attribute relaxation by cyclic AMP to a calcium extrusion that follows phosphorylation of Ca^{2+}–ATPase or to an Na^+–Ca^{2+} exchange carrier. Another hypothesis, prompted by the observation that isoproterenol increases K^+ influx and Na^+ efflux of isolated gastrointestinal smooth muscle cells, postulates an effect on the Na^+/K^+ pump.[22] Enhanced calcium sequestration by the sarcoplasmic reticulum (SR) has also been proposed.

Cyclic GMP (cyclic guanosine-3′,5′ phosphate) is another nucleotide that plays some part in regulating smooth muscle activity, but the experimental evidence about it at present is so confusing that one cannot be certain whether it mediates contraction or relaxation. Relaxing nitro-compounds like nitroglycerine raise the concentration of cyclic GMP in vascular smooth muscle,[19] but so do cholinergic agents that produce contraction. Activation of guanylate cyclase, production of cyclic GMP, and stimulation of a protein kinase are sequentially involved in such responses, and the analogy with cyclic AMP is completed by a specific hydrolyzing phosphodiesterase. In addition, many of the calcium-mobilizing receptors stimulate guanylate cyclase and raise the intracellular level of cyclic GMP. In many classes of receptors, coupling to adenylate cyclase occurs by way of certain guanine nucleotide proteins. These regulatory proteins are apparently key elements in a broad range of receptor–messenger interactions,[9] but at present, few statements about them can be made with certainty, except that they are essential for effective excitation–contraction coupling, include both stimulatory and inhibitory varieties, and regulate the proportions of high and low agonist-affinity states of some receptors.

Phosphoinositides

Metabolic products of membrane polyphosphoinositides act as messengers for a number of receptors,[15] including the $alpha_1$-adrenergic, muscarinic cholinergic, and H_1-histaminergic types. A cascade of reactions begins with receptor-mediated hydrolysis of phosphoinositides to give inositol-trisphosphate and diacylglycerol. Inositol-trisphosphate is apparently a trigger for the release of calcium from intracellular stores and may also affect calcium entry through the membrane. The diacylglycerol effects follow two pathways. One is the activation of protein-kinase-C, which is capable of phosphorylating myosin light chains and other proteins. The other is the release of arachidonic acid from the diacylglycerol molecule. The role of phosphoinositides in the myocardium and vascular smooth muscle is still speculative, but they are clearly affected by such vasoactive transmitters as norepinephrine, acetylcholine, histamine, serotonin, vasopressin, and angiotensin-II.

Receptor selectivity

The *selectivity* of a transmitter or drug for a particular type or subtype of receptor is frequently exploited in research and clinical therapy, and it is important to be aware of the mechanism of such preferential action. Receptor classification expresses the fact that each class has a particularly high affinity for a specific transmitter—adrenergic receptors for norepinephrine and epinephrine, cholinergic receptors for acetylcholine, and so on. Within each class, however, some drugs chemically related to the normal transmitter appear to select one particular type or subtype of receptor. For instance, the functional response to the synthetic drug isoproterenol, which is one of many catecholamines other than norepinephrine that bind to adrenergic receptors, suggests that it acts only on beta-adrenergic receptors. This selectivity arises from the fact that isoproterenol has a much higher affinity for beta-adrenergic than for alpha-adrenergic receptors, and consequently produces mainly those effects that are mediated by the beta variety. The phenomenon is particularly obvious in vascular smooth muscle, where alpha-adrenergic receptors mediate contraction and beta-adrenergic receptors relaxation.

Selectivity is relative, not absolute. The binding of drug D to receptor R is governed by the law of mass action, which in this application can be expressed as follows:

$$\frac{[RD]}{[R_T]} = \frac{[D]}{[D] + K_D} \tag{1.1}$$

All terms in this equation are in molar concentrations. $[RD]$ represents the drug-bound receptors, $[R_T]$ total receptors, and K_D the dissociation constant corresponding to the affinity between drug and receptor.[14,18] For a particular receptor and drug, the higher the drug concentration, the greater the fraction of receptors that it will occupy. For any given drug concentration, the smaller the K_D (i.e., the higher the affinity), the larger the fraction of receptors bound by the drug. The number of drug-bound receptors is a major factor in deter-

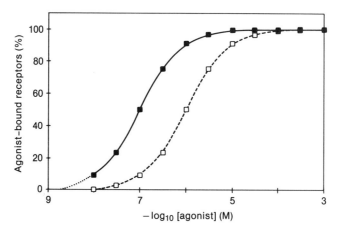

Figure 1.4.   Binding of rwo receptor types by an agonist. *Abscissa,* log agonist concentration. Ordinate, percent of receptors bound. Agonist K_D is 1.0 μM for receptor number 1 (*dashed line*), and 0.1μM for agonist number 2 (*solid line*). The agonist is thus relatively "selective" for receptor number 2, which has a greater affinity for it than receptor number 1 does. Nevertheless, in a tissue that contains both kinds of receptors, a concentration of agonist that binds half the number 2 receptors (0.1 μM) will at the same time bind 9% of the number 1 receptors. To be selective in practice, a drug must have a greater affinity for its preferred receptor type by 2 or 3 orders of magnitude, rather than the factor of 10 illustrated here.

mining the intensity of the cellular response, although not the only one (see below).

Figure 1.4 illustrates the binding of two hypothetical receptor types by a drug that has a higher affinity for one type than for the other, the dissociation constants differing by a factor of 10. In a tissue that contains both kinds of receptors, a drug concentration that activates 50% of the high-affinity type will at the same time bind 9% of the other variety, and the tissue response will be a mixture of the effects mediated by each receptor. Truly selective action is possible only with a drug that has an affinity several hundred- or thousand-fold higher for one class of receptors than for others. The usefulness of many drugs in clinical and experimental work rests on this principle.

Isoproterenol is a selective drug in this sense because it has a much higher affinity for beta- than for alpha-adrenergic receptors, the two K_D's differing by three orders of magnitude. Nevertheless, if the isoproterenol concentration is high enough, it can occupy virtually all of both types. Epinephrine is a relatively selective physiological transmitter, having a greater affinity for beta- than for alpha-adrenergic receptors, although in this case the difference is only a factor of about 10. Consequently, in vascular beds that possess a significant population of both adrenergic types, low epinephrine concentrations cause beta-adrenergic vasodilatation, whereas high concentrations bring alpha-adrenergic receptors into play and produce vasoconstriction. Norepinephrine, on the other hand, has about the same affinity for beta as for alpha-adrenoceptors.

A receptor-mediated response is thus correlated with the drug–receptor affinity, but it also depends on the number of appropriate receptors in the tissue (note $[R_T]$ in equation 1.1). As a rule, the fewer the receptors, the smaller the response. The response is determined, in addition, by the quantitative relationship between receptor occupation and the cell reaction it elicits. A response like muscle contraction, for example, is rarely a simple linear function of the number of drug-bound receptors, and a relatively large response may be produced by drug occupation of only a few receptors. In some cases, a maximum response occurs when only a fraction of the receptor population is bound by an agonist, in which case the tissue is said to have *spare receptors*.[18]

References

Reviews

1. Bernard, C. (1865). *Introduction a l'étude de la médecine expérimentale*. Paris, J.B. Bailliere. (Translation by H.C. Greene, New York, Dover, 1957.)
2. Bylund, D.B., U'Prichard, D.C. (1983). Characterization of α_1 and α_2-adrenergic receptors. *Int. Rev. Neurobiol.* 24:343–431.
3. Campbell, J.H., Campbell, G.R. (1985). Endothelial cell influences on vascular smooth muscle phenotype. *Annu. Rev. Physiol.* 48:295–306.
4. Cryer, A. (ed.) (1983). *Biochemical Interactions at the Endothelium*. Amsterdam, Elsevier.
5. Exton, J.H. (1981). Molecular mechanisms involved in α-adrenergic responses. *Mol. Cell Endocrinol.* 23:233–264.
6. Fishman, A.P., Richards, D.W. (eds.) (1964). *Circulation of the Blood: Men and Ideas*. New York, Oxford University Press.
7. Harvey, W. (1628). *Exercitatio anatomica de motu cordis et sanguinibus in animalibus*. Frankfurt, Guilielmi Fitzeri. (Reproduced with an English translation by C.D. Leake, Springfield, Ill., Charles C. Thomas, 1928.)
8. Kunos, G. (ed.) (1981). *Neurotransmitter Receptors*. New York, Wiley.
9. Rodbell, M. (1985). Programmable messengers: A new theory of hormone action. *Trends Biochem. Sci.* 17:461–464.
10. Schimerlik, M.I. (1989). Structure and regulation of the muscarinic receptors. *Ann. Rev. Physiol.* 51:217–227.
11. Shepro, D., D'Amore, P.A. (1984). The physiology and biochemistry of the vascular wall endothelium. In: *Handbook of Physiology. The Cardiovascular System, Microcirculation*, E.M. Renkin and C. Michel, ed. Bethesda, Md., American Physiological Society, pp. 103–163.

12. Somlyo, A.P., Somlyo, A.V. (1970). Vascular smooth muscle. II. Pharmacology of normal and hypertensive vessels. *Pharmacol. Rev.* 22:249–353.

13. Stiles, G.L., Caron, M.G., Lefkowitz, R.J. (1984). β-Adrenergic receptors: Biochemical mechanisms of physiological regulation. *Physiol. Rev.* 64:661–743.

14. Wold, F. (1971). *Macromolecules: Structure and Function.* Englewood Cliffs, N.J., Prentice-Hall.

Research Reports

15. Berridge, M.J., Irvine, R.F. (1984). Inositol trisphosphate, a novel second messenger in cellular signal transduction. *Nature 312:315–321.*

16. Burton, A.C. (1954). Relation of structure to function of the tissues of the wall of blood vessels. *Physiol. Rev.* 34:619–642.

17. Colucci, W.S. (1986). Adenosine 3′,5′-cyclic monophosphate–dependent regulation of α_1-adrenergic receptor number in rabbit aortic smooth muscle cells. *Circ. Res.* 58:292–297.

18. Furchgott, R.F. (1972). The classification of adrenoceptors (adrenergic receptors). An evaluation from the standpoint of receptor theory. In: *Handbuch der Experimentellen Pharmakologie,* Vol. 33, H. Blaschko and E. Muscholl, eds. Heidelberg, Springer-Verlag, pp. 283–335.

19. Kukovetz, W.R., Holzmann, S., Wurm, A., Poch, G. (1979). Evidence for cyclic GMP–mediated relaxant effects of nitro-compounds in coronary smooth muscle. *Naunyn Schmiedebergs Arch. Pharmacol.* 310:129–138.

20. Mellander, S. (1960). Comparative studies on the adrenergic neuro-hormonal control of resistance and capacitance blood vessels in the cat. *Acta Physiol. Scand.* 50(Suppl. 176):1–86.

21. Palmer, R.M.J., Ferrige, A.G., Moncada, S. (1987). Nitric oxide release accounts for the biological activity of endothelium-derived relaxing factor. *Nature* 327:524–526.

22. Scheid, C. R., Fay, F.S. (1984). β-Adrenergic stimulation of ^{42}K influx in isolated smooth muscle cells. *Am. J. Physiol.* 246 (*Cell Physiol.* 15):C415–C421.

23. Schleier, J. (1918). Der Energieverbrauch in der Blutbahn. *Arch. Gesamte Physiol.* 173:172.

24. Simionescu, N., Heltianu, C., Antone, F., Simionescu, M. (1982). Endothelial cell receptors for histamine. *Ann. N.Y. Acad. Sci.* 401:132–149.

25. Welles, S.L., Shepro, D., Hechtman, H.B. (1985). Vasoactive amines modulate actin cables (stress fibers) and surface area in cultured bovine endothelium. *J. Cell Physiol.* 123:337–342.

2

NORMAL STATE OF THE CIRCULATION

An understanding of the physiological principles that govern cardiovascular function would be of limited value if it were not accompanied by quantitative information about the structures and forces involved. Subsequent chapters will be concerned mainly with the regulatory processes that give the heart and blood vessels their extraordinary ability to adapt to changing circumstances, but first we will define the normal circulatory state. The architecture and dimensions of the system, the volume of blood contained in it, the specific pressures and flows that exist in different parts of the circulation—all of these are parts of the picture the physiologist strives to understand, and a quantitative description of the scene seems a good place to start.

Consider, for example, the bald fact that each ventricle of the heart normally pumps out approximately 100 ml of blood per minute per kilogram of body weight in most resting mammals. No general biological principle is contained in that empirical observation, but it can be a starting point in thinking about heart rate, blood volume, the oxygen-carrying capacity of blood, and tissue metabolism, all of which are interconnected. Information of this kind lends a sense of scale when exploring the functional relationships that are the central theme of physiology, and knowledge of normal circulatory conditions will provide substance for later discussion of physiological signals and mechanisms. The macroscopic, cellular, and molecular phenomena that create the normal state, allowing the living animal to survive and act in a variety of environments, will be considered in later chapters.

Definitions of Normality

Normal limits

Descriptions of the state of the circulation are usually framed in terms of *normal limits,* and a word about the significance of that term is necessary. Such limits are determined by making measurements in a carefully chosen population, the criterion for selection being the apparent absence of any deviation from common standards of good health. The potential for subjective bias at this point is obvious. Data obtained from college athletes, for example, are not the best source of standards for middle-aged subjects of sedentary disposition. Measurements on patients who have been restored to approximately normal function after suffering some previous disorder are sometimes the only available source of data when an invasive procedure is involved, but they are not, of course, the best population for the purpose. Physiological variables are related to sex as well as age in some cases, not to mention diet and other factors.

The word *normal,* then, is sometimes used to mean "free of disease, injury, or defects," but investigators who seek to establish standards also apply it in a mathematical sense. In that context, *normal* distribution of the measurements of a particular variable means that they conform to a specific equation, that of the normal or Gaussian distribution. The values in that case cluster symmetrically around their average in a bell-shaped curve, and a *standard deviation (SD)* can be calculated that describes the proportion of individuals within any selected limits.[10] For instance, 95% of the values fall within the range defined by the mean ± 2 SD.

The average value observed in a test group is no more than a rough indication of the values to be expected in other persons. No two members of a species are identical (*biological variation*), and the conditions of testing cannot be reproduced perfectly every time. Instead, one must identify some range within which the probability of the individual's being similar to the test group can be calculated statistically. The standard deviation is ideal for this purpose, provided that the distribution is indeed mathematically normal. Fortunately, that requirement is met by most cardiovascular variables of interest, as it is in many other biological measurements.

In medical and physiological applications, the goal is usually to identify clinical or physiological disorders, and normal limits or normal range are often defined as the average ± 2 SD, which is the usage adopted throughout this textbook. A narrower range would misdiagnose a considerable fraction of healthy subjects, and a wider range would increase the overlap with values in disease states. The normal standards to be selected thus depend in part on the task in hand, and on the relative importance attached to false positives in contrast to false negatives. Whatever the standards, the inherent conflict between the two different definitions of normalcy must be kept in mind. No matter how healthy a given large population is, 5% of its members will fall outside the ± 2 SD boundaries. The moral is to avoid basing any important decision on just one kind of measurement.

The basal state

Not only must the test population used to establish a standard be carefully selected, but each individual must be studied under the same conditions. Since cardiovascular function is influenced by physical exertion, studies are usually carried out with the subject in a resting state. The requirement is not simply an absence of muscular effort, but an environment as stress free as can be provided. What is sought is a *basal state* in which the subject is completely relaxed, a condition easier to describe than to achieve. A certain amount of apprehension is to be expected in medical patients undergoing an unfamiliar procedure, and the results of many studies are skewed from the normal distribution in a direction that corresponds to less than complete relaxation. Indications of this effect can often be seen in data on cardiac output.

The anesthetics used in many animal experiments have effects of their own on cardiovascular function and may produce results quite different from those achieved in the absence of anesthesia. Sodium pentobarbital, for example, increases the heart rate in the dog to levels above 100 beats/min, whereas the rate in the conscious, relaxed-by-the-fireside dog can be 70 beats/min or even lower. This problem can be avoided and data obtained in the conscious state with surgically implanted transducers. In many cases, the signals can be transmitted by telemetry, so that the animal is under no restraint.

Cardiac Output

The best-known measure of cardiovascular function is *cardiac output,* the volume of blood ejected by the ventricles per minute. The left ventricle propels that amount into the aorta and systemic circulation as the right ventricle pumps an equal volume through the pulmonary circulation. The average cardiac output at rest in large groups of healthy human subjects 16 to 56 years of age is 6.5 liters/min, with a standard deviation of 1.46 liters/min, and the normal range is consequently 3.6 to 9.4 liters/min. These normal values were derived by analysis of reports from seven different laboratories in which cardiac output was measured on a total of 93 healthy subjects, and the distribution of results is shown in Figure 2.1. The papers from which the data were taken are cited in Table 2.1, which also summarizes the normal range (mean ± 2 SD) for other significant variables. Patients with cardiovascular or respiratory disorders were

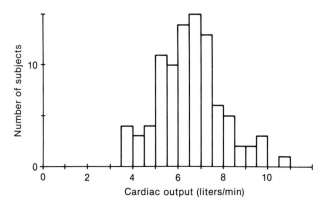

Figure 2.1. Histogram of resting cardiac outputs (*abscissa*) measured in 93 normal adult human subjects.[18,21,23,31,38,41,47]

excluded, as were observations made during anesthesia or accompanied by heart rates greater than 94 beats/min. All subjects were studied in the supine position, an important consideration because cardiac output is affected by posture. Although the heart rate in man tends to be 5 to 10 beats/min faster in the erect than in the supine position, stroke volume is smaller. The end result is that output is about 20% lower when standing or sitting than when lying down (Chapter 13). The selection of the subjects used to establish normal standards and the conditions under which the data were obtained are always relevant, especially when the measurements require cardiac catheterization, a procedure rarely carried out on human subjects unless some disease is at least suspected.

The methods used to determine cardiac output in these subjects were about equally divided among direct Fick, indicator-dilution, and catheter-tip flowmeter techniques (Chapter 14). Other work has shown that there is no systematic difference in the values obtained by these procedures. Most early studies employed the Fick or indicator-dilution methods, but the catheter-mounted flowmeters now available give similar results. For example, measurements of output by catheter-tip velocity sensors in 23 subjects averaged 6.65 (SD ± 1.24) liters/min.[38,41]

The group of 93 patients already referred to included both males and females, but there is no sex difference in the resting cardiac output. Age and body size are significant factors, however, and both must be taken into account. The resting output decreases 0.5 to 1% per year with age,[42] falling from an average of 7.1 liters/min at age 20 to 5.7 liters/min at age 60. In most studies, the resting cardiac output in subjects 15 to 30 years of age appears to depend on body size alone, but beyond that point it declines as a function of age.[19] Resting heart rate does not change systematically, so the stroke volume also becomes smaller with increasing age.

Table 2.1. Normal Hemodynamic Values in Adult Human Subjects in the Basal State

VARIABLE[a]	UNITS	MEAN[b] (± 2SD)	REFERENCE
Heart rate	beats/min	71 (53–89)	18, 21, 23, 31, 38, 41, 47
Blood flow			
Cardiac output	liters/min	6.50 (3.6–9.4)	18, 21, 23, 31, 38, 41, 47
Cardiac index	liters/min m²	3.63 (2.0–5.2)	18, 21, 23, 31, 38, 41, 47
Stroke volume	ml	93 (53–133)	18, 21, 23, 31, 38, 41, 47
Pulsation, Ao, peak	ml/sec	690 (470–910)	38, 41
Pulsation, MPA, peak	ml/sec	628 (420–830)	36
Blood pressures,[c] systemic			
Ao, S/D	mm Hg	122/83	33, 39, 42
Ao, mean	mm Hg	97 (80–113)	33, 39, 42
Ao, pulse	mm Hg	39 (24–54)	33, 39, 42
Large artery,[d] S/D	mm Hg	129/78	26, 33, 42
Large artery,[d] mean	mm Hg	95 (72–118)	26, 33, 42
Large artery, pulse	mm Hg	51 (31–71)	26, 33, 42
Large vein[d]	mm Hg	8 (4–12)	16
Right atrium, mean	mm Hg	5 (0.2–9)	16, 25
Blood pressures,[c] pulmonic			
MPA, S/D	mm Hg	22/11	16, 22
MPA, mean	mm Hg	14.6 (10–19)	22, 25, 37
MPA, pulse	mm Hg	11.4 (6–17)	16, 22
Terminal vein, mean	mm Hg	8 (4–12)	2,[e]
Left atrium, mean	mm Hg	7.9 (2–12)	20
Vascular bed resistance			
Pulmonic	dyn sec/cm⁵	70 (20–120)	16, 37
Systemic	dyn sec/cm⁵	1070 (660–1480)	

[a]Abbreviations: Ao, ascending aorta; S/D, systolic/diastolic; MPA, main pulmonary artery.

[b]For male subjects aged 30 years, weight 68 kg, height 175 cm, surface area 1.80 cm².

[c]Direct measurements through catheters.

[d]For example, brachial or femoral.

[e]Milnor, Nichols, and Walker, unpublished data.

Cardiac output is directly correlated with the overall size of the subject, whether the criterion is height, weight, or body surface area. For reasons to be considered in a later section, most investigators use surface area as the standardizing variable. The ratio of cardiac output to area, called the *cardiac index,* averages 3.6 liters/min m^2 in healthy adults, with a standard deviation of ± 0.82 liter/min m^2. The normal range for the cardiac index is thus 2.0 to 5.3 liters/min m^2.

Relating cardiac output to body surface area has been so widely accepted that more than half of the early studies on normal cardiac output reported only the cardiac index, without specifying the body surface area on which it was based. One weakness of this expression is that the body surface area used in its calculation is never actually measured, but predicted from height and weight by an equation derived from a few early papers in which area *was* carefully determined. Graphs depicting the relationship appear in most textbooks of human physiology. To provide some appreciation of the magnitudes involved, the predicted body surface area of an individual 170 cm in height and 70 kg in weight is 1.80 m^2. The surface area of a typical 10-yr-old is about 1.0 m^2, and smaller values are found in younger children and infants.

The relation between basal cardiac output and body surface area is not linear over the whole range that applies to the human species, although it is almost linear above 1.2 m^2. The relationship, shown in Figure 2.2, suggests that the normal range already cited for the cardiac index applies above 1.2 m^2 and is therefore a satisfactory standard for adults. In children younger than 15 yr, the cardiac output is lower per unit surface area than it is in older individuals. At the lowest extreme, in the period 2 to 15 hours after birth,[46] the cardiac output is about 0.5 liter/min, and newborn infants have a surface area of about 0.25 m^2; their cardiac index averages 2.1 (SD $\pm$ 0.26) liters/min m^2.

The *stroke volume* ejected with each heartbeat, which can be calculated from cardiac output and the heart rate, normally ranges from 50 to 130 ml in adult human subjects at rest, with an average of 93 ml. The human heart rate ranges from 53 to 89 beats/min under basal conditions, and there is a close inverse relation between rate and stroke volume. Long-distance runners, for example, tend to have slow heart rates, but their stroke volume is relatively large and their resting cardiac output is in the range already cited. A stroke volume of 115 ml at a rate of 56 beats/min in one person, and a stroke of 80 ml with a heart rate of 80 beats/min in another, both represent normal variations at rest. The cardiovascular system under resting conditions seems to be set for a particular output, which it can maintain equally well with a small number of large strokes or a larger number of small strokes. The resting situation thus contrasts with the response to exercise, where an increase in heart rate is one of the ways in which the body raises cardiac output.

A direct relation between resting cardiac output and body size exists

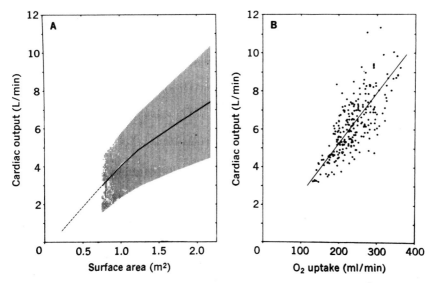

Figure 2.2. **A,** relation between resting cardiac output (*ordinate*) and body surface area (*abscissa*) in man. *Shaded area* includes ±2 standard deviations above and below mean. Surface areas smaller than 1 m² are found in children and infants. Relationship is almost linear for surface areas greater than 1.2 m², lending validity to the use of cardiac index (cardiac output/surface area) as a standard for comparison of different individuals. **B,** relation between cardiac output (*ordinate*) and oxygen uptake (*abscissa*), corresponding approximately to constant arteriovenous oxygen difference of 38.4 ml/l. (Reproduced from Reeves et al.,[47] with permission of the American Physiological Society)

throughout the animal kingdom. Comparisons are best made in terms of output per kilogram of body weight, which amounts to about 100 ml/min kg on the average. as demonstrated by the data in Table 2.2. There are marked variations, however, which probably reflect varying experimental conditions as much as real species differences. The basal cardiac output in dogs is usually 120–130 ml/min kg, for example, whereas in man it is about 102 ml/min kg. A more detailed discussion of the relation between output and body size appears later in this chapter.

The rate of oxygen uptake by the lungs also varies directly with body size. It bears a functional relation to cardiac output, as suggested by one version of the Fick equation (Chapter 14):

$$\text{Cardiac output} = \frac{O_2 \text{ uptake}}{\text{arteriovenous } O_2 \text{ difference}} \tag{2.1}$$

The arteriovenous O_2 difference has been shown to be relatively constant in resting subjects and does not vary with body size. As a result, the relation between output and oxygen uptake is linear, as shown in Figure 2.2B. The best

Table 2.2.   Average Normal Hemodynamic Values in Five Mammalian Species

VARIABLE	COW	MAN	DOG	RABBIT	RAT[a]
Weight (kg)	414	70	20	4.0	0.6
Cardiac output (ml/sec)	680	110	42	5.2	1.2
Heart rate (min^{-1})	71	76	99	288	349
Stroke volume (ml)	570	87	25	1.1	0.21
Mean velocity, ascending aorta (mm/sec)		16	18	32	22

[a]Anesthetized.

Source: data reported in the literature[1,6,45] and unpublished data of Milnor, Nichols, and Yin.

fit to the data in the figure indicates a resting arteriovenous oxygen difference of 38.4 ml of O_2 per liter of blood. This is an overall value, and there are marked variations in different organs. The myocardium, for example, extracts a much greater fraction of the O_2 in its blood supply than do other tissues.

The blood volume of the cardiac chambers is an important physiological variable, and many different techniques have been used to measure it (Chapter 14). The volume of the human left ventricle at the end of diastolic filling is about 125 ml in an average adult in the basal state, and the normal range is 70 to 190 ml. (The ranges observed in healthy individuals do not always correspond to the limits implied by ± 2 SD in data like those of Tables 2.1 and 2.3 because the distribution is not quite symmetric.) The size of the heart increases along with body size as a rule, and chamber volumes are often expressed in relation to body surface area, in which form the average figure for *end-diastolic volume* of the human left ventricle[32] is 70 ml/m^2. The ventricles do not empty completely with each contraction, but leave behind one-third to one-half of the blood that filled them at the end of diastole. The *end-systolic volume* in subjects at rest varies with heart rate and stroke, but 25 to 65 ml is the typical range in man.

Typical stroke volumes for several species are listed in Table 2.2. The strokes of the right and left ventricles are equal except for small beat-to-beat variations, and the amount of blood ejected over a period of minutes is the same for both chambers (Chapter 4). The ratio of stroke volume to end-diastolic volume is called the *ejection fraction* (Table 2.3). Determinations by newer methods of radionuclide scanning agree with those from x-ray angiography in placing the left ventricular ejection fraction at 0.67, with a standard deviation of ± 0.11.[17,32] The fraction is smaller in the right ventricle,[17,28] averaging 0.54 (SD $\pm$ 0.12, $n = 28$). Inasmuch as the stroke volumes of the right and left ventricles are almost identical, this finding suggests that end-diastolic volume is some 20% larger in the right than in the left ventricle, but direct evidence on

Table 2.3.   Left Ventricular Volumes Measured by Angiography in Man

	MEAN ($\pm$ SD)	SOURCE
End-diastolic volume (ml)	125 ($\pm$ 31)	[a]
End-systolic volume (ml)	42 ($\pm$ 17)	[a]
Stroke volume (ml)	82 ($\pm$ 20)	[a]
Ejection fraction	0.67 ($\pm$ 0.11)	[a,b]
Mean wall thickness (mm)	10.9 ($\pm$ 2.0)	[a]

[a]Kennedy et al.,[32] radiopaque medium; $n = 16$.
[b]Berger et al.,[17] radionuclide angiography; $n = 19$.

that point is lacking at present. Although the technically difficult problem of viewing both chambers simultaneously has been overcome, the translation of two-dimensional images into reliable estimates of volume remains an obstacle, and small differences in end-diastolic volumes cannot be detected with certainty. The ejection fraction in both ventricles increases with exercise. At a level of exertion sufficient to double cardiac output, the ejection fraction rises to about 0.81 on the left side and 0.67 on the right side.[17]

All of the blood ejected by the right ventricle flows through the lungs, but the output of the left ventricle is divided among many different pathways and organ systems (Figure 2.3). Approximately 25% of the total output goes to the head and upper extremities, 25% to the lower extremities and pelvic organs, and 50% to the trunk and other viscera. The distribution of the cardiac output in the systemic circulation varies with physiological needs; typical patterns at rest and during exercise are shown in Table 2.4. Skeletal muscle, for example, receives an appreciable fraction of the output in accordance with its large mass, even in basal conditions. With exercise, however, not only does total cardiac output increase but the proportion of it going to muscle rises sharply, whereas the fraction delivered to the splanchnic bed is much lower during exercise than at rest. The figures given for exercise in Table 2.4 are for strenuous but not record-breaking exertion; an output of 42 liters/min has been measured in a world-class long distance runner.[24]

The mechanism that controls the distribution of output is the relative *vascular resistance* of the various organs. Resistance is an expression of the extent to which the physical properties of a vascular bed impede flow (Chapter 6), and local resistances can be altered physiologically to enhance or reduce the share of blood flow delivered to each region. The resistance of the pulmonary vasculature is much lower than that of the systemic circulation. Both carry the same blood flow per minute, but the former typically accomplishes that task with a mean pulmonary artery pressure of about 15 mm Hg, whereas the latter requires a mean aortic pressure of about 96 mm Hg. The vascular properties

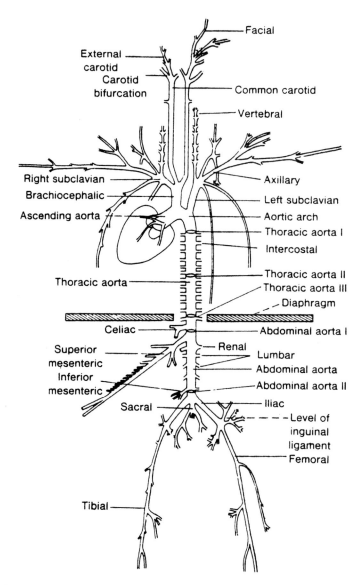

Figure 2.3. Major branches of the arterial tree in the dog. Drawing is to scale, but the scale for diameters is double that for lengths. (Reproduced from McDonald,[5] with permission of Edward Arnold, Ltd)

Table 2.4.   Distribution of Cardiac Output in Normal Human Subjects at Rest and After 10 Min of Strenuous Exercise[a]

VASCULAR BED	BLOOD FLOW (ML/MIN, % OF TOTAL)			
	REST		EXERCISE	
Skeletal muscle	1,200	(21%)	12,500	(71%)
Splanchnic	1,400	(24%)	600	(3%)
Renal	1,100	(19%)	600	(3%)
Cerebral	750	(13%)	750	(5%)
Coronary	250	(4%)	750	(5%)
Skin	500	(9%)	1,900	(11%)
Other organs	600	(10%)	400	(2%)
Cardiac output	5,800	(100%)	17,500	(100%)

[a]From Wade and Bishop.[12]

that determine resistance, and their effects on blood flow and pressure, are discussed in detail in Chapter 6, where the normal values for resistance are also tabulated.

Dimensions of the System

The quantitative attributes of the blood vessels are as important as those of the heart in determining normal circulatory function, and any survey of the normal state must include the dimensions of the vascular system and the amount of blood within it. The systemic and pulmonic vascular trees are, in effect, elastic containers of complex shape filled with blood. The total blood volume varies directly with body weight, averaging 75 (SD ± 8) ml/kg in man (Chapter 13), and the total volume in adults is thus approximately 6 liters. Resting cardiac output tends to be correlated directly with blood volume, the average ratio of output to total volume[31] being 1.2. The total blood volume per unit body weight is species dependent, being lower than the human value in some mammals and higher in others. The distribution of this volume throughout the body is considered in Chapter 12. The fluid properties of the blood that influence the hemodynamic state, such as viscosity and the ratio of cells to plasma, are described in Chapter 13.

The blood-filled vessels range in size from the aorta and main pulmonary arteries down to the capillaries. The diameter of the lumen of the ascending aorta and main pulmonary artery in adult men and women[27,36,41,48] is about 3 cm, giving a cross-sectional area of 7.1 cm^2. There is considerable individual variation, and diameters from 2.2 to 3.4 cm should probably be considered in the normal range.[42] Some studies indicate that the diameter of the aorta is smaller than that of the pulmonary artery, but the two vessels differ at their origins by less than 5%. The caliber of the aorta is scaled to the size of the animal, and it tapers along its length. In a dog weighing 20 kg, the lumen of the aorta has a diameter of about 2.0 cm at its origin, 1.2 cm at the level of the diaphragm, and 0.8 cm just before the branching of the iliac arteries. The outer diameter of the midportion of the femoral artery is typically 0.45 cm in a dog of that size and 0.51 cm in humans.[1]

Although the arteries become smaller and smaller toward the periphery, their numbers increase to such an extent that the total vascular cross section continually increases. The change in vascular cross section at points of vascular branching can be described by a *branching coefficient,* defined as the ratio of the combined areas of the daughter vessels to that of the parent vessel. This coefficient is greater than 1.0 throughout the systemic arterial bed and tends to increase from about 1.10–1.20 in large arteries to higher values in the periphery.[6] Simple bifurcation is common in the arterial tree, but subdivisions do not occur with perfect geometric regularity. At some points, a single small lateral branch may arise from a large vessel, and at others one small artery may divide into many branches.

Systemic circulation

The progressive expansion in the total cross section of the canine systemic circulation is shown in Figure 2.4. The areas of the primary aortic branches add up to scarcely more than that of the aorta itself, but the cross section begins to increase in vessels the size of the femoral and common carotid arteries. Between those vessels and arterioles 100 μm in diameter, the total cross section increases three- to fivefold. The venous tree reverses the process as vessels converge into larger trunks that are individually greater in diameter but fewer in number and smaller in total cross section. Estimates of the total number of capillaries in the systemic circulation[6] range from 2×10^8 to 1.2×10^9, a reasonably close agreement considering the technical problems and assumptions involved. The veins tend to be slightly larger and more numerous than the accompanying arteries at each level in the vascular tree. The increase in numbers begins in the postcapillary region, where there are 2 to 20 times as many small veins as arteries.

There are marked regional differences in the expansion of the arterial area. The data summarized in Figure 2.4 are a composite of studies on several tissues. Much of the information was derived from the canine mesenteric bed, but the lowest portion of the shaded area in the figure comes from measure-

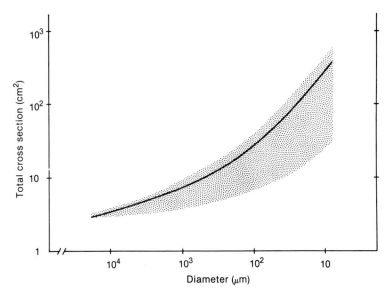

Figure 2.4.   Approximate total cross section of arterial tree (*ordinate*) in relation to vessel diameters (*abscissa*, decreasing toward right), in a 20-kg dog. *Solid* line represents an estimate made by Milnor.[6] *Shaded area* indicates range of other estimates in the literature. (Reproduced from Milnor,[6] with permission of Williams & Wilkins)

ments on vessels of the canine spleen. Differences in tissue vascularity are indicated by the maximum blood flow per unit weight of tissue, which is 5 ml/min per gram of tissue in the salivary gland but 1 ml/min g in skeletal muscle (Chapter 12).

One consequence of the conformation of the arterial tree is that blood velocity falls progressively as the total vascular cross section increases. The whole cardiac output passes through each transverse cross section of the bed, and that output divided by the total cross-sectional area equals average blood velocity, so velocity is inversely proportional to total cross section. The result is that velocity falls from about 16 cm/sec in the ascending aorta to a few tenths of a millimeter per second in the capillaries (Chapter 10), then rises again in the veins. Typical velocities in different parts of the vascular tree are given in Tables 2.2 and 2.5, where a comparison of the values shows that they are similar in different species and consequently are not dependent on body size. The velocity of which we speak here is that of blood moving through the circulation, which should not be confused with *pulse wave velocity,* the speed with which pressure pulsations travel. Wave velocity, like the speed of sound through water, is several hundreds of meters per second (Chapter 6).

Table 2.5.   Typical Blood Velocities in Man and the Dog[a]

	MEAN (SYSTOLIC/DIASTOLIC) VELOCITIES (CM/SEC)	
	DOG	MAN
Systemic vessels		
Ascending aorta	16 (90/0)	18 (112/0)
Abdominal aorta	12 (60/0)	14 (75/0)
Femoral artery	10 (42/1)	12 (52/1)
Femoral vein	5	4
Superior vena cava	8 (20/0)	9 (23/0)
Inferior vena cava	19 (40/0)	21 (46/0)
Pulmonary vessels		
Main artery	15 (60/0)	15 (85/0)
Main vein	18 (30/9)	19 (38/10)

[a]Reproduced with modifications from Milnor,[6] with permission of Williams & Wilkins.

Pulmonary circulation

The main pulmonary artery is of approximately the same diameter as the ascending aorta but extends for only 3 to 4 cm in man before dividing into two main branches. This bifurcation is one of the few places where arterial cross section becomes smaller at a branch point, the branching coefficient being about 0.8. In the next branching the coefficient is about 1.08, and at subsequent junctions it gradually increases[14,30] to 1.20. The main pulmonary artery and the first five generations of branches are elliptical, not circular, in cross section. The ratio of the major to the minor axis is about 1.25 in the main artery, decreases to 1.07 by the fifth order of branching, and is approximately unity thereafter.[14] The pulmonary vessels contain 7 to 10% of the total blood volume in the basal state, and a little more than one-third of that quantity fills the pulmonary capillaries. The pulmonary circulation is described in detail in Chapter 11.

Volume, distensibility, and pressure

The total volume of blood contained in the vascular system is a critical variable because of its influence on blood pressure. Although the energy imparted to the blood by the heart is the principal source of pressure under normal conditions, the relation between blood volume and vascular distensibility also makes an important contribution. In the absence of any cardiac contractions, pressure throughout the circulation reaches an equilibrium at 7 to 12 mm Hg within a few minutes, and this finite MCFP demonstrates that the normal blood volume distends the elastic vasculature slightly (Chapter 6). In other words, the system behaves like an elastic container that has been filled slightly beyond its unstressed capacity. When the force generated by the normal heartbeat is added to this static filling pressure, the result is a mean pressure of about 90 mm Hg in the large systemic arteries and 4 to 10 mm Hg in the veins. The equilibrium established by cardiac pumping thus raises arterial pressure some 80 mm Hg above MCFP but *lowers* venous pressure. The pressure gradient from an antecubital vein to the right atrium averages 2.5 mm Hg, and the drop from vena cava to right atrium is less than 1 mm Hg.[16] Pressures in the microcirculation are between the arterial and venous extremes, as described in Chapter 10.

The distribution of the blood volume among different parts of the system is determined by the relation between local pressure and vascular distensibility. Pressure is high in arteries, but they are not very distensible and the volume of blood in the arterial tree is relatively small. In contrast, a large part of the blood volume resides in the veins, even though their pressure is low, because they are readily distended. The basic measure used to express vascular distensibility is *Young's modulus of elasticity,* the stretching force per unit cross-sectional area required to elongate a strip of vessel wall by 100%. The distribution of elasticity within the arterial tree is discussed in Chapter 6, but some idea of the magnitudes involved is conveyed by the Young's modulus of femoral arteries, which is about 2×10^7 dyn/cm^2, or 20 kg/cm^2.

Virtually all mammalian species exhibit the same vascular pressures under basal conditions,[1] and blood pressure is not related to body size. Small species differences are common enough that investigators must determine normal limits in each case, but the differences are apparently not size dependent. In large and small animals, pressures similar to those found in man supply an adequate blood flow to all tissues. The one prominent exception to this rule is related to body *shape,* specifically the vertical distance between the brain and the heart. The most striking example is the giraffe, which has a mean systemic arterial pressure of at least 220 mm Hg, a high level presumably related to the hydrostatic pressure that must be overcome to move blood from the heart to the head some 3 m above it.[49] The same relationship exists to a lesser degree in cattle, which have a mean arterial pressure of about 135 mm Hg.[45]

Pulsations of Pressure

Measurements of mean values, averaged over an integral number of cardiac cycles, are useful for many purposes, but pressure and flow vary with time throughout each heartbeat, producing characteristic pulsations. The amplitudes of pressure and flow waves are physiologically significant because of the energy involved in producing them, an extra amount of cardiac work that would not be required had evolution devised a steady-flow, nonpulsatile pump (Chapter 4). The simplest quantitative description of such pulsations specifies the highest and lowest values during the cardiac cycle. *Systolic pressure* is the maximum value attained at the peak of the pressure wave, and *diastolic pressure* is the lowest level reached at the end of each cycle. *Pulse pressure* is the difference between systolic and diastolic values. These three measurements are a sufficient description of pressure pulsations in many situations, although a more complete numerical representation can be provided by Fourier analysis (Chapter 6).

Pressures in systemic circulation

The normal range of systolic and diastolic pressures in a large systemic artery (specifically, the brachial artery in the antecubital space) has been studied extensively, thanks to the simplicity of the arm cuff method (Chapter 14). Measurements on literally thousands of healthy persons in a resting state have been reported in various papers, and the results in one such series[9,29] are illustrated in Figure 2.5. The data in this study were obtained from 1988 individuals 15 to 80 years of age, 810 of them male and 1178 female. The results of other studies vary in minor details, but virtually all observations support two general conclusions:

1. Both systolic and diastolic pressure increase with age.
2. The spread of values observed within each cohort becomes greater with age.

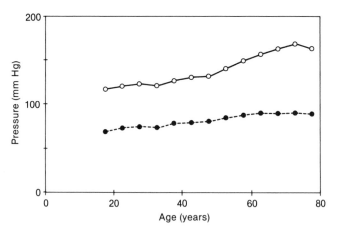

Figure 2.5.   Average systolic and diastolic arterial blood pressure in systemic circulation (*ordinate*) in relation to age (*abscissa*) in 1,988 healthy human subjects. (From data published by Hamilton et al.[29])

Normal standards for pressure must be related to sex as well as age. Average systolic/diastolic values for males,[29] for example, are 118/71 at age 20, 126/77 at age 40, and 150/88 at age 60. Most of the age-related increase in pressure occurs between the ages of 30 and 60, as can be seen in Figure 2.5. The averages in women at the same ages are 118/70, 131/81, and 156/90, respectively, demonstrating that systolic and diastolic pressures are slightly higher in women than in men after the age of 30. For both sexes, the *coefficient of variation* (standard deviation expressed as a percentage of the mean) in systolic and diastolic pressures[9,29] is approximately 11% at age 20, 15% at age 40, and 19% at age 60. Systemic blood pressures are lower in newborns and young children than in adults. The mean arterial pressure is typically 58 mm Hg in the first 24 hr after birth, rises gradually to perhaps 70 mm Hg (88/60) by the age of 4 yr, and reaches the level shown at the beginning of Figure 2.5 by the age of 15 yr (for references, see Chapter 11).

The attention given for many years to the establishment of normal standards in this field has been motivated by the prevalence of human disorders characterized by high blood pressure. The diagnosis of disease is not made from a single reading of a pressure outside normal limits, however. Although statistical limits in large populations can be expressed exactly, the characteristic resting blood pressure in a given human subject cannot always be determined with such precision. Changes of a few millimeters of mercury in systolic or diastolic values over periods of minutes or hours occur frequently, and larger shifts can be caused by emotional stimuli, most of which tend to raise pressure above the basal level. Moreover, there is a certain amount of overlap between values in healthy individuals and those in persons with mild or early stages of disease.

Another potential source of misinterpretation is the practice of defining systolic and diastolic limits separately. Normal standards for *pulse pressure* are also required. To illustrate by an example, the normal ranges for individuals 35 to 40 years of age in the population described by Figure 2.5 are 93 to 159 mm Hg (systolic) and 58 to 100 mm Hg (diastolic). These broad limits must *not* be taken to mean that any systolic/diastolic pair that falls within them is observed in healthy populations. A systolic pressure of 159 mm Hg in the brachial artery is not normally accompanied by a diastolic value of 58 mm Hg. The peripheral arterial pulse pressure in normal human subjects is rarely greater than 70 mm Hg or less than 30 mm Hg.

The pulse pressure, like systolic and diastolic levels, increases with age in the aorta and large arteries. One study on 45 normal subjects[42] has reported that pulse pressure in the ascending aorta averages 31 mm Hg at age 20 and increases steadily, reaching 54 mm Hg at age 60. Figure 2.5 suggests that the same phenomenon occurs in peripheral arteries, although the evidence is indirect because individual pulse pressures were not analyzed in the studies summarized there.

The pulse pressure in large arteries is determined by the elasticity of the vessel and the stroke volume ejected by the heart. Other things being equal, the larger the stroke volume, the greater the pulse pressure. Cardiac output itself does not affect the size of pressure pulsations, although it influences the mean pressure around which the oscillations occur (Chapter 6). The elastic modulus of large arteries increases with age, which is to say that they become stiffer, or less distensible, a change that tends to increase the pulse pressure accompanying a given stroke volume. Inasmuch as the stroke volume actually becomes smaller with age (see above), it is presumably the arterial stiffening that causes the increased pulse pressure in older individuals. Quantitative information about the normal elasticity of arterial walls is given in Chapter 6.

Although *mean* pressure falls by 1 or 2 mm Hg between the ascending aorta and its major branches, *pulse* pressure becomes progressively larger in many individuals. The amplitude of the pulsation increases as it travels down the aorta and into the primary branches because of reflected waves (Chapter 6), which amplify the pulse pressure by about 35% between the aortic arch and the femoral artery in adults under 40 years of age. Direct measurement of pulse pressures by catheterization indicates that pulse pressure averages 39 mm Hg in the ascending aorta and increases steadily along the course of that vessel to about 51 mm Hg in the radial and femoral arteries[16,33,44] (Table 2.1). This amplification diminishes with age; by age 65, the size of the pressure pulsation is about the same in the brachial and femoral arteries as it is in the aortic arch.[44]

The shape of normal pressure pulses in large arteries varies almost as much as their amplitude, because their contours are influenced by reflected waves and reflections are more prominent in some individuals than in others. The concept of pressure and flow wave reflection will be discussed in Chapter 6, but the key fact is that pulsations at any point in the vascular tree are the sum of a forward-moving wave and a pulse that has been reflected back from peripheral sites. The net result depends on the magnitude and timing of the reflected wave, which returns before the peak of the incident wave in some cases and after it in others.

Murgo and his associates[38] have classified arterial pressure waves into three categories based on the timing and prominence of the secondary wave produced by reflections. The type A pulse has a late systolic peak preceded by a slight inflection that marks the onset of the retrograde component (Figure 2.6). Pulse pressure tends to be greater in type A waves than in the other varieties. In type C, the peak systolic pressure is lower and near midsystole, and is followed by a small, early diastolic wave in some instances. Contours that fall between these extremes are designated type B. The population of wave-

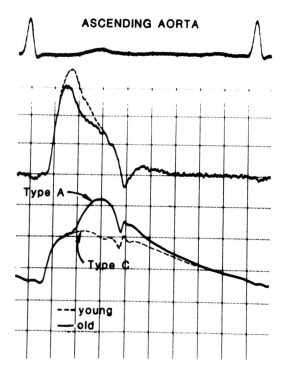

Figure 2.6. Electrocardiogram (*top*), blood flow (*middle*), and pressure (*bottom*) in human ascending aorta. *Solid lines,* type A waves; *dashed lines,* type C waves (see text). (Reproduced from Nichols et al.,[42] with permission of Reed Publishing, USA)

forms is actually a continuum, but this classification is a useful mode of description. Quantitative criteria for defining the categories without ambiguity have been proposed.[38]

The shape of the arterial pressure pulse is closely correlated with age. The intermediate type B predominates in subjects 30 to 50 years of age, type C in younger persons, and type A in older individuals, although there is much overlap. The differences in contour are believed to arise from the size and velocity of the reflected wave in each individual. The type A wave suggests that a relatively large reflection is returning rapidly enough to merge with the early portion of the ongoing pulse. This explanation is consistent with the finding that peripheral resistance rises and arteries become stiffer in older persons, changes that increase reflection and wave velocity, respectively. In contrast, the comparatively low resistance and elastic modulus in younger persons (see below) match the small size and late arrival of the reflected component in type C pulses. It should be emphasized that accurate recording of pulse wave contours requires a high-fidelity manometer system (Chapter 14).

Pressures in the pulmonary circulation

Arterial pressure is lower in the pulmonary than in the systemic circulation. Both carry the same flow of blood per minute (the cardiac output), but the resistance of the pulmonary vasculature is relatively low, in part because of the relatively short length of the system. The average intravascular distance from pulmonic valve to left atrium in humans is about 30 cm, although many shorter and longer paths exist.[6] In the systemic circuit the length of the aorta alone approximates 40 cm in adults, and the longest intravascular pathways from aortic valve to right atrium extend for more than 2 m. This difference, plus the relatively large number of parallel vessels in the pulmonary microcirculation, makes the overall resistance of the pulmonary bed about one-sixth that of the systemic circulation.

Mean pressure in the main pulmonary artery averages about 15 mm Hg under basal conditions, with typical systolic/diastolic values of 22/11 mm Hg (Table 2.1). The pulse pressure is directly related to the stroke volume, just as it is in the systemic arteries. Mean pressure in the terminal pulmonary veins is usually between 4 and 12 mm Hg. In the left atrium, which is the hemodynamic termination of the pulmonary bed, the normal range is 2 to 12 mm Hg. Pressure is usually about 4 mm Hg (range, 1 to 7 mm Hg) higher in the left atrium than in the right.[20]

The values just given apply to adults. Pulmonary arterial pressures undergo a radical change at birth, when the ductus arteriosus, which carries blood from the pulmonary artery to the aorta during fetal life, begins to close. Only a small part of the right ventricular output *in utero* flows through the pulmonary capillaries, a physiologically proper arrangement because the alveoli of the fetus are filled with amniotic fluid and the respiratory exchange of oxygen and carbon dioxide is carried on entirely by the maternal circulation. The fetal lungs are in a semicollapsed state and have a vascular resistance as high as that of the systemic bed, so that pulmonary arterial and aortic pressures are virtually the same, between 50 and 70 mm Hg. With the first breath after birth, the pulmonary vascular resistance falls as the lungs expand and fill with air, and after a few minutes the mean pulmonary arterial pressure has usually fallen to about 30 mm Hg. The pressure continues to decline during the next few months and reaches the normal adult level (Table 2.1) when the ductus arteriosus has completely closed (Chapter 11). After that time, pressure in the pulmonary arteries, unlike that in the systemic arteries, does not rise with age.

The normal sequence of pressures through the pulmonary circulation is discussed in the section devoted to that bed (Chapter 11). The greatest drop in mean and pulse pressures occurs in the microcirculation, as it does in systemic beds (Figure 1.2). A small pressure pulsation of 2 or 3 mm in amplitude persists into the large pulmonary veins, which is not the case in large veins of the systemic circulation. A slight amplification of pulse pressure within the main pulmonary artery can be detected by careful measurement, but it is much smaller than that in the aorta and of no physiological significance.

Pulmonary capillary pressure is about 9 mm Hg at the level of the heart, considerably lower than it is in most systemic beds. Hydrostatic forces play a larger part in determining transmural pressure in the capillaries of the lung than is the case in other organs, especially in human subjects standing erect. A mean pulmonary arterial pressure of 15 mm Hg will just balance the weight of a column of blood 20 cm high, which is about the vertical distance from the right ventricle to the apex of the lungs. For that reason, the transmural pressure is apical regions may not be sufficient to hold the capillaries open, and many of them remain closed under resting conditions (Chapter 11).

Pulsatile Blood Flow

The pulsatile characteristics of blood flow in an artery or vein can be measured by a number of different instruments. The most accurate techniques at present require cardiac catheterization or other invasive procedures, but several useful external methods are also available (Chapter 14). Most sensors measure the average velocity of blood (in centimeters per second), and the cross-sectional area of the vessel lumen must be known to convert velocity into volumetric rate of flow (cubic centimeters per second). The description of pulsatile flows in the human circulation that follows also applies to other mammalian species, given scale factors appropriate to the size of the animal.

Flow in the ascending aorta rises steeply as blood is first ejected from the ventricle; it reaches a peak and then falls slowly until the aortic valve closes (Figure 2.7). It is perhaps worth emphasizing that blood moves forward throughout the ejection period; it continues to move forward after the peak of the flow record, but at a declining rate. During diastole, blood flow in the aortic root and main pulmonary artery is virtually zero, although a small, transient backward flow often appears at the end of ejection in aortic records, because the transducer cuff must be placed a few centimeters distal to the aortic valve and flow into the coronaries occurs during diastole (Chapter 12). The shape of the flow pulse in the aortic root is almost triangular, contrasting with the more rounded contour in the main pulmonary artery (Figures 2.7 and 4.1). The area beneath each curve is the same in both cases, however, because it represents the time integral of volume flow during ejection, that is, the stroke volume. The mean of the pulsatile flow curves, averaged over an integral number of cardiac cycles, is the cardiac output, which in groups of normal human subjects aver-

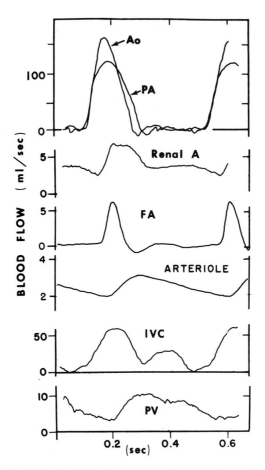

Figure 2.7.   Normal pulsatile blood flow in several canine vessels, scaled for a 20-kg dog. *Ao*, ascending aorta; *PA*, main pulmonary artery; *Renal A*, renal artery; *FA*, femoral artery; *Arteriole* in omentum; *IVC*, inferior vena cava; *PV*, terminal pulmonary vein. Flow units for arteriolar record, 10^{-5} ml/sec; for others, ml/sec. (Reproduced from Milnor,[6] with permission of Williams & Wilkins)

ages 108 ml/sec at rest (Table 2.1). Peak flow is higher in the aorta than in the pulmonary artery, the peak/mean ratio averaging 6.4 in the former and 5.8 in the latter.[6]

The changes in the amplitude, shape, and timing of the flow pulse as it travels along through the main aortic branches and out to the arterioles are indicated in Figure 2.7. At the end of systole the ascending aorta and arch have been distended by the blood ejected from the left ventricle, and the stretched, elastic aortic wall exerts pressure during diastole to move blood into the arterial tree. The systolic distention is not large, about 5% of the diameter in the ascending aorta and 2% in the upper abdominal aorta, but it suffices to maintain flow in the periphery while the ventricles are refilling. For that reason, blood flow usually does not fall to zero between heartbeats in the peripheral arteries, as it does in the aortic root (and main pulmonary artery). Occasionally, however, depending on the length of diastole and the degree of peripheral vasodilatation, flow in some vessels may cease toward the end of diastole, as shown in the femoral arterial record of Figure 2.7. Flow pulsations become smaller as they are transmitted through the arterial tree, but small pulsations persist in the microcirculation and in the pulmonary veins (Chapter 11). The only parts of the systemic venous tree that exhibit pulsatile flow are the terminal segments of the venae cavae near the right atrium, where small retrograde waves are produced by the effects of atrial contraction (Figure 2.7).

Blood does not necessarily move at the same speed at all points across the diameter of a vessel, and the tracings of pulsatile flow discussed thus far are continuous records with time of the *average* rate of flow at a specific vascular cross section. Most flowmeters, including those used to record the flow pulsations shown in Figure 2.7, average the mixture of velocities across the vessel lumen at every instant, but special instruments have been designed to measure local velocity at various sites (Chapter 14), so that the motion of blood at any transverse section can be described by a *velocity profile* (Chapter 6). The velocity profile has a rounded shape in most of the peripheral arterial tree, but in the root of the aorta it is essentially flat (Figure 2.8). As the cylindrical "slug" of ejected blood moves into the aortic arch, the profile becomes skewed so that blood moves more rapidly near the "inner" wall (the side with the smallest radius of curvature) than elsewhere. Beyond the arch and throughout the remainder of the arterial tree, the profile takes on the shape of a parabola, the axial portion of the stream moving most rapidly and the blood near the wall most slowly (Chapter 6).

Pulsations of flow in the pulmonary circulation can be measured in the capillary bed, as well as in the main artery and veins, giving a more complete picture of transmission than is available for other regions. The large vessels can be studied with standard flowmeters, and a unique method has been devised to record pulmonary capillary flow. The subject is placed in a closed chamber, or *body plethysmograph,* and the rate of alveolar uptake of inhaled nitrous oxide is recorded continuously as an indication of capillary blood flow at every instant (Chapter 11). The data so obtained show that flow pulsations are not attenuated as much as pressure waves in passing through the pulmonic circulation. Large pulsations with a peak-to-mean ratio of about 2.0 occur in the pulmonary capillaries, and the ratio is only slightly smaller in the pulmonary veins (Figure 11.5). Most of the venous flow pulsation is transmitted from the main pulmonary artery, although near the end of the veins there can be a small retrograde movement induced by left atrial contraction.[6]

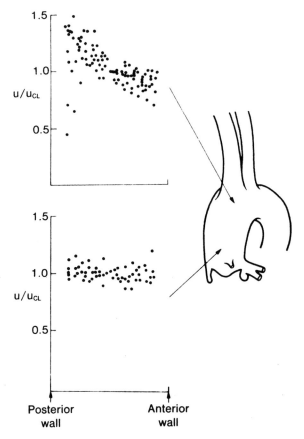

Figure 2.8.   Velocity profiles across diameter of canine ascending aorta at two different sites, at peak systole. Velocities (*u*) expressed in relation to center-line velocity (*u_CL*). *Bottom plot,* flat profile just beyond aortic valve. *Top plot,* skewed profile near the arch, with relatively high velocities near "posterior" wall. (Reproduced from Caro et al.,[2] with permission of Oxford University Press)

Effects of Age

Significant physical changes occur with age in the heart and blood vessels; large arteries dilate and become stiffer, while cardiac muscle undergoes some degree of hypertrophy. The decreasing distensibility of arteries is correlated with specific morphological changes: their collagen content increases, the ratio of collagen to elastin rises, and the medial elastic fibers become fragmented. Increasing stiffness of the aorta is indicated by a rise in the elastic modulus, which more than doubles between the ages of 20 and 60 yr, and a similar change takes place in the pulmonary artery.[40,50] The ascending aorta enlarges in diameter by about 9% per decade[42] the radius averaging 1.0 cm at age 20 as contrasted with 1.8 cm at 60, but thickening of the wall causes the ratio of thickness to diameter to increase. The heart hypertrophies mildly as age advances, with a broadening of myocardial cell diameter and a 50% increase in ventricular wall thickness.[7]

Alterations of blood pressure and flow accompany these structural modifications, as might be expected, and the character of the changes is generally consistent with the predictions of hemodynamic theory. The increment in systemic arterial mean and pulse pressures with age has already been discussed in this chapter, as has the steady decline of resting cardiac output. The elevation of pulse pressure can be explained as the result of increased arterial stiffness, whereas the rising mean pressure in the face of a falling output implies an increase in the peripheral resistance of the systemic circulation. Arteriolar constriction appears to be the cause of the change in resistance, but the stimulus that activates that vasomotor activity has not been identified.

A detailed collaborative study[42] of these changes in normal human subjects shows that systemic resistance increases from 1050 dyn sec/cm^5 at age 20 to 1440 dyn sec/cm^5 at age 60. *Vascular impedance,* a parameter analogous to resistance but derived from the pulsations of pressure and flow (Chapter 6), also increases, the average or characteristic aortic impedance rising from 35 dyn sec/cm^5 to 83 dyn sec/cm^5 between 20 and 60 yr. This age-related change not only is consistent with the increasing arterial stiffness, but also indicates that the effects of stiffening outweigh those of dilatation, which would affect impedance in the opposite direction (see equation 6.23). The possibility that alterations of impedance are related to changes in the function of alpha- and beta-adrenergic receptors with age has been explored by several investigators, but the results are equivocal at present.[13]

The shape of the impedance spectrum is also modified as years pass, the frequency of the first impedance minimum rising from 3.1 to 4.6 Hz.[42] This shift is the result of the increased pulse wave velocity that accompanies a high elastic modulus, which displaces the minimum and maximum of the impedance spectrum to higher frequencies (Chapter 6). The phenomena responsible for these changes in the spectrum also modify the magnitude and timing of reflected waves, altering the contours of pressure waves in the aorta. The development in many older persons of the type A pressure pulsation described in an earlier section is a result of these reflections.

The causes of gradual enlargement of reflected waves with age include not only the increasing peripheral resistance but also a change in the relative amounts of reflection from various sites. This phenomenon has been explained in terms of a *T-tube model* of the arterial tree.[8] In young people, according to this theory, reflections travel back to the heart over relatively short pathways from the upper part of the body and over longer ones from the lower (footward) portions. Waves returning from these two regions arrive out of phase and cancel each other to some extent, reducing net reflection in the ascending aorta. With advancing age, pulse wave velocity increases significantly in the lower parts of the arterial tree but only slightly in the upper regions, making the reflected waves from both areas arrive in the aortic arch at about the same time, so that they reinforce each other. The system then resembles a tube with a single major reflecting site, and prominent maxima and minima appear at appropriate frequencies in the aortic impedance spectrum.

The reasons for diminished cardiac function are less clear. The myocardial hypertrophy can be attributed to the greater load imposed by vascular resistance and impedance, and the reduced cardiac output appears to be related to those same factors. Many investigators doubt that myocardial contractility becomes depressed with age, but the evidence is mixed.[7] The direct relationship between contractile force and myocardial fiber length is curvilinear at all ages (Chapter 4), but with time it becomes steeper and shifts toward the force axis, and cardiac relaxation is prolonged.

All of these age-related changes can be regarded as natural manifestations of maturation and senescence, not disease, although atherosclerosis and hypertension can produce similar effects. An extraordinary series of studies on large numbers of normal subjects in China by Avolio and his associates[15] emphasizes this conclusion. They used a noninvasive sensor to measure arterial pulse wave velocity, an indicator of vessel elasticity, in two populations—one urban, the other rural. Hypertension and a high consumption of salt were prevalent in the urban but not the rural group, and the incidence of atherosclerosis was relatively low in both. Wave velocity increased with age in both populations, but it was lower in the rural group in each age decade. There was a direct correlation between wave velocity and blood pressure, as expected, but the urban–rural differences remained even when subjects with similar blood pressures were compared. The investigators concluded that age, hypertension, and probably salt intake each contribute independently to an increase in arterial stiffness.

Aging of the heart and blood vessels thus modifies their properties significantly and alters the conditions that should be considered normal in each age decade. For the clinician, familiarity with the hemodynamic consequences of aging makes it possible to detect any pathological state that may be superimposed on them. For the investigator, the moral is that the age of experimental animals is a critical variable.

The Influence of Body Size

It seems natural to suppose that the cardiac output at rest should be greater in large animals than in small ones. Blood flow has a nutritional function, and intuition tells us that the more tissue there is to be served, the larger the flow rate required. Comparisons of direct measurements in different mammals and among members of any one species support that hypothesis. What is not clear is whether the output is most closely related to body weight, surface area, or some other measure of body size.

The search for such relationships is founded on the assumption that animals share certain anatomical and physiological properties, in spite of their obvious differences in shape and biological performance. The analytic approach goes back 2 millennia to the time of Euclid and Archimedes, who recognized that the surface area of geometrically defined bodies increases as the square of their linear dimensions. For a cube in which L is the length of each edge, for example, the surface equals $6L^2$ and the volume is L^3. Unlikely as it seems, considering the irregularity and variety of mammalian forms, the assumption that all animals are similar in shape has proved to be approximately correct, *similar* in this context meaning that the number and relative proportions of body parts are the same in all cases. Under such conditions, if blood flow were related directly to the total volume of an animal's tissues, then cardiac output would be proportional to the cube of some linear dimension such as body length or height.

Applications of this *principle of similarity* usually consider the body tissues to be of uniform density, so that weight can be taken as an index of volume, and relationships are expressed as a proportionality between some physiological variable, X, and the body weight (W):

$$X = kW^b \qquad (2.2)$$

The variable k is a proportionality coefficient, and the exponent b is a clue to the relation between X and other bodily dimensions. In two complex structures that differ in magnitude but consist of elements that are similar in number, proportions, and density, both structures will have the same values for k and b with respect to a particular variable (X). Equation 2.2 can be converted to logarithmic form:

$$\log X = \log k + (b \log W) \qquad (2.3)$$

demonstrating that a plot of $\log X$ and $\log W$ should follow a straight line. The proportionality coefficient, k, and the weight exponent, b, can thus be determined from a plot of experimental measurements, although a relatively wide range of weights is required to get reliable estimates. The value of the exponent so determined indicates whether the variable X is proportional to body weight ($b = 1.00$), to surface area ($b = \frac{2}{3}$), or to a linear dimension ($b = \frac{1}{3}$). In practice, the exponent often turns out to have an intermediate value, in which case the result may be empirically useful but its physiological significance remains in doubt.

In the case of cardiac output and body size, observations in a wide range of mammalian species indicate that resting output is a direct linear function of body weight.[6] The relationship, shown in Figure 2.9, extends over four orders of magnitude, and the regression of output (Q, in liters per minute) on weight (W, in kilograms) for the data summarized in that figure is:

$$Q = 0.108 \ W^{0.98} \tag{2.4}$$

Not all investigators agree on this point, however, and various reports[3,6] give weight exponents ranging from 0.7 to 1.0. The lack of agreement arises from the inevitable scatter of measurements obtained from different animals in different laboratories. Determinations of cardiac output are subject to errors of at least ±7%, and surveys include different methods of measurement, various degrees of success in establishing basal conditions, and the presence or absence of anesthesia.

For the present, the expression that seems best to fit all the data available for large and small animals is a linear relationship of 100 ml/min per kilogram of body weight. Although this generalization applies to humans, in whom resting cardiac output in adults averages 102 ml/min per kilogram of body weight, body surface area has come to be the most widely used normalization for output in human subjects. Results are usually reported as a *cardiac index*, the ratio

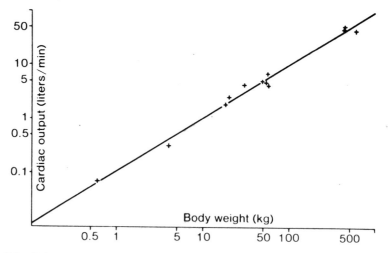

Figure 2.9.   Relation between resting cardiac output (*ordinate*) and body weight (*abscissa*) in 11 mammalian species. Logarithmic scale on both axes. (From data in Table 2.2 for the rat, rabbit, and dog, and measurements on other species reported by Patterson et al.[45])

of output in liters per minute to surface area in square meters. Data in the literature show that surface area and weight are both acceptable factors for correcting output measurements for body size, and that there is little to choose between them. The coefficient of variation is about the same in both cases ($\approx 26\%$), and the correlation coefficients are not very high for either relationship (≈ 0.37).[6]

The emphasis given to body surface area stems from an early belief that metabolic rate is proportional to that variable, an idea that seemed to be consistent with the function of body surface as a regulator of temperature. Metabolic rate was consequently expected to bear the same relation to body weight that surface area does, which is to say that both should be proportional to weight$^{0.667}$, in accordance with the principle of similarity. Proponents of the cardiac index argued as follows: Metabolism is measured by oxygen uptake, and the purpose of cardiac output is to deliver oxygen. Therefore output, like metabolic rate, varies with body surface area. Whatever the merits of that reasoning, there is now convincing evidence that the weight exponent for metabolism is actually closer to ¾ than ⅔; the observed mean basal metabolic rate of animals[4] is

$$\text{Metabolic rate} = 70 \text{ weight}^{0.75} \qquad (2.5)$$

where metabolic rate is in kilocalories per day and weight is in kilograms. This relationship has been confirmed repeatedly, indicating that metabolic rate is not exactly proportional to either surface area or body weight.

A new insight was added to discussions of this subject by McMahon,[34] who drew attention to the fact that dimensional relationships are not really similar in all species. The ratio of girth to body length, or limb diameter to length, is *smaller* in the dog than in the elephant, violating the assumption that proportions among linear dimensions remain constant regardless of body size. Small animals are more slender than large ones, in other words. This difference may be related to the engineering requirements for structural beams and columns, in which diameter must bear a prescribed nonlinear relationship to length in order to avoid buckling or bending. The mathematical nature of this relationship in animals, determined from measurements in a variety of species, leads to the prediction that their surface area, unlike that of regular geometric solids, should be proportional to weight$^{0.75}$, the same as that observed experimentally for metabolic rate.[34]

A number of other attributes of the cardiovascular system are directly correlated with body weight, including blood volume and myocardial mass, although the exact values of the appropriate parameters are debatable.[1,3] Heart rate is inversely related to body size, ranging from 720 beats/min in the mouse to perhaps 24 beats/min in the elephant. Rate is approximately proportional to $W^{-0.33}$, as if it were inversely related to some linear body dimension, but smaller negative exponents have sometimes been reported (-0.25 to -0.29). Evolutionary selection must have played some part in this phenomenon, and one possibility[35,43] is that ventricular work at rest has been minimized by placing the rate at a frequency that matches an optimal fraction of the aortic wavelength (Chapter 6). The species listed in Table 2.2 have aortas approximately one-tenth the fundamental wavelength,[35] placing the heart rate frequency at a relatively low point on the aortic impedance spectrum (Figure 6.16).

Some other variables, notably blood pressure, are independent of body size. Most mammals under truly basal conditions have pressures not much different from those of humans, with the exception, noted earlier, of animals like the giraffe. Blood velocities are also not widely different in animals of different size. Mean velocities of 12 to 32 cm/sec in the ascending aorta have been reported in the rat, rabbit, dog, man, and horse under resting conditions, with no clear relation to body weight. This finding indicates that the relation between aortic cross-sectional area and cardiac output is approximately constant regardless of body size. Arterial elasticity is probably another size-independent property. The elastic modulus of the thoracic aorta is about the same in the rat as in the rabbit and dog,[6] although values reported for the human aorta are higher by a factor of two or three. More detailed examination would take us too far afield, but the reader who finds comparative hemodynamics of interest should consult D'Arcy Thompson's brilliant work, "On Growth and Form,"[11] and the review by Gunther.[3]

References

Reviews

1. Altman, P.L., Dittmer, D.S. (eds.) (1971). *Respiration and Circulation*. Bethesda, Md., Federation of American Societies for Experimental Biology.
2. Caro, C.G., Pedley, T.J., Schroter, R.C., Seed, W.A. (1978). *The Mechanics of the Circulation*. Oxford, Oxford University Press, pp. 315–317.
3. Gunther, B. (1975). Dimensional analysis and theory of biological similarity. *Physiol. Rev.* 55:659–699.
4. Kleiber, M. (1961). *The Fire of Life. An Introduction to Animal Energetics*. New York, Wiley.
5. McDonald, D.A. (1974). *Blood Flow in Arteries*. London, Edward Arnold, p. 48.

6. Milnor, W.R. (1989). *Hemodynamics,* 2nd ed. Baltimore, Williams & Wilkins.

7. Nichols, W.W., O'Rourke, M.F., Avolio, A.P., Yaginuma, T., Murgo, J.P., Pepine, C.J., Conti, C.R. (1987). Age-related changes in left ventricular/arterial coupling. In: *Ventricular/Vascular Coupling. Clinical, Physiological and Engineering Aspects,* F.C.P. Yin, ed. Berlin, Springer-Verlag, pp. 79–114.

8. O'Rourke, M.F. (1982). *Arterial Function in Health and Disease.* Edinburgh, Churchill-Livingstone.

9. Pickering, G. (1968). *High Blood Pressure,* 2nd ed. London, J&A Churchill, pp. 203–228.

10. Snedecor, G.W., Cochran, W.G. (1967). *Statistical Methods,* 6th ed. Ames, Iowa State University Press.

11. Thompson, D'Arcy W. (1917). *On Growth and Form.* London, Cambridge University Press (abridged ed., Cambridge University Press 1966).

12. Wade, O.L., Bishop, J.M. (1962). *Cardiac Output and Regional Blood Flow.* Oxford, Blackwell Scientific.

13. Yin, F.C.P. (1980). The aging vasculature and its effects on the heart. In: *The Aging Heart,* M.L. Weisfeldt, ed. New York, Raven Press, pp. 137–213.

Research Papers

14. Attinger, E.O. (1963). Pressure transmission in pulmonary arteries related to frequency and geometry. *Circ. Res.* 12:623–641.

15. Avolio, A.P., Deng, F.D., Li, W., Lou, Y., Huang, Z., Xing, L., O'Rourke, M.F. (1985). Effects of aging on arterial distensibility in populations with high and low prevalence of hypertension: Comparison between urban and rural communities in China. *Circulation* 71:202–210.

16. Barratt-Boyes, B.G., Wood, E.H. (1958). Cardiac output and related measurements and pressure values in the right heart and associated vessels, together with an analysis of the hemodynamic response to the inhalation of high oxygen mixtures in healthy subjects. *J. Lab. Clin. Med.* 51:72–90.

17. Berger, H.J., Matthay, R.A., Davies, R.A., Zarat, B.L., Gottschalk, A. (1979). Comparison of exercise right ventricular performance in chronic obstructive pulmonary disease and coronary artery disease: Noninvasive assessment by quantitative radionuclide angiocardiography. *Invest. Radiol.* 14:342–353.

18. Bolomey, A.A., Michie, A.J., Michie, C., Breed, E.S., Schreiner, G.E., Lauson, H.D. (1949). Simultaneous measurement of effective renal blood flow and cardiac output in resting normal subjects and patients with essential hypertension. *J. Clin. Invest.* 28:10–17.

19. Brandfonbrener, M., Landowne, M., Shock, N.W. (1955). Changes in cardiac output with age. *Circulation* 12:557–566.

20. Braunwald, E., Brockenbrough, E.C., Frahm, C.J., Ross, J. (1961). Left atrial and left ventricular pressures in subjects without cardiovascular disease. *Circulation* 24:267–269.

21. Cournand, A., Riley, R.L., Breed, E.S., Baldwin, E. deF., Richards, D.W. (1945). Measurement of cardiac output in man using the technique of catheterization of the right auricle or ventricle. *J. Clin. Invest.* 24:106–116.

22. Dexter, L., Dow, J.W., Haynes, F.W., Whittenberger, J.L., Ferris, B.G.,

Goodale, W.T., Hellems, H.K. (1950). Studies of the pulmonary circulation in man at rest. Normal variations and the interrelations between increased pulmonary blood flow, elevated pulmonary arterial pressure and high pulmonary "capillary" pressure. *J. Clin. Invest.* 29:602–613.

23. Doyle, J. T., Wilson, J.S., Estes, E.H., Warren, J.V. (1951). The effect of intravenous infusions of physiologic saline solution on the pulmonary arterial and pulmonary capillary pressure in man. *J. Clin. Invest.* 30:345–352.

24. Ekblom, B., Hermansen, L. (1968). Cardiac output in athletes. *J. Appl. Physiol.* 25:619–625.

25. Fowler, N. O., Westcott, R.N., Scott, R.C. (1953). Normal pressure in the right heart and pulmonary artery. *Am. Heart J.* 46:264–267.

26. Fraser, R.F., Chapman, C.B. (1954). Studies on the effect of exercise on cardiovascular function. II. The blood pressure and heart rate. *Circulation* 9:193–198.

27. Gabe, I.T., Gault, H.J., Ross, J., Jr., Mason, D.T., Mills, C.J., Shillingford, J.P., Braunwald, E. (1969). Measurement of instantaneous blood flow velocity and pressure in conscious man with a catheter-tip velocity probe. *Circulation* 40:603–614.

28. Gentzler, R.D., Briselli, M.F., Gault, J.H. (1974). Angiographic estimation of right ventricular volume in man. *Circulation* 50:324–330.

29. Hamilton, M., Pickering, G.W., Roberts, J.A.F., Sowry, G.S.C. (1954). The aetiology of essential hypertension. I. The arterial pressure in the general population. *Clin. Sci.* 13:11–35.

30. Horsfield, K. (1978). Morphometry of the small pulmonary arteries in man. *Circ. Res.* 42:593–597.

31. Kattus, A.A., Rivin, A.U., Cohen, A., Sofio, G.S. (1955). Cardiac output and central volume as determined by dye dilution curves. Resting values in normal subjects and patients with cardiovascular disease. *Circulation* 11:447–455.

32. Kennedy, J.W., Baxley, W.A., Figley, M.M., Dodge, H.T., Blackmon, J.R. (1966). Quantitative angiography. The normal left ventricle in man. *Circulation* 34:272–278.

33. Kroeker, E.J., Wood, E.H. (1955). Comparison of simultaneously recorded central and peripheral arterial pressure pulses during rest, exercise and tilted position in man. *Circ. Res.* 3:623–632.

34. McMahon, T. (1973). Size and shape in biology. *Science* 179:1201–1204.

35. Milnor, W.R. (1979). Aortic wavelength as a determinant of the relation between heart rate and body size in mammals. *Am. J. Physiol.* 237 (*Regulatory Integr. Comp. Physiol.* 6):R3–R6.

36. Milnor, W. R., Conti, C.R., Lewis, K.B., O'Rourke, M.F. (1969). Pulmonary arterial pulse wave velocity and impedance in man. *Circ. Res.* 25:637–649.

37. Murgo, J.P., Westerhof, N. (1984). Input impedance of the pulmonary arterial system in normal man. Effects of respiration and comparison to systemic impedance. *Circ. Res.* 54:666–673.

38. Murgo, J.P., Westerhof, N., Giolma, J.P., Altobelli, S.A. (1980). Aortic input impedance in normal man: Relationship to pressure wave forms. *Circulation* 62:105–116.

39. Murgo, J.P., Westerhof, N., Giolma, J.P., Altobelli, S.A. (1981). Manipulation of ascending aortic pressure and flow wave reflections with the Valsalva maneuver: Relation to input impedance. *Circulation* 63:122–132.

40. Nakashima, T., Tanikawa, J. (1971). A study of human aortic distensibility with relation to atherosclerosis and aging. *Angiology* 22:477–490.

41. Nichols, W.W., Conti, C.R., Walker, W.E., Milnor, W.R. (1977). Input impedance of the systemic circulation in man. *Circ. Res.* 40:451–458.

42. Nichols, W.W., O'Rourke, M.F., Avolio, A.P., Yaginuma, T., Murgo, J.P., Pepine, C.J., Conti, C.R. (1985). Effects of age on ventricular–vascular coupling. *Am. J. Cardiol.* 55:1179–1184.

43. O'Rourke, M.F. (1967). Steady and pulsatile energy losses in the systemic circulation under normal conditions and in simulated arterial disease. *Cardiovasc. Res.* 1:312–326.

44. O'Rourke, M.F., Blazek, J.V., Morreels, C.L., Jr., Krovetz, L.G. (1968). Pressure wave transmission along the human aorta. *Circ. Res.* 23:567–579.

45. Patterson, J.L., Goetz, R.H., Doyle, J.T., Warren, J.V., Gauer, O.H., Detweiler, D.K., Said, S.I., Hoernicke, H., McGregor, M., Keen, E.N., Smith, M.H., Jr., Hardie, E.L., Reynolds, M., Flatt, W.P., Waldo, D.R. (1965). Cardiorespiratory dynamics in the ox and giraffe, with comparative observations on man and other mammals. *Ann. N.Y. Acad. Sci.* 127:393–413.

46. Prec, K.J., Cassels, D.E. (1955). Dye dilution curves and cardiac output in newborn infants. *Circulation* 11:789–798.

47. Reeves, J.T., Grover, R.F., Filley, G., Blount, S.G., Jr. (1961). Cardiac output in resting man. *J. Appl. Physiol.* 16:276–278.

48. Singhal, S., Henderson, R., Horsfield, K., Harding, K., Cumming, G. (1973). Morphometry of the human pulmonary arterial tree. *Circ. Res.* 33:190–197.

49. Van Citters, R.L., Franklin, D.L. (1966). Telemetry of blood pressure in free-ranging animals via an intravascular gauge. *J. Appl. Physiol.* 21:1633–1636.

50. Yin, F.C.P., Spurgeon, H.A., Kallman, C.H. (1983). Age-associated alterations in vascoelastic properties of canine aortic strips. *Circ. Res.* 53:464–472.

3

PROPERTIES OF CARDIAC CELLS

Cardiac function depends in part on the physiological properties of individual cells and in part on the arrangement and interaction of those cells in the heart as a whole. The physiological characteristics of cardiac cells will be considered here and the overall performance of the four-chambered mammalian heart in the next chapter. The two most important characteristics of the cells are their electrical activity and their ability to contract. The gross and microscopic structures of the tissues play a major role in both phenomena, and morphology is therefore the first topic to be considered.

Morphology

The heart is predominantly a muscular organ, and most of its cells resemble those of skeletal muscle in their striations and microscopic ultrastructure. The cells of certain specialized regions, the *nodes* and *conducting tracts,* differ morphologically and functionally from the rest of the myocardium. Nodal tissue appears in two places, the *sinoatrial node* and the *atrioventricular node* (Figure 3.1). The sinoatrial node lies in the wall of the right atrium in the sulcus terminalis, the junction between the superior vena cava and atrium. The atrioventricular node is located in the lower portion of the interatrial septum, near the membranous portion of the interventricular septum.

The sinoatrial node is the normal pacemaker of the heart, and it is innervated by sympathetic and parasympathetic fibers of the autonomic nervous system. In man, this node is about 2 mm thick and extends along the sulcus for a distance of 2 cm. Its cells are spindle-shaped and smaller than ordinary myo-

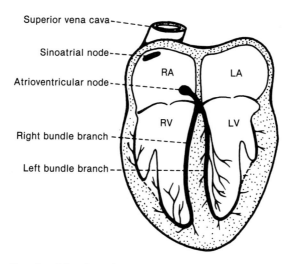

Figure 3.1.   Location of nodal and conducting tissues in mammalian heart. *RA*, right atrium; *RV*, right ventricle; *LA*, left atrium; *LV*, left ventricle.

cardial fibers, and they contain relatively few myofibrils. Small strands of nodal cells extend a short distance out from this region and become continuous with the typical muscle fibers of the atrium.

The atrioventricular node is located in the subendocardial region of the right atrium near the entry of the coronary sinus. It lies along the lower portion of the interatrial septum and contains fibers that closely resemble those of the sinoatrial node. The ventricular end of the node merges with the atrioventricular conducting tract, the *bundle of His*. The atrial border of the node is rather indistinct, as the nodal fibers merge with atrial muscle fibers. The precise morphological characteristics of this junction are unknown at present.

Specialized conducting tracts

The bundle of His is normally the only path by which excitation is carried from the atria to the ventricles. A small amount of connective tissue separates the chambers at all other points on the atrioventricular boundary. Occasionally, one or more additional tracts of conducting tissue between atria and ventricles exist in other locations. Such cases are rare, but the functional effect is to excite some portion of ventricular muscle prematurely. The anomalous excitation is usually detectable in the electrocardiogram and may lead to arrhythmias (Wolfe-Parkinson-White syndrome; Chapter 5).

The bundle of His divides into two main *bundle branches*, and the left main branch travels only a short distance before separating into anterior and posterior subbranches. All these branches subdivide further into a conducting system that travels in the subendocardial regions of both ventricles (*Purkinje fibers*). The system terminates in fine ramifications that extend only a short distance into the ventricular walls. Purkinje fibers have a large diameter (50 to 70 μm) relative to that of the ordinary cardiac muscle fibers. Their sarcoplasm contains a relatively large amount of glycogen and few myofibrils. Specialized ventricular conduction tissue has been identified only in birds and mammals. The degree of differentiation of Purkinje tissue shows marked species variations, being relatively poor in carnivores, rodents, and primates but highly differentiated in ungulates. Fish, amphibia, and reptiles are said to contain no such specialized tissue and apprently rely on ordinary cardiac muscle fibers for impulse conduction.

Muscle cells

The ordinary myocardium that makes up the bulk of the heart consists of elongated, multinucleated cells about 15 μm in diameter and 125 μm in length. The cells are arranged in long columns, with an irregular double membrane marking the place where cells meet end to end. These boundaries, which were originally called *intercalated discs* because of their appearance under light microscopy, are actually continuous, stepwise demarcations between individual cells, replacing the *Z line* wherever they occur. Electron microscopic studies[30,42] have shown that the intercalated disc appears where two cells are opposed end to end and consists of the plasma membranes of the cells (Figure 3.2B). It continues between cells that lie side by side, but in these longitudinal boundaries the cell membranes are often closely opposed in what is called a *gap junction,* or *nexus.*[17] Such junctions are sometimes also found within the transverse disc.

The demonstration of cytoplasmic discontinuity at the level of the intercalated disc was at first disturbing to physiologists, because they were then

Figure 3.2. Ultrastructure of mammalian myocardial cells. **A**, electronmicrograph of one sarcomere (*center*), its ends marked by Z lines approximately 2.2 μm apart, and adjacent parts of two others. Mitochondria are aligned along top and bottom edges of sarcomere. Thin filaments extend from Z line through I band and interdigitate with thick myosin filaments in A band. Dark spots are glycogen particles, found most often in I band and adjacent to M bands. **B**, transverse portion of an intercalated disc. Cell surfaces are 20 to 30 nm apart. *Arrows*, filaments diverging from longitudinal orientation. **C**, sarcoplasmic reticulum in section passing tangentially to a part of the surface of sarcomeres, showing network of anastomosing tubules, continuous across Z lines. **D**, drawing of transverse (T) tubules and sarcoplasmic reticulum. Saccular expansions of the reticulum (subsarcolemmal cisternae) are in close contact with T tubules or with sarcolemma at periphery of muscle fiber. (Reproduced from Fawcett and McNutt,[30] with permission of the Rockefeller University Press)

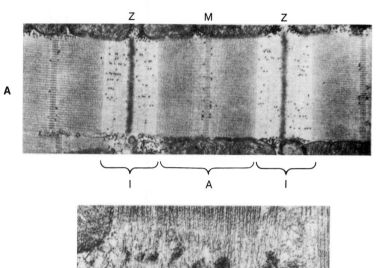

A

Z   M   Z

I   A   I

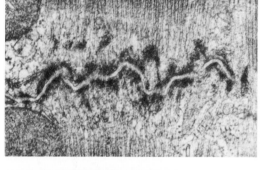

B

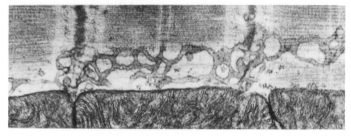

C

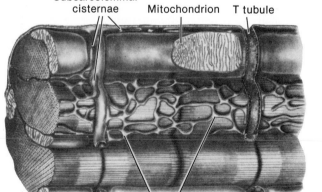

Subsarcolemmal   Mitochondrion   T tubule
cisternae

D

Sarcoplasmic
reticulum

confronted with the problem of explaining how the excitatory impulse was transmitted from one cell to another throughout the heart. Subsequent research showed that transmission is electrical and occurs by means of local current spread from cell to cell via the gap junctions, which are low-resistance pathways between the interiors of adjacent cells.[25,53] Support for this conclusion comes from a variety of experiments. For example, when current is applied across the membrane of one cardiac muscle fiber, the membrane potentials of adjacent fibers are affected. Furthermore, the current spreads about twice as far in the direction of the fiber's longitudinal axis as it does at right angles to that direction. The space constant is approximately 1 mm in heart muscle.[53] Since the average cell length is about 125 μm, a space constant of 1 mm is possible only if cell-to-cell resistance is low, permitting electrical continuity between the individual cells. Finally, when the contacts between cells are disrupted by exposing the muscle to hypertonic sucrose solutions, conduction fails.[25]

The internal structure of the myocardial cells creates the typical striations, or *bands,* which are similar to those of skeletal muscle. Each cell consists of a series of sarcomeres separated by Z lines (Figure 3.2A). Each sarcomere contains the protein filaments that constitute the contractile apparatus, aligned parallel to the long axis of the cell. Thick filaments of myosin, 10 to 12 nm in diameter, lie in the middle of the sarcomere and produce the relatively dark *A (anisotropic) band* (Figure 3.2A). Actin lies in thinner filaments about 5 nm in diameter, which are anchored at the Z lines and extend inward to interdigitate with the thick filaments. The actin of the thin filaments is associated with other essential protein strands, tropomyosin and three types of troponin. The absence of thick myosin strands in the region on either side of the Z line creates a relatively clear *I (isotropic) band.* Actin filaments extend centrally from each Z line, but they do not quite reach the middle of the sarcomere, leaving a relatively light region *(H)* in the center of the A band. A narrow *M band* extends across the center of the A region; its function is not known, but it has an intricate substructure and contains creatine kinase and other enzymes.[22] Large mitochondria are a prominent part of the microstructure of the mammalian myocardium, as are *transverse tubules,* extensions of the plasma membrane into the interior of the cells near the Z line. The cells possess an extensive *sarcoplasmic reticulum (SR,* Figure 3.2C,D), a network that is important in muscular function because it sequesters and releases calcium. At some points, several of these tubes connect with flattened spaces called the *junctional SR.* Circular structures referred to as *corbular SR* (from the Latin word for *basket*) bud from the tubules in some regions.[22,26]

Thin filaments consist mainly of actin, a protein with a molecular weight of about 42,000. The thick filaments are made up of a heavier protein, myosin, which has a molecular weight of about 470,000. The long tail portions of myosin molecules are packed longitudinally in bundles to form the thick filament, while one end of the molecule extends outward to form the "arm" and "head" of the cross-bridge. The head contains two subunits, the myosin light chains, which are essential for the hydrolysis of ATP and thus crucial in cross-bridge function (see below).

This classical description of the sarcomere is accurate as far as it goes, but the organization of muscle cells is now known to be more complex. Early theories of sarcomere function assumed that thick filaments could be connected to Z lines only through attachment of cross-bridges to actin, and that no transverse connections existed between thick filaments. Neither of those assumptions seems to be correct. Some investigators report that connecting *C filaments* extend from each thick filament to the neighboring Z line, and that *side struts* restrict the radial movement of thick filaments.[39] Moreover, some functional studies suggest that large populations of sarcomeres act in unison to produce a *stepwise* muscle response,[46] a phenomenon not explained by anything now known about muscle architecture and still regarded in some quarters as an experimental artifact. Finally, the theory of actomyosin cross-bridges has not been immune to attack. In smooth muscle, at least, cell contraction by an interaction between actin and other proteins (e.g., filamin and desmin), without the formation of cross-bridges, is possible (Chapter 9). Whether this mechanism operates in striated muscle remains to be seen.

New information about the proteins of the contractile apparatus has come to light in studies of molecular polymorphism, slight differences in composition and molecular structure within classes of enzymes or proteins. Cardiac myosin, like its counterparts in skeletal and smooth muscle, has multiple forms. At least five isomyosins have been identified in mammalian hearts by their electrophoretic behavior, physical properties, and amino acid sequence. Several types of myosin light chains, ranging from 16,000 to 27,000 in molecular weight, have been identified in striated and smooth muscles. The structure of actin is more consistent in the many cell types and species where it is found, though not identical in every case. The functional consequences of the various isomyosins are not yet known, but there is reason to believe that they may be of considerable significance. The myosin light chains of atrial muscle, for example, differ from those of the ventricle. Moreover, the proportions of different types of myosin change from infancy to adulthood, and probably in some disease states as well.

Innervation[19]

The heart receives its nerve supply from both major divisions of the autonomic nervous system, sympathetic and parasympathetic. In the intact animal, neural impulses influence heart rate, conduction velocity, and the strength of myocardial contraction. The heart can beat regularly after complete denervation, however, thanks to its inherent pacemaker, and useful experimental information can be gained from the isolated heart, given adequate perfusion through the coronary arteries.

Sympathetic and parasympathetic nerves both exhibit tonic activity under normal conditions; that is, they transmit impulses at some rate at virtually all times (Chapter 8). The parasympathetic nerves are inhibitory in their action, whereas the sympathetic nerves are excitatory, but that generalization must be expanded to take account of the functions of various cardiac tissues. Sympathetic stimulation increases the heart rate, speeds conduction, and increases the force of contraction. Parasympathetic stimulation has the opposite effects, although its influence on contraction is relatively small. At any given moment, all aspects of cardiac function depend quantitatively on the balance between incoming sympathetic and parasympathetic signals.

Heart rate in the intact animal, for example, depends on the action of parasympathetic and sympathetic nerves. The tonic inhibitory activity of the parasympathetic supply is easily demonstrated by severing the vagus nerves, which contain many of the parasympathetic fibers. The heart rate immediately increases. A similar effect is produced by the administration of atropine, which blocks the action of acetylcholine, the chemical mediator liberated by the vagal nerve endings in the heart. Tonic activity of the sympathetic cardiac nerves is demonstrated by the slowing of the heart rate after surgical sympathectomy. The slowing produced by this procedure is by no means as marked as the increase in rate seen when the vagi are cut, however, showing that parasympathetic impulses dominate the resting heart rate.

The parasympathetic preganglionic fibers arise from the vagal nuclei in the medulla and pass via the vagus nerves and their cardiac branches to the cardiac plexus. Here some fibers synapse with postganglionic fibers, whereas others proceed through the plexus and terminate in the intrinsic cardiac ganglia (Chapter 8). From the cardiac ganglia, postganglionic fibers go out to all parts of the heart.[41] The nodal regions are especially rich in parasympathetic innervation, whereas the atrial and ventricular muscles and the conducting network are less well endowed.[43,51]

Terminal autonomic fibers reach the sinoatrial node, the atrioventricular node, the specialized conducting system, atrial muscle, and ventricular muscle except for its most apical portions.[19] The nature of the granules in these terminals suggests that some are adrenergic and a smaller number are cholinergic. *Type C* fibers that persist after complete denervation of the heart have been reported in the free walls of atria and ventricles, lying between myocardial elements.[43] The anatomical relation between myocardial cells and terminations of these nerve fibers is not entirely clear, although the question has been studied by both light and electron microscopy. Neuromuscular junctions like those of skeletal muscle are absent in the heart.

Not all myocardial cells are individually supplied with nerve terminals, suggesting that released neurotransmitters must travel relatively large distances to affect their target cells.[43] Nevertheless, unmyelinated nerve fibers are in immediate contact with some atrial, ventricular, and nodal cells. In the atrioventricular node of the mouse heart, for example, some vesiculated nerve processes travel in sarcolemma-lined tunnels through nodal cells,[51] providing convincing evidence of intimate contact. Afferent fibers also travel in the cardiac nerves, carrying signals from sensors in atrial and ventricular muscles back to the central nervous system (Chapter 8).

Cell Receptors

The cells of the heart, like those of most other tissues, are controlled through intrinsic, membrane-bound proteins called *receptors* (Chapter 1). The principal cardiac receptors are those classed as beta-adrenergic, alpha-adrenergic, and muscarinic cholinergic.

Beta-adrenergic receptors

These receptors have both inotropic and chronotropic effects. Agonists that bind to them increase the force of contraction, reduce the time to peak force, and shorten the relaxation time, in addition to speeding the heart rate. The positive inotropic action contrasts sharply with the beta-mediated relaxation of vascular smooth muscle (Chapter 9). Metabolic effects include stimulation of glycogenolysis and lipolysis.

Beta adrenoceptors have been divided into $beta_1$ and $beta_2$ subtypes that differ in their responses to certain agonists and antagonists. Both kinds are found in the hearts of some animals, but the relative numbers vary in different species.[12] In human ventricles, for example, approximately 80% of the total beta-adrenoceptor pool is of the $beta_1$ variety. There is as yet no clear evidence that the two subtypes serve different functions; $beta_1$ and $beta_2$ types both mediate a positive inotropic effect, although some studies suggest that the $beta_2$ class generates much more adenylate cyclase than the $beta_1$ class per agonist-occupied receptor. Beta receptors in general are prone to *desensitization,* an attenuation of the physiological response on continuous exposure to an agonist, and this reaction may play a part in certain disease states with excessive release of catecholamines.[12] Changes in beta-adrenoceptor number have been found in several clinical disorders. Chronic hypertension is accompanied by decreased cardiac responsiveness to beta stimulation, and decreased numbers of beta receptors in the myocardium. A similar *down regulation* of beta adrenoceptors occurs in myocardial failure. In myocardial ischemia, on the other hand, a rise in beta-receptor numbers and cyclic AMP levels has been reported.

Binding of an agonist to beta-adrenergic receptors causes activation of adenylate cyclase, leading to an increase of intracellular cyclic AMP. The action of cyclic AMP is the same in myocardial as in many other cells, a protein kinase–catalyzed phosphorylation of specific cell proteins. Mechanisms by which cyclic AMP might raise intracellular calcium in heart cells have been suggested but remain speculative, as does the possible involvement of phosphatidylinositol[6,13] (Chapter 1).

Alpha-adrenergic receptors

Some experimental observations make it doubtful that the adrenergic responses of the heart are entirely beta mediated. Although exogenous cyclic AMP, like beta-adrenoceptor stimulation, shortens the duration of contraction, it does not increase the contractile force, as the stimulation of sympathetic adrenergic cardiac nerves does. This lack of response may simply reflect the low permeability of the cell membrane to this messenger, for the more permeable dibutyryl analogue of cyclic AMP *does* increase contractility,[6] although not to the extent that catecholamines do. This fact, together with other evidence, indicates that at least part of the adrenergic effect on contractility derives from alpha-adrenergic receptors. Activation of alpha$_1$ receptors increases the force of contraction, at least in the papillary muscle of the cat,[47] although conflicting evidence has been reported in other preparations. Alpha$_1$ agonists also decrease the rate of automatic firing in Purkinje fibers and cause the release of adenosine from the ischemic myocardium.[38] The existence of calcium channels controlled by alpha-adrenoceptors is well established, but the mechanism of other alpha effects in the heart is not known.

Muscarinic cholinergic receptors

These receptors are the transducers that mediate the negative chronotropic and inotropic actions of acetylcholine on the heart. They act by hydrolyzing phosphoinositides in the membrane. Radioligand studies reveal many more of these receptors per cell in the atria (including sinus and atrioventricular nodes) than in the ventricles.[7] The difference is consistent with the strong effects of parasympathetic stimulation on rate and conduction and with the relatively small changes in contractile force.

Excitation of the Heart

Myocardial contraction is triggered by electrical signals that originate in one part of the heart and travel to all the cardiac chambers. The cell membrane carries an electrical charge on its inner and outer surfaces, like a capacitor, making the interior of a resting cell electrically negative with respect to the extracellular fluid. The resulting difference of potential, or voltage, across the membrane changes abruptly in response to an effective stimulus, creating an *action potential* that is transmitted to adjacent cells (see below).

Resting and action potentials have their origin in the relative concentrations of ions inside and outside the cell and in the selective permeability of the cell membrane. Excitation affects membrane permeability by altering the state of specific channels through which ions move. Modern theories of excitation began with the discovery in nerve axons of critical changes in permeability to sodium and potassium ions, epitomized in the Hodgkin-Huxley[34] model of ion fluxes. More recently, it has become apparent that in cells of the heart and smooth muscle, the movement of calcium ions is equally important. Action potentials in myocardial cells not only transmit a signal, as they do in nerve axons and the atrioventricular conduction system, but also help to supply an essential element in muscle contraction, namely, calcium ions. The process is described in detail later in this chapter. A delightful monograph by Cole[4] describes the experimental and theoretic background of the work on nerves, and the cellular events in the excitation of cardiac muscle have been reviewed at length in a monograph by Noble.[15]

The pacemaker

The regular, rhythmic contractions of the normal mammalian heart originate in its own pacemaker, the sinoatrial node. Impulses arriving through cardiac nerves influence the rate of firing of the sinoatrial node, but it continues to fire regularly after complete denervation. The mechanism for the spontaneous, regular autoexcitation of pacemaker cells consists of a slow depolarization of the membrane in the resting state,[35], the so-called pacemaker potential, which is discussed in a later section.

The tissue of the sinoatrial node represents the remnants of the embryonic sinus venosus, and the early development of cardiac rhythmicity in the embryo[18] is relevant to some aspects of pacemaker activity in the adult. The primordia of the heart are contained in the mesoderm on either side of the foregut invagination of the mammalian embryo. The embryonic cardiac tube is formed by progressive fusion of these paired primordia—the conoventricular region first, the atrial region next, and the region of the sinus venosus last. The first contractions in the embryonic rat heart occur in the ventricular regions at the somite 10 stage, and the atria begin to contract soon thereafter (somite 17). The atria become dominant and initiate contractions that pass from the posterior to the anterior regions of the cardiac tube. These contractions gradually increase in rate and magnitude, blood is set in motion, and the circulation begins.

Later, the sinus venosus forms behind the atrium, starts to contract at a slightly faster rate than the atrium, and thereby assumes control of the cardiac rhythm. This is the final shift of the pacemaker in the developing heart. All these changes occur before any nerve fibers appear in the cardiac muscle and before any specialized conducting system can be identified, demonstrating that a rhythmic and effective heartbeat is possible in the absence of extrinsic control. The shift from ventricle to atrium to sinus venosus also shows that the fastest pacemaker cells tend to capture control of the cardiac rate, a phenomenon that occasionally appears in adult life when some region other than the sinoatrial node begins to fire spontaneously at a rapid rate (Chapter 5).

The location of the normal pacemaker in a sharply circumscribed region, the sinoatrial node, makes it accessible to experimental manipulation. Indeed, one of the observations that led to its discovery was that warming or cooling of the sinus venosus in amphibian hearts produced alterations in the heart rate, whereas local changes in ventricular temperature did not. Other investigators excised or crushed this crucial area and obtained a temporary cessation of the heartbeat, a technique still employed in some research. Electrical recording methods eventually made possible a more precise localization of the pacemaker by demonstrating that the sinoatrial node exhibits electrical potentials before any other region.

Heart rate

The cells of the sinoatrial node normally initiate the sequence of excitation in the heart, and their repetitive discharge consequently determines the heart rate. Autonomic nerve signals to that node modulate its rate of firing by altering one or more of the critical factors, namely, the starting point of the resting potential, the rate of slow depolarization, or the threshold (see below). Most drugs that influence the heart rate do so by changing one or more of these properties. The dominant pacemaking region within the sinoatrial node is not constant, but shifts slightly under the influence of autonomic stimuli.[31]

Under pathological conditions, control may shift to cells in another region, and the heart rate is then determined by the properties of the new pacemakers (Chapter 5). For example, marked slowing or complete suppression of normal sinoatrial pacemaker activity (by experimental stimulation of the vagus nerve or by disease) allows latent pacemakers elsewhere in the heart to assume control. The ectopic pacemaker cells are most frequently located in the atrioventricular node, His bundle, or Purkinje fibers, and their inherent rate is appreciably slower than that of the sinoatrial node. Ischemia or injury of ordinary muscle cells in the atria or ventricles can cause them to become the dominant pacemaker. Even under physiological conditions, a single ectopic beat originating in atrial muscle may on rare occasions interrupt a normal rhythm.

The speed with which excitation is propagated varies greatly in different parts of the heart, ranging from approximately 0.1 m/sec in the atrioventricular node and bundle of His to 10.0 m/sec or more in the Purkinje system. Cell-to-cell conduction in atrial and ventricular muscles has an intermediate speed. The factors that determine propagation velocity are similar to those in nerves and include the rate of initial rapid depolarization, the magnitude of the action potential, and the diameter of the fibers. The electrical phenomena involved in conduction are discussed elsewhere in this chapter.

Within the sinoatrial node itself, excitation spreads at a rate of about 0.05 m/sec, an example of the relatively low speed associated with slow-rising action potentials. When excitation reaches the atrial cells adjoining the sinus node, it spreads through the atria in a uniform radial distribution like fluid poured over a flat surface. This pattern is predominantly the result of spread from one cell to the next, but there are also certain more or less direct conduction paths from the sinus to the atrioventricular node. The existence of such preferential pathways was long doubted because no specialized conducting tracts could be found in the atria. There is now convincing histological and electrophysiological evidence, however, that three internodal bundles of atrial muscle fibers exist in the rabbit, dog, and man.[36] The shortest and probably most important of these is the anterior internodal tract, which leaves the sinus node, curves anteriorly around the superior vena cava, enters the interatrial septum, and terminates at the upper margin of the atrioventricular node. Under normal conditions, conduction through this path brings excitation to the atrioventricular node slightly earlier than would otherwise be the case. The physiological effects of the other internodal, and possibly interatrial, tracts are not known.

Atrioventricular conduction

The time required for excitation to travel from the atrial border of the atrioventricular node to the main branches of the His bundle is surprisingly long, amounting to as much as 0.21 sec in the normal human heart. Much of the delay occurs at the atrial end of the node, over a distance of about 1 mm. Conduction velocity in the junctional area between the atria and the atrioventricular node may be as low as 0.05 m/sec. The resting potentials in this region are lower than those in atrial muscle fibers and sometimes show a slow resting depolarization, thus resembling those of the sinoatrial node cells. There is a gradual transition in the shape of the action potential from the atrial border of the atrioventricular node to the bundle of His, where the potentials resemble those in Purkinje fibers.

As the action potential moves from the atrium into the upper node, it diminishes in size and initial rate of depolarization, which tends to produce slow conduction.[11] These changes are probably the result of a gradual altering of cellular properties along the length of the atrioventricular node. In the lower portion of the node and the bundle of His, the diameter of muscle fibers becomes progressively larger. The fibers of conducting tissue converge to form larger and larger bundles toward the lower end of the node, which tends to produce a faster conduction velocity.[11]

The atrioventricular node transmits atrial impulses only up to a limiting frequency, about 200 impulses/min in humans. If the atrial rate rises above that frequency, some impulses are transmitted and others are not, a condition referred to as *atrioventricular block*. Various types of atrioventricular block are discussed in Chapter 5. The atrioventricular conduction system normally carries impulses in only one direction, from atrium to ventricle. Experimental stimulation of the ventricle produces a spread of action potentials through the ventricular myocardium, but they are not propagated in a retrograde fashion through the bundle of His. As excitation passes from muscle cells into the bundle, the action potentials begin to diminish in size and rate of depolarization, and they die out completely before reaching the lower portion of the atrioventricular node.[48]

Electrophysiological studies on experimental animals have been the primary source of information about atrioventricular conduction, but conduction velocity in different parts of the atrioventricular node and His bundle can now be measured in humans. The electrical signals generated as excitation passes from atrioventricular node to His bundle are extremely small, but they can be detected by applying the analytic method known as *signal averaging* to conventional electrocardiographic records. The deflections observed can then be used to measure conduction time from sinus node to atrioventricular node, His bundle, and ventricular muscle, so that abnormalities of conduction can be localized.[49] Similar records can be obtained during cardiac catheterization from multiple electrodes on a catheter placed near the region to be explored.

Ventricular conduction

Beyond the atrioventricular node and bundle of His, the conduction velocity increases, and the electrical impulse spreads rapidly along the bundle branches and Purkinje network. Although the ultimate ramifications of the Purkinje system extend only a short distance into the endocardial portion of the ventricular wall, and although cell-to-cell conduction from there to the epicardial region is slower, excitation reaches all parts of both ventricles relatively quickly. In the dog heart, impulses arrive at the last region to be activated (the base of the ventricles) only 20 msec after the first cells (in the interventricular septum) have been excited. In man, the corresponding interval is about 70 msec.

The larger Purkinje fibers transmit impulses at a velocity of 2 to 10 m/sec, but as the branches turn inward and terminate in the ventricular muscle proper, the conduction velocity slows to about 0.3 m/sec. Excitation therefore spreads at high speeds along the endocardial surface but more slowly within the ventricular wall. In general terms, activation spreads from left to right in the septum, from apex to base of the free ventricular walls, and from endocardial to epicardial regions. The first impulses to appear at the epicardium are on the surface of the apex of the right ventricle near the thin midseptal region. Ventricular muscle is organized into large bundles, which intertwine in roughly helical patterns, and when impulses leave the Purkinje fibers they follow these bundles. The distribution of the moving boundaries of excitation has been mapped in great detail in the canine heart (Chapter 5).

Excitability and refractory periods

The ability of the intact heart to respond to excitation depends on the time that has elapsed since its last contraction, a finite time being required to recover normal excitability. If, for example, a threshold stimulus is applied experimentally to the ventricle shortly after the beginning of a contraction it will elicit no response, but a short time later the same stimulus will produce a new contraction. The heart is thus refractory to stimulation until it has recovered from previous excitation.

Refractoriness of this kind exists in all cardiac tissues, conducting fibers as well as muscle, and it can be explained in terms of membrane potentials and other cellular events (see below). The consequences affect the heart as a whole, and refractory periods can be demonstrated experimentally in the intact ventricles by measuring the strength of the electrical stimulus needed to elicit a propagated action potential in various phases of the cardiac cycle. This procedure reveals a series of states of refractoriness (Figure 3.3): (1) an *effective refractory period*, (2) a *relatively refractory period*, (3) a period of *supernormality*, and (4) a period of *normal excitability*.

The effective refractory period is defined as that period in the cardiac cycle during which no stimulus, regardless of strength, produces a propagated electrical response. The relatively refractory interval that follows is one in which a propagated action potential can be elicited, but the stimulus required to do so is greater than that needed after complete recovery (i.e., in diastole), and the *latent period* between stimulus and response is longer than it is when excitability has returned to normal. For a short time after the relative refractory period the situation is reversed, and the threshold is slightly *lower* than in diastole; this is the so-called supernormal or vulnerable period. The period of normal excitability extends from the end of the supernormal period to the beginning of the next action potential.

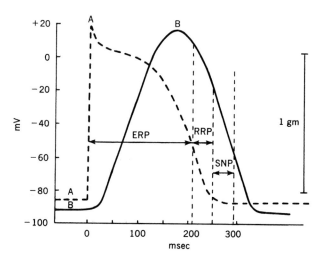

Figure 3.3.   Relation among transmembrane potential (*A, dashed line*), isometric contractile force (*B, solid line*), and refractory periods in isolated feline papillary muscle. *ERP*, effective or absolute refractory period; *RRP*, relatively refractory period; *SNP*, supernormal period. (Reproduced with modifications from Brooks et al.,[2] with permission of Grune and Stratton)

The duration of the refractory periods depends on the time course of re-polarization. Since repolarization is slower in the myocardium than in skeletal muscle or nerve fibers, the refractory period in heart muscle is correspondingly longer. The total refractory period in ventricular muscle of the dog is 250 to 300 msec at normal heart rates, in contrast to 2 to 4 msec for mammalian skeletal muscle and less than 0.5 msec for mammalian nerve fibers. The length of the refractory period also varies in different parts of the heart; ventricular muscle, for example, has a somewhat longer refractory period than do atrial fibers. As the heart rate increases, the muscle recovers its excitability more rapidly and the total refractory period shortens.

Transmembrane Potentials

The excitatory process that triggers contraction has its origin in electrical potentials and ionic movements across the membranes of cardiac cells.[8,14] Analogous potentials exist in all excitable cells and their characteristics are described in general textbooks of physiology, but the phenomena are so central to cardiac function that they will be recapitulated here.

The membranes of myocardial cells are *polarized*, meaning that there is a difference in electrical potential between the inside and outside of the cell. The voltage difference measured between the tip of a microelectrode inserted into the cell and another electrode in the extracellular fluid is about 90 mV in resting

Purkinje fibers. The interior of the cell is negative with respect to the exterior, and the resting potential is therefore said to be -90 mV. To this extent, the membrane behaves like a capacitor with a preponderance of negative charges on its inner side and positive ones on the outer surface. The terms *depolarization* and *reduction of membrane potential* refer to a decrease of the intracellular negativity.

Membrane channels

The charged state arises because the membrane is selective, allowing some ions to enter or leave the cell more readily than others. This discrimination is exercised to a large extent through the opening and closing of *membrane channels*,[10] pores that favor the passage of one or another ion species. These channels are in fact proteins, the structural conformation of which can provide a physical communication, a fluid-filled canal, between the interior of the cell and its external environment.

Modern theory asserts that a channel can be either open or closed, but not in an intermediate state. Each channel opens for a certain length of time, allowing the passage of specific ions, and then closes again. This sequence is repeated at irregular intervals, and the relatively smooth course of electrical activity measured experimentally is an averaging of such events in a vast number of channels. The frequency and duration of opening are modulated by a number of factors, including the membrane potential and the action of membrane receptors. Movement through these channels is passive in the sense that it takes place down an electrochemical gradient when a channel is open. Active pumps that can transfer ions against a gradient also exist in the membrane, functioning to restore resting conditions after any disturbance.

When the opening and closing of a group of channels is voltage dependent, a shift in membrane potential alters the number of channels that are open. The change does not take place instantaneously, however, but takes time to reach a new equilibrium. Any explanation of channel function must account for this combination of time dependence and voltage dependence, and discovering the factors that control the opening and closing (*gating*) of channels has been a challenge to investigators.

Many models have been proposed, and the original theory of Hodgkin and Huxley[34] serves as an illustration. In that prototype, entrance to each channel is controlled by *gates,* which are charged and therefore affected by membrane potentials. In a state of equilibrium, channels are continually opening and closing, but the average number open is constant and depends on the transmembrane voltage. Most channels may be closed at a membrane potential of -80 mV, for example, and the fraction open increases as the voltage is made less negative. The hypothesis describes this relationship in terms of voltage-dependent constants that define the rates of opening (a) and closing (b). If $y(t)$ denotes the fraction of channels open at time t, then the fraction closed is $(1 - y(t))$ and the net rate of change is

$$\frac{dy(t)}{dt} = a(1 - y(t)) - (b \times y(t)) \tag{3.1}$$

When sufficient time has elapsed to establish equilibrium, so that $dy/dt = 0$,

$$y(t = \infty) = \frac{a}{a + b} \tag{3.2}$$

If $a = 0.25$ and $b = 0.50$ at a particular membrane potential, for instance, then 25% of the closed channels open and 50% of the open channels close per unit time, and the net effect when a steady state has been attained (equation 3.2) is that 33% of the total channel population is open at any given instant. The theory thus pictures equilibrium as a dynamic process and gives quantitative expression to the time dependence in terms of rates of change. Each type of ion channel has its own gating rate constants (or, to be exact, rate–voltage curves), corresponding to such differences as the relatively fast development of current through sodium channels and the slower flux through potassium channels (see below).

The Hodgkin-Huxley model assumed two successive gates, m and h, in each channel, so that ions could not pass through unless both were open. Anything that causes the *m-gate* to move to an open position is referred to as *activation*, and closing of the *h-gate* is called *inactivation*. Both are voltage dependent, but with the resting potential at -90 mV, virtually all of the *m*-gates are closed and the *h*-gates open in some types of channels. The extent to which ions move through a channel once it is unobstructed depends on the electromotive driving force (see below). When membrane voltage becomes less negative the *m*-gates open, allowing free passage; later, at some level of depolarization the *h*-gates close, inactivating the channel. As the cell repolarizes, the *m*-gates close again and the *h*-gates reopen. An equation analogous to equation 3.1 expresses time dependence in terms of m and h rate constants. This seemingly complex mechanism was the minimum needed to make the behavior of the model conform to experimental observations on axons. More intricate models have been devised as experimental data have revealed imperfections in the early theory,[4,14,34] but this account indicates the general approach.

Ionic currents

One result of membrane selectivity is a concentration gradient across the membrane for a group of ions that play central roles in cellular function: Na^+, K^+, Ca^{2+}, and Cl^-. The concentration of K^+ in various tissues is 16 to 60 times greater in the cell than it is in the extracellular fluid, for example, whereas the Na^+ concentrations differ by a factor of 4 to 10 in the opposite direction. The equilibrium potential, the voltage gradient that would just prevent movement of an ion across a selectively permeable membrane, can be calculated from the ratio of extracellular to intracellular concentrations of an ion (C_o/C_i) by the Nernst equation:[8,10]

$$E_x = 61.5 \log_{10} \frac{C_o}{C_i} \tag{3.3}$$

where the numerical coefficient takes into account the gas constant (in electrical units), Faraday's constant, unity valence, a temperature of 37°C (converted to the Kelvin scale), and the use of logarithms to the base 10. Equation 3.3 gives the membrane potential, E_x, for a specific ion, x, in millivolts. The nature of logarithmic functions tells us that the potential will be positive if the external concentration is greater than the internal concentration. For example, assuming sodium concentrations of 30 mM inside a cell and 140 mM outside, the Na^+ equilibrium potential is $+41$ mV. The situation is reversed for potassium, $[K^+]_i$ for mammalian cells being about 140 mM and $[K^+]_o$ about 4.0 mM, giving an equilibrium potential of -95 mV for K^+.

Each ion has a contribution to make, but the fact that the resting potential in myocardial cells is close to the K^+ equilibrium potential indicates that K^+ plays an important role under such conditions. Potassium channels are largely open in the resting state, and cells are very sensitive to changes in $[K^+]_o$. Depolarization can be produced by low extracellular K^+ concentrations, or further polarization (hyperpolarization) by high concentrations.

The movement of charged ions constitutes an electrical current, denoted in the case of sodium by the symbol i_{Na}. By convention, membrane currents are described as flowing in the direction traveled by positive charges (not the direction of electron flow, as in physics), thus defining the movement of K^+ ions from cell to external environments as an *outward* potassium current. Highly refined techniques for studying such currents have been developed. *Voltage clamping* employs microelectrodes to inject into a cell a servo-controlled current that holds the membrane potential at a preselected voltage. This method can be applied to multicell preparations, but more exact control is achieved in isolated single cells. *Patch clamping* captures a tiny disc of cell membrane in the tip of a micropipette, making it possible to control ion gradients and potential across a very small patch of membrane, which in many cases contains only one functioning ion channel. Records of current flow through a single channel can be obtained in this way (Figure 3.4). Such records show the intermittent opening and closing of the channel, and provide data for the calculation of its voltage dependence and other properties.[10,40]

The existence of an electrical potential and a current suggests that a membrane resistance for the ion could be calculated by applying Ohm's law. Electrophysiological practice, however, dictates that this property be expressed as the reciprocal of resistance, *conductance*. A current of ions flows when membrane potential (E) differs from the ionic equilibrium potential (e.g., E_K), and the net driving force is then the difference between the two. The potassium conductance, denoted by g_K, is thus given by:

$$g_K = \frac{i_K}{E - E_K} \tag{3.4}$$

Membrane conductance is a convenient concept, even though the relationships among the variables in equation 3.4 are not always linear. Changes in conductance are crucial in cell excitation.

The principal ionic currents in myocardial cells are listed in Table 3.1. In the polarized, resting cell, virtually all sodium channels are closed and potassium channels are open. The fast inward Na$^+$ current (i_{Na}) that corresponds to cell depolarization moves through voltage-regulated sodium channels that activate rapidly and then inactivate quickly when the membrane has become completely depolarized. The inward calcium current (i_{Ca}) probably has two components; one is so rapid that it merges with the rapid upstroke of the action potential, whereas the other is slower and contributes to the plateau. The early influx initiates Ca^{2+} release from the SR (see below).

Open potassium channels in general stabilize the cell in the sense that they move the membrane closer to the K$^+$ equilibrium potential and farther from the firing threshold. They also tend to slow the rate of pacemaker cells. Nu-

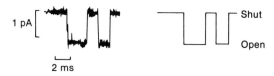

Figure 3.4. *Left,* record of current flow through a single channel in a patch-clamp preparation. *Right,* indication of open and closed states of channel.

merous potassium currents have been postulated,[10,16] but the outward flux i_{K1} listed in Table 3.1 is probably the most important in maintaining resting potentials. The channel bearing this current conducts potassium ions into the cell more readily than in the opposite direction (*inward-going rectification*) and is very sensitive to $[K^+]_o$.

An inward current now designated i_f carries both sodium and potassium ions,[16,28] with Na^+ predominating in the pacemaker behavior of Purkinje fibers. The gating range of i_f channels is in the range -100 to -60 mV. A mixed *outward* current, i_x, is the source of rapid repolarization near the end of an action potential. It consists mainly of K^+ and to a lesser extent Na^+, and is activated in the plateau range of the action potential (-40 to $+20$ mV). The movement of chloride ions is a kind of weak "background" current. The intra/extracellular Cl^- concentration ratio is close to that of the equilibrium potential, and Cl^- channels are thus another stabilizing influence in the maintenance of resting potentials. Not listed in Table 3.1 are three less well-defined channels, two associated with $[Ca^{2+}]_i$-activated K^+ currents[15] (i_{to}, i_{TI}) and the third with a K^+ current induced by acetylcholine by way of muscarinic cholinergic receptors.[20]

The intracellular concentrations of Na^+, K^+, and Ca^{2+} are regulated not only through ion channels but also by active *pumps* in the cell membrane (Fig-

Table 3.1.   Some of the Ion Channels in Cardiac Cell Membranes

CURRENT[a]	IONS CARRIED	ACTIVATION	FUNCTION[b]
Inward currents			
i_{Na}	Na^+	Voltage	AP upstroke
i_{Ca} (i_{si})	Ca^{2+}	Voltage	AP plateau
			E–C coupling
			Pacemakers
i_f	Na^+, K^+	Voltage	Pacemakers
Outward currents			
i_{K1}	K^+	Voltage	Resting potential
			Repolarization
i_x (i_{K2})	K^+, Na^+	Voltage	Repolarization
i_{Cl}	Cl^-	?	?

[a]Earlier symbols in parentheses.
[b]AP, action potential; E–C, excitation–contraction.
Source: Modified from Noble[15] and Reuter.[20]

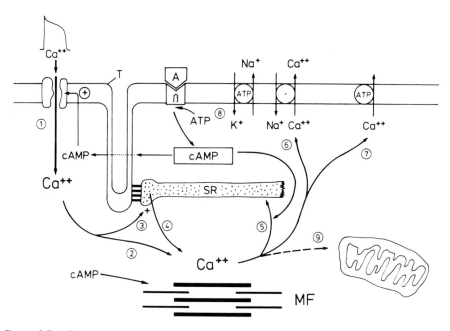

Figure 3.5. Calcium movements in mammalian cardiac muscle. *1*, Ca^{2+} influx through hypothetical cyclic-AMP-regulated calcium channel. *2*, calcium action on myofilaments. *3*, calcium triggering of Ca^{2+} release from sarcoplasmic reticulum (*SR*). *4*, calcium release from SR. *5*, calcium re-uptake into SR. *6*, calcium extrusion from cell by Na–Ca exchange. *7*, calcium extrusion by active membrane pump. *8*, Na–K pump. *9*, mitochondrial calcium uptake. *MF*, myofilaments; *T*, transverse tubule; *A*, agonist binding to beta-adrenergic receptor. Calcium-channel regulation by alpha-adrenergic receptors is not shown (Reproduced from Ruegg,[21] with permission of Springer-Verlag).

ure 3.5). One such regulator is an Na^+–K^+ exchange pump that accumulates K^+ inside the cell and keeps the intracellular concentration of Na^+ low. The Na^+–K^+ pump is blocked by cardiac glycosides, but it is not clear how the beneficial effect of digitalis on the failing heart is related to this mechanism.

Ca²⁺ ions enter the cells mainly through their specific channels,[1,40] but transport across the membrane also occurs by way of two pumping mechanisms. One is an ATP-driven extrusion of Ca^{2+}, the other a Na^+–Ca^{2+} exchanger. Both are calcium dependent in the sense that a rise in $[Ca^{2+}]_i$ stimulates them to expel calcium and a decrease in $[Ca^{2+}]_i$ inhibits them. The stoichiometry of the Na^+–Ca^{2+} exchanger is controversial, but more than two sodium ions appear to be carried for each calcium. It is not blocked by cardiac glycosides. The SR also contains calcium pumps, which move Ca^{2+} into the SR whenever $[Ca^{2+}]_i$ rises.[21] The SR thus has a double function when the muscle cell is excited, first releasing Ca^{2+} to act on the contractile proteins and then promptly reaccumulating it.

Action potentials

The membrane potential of a resting cell can be altered by voltages or currents applied externally or internally, and the effect of a depolarizing stimulus depends on how much it reduces the magnitude of the resting potential. For example, if the membrane potential of a Purkinje fiber cell is reduced experimentally from -90 to -85 mV, that displacement continues as long as the stimulus lasts and then disappears. A sudden change in membrane potential from -90 to -50 mV, however, produces a rapid and complete depolarization. This response, called an *action potential,* is triggered by the initial depolarization, but once started, it follows a preordained course whether the stimulus continues or not. Experiments with stimuli of varying strength show that the action potential becomes inevitable when the membrane has been depolarized to a certain level, called the *excitation threshold.* The condition that initiates an action potential is not, however, the membrane voltage per se but a change from net outward to inward current, a distinction discussed below.

Action potentials follow a characteristic time course (Figure 3.6), although their shape is not quite the same in all cardiac tissues (Figure 3.7). The changes in transmembrane voltage have been divided, for descriptive convenience, into

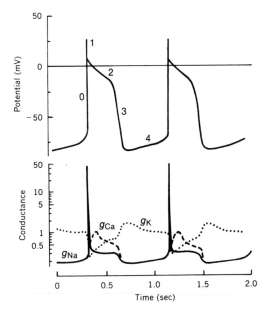

Figure 3.6.   Myocardial cell conductances for sodium, potassium, and calcium (*below,* g_{Na}, g_K, g_{Ca}) in relation to action potentials (*above, mv*). Conductances in millimho/cm². Numerals indicate phases 0–4 in the membrane potential (see text). (Reproduced with modifications from Noble,[15] with permission of Oxford University Press)

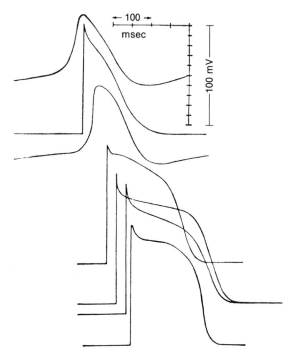

Figure 3.7. Typical action potentials recorded from different regions in the heart. *Top to bottom,* sinoatrial node, atrial muscle, atrioventricular node, bundle of His, Purkinje fiber in false tendon, terminal Purkinje fiber, ventricular muscle. Note sequence of activation, amplitudes, and configuration. (Reproduced from Hoffman and Cranefield,[11] with permission of McGraw-Hill Book Co.)

five successive stages, phase 0 through phase 4, as shown in Figure 3.6. The shifts in membrane conductance that accompany these stages are shown in the same figure. The action potential begins with a very rapid depolarization *(phase 0),* which not only obliterates the negativity of the cell interior but overshoots and transiently reverses the membrane polarity. This fast upstroke is largely the result of activation of sodium channels and an inward sodium current (i_{Na}) driven by the positive Na^+ equilibrium potential (see above). Potassium channels, which were largely open in the resting state, close soon after sodium activation (Figure 3.6) (cardiac cells differ in this respect from the squid axon, where K^+ conductance does not fall at the beginning of the action potential).

Although experimental data indicate that the initiation of an action potential is an all-or-none process, evoked at a specific membrane voltage, the underlying mechanism is probably not a threshold for opening of sodium channels but a consequence of their steep, nonlinear voltage dependence.[10] Even at rest a few channels are open, and a depolarization of only 1 or 2 mV increases their probability of opening. Threshold conditions occur when the inward sodium current caused by depolarization becomes *greater* than the outward currents (K^+, Cl^-). From then on, the decreasing membrane potential causes more and more opening of Na^+ channels, which is why the potential upstroke is said to be *regenerative*. The threshold, in other words, corresponds to the reversal of net membrane current. Because this reversal point depends on rate of activation as well as potential, the specific membrane voltage at which an action potential is generated varies with the duration and shape of the imposed stimulus. Action potentials are produced at a more negative membrane voltage by a square wave than by a slowly rising waveform.

When the inward sodium current has brought the membrane potential to a positive peak, the Na^+ channels inactivate, and g_{Na} quickly falls to a low level (Figure 3.6). The potential falls slightly (*phase 1*) and then remains near zero for a considerable length of time, slowly repolarizing (*phase 2*). The resulting *plateau*, characteristic of myocardial and Purkinje cells and less marked in the nodal tissues (Figure 3.7), contrasts sharply with the short action potentials of nerves. A brief change in chloride conductance early in phase 2 may be involved in the transition from peak to plateau.

The ionic flux that accounts for the plateau is largely a calcium current, with a small contribution by sodium. Most of the Ca^{2+} channels are closed under resting conditions, when the cell is fully polarized, but they open when the membrane depolarizes during excitation. An inward Ca^{2+} current first becomes prominent when the membrane reaches about -30 mV, after which it slowly rises to a peak and then maintains a fairly constant level throughout phase 2. This flux is called the *slow inward calcium current* (i_{Ca} or i_{si}), by contrast with the fast inward sodium current (i_{Na}). Potassium conductance rises, and the balance between the oppositely directed Ca^{2+} and K^+ currents determines the course of the plateau.

Eventually, the Ca^{2+} channels are inactivated, and K^+ conductance reaches its usual high resting level. With the outward K^+ current virtually unopposed, a rapid repolarization develops (*phase 3*), returning the membrane to its previous polarized state and ending the action potential. This does not mean that all other channels are closed, but rather that only those available to K^+ are opening at a significant rate. The total duration of action potentials is about 100 msec in canine ventricular muscle at normal heart rates, and at least twice that long in the human ventricle.

It should be emphasized that the action potential is a sign of changes in the polarization of the cell membrane, a redistribution of electrical charge brought about by the translocation of ions. Intracellular *concentrations* of sodium, potassium, and chloride do not change by more than minute amounts. In the case of calcium, the rise of $[Ca^2]_i$ has an important effect on muscle contraction (see below), but even there a large part of the effect is through the release of intracellular calcium stores rather than the small amount introduced from outside during any one action potential.

Membrane potentials in the sinoatrial and atrioventricular nodes differ somewhat from those in cardiac muscle and the Purkinje system. The action potential rises more slowly, its magnitude is smaller, the overshooting "spike" is less prominent, and resting potentials are lower (Figure 3.7). In these regions the phase 0 depolarization is probably due largely to a slow inward Ca^{2+} current that activates at about -40 mV rather than to a rapid sodium influx. Even in other regions where the fast sodium current dominates phase 0, a similar calcium current may contribute in a small way to depolarization.[44]

Phase 4 is the period between action potentials. The resting potential does not vary in this stage in most cardiac cells, but in pacemaker regions a slow depolarization begins at the end of the action potential and continues until threshold conditions exist and the next firing occurs. The normal cardiac pacemaker, the sinoatrial node, exhibits such *pacemaker potentials,* and their relation to changes in heart rate is discussed below. The same phenomenon can occur in the atrioventricular node and Purkinje system, but pacemaker tendencies in those regions are normally kept in check by the regular arrival of impulses that originate in the sinoatrial node.[45]

Pacemaker potentials

Spontaneous, regular autoexcitation occurs in pacemaking cells because of a slow depolarization of the membrane after each action potential (Figures 3.6 and 3.7). This gradual drift, called the *pacemaker potential,* occurs normally in the cells of the sinoatrial node and is often seen in the atrioventricular node and Purkinje fibers. It can also develop in ischemic or injured myocardium. Cells acting as pacemakers not only exhibit a slow depolarization between action potentials but also have smaller resting and action potentials than other myocardial cells. Within the sinoatrial node, the shape and magnitude of the pacemaker potentials vary to some extent in different cells.[54] The dominant cells have the lowest voltage at the end of the action potential and the most rapid depolarization thereafter. The depolarizing membrane eventually reaches threshold voltage, whereupon sodium conductance increases rapidly and regeneratively and an action potential develops.

The firing rate of a pacemaker depends on the time required for the membrane potential to move from its initial resting values to the threshold for generation of the next action potential. Changes in rate are consequently mediated by alterations in (1) the magnitude of the initial resting potential, (2) the rate of depolarization, and (3) the threshold. If the initial resting potential becomes more negative and all other parameters are unchanged, the interval between action potentials will increase and the rate will be slower than before. Alternatively, an increase in the speed of phase 4 depolarization will increase the pacemaker rate if other factors remain constant. A shift of threshold to a more negative potential will also increase the rate.

The slow depolarization of pacemaker potentials was long thought to arise from a slow decay of potassium conductance from the high level it reaches at the beginning of phase 3 (Figure 3.6), but recent work has caused a radical revision of that view. The directions taken by research in this field over 3 decades make a fascinating story, carefully unfolded in a lecture by Noble.[16] One problem has been that measurements of current themselves do not identify the ions involved, and currents are sometimes temporarily designated by phenomenological names like *slow inward current*. The ion species involved is inferred from the behavior of the current when the extracellular ion concentrations or membrane potential levels are changed. Comparison of the calculated equilibrium potential with the experimentally determined *reversal potential,* the voltage at which a particular current switches from inward to outward (or vice versa), is a common way of judging whether the current consists of Na^+, K^+, or another ion. Active investigation of this field has continued for many years, and the proliferation of currents rivals that of cell receptors or the particles of physics.

Although pacemaker potentials were originally attributed to g_{K+}, it was evident from the beginning that some experimental observations on Purkinje fibers did not quite fit that hypothesis. For one thing, at voltages in the pacemaker range, the current disappears in sodium-free solutions, which, to quote Denis Noble, "is fairly odd behaviour for a highly specific K mechanism."[16] Moreover, the reversal potential of the current is always 5 to 15 mV more negative than reasonable estimates of the K^+ equilibrium potential from the Nernst equation.[8] This evidence, strengthened by other data, forced the conclusion that a pure potassium current could not completely account for the pacemaker phenomenon.

To state the present consensus briefly, it now appears that the pacemaker potential in Purkinje fibers depends on the slow onset of an *inward* current largely carried by *sodium* ions.[28] This current (i_f) moves through a channel that is nonspecific in the sense that it can transmit both Na^+ and K^+ ions, but potassium may play only a small part in the process. Whether the same is true for the cells of the sinoatrial node, where the pacemaker mechanism is known to differ in some respects from that of the Purkinje system, remains uncertain.[16,28] Those who wish to delve more deeply into the literature should be warned that the subscripts applied to channel symbols (i_x, i_{K1}, etc.) change frequently as new experimental data come to light.

Refractoriness

The refractory periods described earlier are an expression in the intact heart of fundamental changes in membrane conductance in individual cardiac cells. A period of unresponsiveness to stimuli, absolute at first and then relative, can be demonstrated in single cardiac cells up to almost the end of the action potential. The sodium channels are primarily responsible for this phenomenon, for once they inactivate, a relatively long time is required for them to recover the ability to be activated again. The recovery is in part voltage dependent,[10] and is thus a function of the extent of membrane repolarization as well as time. The absolute refractory period corresponds roughly to a time when the membrane potential is less negative than −50 mV, which prevents the generation of propagated action potentials. During the relatively refractory period (approximately the latter half of phase 3), action potentials produced by a stimulus of sufficient strength are slow-rising and of small amplitude, presumably because many of the sodium channels are still inactivated.

Under certain abnormal conditions, the recovery of excitability either does not parallel the repolarization of the cell membrane or may extend beyond it. Some metabolic inhibitors, such as dinitrophenol, hasten the repolarization phase of the action potential but increase the total refractory period, and the myocardium remains inexcitable for a considerable time after the membrane potential has returned to its normal level. Alterations in extracellular pH and certain drugs have similar effects.[11]

Mechanisms of Conduction

The mechanisms by which excitation is conducted through the heart are analogous to those in nerve axons. Depolarization of myocardial cells, however, involves the membranes of the invaginating transverse tubules as well as the external cell surface, and the influence of those structures is still not completely known. Apart from that, the extensive and fruitful analyses of impulse transmission in axons[4,14,34] apply equally well to conduction in the tissues of the heart. Conduction velocity varies widely in cardiac tissues, ranging from less than 0.05 m/sec in the atrioventricular node to more than 10 m/sec in the peripheral Purkinje fibers. The velocity in each region is modulated by the autonomic nervous system, and can be altered in addition by pharmacological interventions or disease.

The principal factors related to speed of conduction are the magnitude and rate of rise of the action potential (phase 0) and the diameter of the fibers. The conduction is electrical and depends on the tight junctions or nexuses through which current can pass from one cell to the next. Two phenomena are involved. The first is the flow of current through *local circuits* from a depolarizing region to adjacent muscle still in the resting state. The first region may have been activated by an artificial external stimulus or by conduction from neighboring areas. The result in either case is a current that travels from the interior of the activated cell to that of the adjoining, resting muscle fiber, then through the membrane to the extracellular space, and back over an external path to reenter cell membranes in the first region. Each of these pathways has a finite electrical resistance, and the currents are accompanied by voltage gradients, which act to depolarize to some extent the previously unexcited tissue. The effects of such *electrotonic conduction,* which depends entirely on the passive physical properties of the cells, extend for only a short distance, but they lead to *propagated conduction* in the heart because of a second phenomenon, the action potential generated by cardiac cells whenever they are brought to their threshold. As we pointed out earlier, the specific voltage that constitutes threshold is not a fixed quantity, but varies to some extent with the duration and rate of change of the currents that alter the membrane potential.

The shifts of membrane potential caused by electrotonic local currents decrease sharply with distance, but the effects can establish threshold conditions in the nearest cells, whereupon an abrupt change in membrane conductances and an influx of Na^+ sustain a rapid and complete depolarization, followed by the successive phases of the action potential. This new depolarization, in turn, serves as an electrical source for electrotonic spread to the next cells, and a wave of excitation moves through the tissue. Propagated conduction thus begins with a passive electrotonic event, and then, when the threshold level has been reached, continues as an active regenerative process. The amplitude and rate of rise of the action potentials, and hence the speed of conduction, depend in part of the preexisting membrane potential. Elevation of that potential (i.e., to a less negative value) partially inactivates the sodium channels and slows active phase 0 depolarization. The same effect appears if sufficient time for complete recovery of the sodium channels from the previous beat has not elapsed.

To summarize the overall result, anything that diminishes the amplitude or slows the rate of rise of the action potential slows conduction velocity. This principle applies to physiological as well as pathological states and is consistent with experimental observations on cardiac tissues, where the slowest conduction is found in regions with relative small, slow-rising action potentials (Figure 3.7). Another phenomenon that can be accounted for theoretically is the direct correlation between conduction velocity and the diameter of the fibers involved.[14] The radius of the slow-conducting fibers of the atrioventricular node is about 7 μm, for example, whereas that of the rapidly conducting Purkinje fibers is closer to 50 μm.[15]

The electrical phenomena associated with conduction have been comprehensively analyzed,[4,14] but the resulting equations are extremely complex and will not be presented here in detail. Some idea of their basic form may be gained from the general expression for membrane potentials in a *one-dimensional cable*, a conductive medium enclosed in a cylindrical membrane of constant cross section and infinite length. The relevant variables are the cable radius *(a)*, the intracellular resistivity *(R_i)*, the voltage (potential) across the membrane *(V)*, the capacitance of the membrane *(C_m)*, and the *ionic* current density per unit area of membrane *(I_i)*. The external resistance is assumed to be negligibly small, and the relationships at a longitudinal coordinate *x* are then

$$\left(\frac{a}{2R_i} \cdot \frac{d^2V}{dx^2} \right) - C_m \frac{dV}{dt} - I_i(V,t) = 0 \tag{3.5}$$

This expression must be modified extensively to describe the physiological situation, however, because conducting paths in the heart are finite in length, and the directions of spread in the myocardium are three-dimensional. Moreover, the time and voltage dependence of I_i is not only nonlinear but also a function of active changes in ionic permeability of the membrane, added complications that explain why elaborate theoretic analysis is required to describe the events realistically. Readers who wish to explore the full mathematical treatments should consult the monograph of Jack et al.[14]

Myocardial Contraction

Contraction in cardiac muscle contrasts in several ways with that in skeletal muscle. To begin with, each myocardial contraction is analogous to a single skeletal muscle twitch. The prolonged tetanic contraction that is possible in skeletal muscle cannot occur in the heart under normal conditions, although it can be produced by certain drugs. The mechanical response also takes somewhat longer to develop and declines more slowly in cardiac than in skeletal muscle. Finally, normal variations in the force of cardiac contraction come about through changes in the state of the muscle cells, and not, as in skeletal muscle, through changes in the total number of active fibers. In both types of striated muscle, however, there is a direct correlation between resting muscle length and contractile force.

Much of the information available on myocardial contraction has been gained from observations on the intact heart, but new morphological, biochemical, and physiological data provide insight into the underlying cellular events. Many new techniques have contributed to this progress, including manipulation of membrane potentials[15] and histochemical determinations of the amount and intracellular locations of particular substances. Actual sarcomere lengths in living cells can be measured by methods based on diffraction of light or x-rays.

In some cases the behavior of isolated, individual myocardial cells can be studied. One of the most active fields of research is the connection between an effective stimulus and the resulting mechanical response.

Excitation–contraction coupling

We have seen that cardiac cells are excited by the arrival of a depolarizing stimulus, and we must now ask how such excitation leads to a response in the contractile apparatus.[21,24] The event most essential to contraction is a rise in the concentration of ionized calcium within the muscle cell, and the extracellular environment is one source of this calcium.

As already indicated, the action potential signals a change in cell membrane conductance for Ca^{2+} as well as Na^+, K^+, and other ions, and it is accompanied by calcium influx. At the same time, there is a change in the properties of the sarcotubular membrane such that Ca^{2+} is released from the cisternae of the SR, and possibly from mitochondria and other intracellular structures. The fundamental mechanism of this release *in vivo* is not known, but it can be induced *in vitro* by low Ca^{2+} concentrations (calcium-induced Ca^{2+} release), electrical stimulation, and other maneuvers.[21] In mammalian but not amphibian cardiac muscle, a large part of the calcium involved in contractile activity comes from the SR, but there is also a significant influx through membrane calcium channels during the plateau of the action potential. The Ca^{2+} concentration continues to increase during the early plateau of the action potential, even though some reuptake of free calcium begins almost immediately.

Ionized calcium reaches the troponin molecules on actin filaments by diffusion and releases the inhibitory effect of those molecules on actin–myosin interaction. The essential feature of this interaction is the formation of cross-bridges by the attachment of myosin heads to the actin filaments, and $[Ca^{2+}]_i$ determines the number of actin sites "uncovered," as it were, for bridge attachment. These bridges generate a shearing force that tends to increase the filament overlap, and the basic mechanism of contraction is the asynchronous attachment, hinge-like motion, and detachment of multiple cross-bridges, just as in skeletal muscle. The amount of force developed is a function of the number of active cross-bridges, which in turn depends at every instant on the amount of calcium associated with troponin C. When membrane repolarization begins, the calcium influx subsides, and intracellular Ca^{2+} falls rapidly as some ions are extruded and others rebound to intracellular storage sites.

Excitation thus triggers contraction by giving the contractile proteins access to an appropriate concentration of free calcium. The intracellular concentration of Ca^{2+} in the resting state is about 0.1 to 0.2 μM, and the force-generating interaction of actin and myosin appears when the concentration rises slightly above this level (as in smooth muscle; Figure 9.2). The relatively long plateau of the action potential in myocardial cells is largely attributable to calcium rather than to sodium influx, but membrane transports of these two ions are not totally independent because of the Na^+–Ca^{2+} exchange. Changes in the intracellular concentration and distribution of Ca^{2+} in heart muscle are thus a crucial element in the generation of both the action potential and the contractile process. Modulation of calcium influx by catecholamines appears to occur predominantly by way of beta-adrenergic receptors, which provide cyclic AMP for the phosphorylation of specific intracellular and SR proteins, as discussed earlier in this chapter, but contractility is also significantly affected by the alpha-adrenergic receptors.[6]

Some questions about the relation of free intracellular calcium to myocardial cell contraction remain unanswered. For one thing, the time course of force development does not match the inward calcium current perfectly. Measurements with Ca^{2+}-sensitive dyes or intracellular electrodes show that $[Ca^{2+}]_i$ and force rise together at the onset of a contraction, but Ca^{2+} falls back toward its resting value long before contraction is over.[29] The same observation has been made in vascular smooth muscle, where the triggering of contraction by calcium is not troponin linked (Chapter 9). Inasmuch as the contractile force depends on the amount of ionized calcium that binds to troponin, and not on $[Ca^{2+}]_i$ per se, it may be that the primary function of calcium influx in mammalian and avian hearts is to trigger Ca^{2+} release from the SR and to replenish the SR calcium stores.[21] The intimate relation of the SR to the contractile machinery may then permit SR-released Ca^{2+} to stimulate contraction with relatively little increase in the general cellular level. In any event, it seems clear that the level of free cytosolic calcium is but one element in the coupling of excitation to contraction.

Sarcomere length–force relationship

The force developed by active myocardial fibers is determined by a number of factors, one of which is sarcomere length[3,50] (Figure 3.8). The relationship is qualitatively like that in skeletal muscle, but there are important quantitative differences. First, maximum force is developed at a sarcomere length of about 2.2 μm, but the plateau of force observed in skeletal muscle from 2.0 to 2.2 μm is absent in cardiac muscle. Second, force declines much more steeply at sarcomere lengths above or below 2.2 μm than is the case in skeletal muscle. Third, resting myocardial sarcomere length is rarely less than 1.8 μm, whereas shorter lengths are common in skeletal muscle. Cardiac sarcomeres

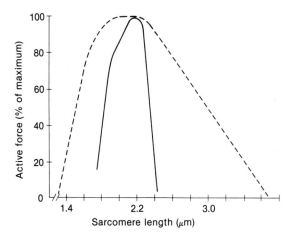

Figure 3.8. Relation between resting sarcomere length (*abscissa*) and peak isometric force (*ordinate*) in papillary muscle from feline heart (*solid line*) and in a skeletal muscle fiber (*dashed line*). (From data reported by Sonnenblick[50] and others)

can shorten to less than 1.8 μm during contraction, but there is a restoring force that extends them again during relaxation.

The sliding-filament model can account for most features of the myocardial force–sarcomere length curve in Figure 3.8. Maximum force is developed when sarcomere length produces optimum overlap of filaments, permitting a maximum number of bridges to form. The smaller force at lengths below 2.0 μm can be attributed to overlapping of the central ends of the thin filaments, which apparently inhibits the formation of cross-bridges, and at very short lengths there may be buckling of the thick fibers at the Z band. At the other end of the curve, a decrease in force as sarcomeres are stretched beyond 2.2 μm is to be expected from the diminishing number of potential cross-bridge sites, but such overextension does not occur under physiological conditions.

Such studies obviously demand high-resolution techniques, and the methods are constantly being improved. Muscle length is not an adequate indicator of sarcomere length, for there is considerable sarcomere shortening in so-called isometric contractions[3] (see below). In addition, the physical site of the *series elastic element* that must be assumed to explain the elastic behavior of muscle (Chapter 9 and Figure 9.7) has not been identified with certainty, although there is strong evidence that much of it resides in the myosin bridge itself.

Filament overlap and the matching of actin binding sites with myosin heads are not the whole explanation of the length–force relationship, however. In addition, the sensitivity of the contractile system to Ca^{2+} increases with sarcomere length.[32] The simplest explanation is that the *affinity* of troponin for

Ca^{2+} increases when the muscle is stretched, but it is also possible that the *effect* of calcium–troponin binding is length dependent. No experimental method of distinguishing between these alternatives has yet been reported.

Studies of papillary muscles

Much of our information about the mechanical behavior of the heart has been obtained from experiments on papillary muscles taken from the ventricle and studied *in vitro*. A typical papillary muscle from the cat is about 12 mm long and 0.7 mm wide, and it can therefore be adequately oxygenated in a bath. Its muscle fibers run longitudinally, and it can be activated as a unit by an electrical stimulus.

In the relaxed state, the only tension in such a muscle is the force that has been applied externally to stretch it to a particular resting length. This resting tension demonstrates the existence in muscle fibers of elastic elements that are stretched as the muscle is passively extended. When the muscle is stimulated, it can develop additional force, or shorten its length, or both, depending on the external constraints imposed on it. If a muscle strip is anchored at both ends so that it cannot shorten, for example, it will nevertheless develop force when effectively stimulated.

The phenomena observed in a papillary muscle preparation consequently depend on the physical setup of the experiment. The four most common arrangements are shown in Figure 3.9. In an *isometric* experiment (Figure 3.9A) the muscle is first stretched to a chosen resting length, and both ends are then anchored so that the muscle cannot shorten. When stimulated, the muscle develops force while maintaining a constant length. In an *isotonic* contraction (Figure 3.9B) the upper end of the muscle is anchored, and a weight *(preload)* is suspended from the lower end. The resting force is then equal to the weight attached, and this force remains constant when the muscle is stimulated and shortens.

Isometric contraction resembles the isometric periods at the beginning and end of contraction of the intact ventricle *in vivo* (Chapter 4), during which ventricular volume remains constant. Simple isotonic contraction (Figure 3.9B) is like the ventricular ejection period (Figure 4.1) in the sense that the muscle is shortening, but there is no variation in force. To provide conditions that resemble those of ventricular contraction more closely, these two modes can be combined in a preparation that is both preloaded and afterloaded (Figure 3.9C). The lower end of the muscle is anchored, the upper end is attached to a lever, and the preload is suspended from the opposite end of the lever, stretching the muscle to a preselected resting length. A stop is then placed above the

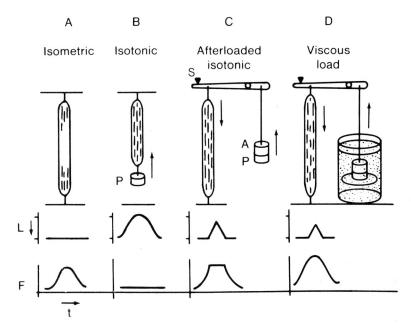

Figure 3.9. Four experimental arrangements for studying papillary muscles *in vitro* (*above*), and the changes in length (*L*) and force (*F*) developed on stimulation (*below*). Upward deflection in length records denotes shortening. **A**, isometric contraction. **B**, isotonic contraction. **C**, isotonic afterload. **D**, viscous afterload (see text).

muscle end of the lever, so that it is impossible for the muscle to lengthen further. An additional weight (the *afterload*) is then added, but the muscle does not yet bear that weight and the resting force remains equal to the preload.

When the muscle is stimulated, it begins to develop *active force* but does not shorten until the force generated exactly equals preload plus afterload. Thereafter, the muscle shortens, pulling down the lever, lifting the load, and maintaining a constant force. After reaching maximum shortening (which depends on the condition of the muscle, the chemical environment, and the load) the muscle begins to lengthen again, and eventually returns to its resting length. At that point, the muscle force becomes less than the total load and gradually falls until it equals the preload. The response is thus isometric at the beginning and end of contraction and isotonic in the midportion.

This preparation (Figure 3.9C) is still not a realistic model of ventricular contraction. In the living animal, wall force and pressure vary with time as blood is ejected (Figure 4.1), because the ventricle is not called on to lift a weight, but rather to move a viscous fluid into a viscoelastic arterial tree. The analogous conditions for a papillary muscle experiment would be those shown in Figure 3.9D, where a *viscous afterload* has been added. Preload and after-load weights are the same as in Figure 3.9C, but a circular plate submerged in a viscous fluid (a *dashpot*) constitutes an additional afterload.

As before, the muscle develops force when stimulated, and it does not shorten until it generates enough force to lift the weights of preload and after-load. When it does begin to shorten, however, a new phenomenon appears. The muscle must not only lift the weights, but also pull the plate through the viscous medium, which requires additional force. The amount of extra force is a function of the fluid viscosity, the diameter of the plate, and the *velocity* with which the muscle shortens. The muscle must "choose," so to speak, whether to shorten rapidly, which requires relatively great force, or to shorten more slowly with less force. The particular time course of force and shortening velocity that the muscle exhibits under these conditions depends on inherent properties of the muscle and on its chemical environment in some way that is not yet entirely clear.

The dashpot in Figure 3.9D is analogous to the elements that oppose ejection of blood from the ventricle, namely, the viscosity of blood and the elasticity of arteries (Chapter 6). The viscous nature of the afterload *in vivo* has received little attention until recently, and few experiments of this kind have been reported. A large body of information about myocardial contraction has been obtained, however, by the other three kinds of experiments illustrated in Figure 3.9.

Length–tension–velocity relations

The relationship between sarcomere length and contractile force is the source of a fundamental property of both skeletal and cardiac muscle. When resting cardiac muscle is stretched to progressively greater lengths, the force developed when it is stimulated under isometric conditions increases (Figure 3.10A). The total tension developed is the sum of the resting tension induced by passive stretching and an active force generated by the muscle. The same relationship can be demonstrated in intact ventricles, and it is the basis for what has to come to be known as the *Frank-Starling law of the heart,* which states that the work performed by the ventricle is a function of end-diastolic fiber length (Chapter 4).

An equally important relationship exists between the force and shortening velocity of myocardial fibers. As Figure 3.10B indicates, the shortening velocity of an isotonically contracting papillary muscle (in a constant physicochemical environment) is inversely related to the weight the muscle is required to lift. If the weight is sufficiently large, the muscle is unable to shorten, but develops a *maximum isometric force* (P_0). Lesser weights will be lifted at a ve-

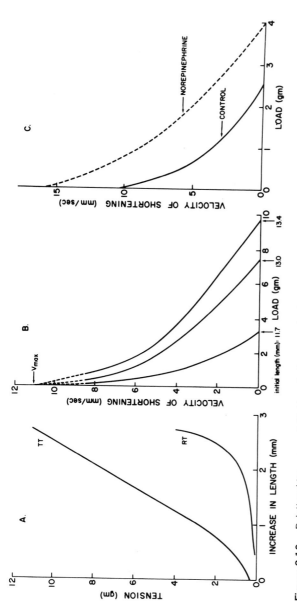

Figure 3.10. Relationships among initial length, force, and velocity of shortening in isolated feline papillary muscle. **A**, both isometric resting force (*RT*) and total developed force (*TT*) are directly correlated with initial (resting) muscle length. **B**, relation between isotonic force (load, *abscissa*) and velocity of shortening (*ordinate*) for three initial muscle lengths (from left to right, 11.7 mm, 13.0 mm, and 13.4 mm). Velocity of contractile elements is inversely related to load in each case. The greater the initial length, the greater the load at which no shortening occurs (P_0, arrows, velocity = 0), but maximum unloaded velocity (V_{max}, determined by extrapolation to the ordinate) is approximately the same in each case. **C**, effect of norepinephrine on force–velocity curve (initial length constant). P_0 and V_{max} are both increased. (From data reported by Sonneblick[50])

locity characteristic of the load. Extrapolation of the curve to the velocity axis gives an estimate of the *maximum unloaded velocity of shortening* (v_{max}).

An interaction between the force–length and force–velocity properties is also evident in Figure 3.10B. The greater the preload, and hence the greater the initial muscle length, the greater the P_0. It has been argued that v_{max} is independent of preload and afterload and is therefore a useful index of the myocardial state, but such independence is not demonstrable under all conditions. The various neural and humoral influences that control myocardial behavior in the living animal alter both v_{max} and P_0, thus establishing new force–length and force–velocity relationships. Norepinephrine, for example, increases both parameters (Figure 3.10C), so that the tension developed and the velocity of shortening are greater at any length than before.

All these relationships can be demonstrated in the heart *in vivo*, although it is more difficult to measure the relevant variables because of the complex shape of the ventricle, the arrangement of its muscle fibers, and the nonhomogeneous distribution of force within its walls. Nevertheless, the knowledge gained from observations of papillary muscles *in vitro* has proved to be a reliable foundation on which to build an understanding of ventricular function (Chapter 4).

All-or-none nature of contraction

Suprathreshold electrical stimulation of cardiac muscle gives rise to a maximal contraction; stronger stimuli do not produce a greater force. This *all-or-none law,* which also applies to skeletal muscle, does not mean that the contractile response is always the same, but only that the magnitude of the contraction does not depend on the strength of the stimulus (provided that the stimulus is of at least threshold amplitude). The contraction is always the maximum possible under the existing conditions, but the conditions, which include temperature, pH, ionic concentration, and a host of other factors, determine what that maximum is.

Stimulus frequency and force of contraction

The frequency and regularity of contraction also influence myocardial performance. The relationship is manifested in three ways: (1) the staircase or *treppe* phenomenon, (2) posttetanic potentiation, and (3) postextrasystolic potentiation.

1. The *staircase* phenomenon can be demonstrated by suddenly increasing the heart rate (by direct stimulation), which causes the amplitude of

each successive contraction to increase until a maximum steady level is reached. This response is readily demonstrated in the isolated heart, but not *in vivo*.[2] The mechanism is not entirely clear, but an increase in the rate of calcium influx into the muscle cell accompanies the increase in force.[24] Calcium efflux lags behind influx at first, tending to raise $[Ca^{2+}]_i$. The force–frequency relation may also depend on the time available between contractions for retrieval of Ca^{2+} by internal storage sites.

2. *Posttetanic potentiation* occurs when the rate of stimulation is suddenly decreased. The first few contractions at the slower rate are much stronger than before, but then the amplitude of the contractions progressively declines to a steady level as the slower stimulation continues. Again, a temporary imbalance between the mechanisms of Ca^{2+} supply and withdrawal is the probable explanation.

3. *Postextrasystolic potentiation* consists of an increased strength of contraction after an extrasystole or premature beat (Chapter 5), a response that has been observed in intact hearts as well as in isolated preparations. The first few contractions following the extrasystole are much more forceful than normal, although the strength of the extrasystole itself is less than that of the preceding contraction.

An early explanation of postextrasystolic potentiation attributed it to changes in initial fiber length. The premature contraction occurs at a time when the heart is incompletely filled, and the force–length relationship predicts that under such conditions a weak contraction should occur. A premature beat is ordinarily followed by a longer than normal interval before the next beat, and this *compensatory pause* allows greater filling and increased end-diastolic fiber length. Later evidence showed that this explanation is at best incomplete, because postextrasystolic potentiation is also seen in isolated hearts maintained at *constant* initial volume, and hence constant end-diastolic fiber length. Moreover, the potentiation resulting from an extrasystole is always greater than that resulting from a single "dropped" beat, although the ventricular filling time is longer after the dropped beat than after an extrasystole.[2] It seems reasonable to conclude that the postextrasystolic potentiation is not entirely due to a change in the initial length of the muscle fibers.

A more plausible hypothesis[55] that would account for all of the frequency–force relationships assumes that calcium rebinds to intracellular sites at an exponentially decreasing rate after the onset of the action potential. According to this theory, the longer the interval between action potentials (up to a limit of several seconds), the greater the amount of calcium stored and hence the greater the "package" of calcium available for release by the next stimulus.

The relatively long interval following a premature contraction would provide a large intracellular Ca^{2+} store for release in the next beat, and once a dynamic balance between the factors regulating $[Ca^{2+}]_i$ was achieved, the force of contraction would return to a level characteristic of the basic frequency. Speeding up the heart rate and thus shortening the interval between beats would have the opposite effect.

Myocardial contractility

The concept of *contractility* is one of the oldest notions in myocardial mechanics and one of the most important. The underlying idea is significant, even though investigators cannot agree on a definition of contractility, much less on how to measure it. The position usually taken is that expressed by an eminent jurist with regard to obscenity: "I can't define it, but I know it when I see it."

The literal definition, "ability to contract," does not suffice because the ability of muscle to develop force is as fundamental as its ability to contract, or shorten. Indeed, isometric and isotonic responses demonstrate that shortening and force development are in some sense equivalent. The basic premise on which the concept of contractility is founded is that the response of cardiac muscle is controlled by the structure of the myocardial cell and by its physical and chemical environments. As long as the environmental conditions remain constant, the characteristics of myocardial contraction should remain constant. What troubles cardiac physiologists is an apparent exception to that rule, namely, that myocardial performance seems to change with the degree of external constraint on the muscle (the *load*), even when all other conditions are kept constant. There is a difference between what the muscle is *capable* of doing (its contractility) and what it actually does under a specific set of circumstances.

The solution has been to assume that this apparent anomaly would vanish if an appropriate measurement could be discovered, and various parameters of cardiac function have been nominated for this role. The search is not made easier by the long list of relevant environmental conditions, which include the intracellular concentrations of ions, enzymes, and energy substrates; the polarization of cell membranes; and the physical state of organelles, to list but a few. The lack of a generally accepted measure of muscle contractility is particularly awkward because of the need to evaluate myocardial performance in research and clinical settings. Many indices of contractility have been proposed, all aimed at learning to what extent the heart is being influenced by the cellular environment, by the load, or by myocardial disease. Some such indices are empirically useful (Chapter 4), but none is entirely satisfactory.

As always, our understanding of phenomena is limited by the nature of the variables we can measure—in this case, muscle length and force as functions of time. Unfortunately, there is abundant experimental evidence to show that these variables are not independent of load. Muscle length, shortening velocity, and force (or ventricular volume, outflow, and wall stress) are all affected by preload and afterload. If, as many believe, myocardial contractility should be defined as the ability to respond mechanically in a way that depends on environmental conditions but not on load, then some other approach must be sought. Nevertheless, the force–length–velocity relationships (Figure 3.10) are sometimes used as a basis for determining myocardial contractility. Although these relations reflect fundamental properties of cardiac muscle, they fall short as a description of myocardial function *in vivo*. For one thing, they vary with time in each cardiac contraction, a fact omitted from conventional force–length and force–velocity curves. The total force plotted in Figure 3.10A is the peak value, and the velocities in Figure 3.10B and 3.10C are early velocities. This difficulty can be circumvented by assuming that the relationships vary with time only at the very beginning and end of contraction, but the evidence offered to support this assumption is unconvincing.

Inconsistencies in our preconceived ideas may be at the root of the difficulties encountered in trying to find a rigorous, practical definition and measure of myocardial contractility. To be specific, insisting that contractility is independent of load may be incompatible with the way the muscle cell actually works. For example, the availability of intracellular Ca^{2+} depends to some extent on sarcomere length,[3] as noted earlier. Resting muscle length depends on preload. Given those facts, it seems paradoxical to assert that the concentration of calcium ions is one of the determinants of contractility but that fiber length is not.

All the reservations noted above with respect to myocardial contractility apply with equal force to attempts to measure what has been called the *intensity of the active state*.[3] Such attempts are based on the idea that excitation produces a change in the contractile apparatus that cannot be directly measured in the shortening or force that follows. Hill[33] first proposed that the *active state* be measured by the tension that the contractile element can just bear without either lengthening or shortening, and determining its intensity therefore required a series of experimental force steps. Alternative definitions in terms of shortening velocity have been proposed.[3] The concept of an active state is complicated by the fact that the ability to shorten and the ability to develop force do not follow the same time course.[3,37] In cardiac (and skeletal) muscle, the capacity for shortening begins and reaches a maximum much earlier than that for the generation of force. The reason for this difference is not known, but the important point is that contraction is a time-varying process that cannot be expressed in a single variable. Methods that have been used to derive some practical estimate of myocardial contractility are considered in Chapter 4.

Cardioactive Agents

A variety of substances affect cardiac function and are consequently said to be *cardioactive*. Many of the ions normally present in body fluids fall into this category, along with the neurotransmitters released by autonomic nerves and the adrenal medulla. Two kinds of actions may be distinguished. Effects on the contractility of the myocardium are called *inotropic,* and those on pacemaker or conduction rates are designated *chronotropic*. The cardiac effects of most of these agents were discovered empirically, but many of their actions can now be explained in terms of cellular mechanisms. Drugs used to treat disturbances of cardiac rhythm are discussed in Chapter 5.

A *positive* inotropic effect, which is one that increases the force of contraction, can be brought about by any mechanism that makes a greater number of free intracellular calcium ions available to the troponin on actin filaments. In cardiac muscle, this occurs when the SR, triggered either by electrical potentials or by Ca^{2+} influx through membrane channels, releases Ca^{2+} within the cell. Both voltage-regulated and cyclic AMP–activated calcium channels can be involved, the latter brought into action through the stimulation of beta-adrenergic receptors and the resulting rise in cyclic AMP. Ca^{2+} channels controlled by alpha-adrenoceptors may also play a part, but that mechanism has not been thoroughly explored in the heart. An increase in heart rate, or *positive* chronotropic action, may be associated with any of the three kinds of change in membrane potentials discussed earlier in this chapter, namely, decreased early resting potential, more rapid resting depolarization, or lowering of the excitation threshold.

Catecholamines

The myocardium is exposed not only to *norepinephrine* released from sympathetic adrenergic terminals throughout the heart, but also to *epinephrine* released along with norepinephrine from the adrenal medulla into the bloodstream. The two catecholamines have similar positive inotropic and chronotropic effects on cardiac cells. They enhance contractility, increase the heart rate, accelerate conduction, and shorten the action potential. Purkinje fibers become more excitable and tend to develop spontaneous pacemaker activity.

A complete explanation of the cardiac effects of norepinephrine and epinephrine in terms of ion channels and currents is not yet possible, but some relevant facts have been established. First, these agents cause an increase in i_{Ca} and a consequent rise in $[Ca^{2+}]_i$, which is sufficient to account for the positive inotropic response. Second, the chronotropic actions of catecholamines are consistent with their effects on membrane potentials, even though some uncertainty remains about the ion movements that support the potential changes.

The faster sinoatrial nodal rate induced by catecholamines, for example, fits with the simultaneous increase in the rate of resting depolarization. The faster conduction velocities that are observed are in line with the increased rate of initial depolarization observed with norepinephrine and epinephrine (at least in Purkinje fibers), although the mechanism is not clear because sodium conductance is not affected.[15] The tendency to develop extrasystoles is consistent with a lowering of the firing threshold in Purkinje fibers. How other membrane effects of catecholamines impinge on the contraction process is a matter of speculation. Mechanical systole becomes shorter along with the action potential duration, and this change has been attributed to stimulation of the SR calcium-reabsorbing mechanism and to reduced troponin affinity for Ca^{2+}.

The influence of norepinephrine on the mechanical function of the heart may be partly the result of enhanced SR storage of Ca^{2+}, although unequivocal evidence for this process is lacking. Discussions of Ca^{2+} influx in myocardial cells usually center on the inward current during each action potential, but the background level of catecholamines in the cellular environment probably modulates contractility continuously. Plasma norepinephrine and epinephrine supplied by the adrenal medulla have access to cell receptors via the extracellular space, and adrenergic receptors increase flux through Ca^{2+} channels, the beta type through the mediation of cyclic AMP and the alpha type by a seemingly direct action. Norepinephrine is also released in the heart by the continuous impact of several impulses per second in sympathetic adrenergic nerves, and the result may be a slow subthreshold influx of Ca^{2+} during resting potentials. Although Ca^{2+} pumps would tend to counteract this inflow, some of it might be taken up by the SR, adding to the stores in that structure and making the next SR release of Ca^{2+} greater than it otherwise would have been.

The direct actions of *epinephrine* on the heart are essentially the same as those of norepinephrine.[2,11] Small differences in their effects on intact animals are the result of the beta-adrenergic receptor's higher affinity for epinephrine, which tends to make peripheral vasodilatation more prominent with that catecholamine. *Isoproterenol,* a synthetic drug often used in clinical medicine and research, is a powerful stimulant of myocardial contractility and at the same time a general vasodilator, as one might expect from its high affinity for beta-adrenergic receptors.

Acetylcholine

The cardiac actions of acetylcholine can be demonstrated by stimulating the vagus nerves, which carry parasympathetic fibers to the heart.[9] The resulting release of acetylcholine at the nerve terminations causes (1) slowing of the heart rate, (2) marked reduction of conduction velocity through the atrioventricular node, and (3) decreased strength of contraction. Low-frequency stimulation of the vagus nerve reduces the pacemaker rate by slowing phase -4 depolarization, and if the frequency of vagal stimulation is high enough, the sinoatrial node stops firing altogether. After a short period of arrest, an ectopic pacemaker usually appears and drives the heart at its own rate.

Slowing of atrioventricular conduction by vagal stimulation is evident in lengthening of the electrocardiographic P–R interval (Chapter 5). If the stimulation frequency is increased, conduction slows even more, and 2 : 1 atrioventricular block may occur, meaning that impulses from the atria alternately succeed and fail in traveling through the atrioventricular node to the ventricles. The contraction rate of the ventricles in such a case is only half that of the atria. The block occurs at the atrial border of the node,[11] the same region in which most of the normal atrioventricular delay appears.

The refractory period of atrial muscle fibers is also shortened, and their conduction velocity slightly increased, by vagal stimulation. Moreover, the atria become more excitable, and direct electrical stimulation of the atria during vagal stimulation often elicits atrial fibrillation. Vagal stimulation also has a negative inotropic action on ventricular contraction, but this effect is so weak that it can be demonstrated only under carefully controlled experimental conditions. Acetylcholine applied to the atria mimics the effects of vagal stimulation,[35] but the ventricles and Purkinje system are relatively insensitive to direct application.

Studies with radioactive potassium provide clear evidence that acetylcholine increases permeability to potassium ions, especially in the sinus region. The large increase in outward potassium current increases the net repolarizing current and thus shortens the action potential,[15,35] a reduction that accounts in part for the negative inotropic effect. Some evidence suggests that acetylcholine may also inhibit iC_a and reduce contractile force in that way.[15] The membrane becomes hyperpolarized at a potential about 10 mV more negative than in the control state, which reinforces the tendency to slow the rate of pacemakers.

The effect of acetylcholine at parasympathetic endings in the heart differs from its action at the myoneural junction of skeletal muscle. In both instances the permeability of the postjunctional muscle fiber membrane is increased, but the increase is nonselective in the myoneural junction, and the membrane potential therefore tends to fall toward the low level that would be assumed if sodium and other ions were free to diffuse;[27] the result is a depolarizing, excitatory action. In the sinus node cells, on the other hand, acetylcholine induces a highly selective increase in permeability to potassium, resulting in hyperpolarization.

Ions

It has long been known that the cations sodium, potassium, and calcium must be present in the proper proportions in any solution bathing the heart if its activity is to be preserved for any length of time. The oxygenated fluids devised for perfusion of the frog heart contain the cations Na^+, K^+, and Ca^{2+} and the anions Cl^- and HCO_3^-. Solutions for the perfusion of mammalian hearts also contain dextrose and sometimes inorganic phosphate and $MgCl_2$. The composition of some widely used physiological salt solutions is shown in Table 3.2. The dependence of normal cellular function on certain ions[23] becomes evident when their concentration is changed, as the following summary indicates.

Sodium

The extracellular concentration of sodium is closely regulated in the intact animal, and the small changes that normally occur have little effect on cardiac function. In experiments on the isolated heart, however, raising the external sodium ion concentration reduces the myocardial force, provided that the calcium concentration is kept constant. This response has its origin in a competition between calcium and sodium ions, as indicated in earlier comments on the Na^+–Ca^{2+} exchanger. A decrease in external Na^+ permits a greater influx of calcium in subsequent action potentials,[3] and as a result, the force developed depends (in part) on the ratio of calcium to sodium ions.

Chronotropic effects of very low Na^+ concentrations include slowing of the heart and of conduction. A slower velocity of conduction is to be expected

Table 3.2. Physiological Salt Solutions (percentages of anhydrous salts)

AUTHOR	SPECIES	NACL	KCL	CACL₂	NAHCO₃	OTHER SALTS	
Ringer	Frog	0.6	0.0075	0.01	0.01	—	
Locke	Mammals	0.92	0.042	0.018	0.015	Dextrose	0.1
Tyrode	Mammals	0.8	0.02	0.01	0.1	Dextrose	0.1
						$MgCl_2$	0.01
						NaH_2PO_4	0.005

because the initial inward sodium current, which is responsible for the fast-rising phase of the action potential, depends in part on the chemical gradient across the membrane. The lower the external sodium ion level, the slower the upstroke and the smaller the amplitude of the action potential, conditions that tend to slow propagation. Continued exposure to sodium concentrations of less than 0.1 N suppresses pacemaker activity completely, and the heart stops in a relaxed state.[11]

Potassium

Changes in extracellular potassium concentration produce marked chronotropic effects. A twofold increase in serum potassium concentration, for example, slows the heart rate and decreases the conduction velocity. Impaired conduction is especially prominent in the atrioventricular node and may result in varying degrees of block. Higher levels of potassium can lead to arrhythmias, including fibrillation. Most, but not all, of these actions can be attributed to known actions of potassium on membrane potential. Deviations of potassium levels from normal can often be detected by electrocardiographic signs of conduction disturbances.

The two major membrane effects of an increase in extracellular potassium are (1) a decrease in resting potential (partial depolarization) and (2) a shortening of action potential duration.[2,5,11] The resting potential decreases (i.e., becomes less negative) because the electrochemical gradient of K^+ has been made smaller. The rate of rise and the overall amplitude of the propagated action potential consequently diminish, which slows conduction velocity and may, in an intact animal, produce atrioventricular block. In addition, as the resting potential in pacemaker cells becomes less negative it approaches the threshold potential, which tends to increase the rate of firing. When the resting potential is very close to or beyond the threshold level, excitability becomes depressed or is abolished.

The shortening of action potentials by high extracellular K^+ levels is more difficult to explain, for one might expect that the repolarizing outward potassium current would be reduced in these circumstances, prolonging repolarization. The evidence for shortening of the action potential is unequivocal, however, and a hypothesis involving inward rectification of potassium currents has been devised to account for it.[3] The ratio of external K^+ to Ca^{2+} is also a critical factor in these effects, and the influence of elevated K^+ on isolated ventricular muscle can be reduced if external Ca^{2+} is lowered concomitantly.[2,11] This interaction, unlike the Na^+–Ca^{2+} competition, probably does not depend on membrane binding sites, but rather on the duration of the action potential. The shorter the action potential, the less the net calcium influx.

Calcium

Calcium ions have a positive inotropic effect, which is to say that an increase in the extracellular concentration of Ca^{2+} produces an increase in maximum isometric force. The mechanism of this action was indicated in the earlier discussion of the contractile process. Elevated extracellular Ca^{2+} tends to produce a greater calcium influx during the action potential, making available more free calcium to bind troponin and thereby increasing the force of the contraction. Very low extracellular calcium levels reduce myocardial force until there is almost no contractile response, although action potentials still appear.[2] Cardiac muscle is much more sensitive than skeletal muscle in this respect.

Calcium is also a chronotropic agent[5,11,23] and elevations of plasma calcium levels slow the heart rate, primarily by raising the excitation threshold. Low calcium concentrations tend to increase the rate, although the effects are small unless Ca^{2+} is reduced to about one-tenth the normal level. This effect is mediated by an increase in the rate of diastolic depolarization, the *pacemaker potential*. Purkinje tissue is especially sensitive to low calcium concentrations and often develops spontaneously firing ectopic foci under such conditions.

Cardiac glycosides

The active components of digitalis, known as *cardiac glycosides,* exert a positive inotropic action when myocardial contractility is depressed. This effect is of great importance in medical therapy, although excessive doses of such drugs can produce arrhythmias and conduction block (Chapter 5). The mechanism of action has not been fully explained, but one hypothesis asserts that low (therapeutic) concentrations potentiate the activity of Na^+, K^+-ATPase, whereas high (toxic) concentrations inhibit it.[23]

References

Reviews

1. Bean, B.P. (1989). Classes of calcium channels in vertebrate cells. *Ann. Rev. Physiol.* 51:367–384.

2. Brooks, C. McC., Hoffman, B.F., Suckling, E.E., Orias, O.O. (1955) *Excitability of the Heart.* New York, Grune & Stratton.

3. CIBA foundation Symposium (1974). *The Physiological Basis of Starling's Law of the Heart*. Amsterdam, Associated Scientific Publishers, pp. 57–91, 123–128.

4. Cole, K.S. (1968). *Membranes, Ions and Impulses*. Berkeley, University of California Press, pp. 274–369.

5. Cranefield, P.F. (1975). *The Conduction of the Cardiac Impulse*. Mt. Kisco, N.Y., Futura.

6. Drummond, G.I., Severson, D.L. (1979). Cyclic nucleotides and cardiac function. *Circ. Res.* 44:145–153.

7. Fields, J.Z., Roeske, W.R., Morkin, E., Yamamura, H.I. (1978). Cardiac muscarinic cholinergic receptors. Biochemical identification and characterization. *J. Biol. Chem.* 263:3251–3256.

8. Fozzard, H.A., Arnsdorf, M.F. (1986). Cardiac electrophysiology. In: *The Heart and Cardiovascular System*, H.A. Fozzard et al., ed. New York, Raven Press, pp. 1–30.

9. Higgins, C.B., Vatner, S.F., Braunwald, E. (1973). Parasympathetic control of the heart. *Pharmacol. Rev.* 25:119–155.

10. Hille, B. (1984). *Ionic Channels of Excitable Membranes*. Sunderland, Mass., Sinauer.

11. Hoffman, B.F., Cranefield, P.F. (1960). *Electrophysiology of the Heart*. New York, McGraw-Hill.

12. Hoffman, B.B., Lefkowitz, R.J. (1982). Adrenergic receptors in the heart. *Annu. Rev. Physiol.* 44:475–484.

13. Homcy, C.J., Graham, R.M. (1985). Molecular characterization of adrenergic receptors. *Circ. Res.* 56:635–650.

14. Jack, J.J.B., Noble, D., Tsien, R.W. (1983). *Electric Current Flow in Excitable Cells*. Oxford, Clarendon Press.

15. Noble, D. (1979). *The Initiation of the Heartbeat*, 2nd ed. Oxford, Clarendon Press.

16. Noble, D. (1984). The surprising heart: A review of recent progress in cardiac electrophysiology. *J. Physiol.* 353:1–50.

17. Page, E., Shibata, Y. (1981). Permeable junctions between cardiac cells. *Annu. Rev. Physiol.* 43:431–441.

18. Patten, B.M. (1949). Initiation and early changes in the character of the heartbeat in vertebrate embryos. *Physiol. Rev.* 29:31–47.

19. Randall, W.C. (1977). *Neural Regulation of the Heart*. New York, Oxford University Press.

20. Reuter, H. (1984). Ion channels in cardiac cell membranes. *Annu. Rev. Physiol.* 46:473–484.

21. Ruegg, J.C. (1986). *Calcium in Muscle Activation*. Berlin, Springer-Verlag.

22. Sommer, J. R., Jennings, R.B. (1986). Ultrastructure of cardiac muscle. In: *The Heart and Cardiovascular System*, H. A. Fozzard et al., ed. New York, Raven Press, pp. 61–100.

23. Van Winkel, W. B., Schwartz, A. (1976). Ions and inotropy, *Annu. Rev. Physiol.* 38:247–272.

24. Winegrad, S. (1979). Electromechanical coupling in heart muscle. In: *Handbook of Physiology, Section 2: The Cardiovascular System. Vol. I, The Heart*. Bethesda, Md., American Physiological Society, pp.393–428.

Research Reports

25. Barr, L., Dewey, M.M., Berger, W. (1965). Propagation of action potentials and the structure of the nexus in cardiac muscle. *J. Gen. Physiol.* 48:796–823.

26. Bossen, E., Sommer, J.R., Waugh, R.A. (1978). Comparative stereology of the SR of the mouse and finch left ventricle. *Tissue Cell* 10:773–784.

27. Del Castillo, J., Katz, B. (1955). Local activity at a depolarized nerve–muscle junction. *J. Physiol.* 128:396–411.

28. DiFrancesco, D. (1981). A study of the ionic nature of the pace-maker current in calf Purkinje fibers. *J. Physiol.* 314:377–393.

29. Fabiato, A. (1981). Myoplasmic free calcium concentration reached during the twitch of an intact isolated cardiac cell and during calcium induced release of calcium from the sarcoplasmic reticulum of a skinned cardiac cell from the adult rat or rabbit ventricle. *J. Gen. Physiol.* 78:457–497.

30. Fawcett, D.W., McNutt, N.S. (1969). The ultrastructure of the cat myocardium. I. Ventricular papillary muscle. *J. Cell Biol.* 42:1–45.

31. Goldberg, J.M. (1975). Intra-SA-nodal pacemaker shifts induced by autonomic nerve stimulation in the dog. *Am. J. Physiol.* 229:1116–1123.

32. Hibberd, M.G., Jewell, B.R. (1982). Calcium- and length-dependent force production in rat ventricular muscle. *J. Physiol.* 329:527–540.

33. Hill, A.V. (1949). Abrupt transition from rest to activity in muscle. *Proc. R. Soc. Lond. (Biol.)* 136:399–420.

34. Hodgkin, A.L., Huxley, A.F. (1952). A quantitative description of membrane current and its application to conduction and excitation in nerve. *J. Physiol.* 117:500–544.

35. Hutter, O.F., Trautwein, W. (1956). Vagal and sympathetic effects on the pace-maker fibers in the sinus venosus of the heart. *J. Gen. Physiol.* 39:715–733.

36. James, T.N., Sherf, L. (1971). Specialized tissues and preferential conduction in the atria of the heart. *Am. J. Cardiol.* 28:414–427.

37. Julian, F.J., Moss, R.L. (1976). Active state in striated muscle. *Circ. Res.* 38:53–59.

38. Kitakaze, M., Hori, M., Tamai, J., Iwakura, K., Koretsune, Y., Kagiya, T., Iwai, K., Kitabatake, A., Inoue, M., Kamada, T. (1987). α_2-Adrenoceptor activity regulates release of adenosine from the ischemic myocardium in dogs. *Circ. Res.* 60:631–639.

39. Magid, A., Ting-Beall, H.P., Carvell, M., Kontis, T., Lucaveche, C. (1984). Connecting filaments, core filaments, and side struts: A proposal to add three new load-bearing structures to the sliding filament model. In: *Contractile Mechanisms in Muscle,* G.H. Pollack and H. Sugi, eds. New York, Plenum Press, pp. 307–328.

40. McDonald, T.F., Cavalié, A., Trautwein, W., Pelzer, D. (1986). Voltage-dependent properties of macroscopic and elementary calcium channel currents in guinea pig ventricular myocytes. *Pfluegers Arch.* 406:437–448.

41. McKibben, J.C., Getty, R. (1968). A comparative morphologic study of the cardiac innervation in domestic animals. I. The canine. *Am. J. Anat.* 122:533–543.

42. McNutt, S.N. (1970). Ultrastructure of intracellular junctions in adult and developing cardiac muscle. *Am. J. Cardiol.* 25:169–183.

43. Napolitano, L.M., Willman, V.L., Hanlon, C.R., Cooper, T. (1965). Intrinsic innervation of the heart. *Am. J. Physiol.* 208:455–458, 1965.

44. New, W., Trautwein, W. (1972). Inward membrane currents in mammalian myocardium. *Pfluegers Arch.* 334:1–23.

45. Noma, A., Irisawa, H. (1976). A time- and voltage-dependent potassium current in the rabbit sinoatrial node. *Pfluegers Arch.* 366:252–258.

46. Pollack, G.H. (1986). Quantal mechanisms in cardiac contraction. *Circ. Res.* 59:1–8.

47. Rabinowitz, B., Chuck, L., Kligerman, M., Parmley, W.W. (1975). Positive inotropic effect of methoxamine: Evidence for alpha-adrenergic receptors in ventricular myocardium. *Am. J. Physiol.* 229:582–585.

48. Sano, T., Ohtsuka, E., Shimamoto, T. (1960). "Unidirectional" atrioventricular conduction studied by microelectrodes. *Circ. Res.* 8:600–608.

49. Scherlag, B.J., Lau, S.H., Helfant, R.H., Berkowitz, W.D., Stein, E., Damato, A.N. (1967). Catheter technique for recording His bundle activity in man. *Circulation* 39:13–18.

50. Sonnenblick, E.H. (1966). The mechanics of myocardial contraction. In: *The Myocardial Cell: Structure, Function and Modification by Cardiac Drugs*, S.A. Briller and H. L. Conn, Jr., eds. Philadelphia, University of Pennsylvania Press, pp. 173–250.

51. Thaemert, J.C. (1970). Atrioventricular node innervation in ultrastructural three dimensions. *Am. J. Anat.* 128:239–263.

52. Vassort, G. (1973). Existence of two components in frog cardiac mechanical activity. *Eur. J. Cardiol.* 1:163–168.

53. Weidmann, S. (1969). Electrical coupling between myocardial cells. *Prog. Brain Res.* 31:275–281.

54. West, T. C. (1955). Ultramicroelectrode recording from the cardiac pacemaker. *J. Pharmacol. Exp. Ther.* 115:283–290.

55. Wood, E.H., Heppner, R.L., Weidmann, S. (1969). Inotropic effects of electric currents. I. Positive and negative effects of constant electric currents or current pulses applied during cardiac action potentials. II. Hypotheses: Calcium movements, excitation–contraction coupling and inotropic effects. *Circ. Res.* 24:409–445.

THE HEART AS A PUMP

The four-chambered mammalian heart is a complex pump that moves blood through the vascular system. The left heart chambers maintain a circulation through the systemic vascular bed, and those on the right simultaneously perfuse the pulmonary vessels. The special properties of cardiac cells that are the basis for the operation of this pump were discussed in the preceding chapter. Here we are concerned with excitation, conduction, and contraction in the heart as a whole.

Events of the Cardiac Cycle

Each heartbeat, or cardiac cycle, is an intricate sequence of electrical and mechanical events. A comprehensive view of this sequence is given in Figure 4.1, where pressure in the various chambers is shown in relation to valve actions and ventricular outflow. The deflections of the electrocardiogram are a useful time reference; the beginning of the P wave marks the first excitation of the atria, and the onset of the QRS complex shows the earliest activation of ventricular muscle. Pressure variations in the right heart chambers are similar in contour to those on the left side but smaller in magnitude.

A step-by-step review of events on the left side of the heart is instructive, and mid-diastole is a reasonable place to start. Shortly after the beginning of the P wave, atrial contraction causes a small increase of pressure in that chamber, the *a* wave. The delay corresponds to a latent period between electrical and mechanical responses. A similar wave appears in the ventricle because the atrioventricular valve is open. The large area of the normal mitral valve open-

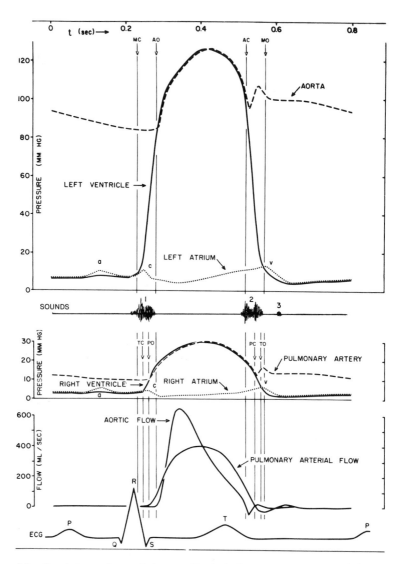

Figure 4.1. Events in cardiac cycle in man. *Top to bottom;* pressure in aorta, left ventricle, and left atrium; heart sounds; pressure in pulmonary artery, right ventricle, and right atrium; blood flow in aorta and pulmonary artery; electrocardiogram. Valve opening and closing indicated by *AO* and *AC*, respectively, for aortic valve; *MO* and *MC* for mitral valve; *PO* and *PC* for pulmonic valve; *TO* and *TC* for tricuspid valve. (Reproduced with modifications from Milnor,[7] with permission of Williams & Wilkins)

ing offers very little resistance to flow. The aortic valve remains closed throughout the diastolic period.

With the onset of ventricular contraction, the mitral valve closes, and intraventricular pressure starts to rise. The aortic valve remains shut for a time, and the ventricle contracts isometrically, or, to be exact, isovolumetrically. This *isovolumic contraction period* normally lasts for 0.04 to 0.05 sec in humans and ends when ventricular pressure equals that in the aorta, at which time the aortic valve opens and blood is ejected rapidly. Here, too, the normal valve opens widely, and the minute pressure gradient across it is undetectable in routine measurements. Aortic and ventricular pressures rise and fall together in the *ejection period,* following a trajectory dictated by the time course of muscle contraction and the systemic arterial input impedance (Chapter 6).

Ventricular force reaches a peak and begins to decline, but the myocardial fibers continue to shorten, and blood flow into the aorta continues. In the latter part of ejection, the momentum already acquired by the blood contributes to its motion, and as a result, pressure may be slightly higher in the aorta than in the ventricle. Eventually, ventricular pressure starts to fall more sharply, and the aortic valve immediately closes. An *isovolumic relaxation period* follows, with no change in volume until pressure in the ventricle falls below that in the atrium, whereupon the mitral valve opens again.

In the diastolic period that follows, some of the blood that has been accumulating in the left atrium flows into the ventricle, along with blood returning through the pulmonary veins. The ventricle is not completely empty after the ejection period, but contains a finite end-systolic *residual volume.* Inflow from the atrium adds to that volume, slowly increasing it to the *end-diastolic volume* that precedes the next ventricular contraction. The diastolic compliance of the normal ventricle allows a relatively small pressure to accomplish this filling. The ratio of stroke volume to end-diastolic volume is called the *ejection fraction.*

The lengths of ventricular diastole and systole vary with the heart rate. At a rate of 75 beats/min, diastole occupies about two-thirds of the full cycle. Faster heart rates shorten both periods, but diastole is affected more than systole, and very rapid heart rates can reduce stroke volume by causing excessive shortening of diastole. Diastolic filling of the ventricle consists of an early, rapid inflow from the atrium followed by a relatively long, more gradual phase (*diastasis*).

Three small but usually detectable atrial pressure waves occur in each cardiac cycle. Contraction of the atrium toward the end of diastole not only produces the *a* wave but also adds a small increment to the ventricular volume, slightly increasing myocardial fiber length. Following closure of the mitral valve the atrial and ventricular pressures no longer coincide, but the sharp rise in pressure that accompanies ventricular contraction causes the valve to bulge into the atrium, producing the atrial *c* wave. Venous filling of the atrium during the remainder of ventricular systole causes a gradual increase in atrial pressure, which ends when the mitral valve reopens. The relatively sudden drop in pressure at that instant creates the atrial *v* peak.

Pressure changes in the right atrium are transmitted back into the veins for a short distance, and the characteristic a, c, and v waves are often visible as small outward pulsations of the external jugular vein. These excursions are not simultaneous with those in the atrium, but are delayed for about 0.2 sec by the time required for transmission. The waves can normally be seen only with the subject supine, because the vein collapses in the erect posture. The superior vena cava and external jugular act as a kind of vertical manometer tube in the erect position, and the jugular is not distended and clearly visible unless right atrial pressure is abnormally high, that is, high enough to support a column of blood that extends above the clavicle.

Action of valves

The four cardiac valves—mitral, tricuspid, aortic, and pulmonic—direct the flow of blood through the heart and normally prevent backward movement of blood from one chamber to another. The valves open or close in response to pressure differences between the chambers they separate. The rise of left ventricular above atrial pressure closes the mitral valve, for example, and the aortic valve opens when ventricular pressure begins to exceed aortic pressure. The shape and structure of the valves prevent retrograde flow.

Certain features of cardiac anatomy contribute to the efficient operation of the valves. The aortic root and sinuses of Valsalva are somewhat wider than the aortic valve orifice, and this difference has a significant hemodynamic effect. Forcing blood through an orifice into a larger chamber sets up eddy currents, and these currents tend to keep the valve cusps from being pressed against the aortic walls, where they might obstruct coronary inflow. In the case of atrioventricular valves, the chordae tendineae, which extend from the papillary muscles in the ventricle to the edges of the valve, allow it to close but keep it from prolapsing into the atrium.

Ventricular outflow

The rates of blood flow into the aorta and pulmonary artery are also shown in Figure 4.1. The contours of the flow pulse differ in these two arteries, but the area under the curve is proportional to the stroke volume and hence is the same in both cases. The right ventricle begins to contract a little before the left, a consequence of slight differences in the excitation paths, so that outflow into the pulmonary artery leads that into the aorta by approximately 0.02 sec. The left ventricular discharge rises rapidly to a peak and then falls, whereas the right outflow increases and declines more smoothly and has a lower maximum. Ejection ends a little earlier in the left than in the right ventricle.

Heart sounds

Mechanical vibrations that create two separate sounds accompany each heartbeat, and both are clearly audible when an ear or a stethoscope is applied to the chest wall. The first sound marks the beginning of ventricular systole, and the second sound signals its end (Figure 4.1). A third sound is sometimes heard in diastole. A large body of empiric knowledge relating heart sounds to cardiac function has been acquired over the years, and auscultation of the heart consequently occupies a prominent place in medical diagnosis. For example, some kinds of cardiac murmurs, prolonged vibrations in part of the cycle, are a sign of pathological conditions, whereas other types may be heard in normal subjects and have no pathological significance.

The *first heart sound* occurs as ventricular contraction begins, during the latter part of the QRS complex, and is most prominent near the apex of the heart. The sound is low-pitched, with frequencies in the range 30 to 45/sec, although the vibrations are not perfectly regular. It originates in vibrations of the atrioventricular valves as they close, and in vibrations in the muscle itself as it develops tension. In addition, the cusps of the opening aortic valve may vibrate as eddies form behind them. Atrial contraction produces a faint sound that usually blends with the onset of the ventricular first sound.

The *second heart sound* is generated by closing of the aortic and pulmonic valves. It can be heard most distinctly over the anatomical location of these valves, the level of the second intercostal space near the sternum. The second heart sound happens to fall near the end of the T wave, but the relationship is not exact, and the termination of this electrocardiographic wave should not be regarded as an indicator of any mechanical event. The sound is sharper in character than the thudding first heart sound and somewhat higher in pitch (50 to 70 vibrations/sec). It has two components, aortic and pulmonic, because the two valves do not close at exactly the same instant. The interval between the two events is normally very short, less than 0.1 sec, but the difference is some-times audible. Closing of either valve under abnormally high pressure increases the intensity of its contribution. In some normal individuals, a distant *third heart sound* is heard early in diastole 0.1 to 0.2 sec after the second heart sound. Its mechanism is uncertain, but it occurs at the end of the rapid-filling phase of ventricular diastole and may originate in vibration of the ventricular structures when inflow decelerates rather suddenly.

Phonocardiography is the recording of heart sounds and murmurs through a microphone and an electrical amplifier. The timing of heart sounds and their correlation with other physiological events are clearly evident in such records. The human auditory system is very efficient at analyzing the timing and quality of heart sounds, however, not to mention filtering out ambient noise. For that reason, phonocardiography is not widely employed in clinical work, but is applied when the exact timing of a murmur or heart sound is critical. The second heart sound, for example, is recorded in some research work to indicate the instant of aortic or pulmonic valve closing.

Determinants of Ventricular Function

The function of the ventricle as a pump is, in effect, an extension of the physiological properties of cardiac cells (Chapter 3), organized by the sequence of excitation discussed in Chapter 3. The gross structure of the ventricles is formed by layers of large muscle bundles, the fibers of which fan out in patterns that have been recognized gradually over many years of study. The bundles follow figure-of-eight pathways, rather like broad straps that encircle the ventricular chambers, a morphological arrangement described meticulously by Streeter.[14]

Information about ventricular function has been gained from experiments on isolated hearts, as well as from studies of living animals and human subjects. A mammalian heart can continue to beat for hours after removal from the body if it is supplied with the proper cellular environment by perfusion with blood or appropriate salt solutions. The solutions can be oxygenated by the animal's own lungs or by an artificial device. Such experiments show that in most respects the ventricles behave in exactly the way one would predict from experiments on papillary muscles (Chapter 3).

The most important factors that enter into the regulation of cardiac function[3] are listed in Table 4.1. One group, of which the Starling mechanism is a prominent example, can be considered *intrinsic* because they are inherent in the function of cardiac cells. These intrinsic properties provide the heart with a certain degree of *autoregulation,* enabling it to respond to a variety of physiological demands without the intervention of external controls. Other influences may be classed as *extrinsic.* Stimuli that reach the myocardium through the nervous system or bloodstream are obvious examples, but external constraints on ventricular compliance and the control of orderly excitation by the specialized conducting system belong in the same category.

Table 4.1.   Determinants of Ventricular
Function

Intrinsic (autoregulation)
    End-diastolic fiber length, which depends on:
        Filling pressure (preload)
        Duration of diastole
        Diastolic compliance
        Pericardial constraint
    Afterload
    Frequency of contraction

Extrinsic
    Autonomic nerve signals and transmitters
    Blood-borne agents
        Oxygen, carbon dioxide
        Catecholamines, etc.
    Locally produced agents.
    Coordination of contraction
        Timing of atrial systole
        Sequence of ventricular excitation

Intrinsic regulatory mechanisms

Length–force–velocity relationships

Although the force–length relationships observed in papillary muscle preparations (Figure 3.10A) also exist in the intact ventricle, the relevant variables
are more difficult to measure in a three-dimensional structure. The longitudinal
length and force in the essentially one-dimensional papillary muscle are replaced in studies of the intact ventricle by circumferential fiber length and tangential force. The variables that are actually measured are the intraventricular
pressures and volumes as functions of time. To translate such data into the
appropriate force, length, and velocity of shortening, the ventricle is assumed
to have the shape of a sphere or some other regular geometric body.[8]

The circumference of a perfect spherical shell, for example, can be calculated from its volume. Tangential force in the wall of such a shell can be
calculated from the area of its surface and the transmural pressure (force/area)
by way of the law of Laplace. If wall thickness is known, the gradient of force
through the wall can be determined. These principles offer a way of estimating
ventricular fiber length and force from pressure and volume, although the results are no more than a practical compromise with the irregular shape of the
real ventricle. Conical or ellipsoidal models are frequently used for this purpose; the ventricular chamber resembles a half-cone more than any other geo-

metric figure, its apex corresponding to the apex of the heart. Contraction reduces the radii of the cone without causing much change in its height. Data obtained by such approximations show relationships among force, length, and velocity of shortening similar to those found in papillary muscle.

Preload

Preload, the force just prior to contraction (Chapter 3), is related in the ventricle to end-diastolic pressure. Ventricular compliance as well as pressure determines fiber length at the end of diastole, however, and the compliance can vary with coronary perfusion pressure, intrapleural pressure, constraint by the pericardium, and conditions in the opposite ventricle.[8,21] Only when these variables are in the normal range can changes in diastolic pressure be treated as if they had the same significance as changes in volume.

Afterload

The functioning ventricle faces an afterload, but it is more difficult to define that load than it is in the case of an isolated papillary muscle (Chapter 3). In an isotonic muscle strip the investigator loads the tissue by suspending a weight from it, and the force on the muscle is at all times equal to that weight (Figure 3.9). The ventricle, however, is not called on to lift a weight, but to move a viscous fluid into a viscoelastic system. The afterload on an intact ventricle is consequently not a simple quantity, and authorities do not agree on how it should be measured or expressed. Some, using the analogy of the muscle strip, argue that aortic pressure *is* the afterload. One awkward result of this view is the implication that the ventricle plays a part in determining its own afterload, because ejection pressure depends in part on how rapidly the ventricle ejects blood into the arteries (see below).

An alternative and more consistent approach regards the arterial system itself as the ventricular afterload, and the problem then becomes one of expressing the arterial properties. Vascular resistance is one way of doing so, but it is a very incomplete one. Strictly speaking, the factors that oppose ventricular ejection are the viscosity of blood and the viscoelasticity of the aorta or pulmonary artery; the hemodynamic result cannot be expressed in a single number. The input impedance of the systemic or pulmonic arteries is the most appropriate measure of ventricular afterload,[24] but it is complicated to analyze and takes the form of a frequency-dependent spectrum (Chapter 6). The choice is thus between a simple variable like mean aortic pressure, which is an indirect, partial representation of the real afterload, and the more complete but complicated analysis involved in computing impedance. The first is adequate for some investigative purposes, whereas the second is required for others.

Starling's law of the heart

The influence of resting fiber length on force of contraction is a major element in our understanding of ventricular function, thanks to the early investigations of Frank and subsequent work by Starling.[13] They both used isolated heart preparations, in which filling pressure of the atrium, and hence of the ventricle, can readily be controlled by varying the height of a fluid reservoir. Starling concluded, from Frank's observations on the frog and his own on the canine heart, that end-diastolic fiber length largely determines the energy imparted to the blood by ventricular contraction. Ventricular work increases along with initial length up to a certain point, he asserted, and then decreases at greater lengths. This phenomenon, now amply confirmed in animals and in man, is known as *Starling's law,* although it should perhaps be called the *Frank-Starling law.*[5] The relationship arises from the degree of filament overlap and the sarcomere length–dependent availability of Ca^{2+} (Chapter 3).

Although Starling identified *energy* as the dependent variable in this relationship, his early papers actually demonstrated the relation of ventricular ejection *pressure* to end-diastolic volume. Pressure–volume curves are a convenient way of expressing ventricular function, and Figure 4.2 illustrates the form they usually take. The relationships when the muscle is inactive (i.e., not contracting) can be determined experimentally by varying the filling pressure and

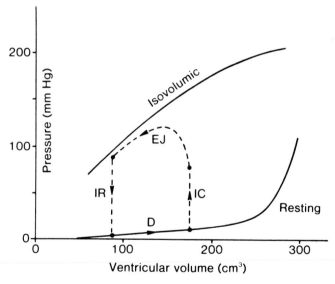

Figure 4.2.   Example of pressure–volume relationships in human left ventricle. *Lower solid line,* resting, noncontracting state. *Upper solid line,* maximum pressure reached under isovolumic conditions. *Dashed line,* sequence in typical normal beat. *D,* diastole; *IC,* isovolumic contraction; *EJ,* ejection; *IR,* isovolumic relaxation. (Reproduced from Milnor,[7] with permission of Williams & Wilkins)

measuring the resulting ventricular volume. The ventricle is quite distensible in this relaxed state, and small increments in pressure produce relatively large increments in volume. The passive compliance is nonlinear, however, and the chamber becomes stiffer as it is distended, as indicated by the steep rise of the relaxed curve above 200 cm^3 in the figure.

The pressure–volume relationship in the active, contracting state can be measured in a similar way. The uppermost curve in Figure 4.2 represents the peak pressure developed in *isovolumic* contractions, where the experimental arrangement prevents the ventricle from ejecting blood. These are the highest pressures that can be developed in the existing state of contractility (which is kept constant in such experiments), and lower peaks would be reached if the ventricle were allowed to expel blood in a normal manner. The greater the relaxed volume when contraction begins, the higher the peak isovolumic pressure, demonstrating the ventricular equivalent of the force–length relationship discussed in Chapter 3. In some experiments on isolated hearts, the active curve has been seen to *fall* at very high volumes, but that does not occur under physiological conditions. The work per stroke (not shown in the figure) also rises as filling pressure is increased, an expression of Starling's law of the heart.

The loop shown in Figure 4.2 is an example of a single normal, ejecting contraction, starting in this case from an end-diastolic volume of 175 cm^3, proceeding through isovolumic contraction until the aortic valve opens, ejecting a stroke volume (at a lower than isovolumic pressure), relaxing isovolumically after aortic valve closure, and filling again in diastole. The dimensions of the loop depend on the initial end-diastolic volume, myocardial contractility, and afterload. The area within the loop is proportional to the ventricular external stroke work (see below).

Recognition of Starling's law as a fundamental physiological principle led to the introduction of the *ventricular function curve*,[11] a plot of the relation between stroke work and end-diastolic fiber length or some indirect indication of it, such as ventricular filling pressure (Figure 4.3). Such curves are a convenient graphic display of cardiac function, showing the changes in stroke work to be expected in response to changes in preload as long as the state of the myocardium is unaltered. Ventricular and atrial end-diastolic pressures are virtually the same when the valve between them is normal, and for practical reasons, mean atrial pressure is sometimes accepted as an index of ventricular fiber length, as in Figure 4.3. The use of pressure as an indication of fiber length assumes constant compliance, but for any one set of observations, that is usually a reasonable assumption.

Ventricular function curves are sometimes used as a measure of myocardial contractility (see below), in effect defining contractility as the relation between work and fiber length. Upward displacement of the plot by any interven-

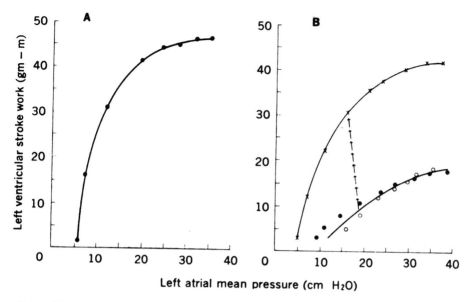

Figure 4.3. Left ventricular function curves in open-chest dog, showing relation between mean left atrial pressure (ventricular filling pressure, *abscissa*) and ventricular stroke work (*ordinate*). Data were obtained by measuring responses at a number of experimentally controlled left atrial pressures. **A**, initial control state; increasing filling pressure stretches ventricular fibers to greater end-diastolic length, hence greater work per stroke. **B**, control curve (*open circles*, lower than in **A**), effect of infused epinephrine (*crosses*), and later control in the absence of epinephrine (*closed circles*). The upward shift of the curve by epinephrine is an indication of increased myocardial contractility. (Reproduced from Sarnoff,[11] with permission of the American Physiological Society)

tion is then considered an increase in contractility (Figure 4.3B), and vice versa. The function curve does not fall at high filling pressures in normal intact animals, but it may do so when the myocardium is diseased or its coronary blood supply is inadequate.

Starling's law is now accepted as one of the fundamental mechanisms in cardiac regulation, but it is not the only one, and its operation is not evident in all physiological responses. During exercise, for example, cardiac work increases but no change in end-diastolic pressure may be detected. This fact does not disprove Starling's law, but merely demonstrates the existence of other important mechanisms. Exercise, moreover, is accompanied by changes in autonomic stimuli, peripheral resistance, and a number of other variables.

The velocity of fiber shortening[12,18,26] does not appear in ventricular function curves, but this variable can be added to create a three-dimensional plot (Figure 4.4). Myocardial function is then represented by a surface, which is constructed from the observed pressure–volume, pressure–velocity, and volume–velocity relationships. This surface has been recommended as an al-

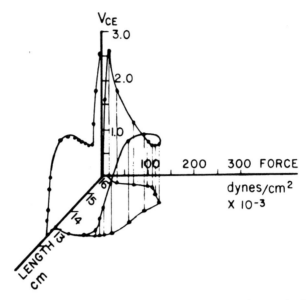

Figure 4.4. Force, length, and contractile element velocity (v_{ce}) in left ventricle of an anesthetized dog. Ventricular volume measured by biplane cineradiography was used to estimate circumference (length). Points are plotted at intervals of 14.8 msec, showing sequence of events in one cardiac cycle. Force in kilodyn/cm², length in cm, and velocity in circumferences per sec. Each beat follows a path that begins by rising to a peak in the back plane of the figure during the isovolumic contraction period, moves out to vary in three dimensions during ejection, and travels in the bottom plane during diastole. (Reproduced from Bove and Lynch,[17] with permission of the American Physiological Society)

ternative way of expressing contractility,[3,18,20] but it shares with other methods a number of defects. The main deficiency is a tendency for the force–velocity relation to deviate from a simple curvilinear relationship during ejection, when the events observed depend on aortic (or pulmonic) impedance (Chapter 6) as well as on myocardial function. Such deviations also suggest that the velocity to be considered is that of the sarcomeric *contractile element*, not the muscle fiber as a whole. Muscle behaves as though it contained passive elastic as well as contractile components, and some theoretic model of the myocardium must be assumed in order to calculate the length and velocity of the active element. Many different models have been described,[7] and some are discussed in Chapter 9.

Other intrinsic mechanisms

Not all forms of intrinsic regulation depend on fiber length. Control mechanisms that do *not* involve changes in end-diastolic volume have been called *homeometric,* to contrast them with the *heterometric* Starling mechanism.[11]

The relation between myocardial force and velocity of shortening (Figure 3.10B and one plane of Figure 4.4) is an example of homeometric regulation, for it expresses a myocardial property that is independent of initial length. Afterload, however, influences the force–velocity relationship and the stroke volume. Increasing the load by sudden partial occlusion of the aorta leads to a higher pressure in the next beat, but less blood is ejected at a lower velocity.

Frequency of contraction acts through intrinsic attributes of the myocardium to affect cardiac function in two different ways, one homeometric, the other heterometric. One is illustrated by the staircase phenomenon, in which an increase in rate enhances contractility transiently (Chapter 3). The other has to do with the relation between heart rate and length of diastole. As the interval between beats becomes shorter with tachycardia, diastole is abbreviated more than systole, decreasing the filling time even more than would otherwise be the case. The resulting decrease of end-diastolic volume reduces cardiac output, but the effect is significant only at very high rates.

Extrinsic control of myocardial function

Nerve impulses and cardioactive substances borne by the blood are the two principal means of extrinsic control. Stimulation of sympathetic cardiac nerves increases ventricular force of contraction, speeds the velocity of shortening, and shortens the ejection period. Cardiovascular reflexes that evoke a higher frequency of sympathetic adrenergic impulses have the same effect. These stimuli combine to provide a graded cardiac control system, although they do not produce a constant level of muscular tone like that in vascular smooth muscle. The same kinds of responses are modulated by the catecholamines released into the bloodstream by the adrenal medulla, although the responses of intact animals to epinephrine and norepinephrine are modified by peripheral vascular actions of those transmitters. Parasympathetic nerves are also active in cardiac control. The principal effects of parasympathetic stimuli are on heart rate and atrioventricular conduction, but there is also some modulation of ventricular muscle function. When all other factors are strictly controlled, stimulation of the distal end of transected vagal nerves causes a slight depression of contractility, in addition to slowing the heart rate and conduction velocities.

The partial pressure of oxygen and carbon dioxide in the environment of myocardial cells is another extrinsic source of regulation. Hypoxia and hypercapnia depress contractility. Hypoxemia induced by breathing 12% oxygen in nitrogen, for instance, reduces cardiac output, as does hypercapnia brought on by inhalation of high concentrations of carbon dioxide. Reflexes mediated by the arterial chemoreceptors (Chapter 7) in intact animals minimize such effects in all but extreme cases.

The sequence of atrial and ventricular contraction is an additional extrinsic determinant of cardiac function, or at least one that is imposed by the pacemaker and conduction system. Near the end of diastole, atrial contraction pumps a small increment of blood into the ventricles, adding to ventricular volume and thus enhancing contractile force in the next beat. Atrial fibrillation or complete atrioventricular block does away with this marginal effect, although both conditions are compatible with adequate cardiac function. The normal sequence of ventricular excitation dictated by the bundle of His and Purkinje system is a more important factor in the efficient ejection of blood. When this sequence is lacking, as when the heart is stimulated experimentally at a point on the ventricular free wall, stroke work is decreased. In the profound disorganization of response represented by ventricular fibrillation (Chapter 5), the heart ceases to pump blood at all.

Ventricular compliance can be affected by extrinsic factors, thus invoking the intrinsic regulation connected with end-diastolic fiber length. The fact that ventricular distensibility is subject to change means that inferences about fiber length based on pressure or volume must be made with caution. Pressure in the coronary arteries is one factor that can alter ventricular compliance, the coronary vascular tree acting as a kind of flexible skeleton in cardiac muscle. The pericardium is also a determinant of ventricular distensibility, although its influence is normally minimal. The normal heart can function perfectly well in the absence of the pericardium, but its removal leads to an increase in diastolic volume with normal filling pressures. Pressure within the intact pericardial sac varies slightly with that in the ventricle, a fact to be taken into account when estimating transmural ventricular pressure.[21] Thickening of the pericardium by disease can reduce the effective ventricular compliance to a marked degree. The pericardium not only influences pressure–volume relations in the cardiac chambers but also acts to limit total heart volume, enhancing the mechanical interaction between the two ventricles. Increased diastolic volume in one ventricle, for example, tends to raise diastolic pressure in the other.[21]

Myocardial contractility

In research and clinical medicine, it is often important to evaluate the functional ability of the heart. For example, if an abnormally low cardiac output is found in a patient with stenosis of the aortic valve, is it low because the heart muscle is diseased or because the muscle is healthy and doing as well as could be expected considering the outflow obstruction? We have already seen that the performance of the heart in a given situation does not necessarily reflect its ability to function were it free of the constraints imposed by preload and afterload (Chapter 3). The concept of contractility is an attempt to express what the myocardium is capable of doing, in contrast with what it actually does. Contractility is an expression of the physicochemical state of the myocardial cells, but performance depends on contractility *plus* filling pressure and the opposition to outflow. For that reason, investigators have long tried to find some hemodynamic parameter that is not affected by preload or afterload.

Many indices of myocardial contractility have been proposed, and their very number indicates that none is entirely satisfactory.[3,6,10] The search for such indicators concentrated at first on the rate of rise of intraventricular pressure *(dP/dt)* and peak pressure, because stimuli that were believed to improve contractility increased these parameters. Measurements of the rising phase during the isovolumic contraction period might be thought to be immune to afterload effects, but it soon became apparent that initial *dP/dt* varied with preload. The maximum *dP/dt* divided by the simultaneous "developed" pressure (observed minus end-diastolic) to give *dP/Pdt* has been proposed as a number that avoids preload effects, but it does not do so completely.

Other indices have been derived from measurements of blood flow during the ejection period, examples being the ejection fraction and the maximum acceleration of blood.[27] Although the ejection fraction is load dependent to some extent, values below 0.4 are usually a sign of ventricular dysfunction regardless of load. Maximum acceleration occurs early in the ejection period, when the main opposition to flow is inertial, so it may be relatively unaffected by the resistance and compliance of the arterial tree.

Indicators of contractility calculated from both pressure and flow during ejection constitute still another group; ventricular function curves fall into this category (Figure 4.3). Maximum unloaded velocity of fiber shortening is another such parameter (v_{max}, Chapter 3), even though its application is restricted by the need for multiple determinations of velocity at various loads, the complexities of estimating fiber length and wall force in the ventricle, and the uncertainties involved in extrapolation. In addition, v_{max} varies with preload and with the model used to compute it.[28]

One original and promising method of evaluating myocardial contractility has been developed by Suga[32] and Sagawa et al.,[10] who express ventricular contraction and relaxation as changes in ventricular compliance or its reciprocal, elastance. In experiments on isolated hearts pumping into a mechanical impedance, they showed that in a constant state of contractility the *end-systolic* pressure and volume tend to fall along a straight line, which intercepts the volume axis at a finite value, V_d (Figure 4.5A). Changes in resistance or characteristic impedance altered V_d but had little effect on the slope of the line,[10] at least when the ejection fraction was in the neighborhood of 0.5. Actually, a set of such lines exists, one for each instant after the beginning of ejection; these lines become steeper as contraction progresses, finally reaching a maximum at end-

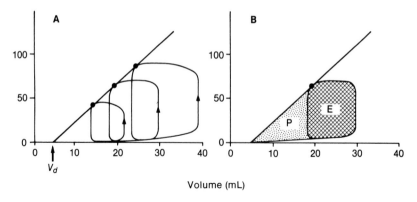

Volume (mL)

Figure 4.5. Left ventricular pressures (*ordinate*) and volumes (*abscissa*) in isolated canine heart pumping into a constant artificial arterial resistance and impedance. **A**, three beats, each starting from a different end-diastolic volume. End-systolic points tend to fall on a straight line, which intercepts the volume axis (*arrow, V_d*). (Reproduced with modifications from Maughan et al.,[23] with permission of the American Heart Association) **B**, middle loop from **A**, illustrating the two kinds of mechanical work done by ejecting beats. *External work (E)*, the energy manifested as blood pressure and flow, is proportional to the area within the loop. *Potential work*, or energy, is related to the pressure remaining at the end of systole, and is proportional to area labeled *P* beneath the end-systolic pressure–volume line. (Reproduced with modifications from Sagawa et al.,[10] with permission of Oxford University Press)

systole (*maximum elastance, or E_{max}*). The value of E_{max} increases (i.e., the slope becomes steeper) in the presence of agents that increase contractility.

Ventricular behavior can, therefore, be characterized as that of a *time-varying elastance,* a concept that has not only provided a well-defined function to describe ventricular performance but has also stimulated many new lines of research. The variable E_{max} appears to be valid as an indicator of contractility over a wide but not unlimited range of conditions. It is not a reliable guide in the presence of extreme deviations from normal afterload, stroke volume, ejection fraction, or coronary perfusion pressure. The same restriction applies to every index of myocardial contractility that has been tested, and the evidence suggests that no functional measurement can be completely independent of afterload. Indeed, the fact that fiber length influences the availability of ionized calcium to the contractile apparatus argues strongly against such independence (Chapter 3). Changes can be detected in virtually all indices in the beat following an abrupt change of load, and a new stable state is not reached for 10 to 15 min.[22]

Unfortunately, the best experimental test that can be designed at present for parameters intended as a practical measure of contractility is their ability to distinguish between normal subjects and patients with clear signs of cardiac malfunction, whereas the goal is a measurement that will detect the subtle changes that precede overt abnormalities. Most indices change in the appropriate direction in response to experimental procedures, but they often fail to identify a particular case as normal or abnormal because the measurements in those populations overlap. The best solution is probably to judge contractility from as complete a collection of data on pressure, flow, and cardiac dimensions as possible, not from a single number. As Blinks and Jewell[1] have pointed out, "If the index is really simple, its informational content is unlikely to be adequate."

Cardiac Output and Work

Cardiac output

The volume of blood ejected per minute by each ventricle is referred to as the *cardiac output;* this variable is one of the most common measures of cardiac function. Right and left ventricles eject the same amount of blood if their outputs are averaged over several minutes, although there are small beat-to-beat differences from time to time. Right and left ventricular stroke volumes obviously could not differ for long, or the pulmonary or systemic vascular beds would become overdistended. The ventricle does not eject all of the blood it contains with each beat but leaves behind a residual amount, about 30 to 40% of end-diastolic volume. The *ejection fraction,* or ratio of stroke to end-diastolic volume, is thus normally 0.6 to 0.7 (Chapter 2).

The average cardiac output in adult humans is 6.5 liters/min, corresponding to an average stroke volume of 90 ml and a heart rate of 72 beats/min. As with all hemodynamic variables, the normal range is relatively broad, approximately 4 to 9 liters/min. Cardiac output is directly correlated with body size; its relation to age, body surface area, and other factors is described in Chapter 2.

Cardiac work

The myocardium is, in effect, a machine that converts chemical into mechanical energy, and the physical work done by the heart is an important aspect of cardiac function. The contracting ventricle imparts a certain amount of mechanical energy to the blood, and this energy can be calculated from records of blood pressure and flow throughout the ejection period.[7,25] Ventricular power, or the rate of doing work, equals the product of pressure and flow at every instant (Figure 4.6). Stroke work is consequently the integral of that product, $\int PQ\ dt$, where P is pressure in the outflow artery, Q is the volumetric rate of flow (e.g., in milliliters per second), and integration is carried out from

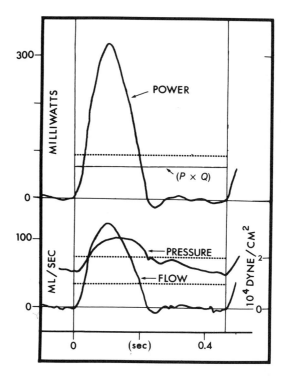

Figure 4.6. Pulsatile pressure, blood flow, and their product, hydraulic power, in the main pulmonary artery of an anesthetized dog. Power was recorded by continuous electronic multiplication of pressure by flow. *Abscissa*, time in sec. *Above*, mechanical power supplied by the right ventricle (omitting kinetic energy). *Below*, pressure (*ordinate on right*, 10^4 dyn/cm^2) and flow (*ordinate on left*, ml/sec). *Dashed lines*, averages of each curve over one cardiac cycle. Product of mean pressure and mean flow, shown by *solid horizontal line* in upper panel ($P \times Q$), is smaller than true average power indicated by dashed line in upper panel; difference is the extra energy entailed in pulsations (see text). (Reproduced from Milnor,[7] with permission of Williams & Wilkins)

the beginning to the end of ejection. The result of this calculation, which is called *external stroke work*, is implicit in the pressure–volume "loop" representing a cardiac cycle (Figure 4.5), because external work is proportional to the area of the loop. Such calculations do not include kinetic energy, which can be computed from the mass *(m)* and velocity *(v)* of the moving blood (kinetic energy $= mv^2/2$). Only a small portion of external cardiac work, 2 to 7%, is kinetic in nature.

The relation between the energy involved in cardiac work and the mechanical performance of the heart raises many problems that have yet to be solved. The energy liberated by muscular contraction can be determined directly by measuring the heat produced, but it is technically easier to determine myocardial oxygen consumption. In terms of a standard physical unit of energy, the joule (J), myocardial consumption of 1 ml of oxygen is equivalent to about 20 J, a value that remains constant within ±5% whether fatty acids or carbohydrates are the energy substrate.[10] A typical resting uptake of 0.5 ml O^2/sec by the muscles of both ventricles in humans would therefore correspond to 10 J/sec.

Three components[10] account for about half of the total myocardial oxygen consumption under resting conditions with normal preload, afterload, and contractility:

1. External mechanical work.
2. Basal metabolism.
3. Potential mechanical energy.

Each of these three activities employs approximately 10 to 20% of the oxygen uptake of the heart. The remainder is dissipated in excitation–contraction coupling and other processes not yet clearly identified.

A relatively small part of the total energy involved in contraction transmits movement and pressure to the blood and hence appears as *external* work (e.g., 1.9 J/sec for the right and left ventricles combined in human subjects at rest[7]). The *basal* energy is that required to maintain the basal metabolism of the cardiac tissues, apart from the ejection of blood. This nonmechanical component can be determined only by measuring heat production or oxygen consumption in an arrested, noncontracting heart.

Potential energy, like external work, is calculated from measurements of ventricular pressure and volume. This component is called *potential* because it is the result of mechanical action revealed by the pressure that remains in the ventricle at the end of ejection—for example, the end-systolic pressure in the pressure–volume loop of Figure 4.5B. Contraction has stored in the wall at that time an amount of energy proportional to the area labeled *P* in that figure. If the afterload were suddenly reduced to zero at this point, pressure and volume would travel down the end-systolic line, converting the potential energy into actual mechanical energy. Under ordinary conditions, however, the potential energy is dissipated as heat during isovolumic relaxation. In an isovolumic beat, where experimental conditions prevent the ventricle from ejecting blood, all the mechanical work is of the potential kind. Recognition of this component is an important by-product of the intensive examination of pressure–volume relationships by Suga and by Sagawa's group.[10] The basal energy component is not affected by load, but external and potential work are sensitive to both afterload and inotropic state.

In any machine that harnesses energy, the ratio of useful work to total energy expended is called its *efficiency;* this term can be applied to the ratio of cardiac work to oxygen consumption. With respect to external work, myocardial efficiency is not constant. For example, a given stroke volume ejected at high pressure consumes more oxygen per unit of external work than the same stroke at low pressure does.[31] The myocardium is less efficient, in other words, when pumping against a high resistance. Furthermore, it can increase stroke volume more efficiently than it can raise outflow pressure. This fits with clinical observations that the high *volume load* of an intracardiac shunt is better tolerated by the heart than the excessive *pressure load* of aortic stenosis. In spite of these variations in the oxygen cost of the external and potential components considered separately, the efficiency of combined external and internal mechanical work—that is, (external plus potential work)/(total oxygen consumption minus that attributable to basal energy)—appears to be constant[10] at about 30%. The physiological meaning of this constancy has yet to be worked out.

The pressure dependence of oxygen usage has led investigators to predict myocardial oxygen consumption from various attributes of ventricular pressure, including the maximum pressure, the corresponding wall force, or the time integral throughout systole (the *tension–time index*[10,31]); all of these predictors are empiric in the present state of knowledge. Other connections between myocardial energetics and mechanical performance have been investigated actively, but their conclusions remain tentative. The velocity of muscle shortening, for example, is directly related to ATPase activity in organisms ranging from molluscs to mammals and varies with the inotropic state in mammalian species. For that reason, unloaded velocity (v_{max}) is often interpreted as an index of the rate of cross-bridge cycling in smooth as well as striated muscle. Another approach uses measurement of ATP turnover to estimate the thermodynamic efficiency of the contractile machinery. Some experiments of this kind suggest that 60 to 70% of the available free energy of ATP is converted into mechanical work in the ventricular cross-bridges.[10] In addition, the possibility of shifts in the efficiency of cross-bridge function has been suggested by changes in ATPase isoenzymes (various combinations of the same polypeptides) observed in myocardial hypertrophy and other conditions.[16]

Power

The total hydraulic power, or external work per unit time, averages 240 mW for the right ventricle of adult human subjects at rest and about seven times that value for the left ventricle. The power exerted varies with cardiac output and arterial pressure, among other things, and it changes during exercise and other physiological responses. Left ventricular power increases about threefold in dogs running at a speed sufficient to raise output by a factor of 2.5, for example.[7] The relationship is nonlinear and is affected by heart rate and arterial impedance. Myocardial disease reduces the ability of the heart to increase its power and output.

Since the work demanded of the heart depends strongly on the mixture of arterial properties that retard the motion of blood, it is sometimes useful to look at blood pressure and flow as if they were each the sum of two parts, the time-averaged mean value and the pulsations around that mean. Cardiac power can then be separated into two components: (1) the amount that would be required to produce steady, nonpulsatile flow at the observed mean value and (2) the power exerted to produce the pulsations.[25]

Steady-flow power is expended principally in moving blood through arterioles, and hence depends to a great extent on peripheral resistance. The *oscillatory power* exerted in pulsations is largely determined by the viscoelasticity of the largest arteries, which can be expressed as arterial input impedance (Chapter 6). The oscillatory component is an extra expenditure of energy, a price imposed by the pulsatile nature of the heart's activity. A steady-flow pump would use less power to provide the same cardiac output.

Oscillatory power amounts to about one-third of total right ventricular power at rest, a proportion consistent with the ratio of pulsatile to mean pressure and the relatively low peak flow in the pulmonary artery (Figure 4.1). In the left ventricle, oscillatory power is approximately one-sixth of the total.[7] Stiffening of the aorta by disease or age, which elevates the impedance faced by the left ventricle, increases the oscillatory power required to maintain a normal cardiac output. Hypertension associated with high peripheral resistance, on the other hand, increases steady-flow power if all other factors are constant.

Modern diagnosis and treatment of cardiac disorders are based in part on recognition of all these facts. Disease processes often lead to high peripheral resistance or aortic impedance, creating an arterial system that demands excessive cardiac work if blood flow is to be kept normal. Abnormally high or low expenditures of cardiac power are undesirable, whether steady-flow or oscillatory in nature. Nevertheless, the absolute level of cardiac power does not necessarily indicate the state of the myocardium. An elevation of cardiac power may simply mean that a normal myocardium is generating enough power to move a normal output through an outflow obstruction.

Interaction Between Heart and Circulation

Dynamic equilibrium in the circulation

The fact that blood moves in a circle, traveling through the vascular tree and returning to the heart, has many hemodynamic implications. The principal one is that pressures and flows in all parts of the system are interdependent and exist in a kind of dynamic equilibrium. The simplest statement of this interaction is one developed by Guyton and his associates[4] based on an elementary model in which there are certain inevitable relationships among cardiac, arterial, and venous properties. More complex models of the cardiovascular system have been devised by many investigators, almost always as a way of making clear the relationship of one phenomenon to another. Such efforts are necessary because biological systems characteristically involve a large number of variables, and their interaction is most readily expressed in mathematical equations. The more elaborate models are applied principally in solving specific research problems.

Guyton's model makes cardiac output a function of filling pressure only, eliminates all reflex responses, and considers mean, not pulsatile, pressure and flow. The starting point for the analysis is the pressure that exists in all parts of the circulation when the heart is *not* functioning, a pressure that depends on the total blood volume and the overall compliance of the system. This mean circulatory filling pressure (MCFP), which can be determined in experimental animals by transient arrest of the heart (e.g., by ventricular fibrillation), is ordinarily 7 to 10 mm Hg. When the heart is beating normally, pressure is greater than this value in arteries and less in veins, while pressures equal to the MCFP exist in the neighborhood of the distal capillaries or venules.

The amount of blood flowing through the venous system and into the atrium, the *venous return,* is a function of right atrial pressure, MCFP, and venous resistance. Atrial pressure also determines cardiac output in this model, and output must equal venous return by definition. Two relationships are thus established, and they can be plotted against atrial pressure as a *Starling curve* and a *venous return curve* (Figure 4.7). The intersection of the lines indicates the only cardiac output value that will satisfy the given set of conditions. The conditions include the MCFP, which is a determinant of the venous return curve, and a specification of myocardial contractility in the form of a particular Starling curve. Guyton showed the empiric validity of the concept in animal experiments and described the appropriate equations for theoretic treatment.[4] The pulmonary circulation can be analyzed in the same way as the systemic.

This model is a greatly simplified approach to cardiovascular function, but it does promote an understanding of the interdependence of various parts of the system. It is necessary to remember that the heart and blood vessels are subject to the influence of the regulatory mechanisms already discussed, which modify the curves shown in Figure 4.7. When reasoning about cardiovascular responses, it is also essential not to mistake equations for statements of cause and effect. The effects of changes in atrial pressure are emphasized in this particular analysis, but the cause of such changes is an equally important physiological question.

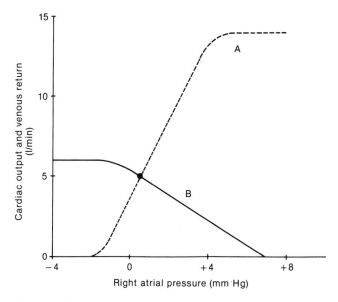

Figure 4.7. Example of theoretic steady-state relation between right atrial pressure (*abscissa*) and blood flow (*ordinate*) in the systemic circulation, assuming constant myocardial contractility and vascular conditions. Starling curve (*A*) defines cardiac function (cardiac output, *dashed line*). Mean circulatory filling pressure and resistance of the venous tree determine curve *B* (venous return, *solid line*). Outflow from left ventricle must equal flow returning to the right atrium, so operating point is intersection of *A* and *B*. (Reproduced with modifications from Guyton et al.,[4] with permission of W.B. Saunders Co.)

Ventricular–arterial coupling

Ventricular performance is strongly influenced by afterload, and changes in arterial resistance or impedance have characteristic effects on the ejection of blood. The typical relation between afterload and the waveforms of pressure and flow is illustrated in Figure 4.8. The records shown in that figure were obtained from an isolated heart[19] in experiments where the aorta was replaced by an adjustable mechanical resistance and capacitance, and those two variables clearly have different effects on the function of the ventricle. When the resistance was raised, ventricular outflow diminished and intraventricular pressure increased. When capacitance was reduced (analogous to stiffening of the aorta), flow decreased and peak pressure rose. The shape of the waves changed with both maneuvers. The environmental conditions that influence myocardial contractility were kept constant throughout the experiments, so that the alterations in pressure and flow represent an inherent response of ventricular muscle to afterload, the mechanism of which has yet to be discovered.

Myocardial and arterial properties thus combine to influence cardiac func-

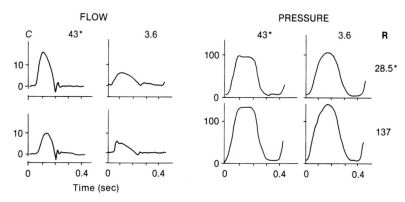

Figure 4.8.   Responses of left ventricle of isolated feline heart to alterations of the resistance and capacitance of a hydraulic model that replaced the aorta and arterial tree. *Left*, ventricular outflow (ml/sec); *right*, intraventricular pressure (mm Hg). *Abscissas*, time in sec. Numbers above the curves indicate capacitance of the model (C, in 10^{-6} cm^4 sec^2/g mass). Numbers on the right represent model resistance (**R**, in 10^3 g/cm^4 sec). *Asterisks* indicate approximate normal values *in vivo*. A capacitance of 43×10^{-6} cm^4 sec^2 /g is equivalent to volume distensibility of about 0.06 cm^3/ mm Hg. (Reproduced with modifications from Elzinga and Westerhof,[19] with permission of the American Heart Association)

tion, and it is natural to wonder whether some combinations may be more efficient than others. This idea is related to the engineering process of *optimization,* in which the interacting parts of a system are matched in a way that produces the best results. Following this line of thought, investigators have sought to define the conditions for optimum coupling of ventricle to arterial tree.[9,15]

The first step is the daunting task of deciding which variables nature has chosen to protect most carefully. Questions immediately arise that cannot be answered unequivocally. Is the cardiovascular system optimum for basal conditions or for physical exertion? Are pulsations of pressure and flow really wasteful accidents of intermittent cardiac contraction, or are they physiologically desirable? In spite of these uncertainties, it seems reasonable to guess that optimal coupling of the heart to the vascular tree should achieve four goals:

1. A cardiac output sufficient to meet the metabolic needs of all organs.
2. Microcirculatory pressures suitable for capillary exchange.
3. Atrial pressures sufficient to operate the Starling (fiber length) mechanism.
4. Minimum expenditure of energy.

In other words, the heart should circulate an adequate supply of blood, the pressure drop along the vascular tree should meet certain requirements, and these tasks should be accomplished as economically as possible.

From this point of view, what can be said about the mammalian cardio-vascular system? Consider mean pressures in the systemic circulation. With a normal cardiac output, the resistance proximal to the capillaries is such that blood enters them at a pressure of about 20 mm Hg, a level entirely suitable for physiological exchange across the capillary membrane (Chapter 10). The total decrement in mean pressure from aortic valve to right atrium is typically 85 mm Hg, leaving about 5 mm Hg for atrial filling. The pressure gradients, then, appear to be optimal. They are determined by the dimensions, architecture, and tone of the blood vessels, and given such a vascular system, the steady-flow power generated by the heart is adequate but no greater than needed. Any decrease in that power, however, would make all pressures lower than desired unless compensatory vasomotor responses intervened. Conversely, any change in vascular resistance would alter blood flow unless steady-flow cardiac work changed appropriately at the same time.

Pulsations of pressure and flow are another matter. If these oscillations serve no physiological purpose (which is no more than an assumption in the present state of knowledge), but are merely an unavoidable result of intermit-tent cardiac contraction, then an optimal system should make them as small as possible. The smaller the oscillatory power component, the better. This re-quirement implies low aortic input impedance or, in other words, a wide and highly distensible aorta.[9] Diastolic pressure would then not fall much below the mean, satisfying a criterion not stated above, namely, high diastolic pressure to perfuse the coronary arteries (Chapter 12).

One further consideration is the frequency dependence of aortic and pul-monic impedance,[15,29] which is caused by reflection of waves from peripheral sites (Chapter 6). The greater the magnitude of such reflections, the higher the impedance at the low frequencies where most of the pulsatile energy is concen-trated, which suggests that reflection should be minimized. Peripheral vaso-constriction increases reflection, and vasodilatation decreases it. The ideal pe-ripheral resistance must, therefore, be a compromise between that needed to produce normal pressure gradients and the conditions that cause least reflec-tion. Whether evolution can do even better along these lines remains to be seen.

Cardiac Failure

The heart is able to cope with abnormal conditions in the vascular system, and even in its own structure, to a remarkable degree. Resting blood pressure and cardiac output may be kept at normal levels in spite of marked pathological disturbances. There are limits, however; when the abnormality is too severe, the heart may no longer be able to meet the body's needs, a condition known as *heart failure*.[3] This name is applied to the clinical state that ensues, *conges-*

tive heart failure, and also to the pathophysiological events that accompany the disorder.

One early physiological sign of myocardial failure is an increase of end-diastolic pressure in the affected ventricle. The ventricular function curve (Figure 4.3) is depressed, and increased filling pressure may or may not succeed in producing a normal stroke volume. Eventually the ventricle dilates, the residual volume increases, and the ejection fraction becomes smaller. Under some conditions the myocardium hypertrophies, thickening the ventricular wall and increasing the muscle mass. Venous pressure tends to rise upstream, and it may reach levels that affect function adversely in various organs. With left ventricular failure, an elevation of pulmonary venous and capillary pressures leads to fluid accumulation in the alveoli of the lung, interfering with gas exchange. Right ventricular failure leads to high systemic venous pressure and edema of peripheral tissues.

The cellular basis of myocardial failure is unknown. The disorder is brought on by burdens imposed on the heart, but what exactly is it that fails? Some derangement of cellular function is probably involved; otherwise, it would be difficult to understand the gradual development of failure in the face of an essentially constant mechanical overload. The properties of the contractile proteins, the supply and utilization of energy, and the coupling between excitation and contraction have been investigated from this point of view, but the results are equivocal.

Exhaustion of the various compensatory mechanisms has been offered as a possible explanation. Sympathetic stimulation is increased in heart failure, and local catecholamine stores may be depleted after a time. Some investigators have found an initial increase in the number of myocardial beta-adrenoceptors, followed by a decrease in the end stages of failure. An alternative possibility is that some kinds of compensation are actually harmful in extreme form. Increased end-diastolic volume, for example, brings the beneficial action of Starling's law into play, but overdistention has deleterious effects on the muscle.

The disturbances in heart failure are not limited to the heart, although cardiac malfunction is the initial cause of the problems in other organ systems. Total extracellular fluid rises and total plasma volume increases at the same time, which tend to exacerbate the consequences of an already distended vascular system. The source of this fluid imbalance is the kidney's failure to manage salt and water excretion in the normal way; the causes of this renal disturbance are only partly known.

The salt and water retention of heart failure is associated in some way with overactivity of the renin-angotensin system (Chapter 8). Cells in the juxtaglomerular portion of the afferent renal arterioles increase their production of renin in the early stages of heart failure, leading to an increase in circulating angiotensin-II and aldosterone. The stimulus that acts on these cells is obscure, but many investigators believe it to be a decrease in renal blood pressure or flow. If so, either a redistribution of flow within the kidney or localized changes in pressure must be involved, because the first signs of cardiac failure are sometimes seen when cardiac output and arterial pressure are still normal. Pomeranz and his colleagues[30] have shown that low-intensity stimulation of renal nerves reduces flow in the cortical region and increases it in the renal medulla, demonstrating that neurally mediated redistribution can occur. The blood level of atrial natriuretic peptide is elevated in congestive heart failure, as would be expected with increased blood volume, suggesting that this element of the sodium and water regulating system, at least, is working properly (Chapter 7).

The relevant action of aldosterone in this context is the promotion of sodium resorption in the distal renal tubules. Angiotensin-II doubtless contributes to the peripheral vasoconstriction, which would tend to maintain normal pressure in the face of diminished cardiac output, but vasodilating prostaglandins may appear at the same time. Evidently, the hormonal disturbances that accompany cardiac failure induce a mixture of compensatory and deleterious effects, a complex web of responses that has yet to be untangled. Fortunately, the clinical disorder can often be relieved for long periods of time by therapy that includes cardiac glycosides and diuretics.

References

Reviews

1. Blinks, J.R., Jewell, B.R. (1972). The meaning and measurement of contractility. In: *Cardiovascular Fluid Dynamics, Vol. 1,* D.H. Bergel, ed. London, Academic Press, pp. 225–260.

2. Braunwald, E., Ross, J., Jr. (1979). Control of cardiac performance. In: *Handbook of Physiology, Section 2: The Cardiovascular System. Vol. I, The Heart,* R.M. Berne, N. Sperelakis, and S.R. Geiger, eds. Bethesda, Md., American Physiological Society, pp. 533–580.

3. Braunwald, E., Ross, J., Jr., Sonnenblick, E.H. (1967). *Mechanisms of Contraction of the Normal and Failing Heart.* Boston, Little, Brown.

4. Guyton, A.C., Jones, C.E., Coleman, T.G. (1973). *Circulatory Physiology: Cardiac Output and Its Regulation,* 2nd ed. Philadelphia, W.B. Saunders.

5. Lakatta, E.G. (1986). Length modulation of muscle performance: Frank-

Starling law of the heart. In: *The Heart and Cardiovascular System. Scientific Foundations,* H.A. Fozzard et al., eds. New York, Raven Press, pp. 819–843.

6. Mason, D.T., Spann, J.F., Jr., Zelis, R., Amsterdam, E.A. (1970). Alterations of hemodynamics and myocardial mechanics in patients with congestive heart failure: Pathophysiologic mechanisms and assessment of cardiac function and ventricular contractility. *Prog. Cardiovasc. Dis.* 12:507–557.

7. Milnor, W.R. (1989). *Hemodynamics,* 2nd ed. Baltimore, Williams & Wilkins.

8. Mirsky, I., Ghista, D.N., Sandler, H., eds. (1974). *Cardiac Mechanics: Physiological, Clinical, and Mathematical Considerations.* New York, Wiley.

9. O'Rourke, M.F., Yaginuma, T., Avolio, A.P. (1984). Physiological and pathophysiological implications of ventricular/vascular coupling. *Ann. Biomed. Eng.* 12:119–134.

10. Sagawa, K., Maughan, L., Suga, H., Sunagawa, K. (1988). *Cardiac Contraction and the Pressure–Volume Relationship.* New York, Oxford University Press.

11. Sarnoff, S.J. (1955). Symposium on regulation of performance of heart; myocardial contractility as described by ventricular function curves; observations on Starling's law of heart. *Physiol. Rev.* 35:107–122.

12. Sonnenblick, E.H. (1966). The mechanics of myocardial contraction. In: *The Myocardial Cell: Structure, Function, and Modification by Cardiac Drugs,* S.A. Briller and H. L. Conn, Jr., eds. Philadelphia, University of Pennsylvania Press, pp. 173–250.

13. Starling, E.H. (1918). *Linacre Lecture on the Law of the Heart.* New York, Longmans, Green.

14. Streeter, D.D., Jr. (1979). Gross morphology and fiber geometry of the heart. In: *Handbook of Physiology, Section 2: The Cardiovascular System. Vol. I, The Heart.* Bethesda, Md., American Physiological Society, pp. 61–112.

15. Yin, F.C.P. (ed.) (1987). *Ventricular/Vascular Coupling. Clinical, Physiological, and Engineering Aspects.* New York, Springer-Verlag.

Research Papers

16. Alpert, N.R., Mulieri, L.A. (1982). Increased myothermal economy of isometric force generation in compensated cardiac hypertrophy induced by pulmonary artery constriction in the rabbit. A characterization of heat liberation in normal and hypertrophied right ventricular papillary muscles. *Circ. Res.* 50:491–500.

17. Bove, A.A., Lynch, P.R. (1970). Radiographic determination of force–velocity–length relationships in the intact dog heart. *J. Appl. Physiol.* 29:844–888.

18. Brutsaert, D.L., Claes, V.A., Sonnenblick, E. (1971). Effects of abrupt load alterations on force–velocity–length and time relations during isotonic contractions of heart muscle: Load clamping. *J. Physiol.* 216:319–330.

19. Elzinga, G., Westerhof, N. (1973). Pressures and flow generated by the left ventricle against different impedances. *Circ. Res.* 32:178–186.

20. Fry, D., Griggs, D., Greenfield, J. (1964). Myocardial mechanics: Tension-velocity–length relationships of heart muscle. *Circ. Res.* 14:73–85.

21. Janicki, J.S., Weber, K.T. (1980). The pericardium and ventricular interaction, distensibility and function. *Am. J. Physiol.* 238:H494–H503.

22. Jewell, B.R., Hanck, D.A. (1987). Effects of inotropic interventions on end systolic length–force curve of cat ventricular muscle. *Cardiovasc. Res.* 21:559–564.

23. Maughan, W.L., Sunagawa, K., Burkhoff, D., Sagawa, K. (1984). Effect of arterial impedance changes on the end-systolic pressure–volume relation. *Circ. Res.* 54:595–602.

24. Milnor, W.R. (1975). Arterial impedance as ventricular afterload. *Circ. Res.* 36:565–570.

25. Milnor, W.R., Bergel, D.H., Bargainer, J.D. (1966). Hydraulic power associated with pulmonary blood flow and its relation to heart rate. *Circ. Res.* 19:467–480.

26. Noble, M.I.M., Bowen, T.E., Hefner, L.L. (1969). Force–velocity relationship of cat cardiac muscle, studied by isotonic and quick-release techniques. *Circ. Res.* 24:821–833.

27. Noble, M.I.M., Trenchard, D., Guz, A. (1966). Left ventricular ejection in conscious dogs: Measurement and significance of the maximum acceleration of blood from the left ventricle. *Circ. Res.* 19:139–147.

28. Parmley, W.W., Chuck, L., Sonnenblick, E.H. (1972). Relation of V_{max} to different models of cardiac muscle. *Circ. Res.* 30:34–43.

29. Piene, H., Sund, T. (1981). Does normal pulmonary impedance constitute the optimum load for the right ventricle? *Am. J. Physiol.* 242:H154–H160.

30. Pomeranz, B.H., Birtch, A.G., Barger, A.C. (1968). Neural control of intrarenal blood flow. *Am. J. Physiol.* 215:1067–1081.

31. Sarnoff, S.J., Braunwald, E., Welch, G.H., Jr., Case, R.B., Stainsby, W.N., Macruz, R. (1958). Hemodynamic determinants of oxygen consumption of the heart with special reference to the tension–time index. *Am. J. Physiol.* 192:148–156.

32. Suga, H. (1971). Left ventricular time-varying pressure/volume ratio in systole as an index of myocardial inotropism. *Jpn. Heart J.* 12:153–160.

5

ELECTRICAL ACTIVITY OF THE HEART

The orderly spread of excitation through the heart generates an electrical field in the body, thus creating differences of electrical potential between points on the body surface. These voltages can be measured with a sensitive meter called an *electrocardiograph,* and the electrocardiograms produced by such instruments display waves that reflect the sequence of excitation as it moves through the atria and ventricles. Because the electrocardiogram is an accurate and non-invasive method of following this sequence, it is widely used in clinical diagnosis and research. Deviations from the normal cardiac rhythm and paths of conduction can be detected readily, and various pathological states can be recognized.

Interpretation of the electrocardiogram requires a clear understanding of the anatomy of the heart, the formation and conduction of electrical impulses within it, and the changes in permeability of the cell membranes that lie behind those phenomena. The relation between the electrical activity in myocardial cells and the electrical field that is generated throughout the whole body is another essential part of the information needed, making it necessary to consider the physical principles that govern the flow of electrical currents in a volume conductor.

The Cardiac Electrical Field

Transmembrane potentials are, by definition, differences in voltage between the inside and outside of a cell, but the voltage measured by an electrocardiograph is quite another matter. The electrocardiogram records differences of

140

potential in an electrical field at a distance from the heart, and that electrical field exists because excitation spreads sequentially from one part of the heart to another. At every instant, from the beginning of an action potential in the first myocardial cell to be excited until the complete repolarization of the last one, it is possible to identify a line of demarcation that separates cells that have just been activated from those still in a resting state. This advancing *wave front* is the source of the electrical field, because the surface of cells just depolarized is electrically negative with respect to the exterior of those not yet activated.

The potential difference arises from local currents (Chapter 3), and the wave front can be likened to a row of electric batteries, lined up with their positive poles pointing in the direction of spread and their negative poles toward the tissue just activated. The field generated by such dipoles extends in all directions, causing currents to flow in a pattern like that of iron filings in a magnetic field, and the voltage gradients produced by a dipole in a three-dimensional conductive medium, or *volume conductor,* conform to known equations. Consequently, if the location, orientation, and magnitude of the dipole are known, it is theoretically possible to predict the potential difference between any two points in the field. Conversely, given a measurement of the potentials at several such points, the properties of the dipole can be deduced; this method of reasoning is the basis for interpreting electrocardiograms. The electrical field of the heart is complex because the excitation front is equivalent to a great number of dipoles, which vary in their orientation.[11] Moreover, the dipoles are not exactly perpendicular to the advancing front, but tend to align themselves along each cell's longitudinal axis.[18] Nevertheless, the general principles that apply in this situation are the same as those that govern the potentials generated by a single dipole.

The relation between dipoles and the electrocardiogram is illustrated in Figure 5.1, which represents a strip of atrial tissue isolated in a bath of physiological saline. A voltmeter is connected to electrodes a and b at the edges of the bath to record the difference in voltage that develops between them. In this example, the two electrodes are positioned so that a line between them is parallel to the longitudinal axis of the muscle strip, for reasons that will become apparent. The voltmeter is connected in such a way that the recording pen moves upward when b is electrically positive with respect to a. A suprathreshold stimulus is now applied to the left-hand end of the strip, depolarizing the cells in that region (1), and excitation proceeds to spread from left to right (2). A relatively narrow, homogeneous strip has been chosen to ensure that the excitation will advance as a more or less even front.

The strip contains many cells, of course, and each one eventually exhibits an action potential, but the key fact for our present purpose is that the advancing wave front resembles at every instant an array of dipoles, each oriented with its *positive* pole pointing to the right. The resulting electrical field makes

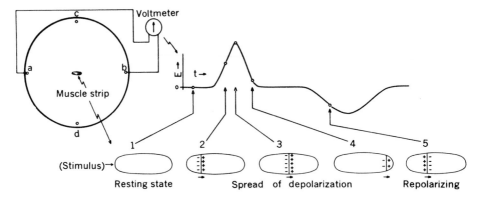

Figure 5.1.   Excitation and recovery of a small strip of myocardial tissue in a volume conductor (saline bath), and the resulting electrical potential between two electrodes, *a* and *b*, at a distance from the strip. *1*, strip in resting state. Left end of strip is stimulated, so that a front of excitation moves from left to right (*2–4*). The advancing front of excitation is electrically equivalent to a row of batteries, or dipoles, with their positive poles oriented toward the direction of advance. Subsequent repolarization, assumed in this example to proceed in the same left-to-right sequence, is equivalent to a row of reversed dipoles (*5*). For relation to voltmeter readings, see text. (Reproduced from Milnor,[9] with permission of C.V. Mosby Co.)

electrode b positive with respect to a, giving an upward deflection in the record. When the front is halfway across the strip in this example, a maximum number of cells is involved and the recorded voltage reaches its highest value (3). As the width of the strip diminishes beyond that point, fewer cells are involved and the voltage magnitude decreases (4), reaching zero when the last cells at the right end undergo depolarization.

We now assume that the first cells to be depolarized are also the first to repolarize, giving a wave of repolarization that spreads from left to right; this time the wave front is like an array of dipoles with their *negative* poles pointing to the right (5). The sequence of repolarization thus causes a downward (*negative*) wave in the electrocardiogram, more spread out in time than the first wave because the action potentials are not all exactly the same in length and cells complete their repolarization at different times. (To anticipate for those familiar with clinical electrocardiograms, the fact that ventricular depolarization and repolarization waves are not usually opposite in direction in humans indicates that the two processes do not follow the same sequence in our species.)

A simple equation that describes the electrical field in this illustration is

$$E = kV \cos \alpha \qquad (5.1)$$

where E is the voltage measured between two electrodes equidistant from the dipole, k is a proportionality constant that depends on the conductivity of the medium and the distance between dipole and electrodes, V is the magnitude of the dipole voltage, and α is the angle subtended by two lines, one passing through the electrodes and the other through the positive and negative poles of the source. If electrodes a and b were reversed, the record would be an inverted image of the one shown in Figure 5.1. If the voltmeter were connected to electrodes c and d, angle α would be 90° and no voltage would be recorded. No potential is detected by a lead that is oriented at right angles to the dipole, although other leads record a positive or negative deflection.

In spite of its simplicity, this example illustrates all the basic principles of electrocardiography. The human body is certainly not a symmetric, homogeneous conductor, yet that model is approximately valid. The torso as a whole is a volume conductor, while the arms and legs act like simple linear conductors attached to the torso for the electrocardiographer's convenience. The advancing excitation front in the mammalian heart is not straight but irregular, sometimes moving in opposite directions in different parts of the heart (e.g., the free walls of the right and left ventricles), yet the net effect of this diverse orientation is like that of a single equivalent dipole centered in the heart. The body surface is sufficiently far away from the myriad dipoles for their effects to be averaged by a kind of vectorial addition. This is not to say that signs of multiple dipole activity are totally absent, for they can be detected by careful measurements over the precordium and have been the subject of much research,[11] but only that the single equivalent dipole hypothesis suffices for most purposes as a description of the voltage source.

As far as the electrocardiogram is concerned, then, the heart behaves approximately as if it were a single dipole that changed its orientation and the magnitude of its voltage throughout the cardiac cycle. To the extent that the normal sequence of activation and the relative masses of muscle involved at each moment are known, it is possible in principle to predict the gyrations of this dipole, and thus the electrocardiographic waves to be expected from any pair of electrode positions of the body surface. Conversely—and this is the source of practical applications—the sequence of activation in a particular subject can be deduced from his or her electrocardiogram.

Electrocardiography

The potential differences in the electrical field of the heart are in the millivolt range, and only with the advent of instruments that could measure such small voltages did electrocardiography become possible. The first accurate recordings of electrocardiographic waves were made by Einthoven[20] in 1903, although primitive measurements had been made in the late nineteenth century with slowly responding devices that distorted the signals.[1] Einthoven used a string galvanometer, in which the electrocardiographic electrodes were connected to a gold-plated thread suspended between the poles of a large electromagnet, and the optical shadows of the thread's movements were recorded photographically. This instrument was a massive structure the size of a grand piano, but it had a high-frequency response and produced records better than some of those published today. Advances in electronics have progressively reduced the size of electrocardiographs, and some modern devices can be carried in a pocket. Electrocardiographic signals can also be transmitted to remote receiving stations over telephone lines or by telemetry. Computers are now widely used to measure the amplitude and duration of electrocardiographic waves, compare the results with stored information about specific clinical abnormalities, and print out the probable significance of the electrocardiogram that has been analyzed.[10]

Einthoven introduced the standard *limb leads* that are still in use, an electrocardiographic lead being any pair of anatomical sites for placement of the electrodes. He also postulated that electrodes on the right arm, left arm, and one leg could be considered the points of an equilateral triangle in a volume conductor, the torso. The electrical activity of the heart at any instant was assumed to produce an equivalent dipole at the center of this triangle, which could be plotted as a vector, and the voltage recorded by any lead at that instant could then be calculated by projecting the vector onto the lead (Figure 5.2). *Projection* in this context means extending lines perpendicular to the lead from the origin and tip of the dipole to the line representing the lead, a geometric method of solving equation 5.1. Although this concept, referred to as the *Einthoven hypothesis,* is only an approximation of the conditions *in vivo,* it remains the basic principle for interpretation of the electrocardiogram.

The standard limb leads are designated by the Roman numerals I, II, and III, as indicated in Table 5.1. One electrode of each lead is called *positive* and the other *negative,* but these terms merely indicate the connections to the recording device. In lead I, for example, the identification of the left arm electrode as positive means that an upward, or positive, wave will be recorded in that lead whenever the left arm is electrically positive with respect to the right arm. Because of the relationships among the three leads, the deflection in lead II at any instant equals the sum of those in leads I and III, a rule that can serve as a check on proper connection of the electrocardiographic cables. One wire from each electrode to the electrocardiograph is sufficient to record the three limb leads, but a fourth wire is usually attached to an electrode on the remaining leg to act as a ground. As with other electrical instruments used on human subjects, considerations of safety enter into the design of electrocardiographs,[14] and standards in the United States are prescribed by federal law.

Figure 5.2A shows the Einthoven triangle and limb leads, and a vector representing the equivalent cardiac dipole at one instant in the middle of ven-

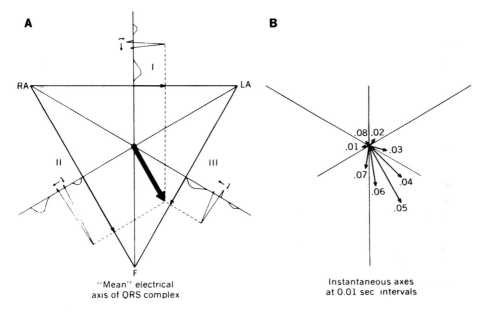

A   "Mean" electrical
axis of QRS complex

B   Instantaneous axes
at 0.01 sec intervals

Figure 5.2. Electrical axes of QRS complex, derived from standard limb leads. **A**, axis at one instant near QRS peak, plotted in Einthoven triangle. **B**, instantaneous electrical axes at intervals of 0.01 sec throughout the QRS complex, showing changing orientation and magnitude. For details, see text. (Reproduced from Milnor,[9] with permission of C.V. Mosby Co.)

tricular depolarization. The point chosen corresponds to the peak of the greatest deflection in this example, but the peaks are not simultaneous in all leads in every subject. Note that the electrocardiogram tracings are plotted in directions that match the positive-negative designations of each lead; leads II and III are "upside down," so to speak, in the figure because a positive deflection in those leads represents relative positivity of the leg at the lower end of the triangle.

A plot like that in Figure 5.2A could be made for any instant in the cardiac

Table 5.1.   Electrode Positions for Electrocardiographic Leads

LEAD	POSITIVE	NEGATIVE
Standard limb leads		
I	Left arm	Right arm
II	Leg	Right arm
III	Leg	Left arm
Unipolar leads		
V_1, V_2, etc.	Exploring electrode	Central terminal[a]

[a]Right arm, left arm, and leg connected through resistors.

cycle, and a series of cardiac dipole vectors during ventricular depolarization is shown in Figure 5.2B. At 0.01 sec after the beginning of depolarization, for example, a front of excitation is spreading through the interventricular septum from left to right. The equivalent vector at that moment points to the right, and it is small because relatively few cells are involved. The lead I deflection at this time would be small and negative (downward). At 0.05 sec, a wide front is spreading through the free walls of the left and right ventricles, but the dominant muscle mass of the left side pushes the net vector toward the left as well as footward. (The caudad direction arises because much of the posterior wall of the left ventricle lies on the diaphragm, emphasizing that the anatomy of the heart *in situ* must be kept in mind.) The sequence of vectors in another normal individual would differ to some extent in direction and amplitude.

As we have already suggested, the practical application of electrocardiography consists of inspecting the recorded leads to learn what is happening in the heart, rather than the inverse process described here for didactic purposes. Vectors representing atrial depolarization or ventricular repolarization are not shown in the figure but could be plotted in a similar way, or the whole cardiac cycle could be displayed on an oscilloscope as a vectorcardiogram (see below).

Waves of the electrocardiogram

From the discussion thus far, it should be evident that the direction, magnitude, and shape of the waves in any one lead may not be the same as in other leads. They differ because each lead "looks at" the heart from a different point of view. Nevertheless, the normal sequence of deflections is similar in all leads, and a standard terminology is applied to them. A typical sequence in one normal human heartbeat is shown in Figure 5.3. This diagram is merely an example, and a wave shown as upright in this figure might appear as a downward deflection in other leads. Atrial depolarization is the first event, and the spread of excitation over the atria is reflected in the electrocardiogram as a small, slow deflection called the *P wave*. Ventricular depolarization is signaled by a larger, multiphasic wave called the *QRS complex,* which is followed by a slower *T wave* generated by ventricular repolarization. A normal P–QRS–T sequence shows that the usual pacemaker is in control; the effects on the electrocardiogram of abnormal pacemakers or conduction are discussed in a later section. In human electrocardiograms, the QRS complex and T wave usually have the same direction (although the T wave is sometimes biphasic), indicating that repolarization does not develop in the same spatial sequence as depolarization. Experimental evidence supports this conclusion by showing that the subendocardial layers of ventricular muscle are the first to be depolarized but the last to recover.

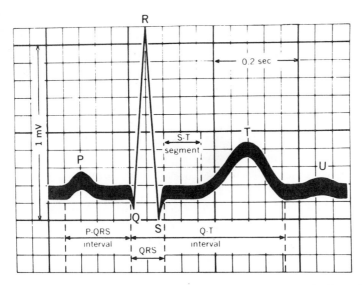

Figure 5.3. Conventional terms for electrocardiographic waves and intervals. (Reproduced from Milnor,[9] with permission of C.V. Mosby Co.)

The P wave ends when the last atrial cell has been activated, but as a rule, nothing corresponding to atrial repolarization appears in the electrocardiogram, presumably because the voltages are small and spread over a considerable period of time, overlapping the QRS complex. After the P wave comes a flat segment, or *isoelectric period,* during which excitation is entering the atrioventricular node and moving through the His bundle, its branches, and the Purkinje system (Chapter 3). This special conducting system, being insulated and relatively small in cross section, produces no deflections in electrocardiograms from the body surface.

The QRS complex begins when the first ventricular muscle cell is depolarized and ends when an action potential rises sharply in the last cell. The various spikes of the QRS complex are given individual names to facilitate description. If the first deflection of the complex is negative (i.e., downward), it is called a *Q wave;* the first positive deflection, whether preceded by a Q wave or not, is called an *R wave;* a negative deflection preceded by a positive one is called an *S wave.* If additional deflections are present, they are designated R′, S′, and so on. This terminology is merely a convention and carries no implication about the part of the ventricles being depolarized when the deflection occurs. Events in the heart that produce an R wave in one lead may produce an S wave in another, for example. Q waves are not usually present in every lead; indeed, the QRS complex may be entirely positive or entirely negative in some leads.

Note that there is no such thing as a positive Q wave or a negative R wave in this terminology.

The components of the QRS complex are rapid, and the performance of the electrocardiograph should be good enough to reproduce them faithfully. A frequency response that is flat ($\pm 5\%$; Chapter 14) to 100 Hz is more than sufficient to record all the components that are known to be of significance. Although low-frequency components include some unvarying isoelectric periods, the response need not extend down to 0 Hz. Actually, there are practical advantages in a finite cutoff at the low end because of the slow baseline wandering caused by drying out of electrode paste and changes in skin resistance. A uniform response down to 0.2 Hz is a satisfactory compromise. The square-wave signal available in most electrocardiographs for calibration provides a simple test of the frequency response.

The duration of the P wave indicates the time required for all atrial cells to undergo the rising phase of depolarization, which is normally about 0.10 sec in man. The interval between the onset of the P wave and the beginning of the QRS complex is usually referred to as the *PR interval*, although it is more properly designated the *P-QRS interval*. Although the PR interval includes atrial depolarization as well as atrioventricular conduction time out to the Purkinje system terminations, it is usually employed to detect delays of conduction in the atrioventricular system because the onset of depolarization within the atrioventricular node cannot be identified without special techniques. The PR interval is inversely related to the heart rate and normally ranges in humans from 0.13 to 0.21 sec. The overall duration of the QRS complex represents the time taken for all ventricular cells to be depolarized and is therefore a clue to conduction disturbances within the muscle. The normal human range is 0.06 to 0.11 sec. The principle that a lead does not detect voltages from an excitation front moving at right angles to it (equation 5.1) can affect the apparent QRS duration in some (never all) leads. If this conduction exists for a given lead at the beginning or end of ventricular depolarization, the QRS complex will be isoelectric for a moment and will appear to be shorter in duration than it is elsewhere.

The process of ventricular repolarization, beginning early in the QRS complex for some cells and later for others, continues until the end of the T wave signals that the whole population has returned to resting potential. The T wave results from asynchronous repolarization in a multitude of cells. It is difficult to account for its shape in any systematic way, although the contours have been found empirically to be a sign of electrolyte abnormalities and other pathological disturbances. A small *U wave* occasionally appears after the T in some leads; its origin is not known.

The ST segment, the relatively flat tracing between the end of the QRS complex and the onset of the T wave, is fortuitous in the sense that it arises as the sum of widely distributed phenomena, including the contributions of many cells at the plateau of their action potential. Clinical observations have shown that certain abnormalities of the ST segment are sensitive indicators of myocardial ischemia.[6] The *QT interval,* defined as the time from beginning of the QRS complex to end of the T wave, indicates the total ventricular depolarization and repolarization time. Like most other electrocardiographic functions of time, this interval varies with heart rate, normally ranging from 0.32 to 0.41 sec. Shortening or lengthening of the QT interval is usually associated with abnormal ion concentrations, drugs, or disease, as might be expected from the activities of the cell membrane that are responsible for action potentials. Normal limits for all these variables, related to age, sex, and heart rate, are given in many textbooks of electrocardiography[6,8] and in a definitive work by Simonson.[12]

Unipolar leads

According to the Einthoven hypothesis, the standard limb leads reflect activity in all parts of the heart, summed vectorially by the distance between the electrodes and the source. At a later point in the history of electrocardiography, new leads—the *unipolar leads*—were devised with the intention of measuring electrical events limited to specific regions of the heart. The reasoning was as follows: What was needed was an "indifferent" electrode that was not affected by the heart at all, which could be paired with an exploring electrode placed over the right ventricle, left ventricle, or any other selected region. To create an indifferent point, the right arm, left arm, and leg were connected (through resistors) to a common junction in the electrocardiograph, named the *central terminal.* This terminal, it was argued, would sum potentials from the three standard limb electrodes, giving a net voltage of zero regardless of the direction of the wave fronts in the heart. The potential difference between the central terminal and an electrode placed over the anterior wall of the right ventricle would then reflect predominantly the electrical activity in that particular region.

Such leads were designated *V leads* (for *voltage*), and six standard positions for the exploring electrode were adopted, beginning with the fourth intercostal space at the right margin of the sternum (V1) and continuing across the precordium to the midaxillary line (V6). An enormous body of empiric knowledge of the waves that appear in such leads under normal and pathological conditions has been acquired, and the unipolar precordial leads are now indispensable in clinical work.[6,8] Combined with the three standard limb leads (Figure 5.4), they provide detailed information about electrical events in the heart.

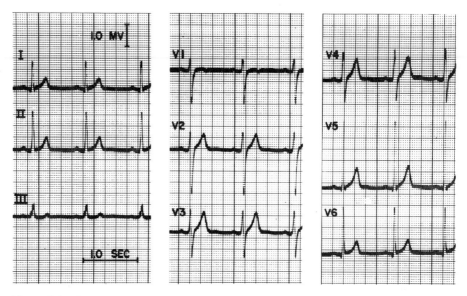

Figure 5.4. Electrocardiogram in normal adult human subject. *Left to right,* standard limb leads, I, II, and III; precordial leads V1, V2, V3; precordial leads V4, V5, V6.

Unipolar limb leads have also been introduced, VR, for example, being a lead between the central terminal and the right arm electrode. Unipolar limb leads provide exactly the same information as the standard limb leads—after all, they employ the same electrode positions—and the choice is a matter of personal preference.

Successful as the unipolar leads have been in practice, investigation has shown that they do not detect local events exclusively. If bipolar electrodes were placed directly on the surface of the heart, the principal deflection observed would, indeed, correspond to the arrival of excitation between them. On the surface of the body, however, an electrode is a considerable distance from cardiac muscle, and it is influenced by excitation in most regions of the heart. A unipolar lead with the exploring electrode over the right ventricle, for example, records waves that originate in the atria and the left ventricle, as well as in the right ventricle, although not with exactly equal sensitivity. Ischemia of the anterior wall of the right ventricle causes a larger abnormality in a unipolar lead from the fourth right interspace than in one from the back, for example, but if the effects were strictly local, no change at all would be detected at the more remote site. Moreover, the deflections in the unipolar precordial leads can be predicted with considerable accuracy from an orthogonal arrangement of electrodes on the shoulders and abdomen,[24] demonstrating that the waves do not represent purely local events.

Such evidence argues that unipolar leads do not record selectively from a small area of muscle near the exploring electrode, but behave like bipolar leads oriented along a special axis in the field. The waves observed in unipolar leads are consistent with a view of the central terminal as a point in the anatomical center of the four-chambered heart, and the orientation of the lead is defined by a line between that point and the exploring electrode, the latter being considered the positive end of the lead. Consequently, the principal value of unipolar precordial leads is that they sample the electrical field in directions not covered by the limb leads. The electrical field of the heart exists in three dimensions, but the Einthoven triangle is two-dimensional. The standard limb leads lie in a frontal plane and are not affected by wave fronts moving in a sagittal direction. This defect could be remedied by adding a lead between one electrode on the chest wall and another on the back, but that solution has not been adopted in routine electrocardiography. The unipolar precordial leads are an alternative solution, providing not local information but a different point of view.

Many other electrocardiographic techniques are used for research or specific clinical purposes. For example, electrodes mounted on a cardiac catheter can be positioned near the atrioventricular junction to detect His bundle activity.[28] In standard electrocardiograms, no waves appear during the interval between the end of the P wave and the beginning of the QRS complex, but intracardiac records show deflections corresponding to arrival of excitation at the beginning of the atrioventricular node and at the His bundle, providing useful information on certain arrhythmias or anomalies of conduction. These same deflections, which are too small to show up in conventional records, can also be recorded from the body surface by a technique known as *signal averaging*. This procedure offers a noninvasive way of observing the details of atrioventricular conduction by adding the voltages in a series of successive cardiac cycles, which causes the truly repetitive events to become larger and larger while random noise tends to be canceled out.

Vectorcardiography

The continuous motion of the tip of the equivalent cardiac vector can be traced out by connecting a horizontal and a vertical lead to the X and Y amplifiers of an oscilloscope (Figure 5.5). The vectorcardiogram recorded by the oscilloscope beam describes one small loop for the P wave, another larger one for the QRS complex, and a third for the T wave. The QRS loop is a continuous representation of the ventricular depolarization that is represented in the vector diagram of Figure 5.2B by discrete samples. The same events can be reconstructed in three dimensions by adding a sagittal lead, giving a complete spatial

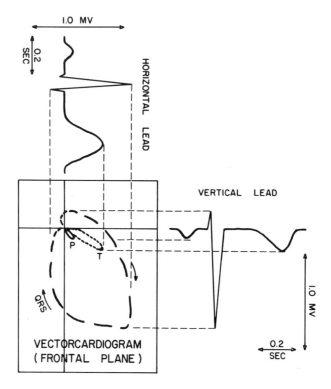

Figure 5.5. Frontal plane vectocardiogram, recorded by connecting a left-to-right lead (lead I) to the horizontal amplifier of an oscilloscope, and a vertical (head-to-foot) lead to the vertical amplifier. Oscilloscope beam traces out loop corresponding to P, QRS, and T waves, representing continuous measurements of instantaneous electrical axes. Series of QRS vectors shown in Figure 5.2B illustrates eight points on a similar loop. Tracing is blanked at regular intervals (0.004 sec) to indicate timing. (Reproduced from Milnor,[9] with permission of C.V. Mosby Co.)

record of the electrocardiographic phenomena in one cardiac cycle, although the time dimension can be shown only by interrupting the beam at specified intervals. Three-dimensional models of the vectorcardiogram show that the contours of the loops and their relations to each other are fairly constant in normal individuals. The wide range of normal limits for any one electrocardiographic lead is the result of slight differences in the orientation of the whole set of loops in space.

Vectorcardiography is occasionally useful in clinical situations, but its greatest value is as a teaching device, making it easier to acquire the habit of imagining the cardiac vectors that must have been present to produce a given electrocardiogram. Because the same information is contained in conventional electrocardiograms—once one has learned to extract it—and because time relationships are depicted more clearly in the electrocardiogram, vectorcardiography will probably continue to supplement standard electrocardiography rather than replace it.

Disturbances of Conduction

The normal pathways by which action potentials are conducted through the heart and the cellular basis of conduction have already been described (Chapters 3 and 4). Conduction in any part of the heart can be slowed or blocked by abnormal conditions, and the electrocardiographic PR interval, QRS duration, and QRS waveform are clues to the sites affected.

Atrioventricular block

Conduction proceeds more slowly in the atrioventricular node and bundle of His, taken as a whole, than anywhere else in the heart. An indication of the time occupied by this process is given by the PR interval, although such a measurement includes conduction through the right atrium as well as the atrioventricular system. The velocity of atrioventricular conduction, like the heart rate, is continuously modulated by autonomic nerves; the PR interval shortens when the heart rate increases and lengthens when it slows. These changes are relatively small, but they must be taken into account, and tables of normal limits[6,12] for the PR interval always specify the heart rate at which they apply. The potential effects of neural control on atrioventricular conduction are evident in the marked prolongation of the PR interval that can be produced by vagal stimulation.

Excitation reaches the atrioventricular node shortly before the end of the P wave, while depolarization is still advancing through the left atrium, and a relatively long time elapses before conduction through the atrioventricular node and His bundle excites the first ventricular muscle cells. Experimental measurements have shown that a large part of this delay occurs at the upper edge of the atrioventricular node, the interface between atrial muscle and the node. The apparent conduction velocity is less than 0.05 m/sec, a slowness consistent with the small diameter of atrioventricular nodal fibers. Activation reaches the His bundle during the middle third of the PR interval. In the bundle of His the velocity rises to about 0.8 m/sec, a rate similar to that in some parts of the atrium. Conduction travels at a rate of 2 to 10 m/sec in the Purkinje system and at 0.2 to 0.4 m/sec in ventricular muscle. The data available on conduction have been obtained largely from canine hearts, but the velocities are probably not radically different in man. The values are not the same in all other species, however.

Disease or the administration of drugs can slow the velocity of conduction from atria to ventricles and can extend the refractory period of the cells involved. The effects range from slowing of atrioventricular conduction to a persistent failure to conduct at all; this whole range of phenomena is called *atrioventricular block*. Slowing of conduction that merely prolongs the PR interval is called *first-degree atrioventricular block*. Failure to transmit some but not all impulses arriving at the junction is referred to as *second-degree atrioventricular block*, and refractoriness to all incoming excitation is called *third-degree* or *complete atrioventricular block*. In complete block, the ventricles are driven by some focus below the obstruction. An intermediate form of block, called the *Wenckebach phenomenon*, consists of a PR interval that gradually increases over successive beats until one P wave is finally blocked completely and hence is not followed by a QRS. Many other variants of atrioventricular block are described in specialized texts.[5,6,8]

Bundle branch block

Complete block of conduction through one of the branches of the His bundle deprives the affected region of its normal sequence of activation. In right bundle branch block, for example, excitation does not reach the right ventricle through its Purkinje system but rather by spread from the left ventricle, which is activated in the normal way. A propagated wave advances from the left ventricular to the right ventricular muscle, confined to the muscle cells because the Purkinje terminations do not usually support retrograde conduction. Intramuscular conduction is relatively slow, and the spread of depolarization through the right ventricle therefore takes longer than usual, prolonging the overall time required for initial depolarization. In left bundle branch block the situation is reversed, and it is the left ventricle that undergoes delayed depolarization.

An increase in QRS duration beyond the upper normal limit of 0.11 sec is consequently one of the signs of bundle branch block, and analysis of the late portion of the QRS complex in various leads reveals which branch is affected. In uncomplicated bundle branch block, each QRS complex is preceded by a P wave and a conventional PR interval, indicating that each ventricular response is caused by normal atrial excitation conducted through the atrioventricular node. The QRS complex is also prolonged in ventricular tachycardia, however, and for a similar reason. The ectopic focus is located in one ventricle, and activation in the contralateral chamber is delayed. Identification of the disturbance as ventricular tachycardia rests on the absence of any electrocardiographic evidence that the ventricles are being driven from a higher center. Atrial tachycardia combined with bundle branch block is sometimes impossible to distinguish from ventricular tachycardia. The functional effects of bundle branch block on cardiac pumping are negligible, although stimulation of one ventricle to produce an analogous situation in experimental animals reveals a small decrease in stroke volume.

Disturbances of Rate and Rhythm

The clinical features of abnormalities of cardiac rate and rhythm are described in appropriate textbooks,[6,7] but the kinds of disturbance that can occur throw some light on normal function and will be discussed briefly here. Variations in heart rate occur physiologically, of course, and such changes must be distinguished from abnormal conditions. *Tachycardia,* defined as a heart rate greater than 100 beats/min, is part of the physiological response to exercise, for example. Abnormal tachycardias, driven by a pacemaker other than the sinoatrial node, are usually characterized by an abrupt onset and the absence of an appropriate physiological stimulus. Heart rates slower than 60 beats/min are called *bradycardia*. Sinus bradycardia at rates between 50 and 60 beats/min is physiological, and is often found in athletes trained for endurance events like long-distance running.

Another instance of an entirely normal response is a waxing and waning of heart rate in phase with respiration. This phenomenon is called *sinus arrhythmia* because the sinus node remains in control, its rate being modulated by pulmonary stretch receptors. Inflation of the lung activates these mechanoreceptors, and their afferents travel in the vagus nerves (Chapter 11). The regular increase and decrease in the interval between heartbeats is readily detected in the electrocardiogram, but the maxima and minima do not coincide exactly with peak inspiration or expiration.

Mechanisms of arrhythmia

Most disturbances of cardiac rhythm arise when a small group of cardiac cells competes with or replaces the normal pacemaker. Any circumscribed region that acts in such a way is called an *ectopic focus,* meaning that it is not located in the usual pacemaking region, the sinoatrial node. Arrhythmias may consist of a few extra beats that interrupt normal events only briefly *(extrasystoles),* or they may impose a rapid, ectopically controlled heart rate for long periods of time. The location of the ectopic site and its mechanisms can often be diagnosed from the electrocardiogram. On rare occasions, the sinoatrial node and an ectopic site may both elicit cardiac responses, a state called *parasystole*. Three different phenomena account for most abnormal cardiac rhythms: automaticity, triggered activity, and reentry.

Automaticity

This term describes the ability of a cell to produce action potentials spontaneously and regularly without extraneous stimuli, a behavior that arises from slow depolarization of the membrane to threshold voltage after each action potential (Chapter 3). Spontaneous depolarization of this kind is characteristic of the sinoatrial node, the normal cardiac pacemaker, but it can also appear in the junction of the His bundle with the atrioventricular node (atrioventricular junction), in the bundle itself, in the bundle branches, or in the Purkinje system. A similar automaticity has been observed in some cells of the coronary sinus and at the base of the atrioventricular valves. Other cardiac cells do not have this ability; their resting membrane potential remains constant until it is displaced by current from an adjacent cell that has been activated in some way. Atrial and ventricular muscle fibers do not normally develolp automaticity, but they can do so under the influence of anoxia, injury, catecholamines, aconitine, or digitalis derivatives.

The inherent firing rate of potentially automatic cardiac cells is not the same in all regions. The sinus node fires at a rate of 60 to 80 impulses/min under basal conditions, although physiological controls can raise the rate to 200 or lower it to 50 beats/min. The His bundle and its atrioventricular junction are capable of generating 40 to 60 impulses/min, whereas the intrinsic rate of the ventricular Purkinje system is only 20 to 45/min. A hierarchy exists, in other words, and the fastest site is the sinoatrial node. The sinoatrial pacemaker consequently suppresses any tendency to automaticity in the lower centers because the normal spread of excitation discharges them more rapidly than they can generate new impulses.

As a result, an ectopic focus can gain control of the heartbeat only if higher cardiac centers of impulse formation fail or if the ectopic site fires at a very fast rate. The first alternative can be observed in the classical student experiment of stimulating the vagus nerve at an intensity that arrests the sinus node for a long period. After a time some ectopic site, usually in the His bundle or Purkinje fibers, escapes and begins to fire at its intrinsic rate. The second alternative, an ectopic focus that generates impulses more rapidly than the higher centers, occurs only when the heart has been subjected to pathological or pharmacological stimuli such as anoxia, injury, high levels of catecholamines, or digitalis.

Triggered activity

This name is given to a condition marked by one or more beats from a focus that does not fire spontaneously, but only when driven by an action potential arriving from some other site.[2] Such a focus is not truly automatic because it does not exhibit resting (phase 4) depolarization in the absence of an external stimulus. When an effective stimulus arrives, however, the action potential it evokes is followed by afterpotentials that first hyperpolarize and then depolarize the cell (Chapter 3). If the afterdepolarization reaches threshold, the result is a triggered action potential that evokes either a single beat or a succession of self-triggered responses. The effects of a triggered focus may thus be a single extrasystole, several rapid beats, or even a prolonged tachycardia. Any tendency of a cell to manifest triggered activity is enhanced by the same pathological and pharmacological conditions mentioned above for automatic ectopic sites. The ionic basis of the afterpotentials is not known but may be an oscillatory intracellular release[27] of Ca^{2+}.

Reentry

This is the term applied to the progress of a self-sustaining excitation along a restricted path that eventually returns to its starting point, whereupon the excitation reenters the path to repeat the circle. This abnormal process arises from an unusual combination of circumstances in which (1) excitation is forced to follow unidirectionally a path that may be irregular and tortuous but is in effect circular and (2) the refractory period and conduction velocity of the tissue involved are such that the returning impulse finds the initial site ready to respond again. The conditions needed for reentry do not normally exist in the heart, but they can be produced experimentally and develop in some pathological states. For example, stimulation of a ventricle at a time when the refractory period has ended in some cells, but not all of them, can produce ventricular fibrillation (see below).

The circus movement involved in reentry implies that the path leads around an inexcitable center. It was first invoked as an explanation of atrial fibrillation (see below), where the muscle around the openings of the vena cava into the right atrium seemed to provide the right conditions. Early investigators showed that excitation could be made to circle continuously around rings cut from a jellyfish; they reported that this response continued without further stimulation for 11 days in one experiment! Similar observations demonstrated that unidirectional block is a prerequisite for circus movements. A single stimulus caused excitation to travel in both directions and die out when the two waves met at the far side of the ring, but the application of several stimuli in succession produced continuous movement in one direction, apparently by creating asymmetric refractoriness.[25]

Recent research makes it clear that the center of the circle need not be physically blocked by an anatomical structure or absence of tissue. A reentrant pathway can be established experimentally in a sheet of atrial muscle. Careful mapping of potentials shows that excitation then spreads toward the center, as well as along the circular path. Excitation does not cross the center and thus interfere with the circus movement, however, because of mutual blocking of the centripetal advance. An inexcitable *vortex* thus creates one of the conditions for continued reentry, and this phenomenon can be produced in a space no greater than 6 mm in diameter.[15] A small reentrant circle of this kind can serve as an ectopic site, and precise electrophysiological measurements would be needed to distinguish it from an automatic focus. Reentry also requires that path length and conduction velocity be matched so that the "head" of the excitation process completes one circuit in exactly the right time, never quite reaching its refractory "tail." Local blocks must also protect the circuit from external activation. Therapeutic drugs rarely satisfy all the theoretic requirements for eliminating reentrant circuits, but agents that prolong refractory periods are often effective.

Although the processes described above can be demonstrated experimentally, modern research has made us less certain about the physiological mechanisms involved in specific arrhythmias than was the case some years ago. Experiments on cardiac tissues and isolated cells, together with computer simulations, have shown that extrasystoles and tachycardias need not always arise from the automaticity of a single ectopic focus, as was thought at first, and that fibrillation is not necessarily caused by a reentrant circus movement. The information now available has made it possible not only to recognize alternative explanations but also to develop rational therapy for each kind of disturbance.

Specific arrhythmias

An understanding of the normal process of cardiac excitation and of the events that can interfere with it makes it easy to recognize the simple arrhythmias. More than one disturbance may be present, however, and combined abnormalities of conduction and impulse formation can become extremely complicated. Not without reason did Louis Katz, in his classical text on electrocardiography,[5] label many illustrations "complex arrhythmia, not suitable for beginners." Most students of physiology need do no more than be aware of such possibilities and of monographs in which they are described.[5-7] The descriptions given below apply to situations where only one kind of arrhythmia exists.

Extrasystoles

A single action potential from an ectopic focus almost anywhere in the heart can produce an extra heartbeat, or extrasystole. Such beats are premature in the sense that they occur before the next normal beat would be expected. Extrasystoles of atrial origin produce a premature P wave, slightly different in shape from the normal ones, followed after the usual interval for atrioventricular conduction by a ventricular response (QRS-T) no different from that in the regular, normal beats (Figure 5.6A). Excitation from the extrasystole spreads back to the sinoatrial region as well as to the atrioventricular conduction pathway, and it discharges the normal pacemaker cells so that their characteristic slow depolarization to threshold begins all over again. For that reason, the next normal beat occurs only after a *compensatory pause,* a period equal to the duration of the normal cardiac cycle. Atrial extrasystoles are common and probably occur in all normal individuals at one time or another. The hemodynamic consequences are trivial, amounting to no more than a slight fall in pressure during the compensatory pause and a modest increase in the stroke volume of the next beat.

Extrasystoles arising from the atrioventricular node or bundle of His are less common but can also occur in normal hearts. The impulse travels in two directions simultaneously, upward to the atria and downward through the conduction system to the ventricles. The P wave and QRS complex are consequently not separated by the usual time delay; depending on the location of the ectopic focus, the extrasystolic P may precede the QRS complex by a small interval, overlap it, or even follow it. Such retrograde P waves are frequently abnormal in shape, and their polarity in limb lead II indicates that atrial exci-

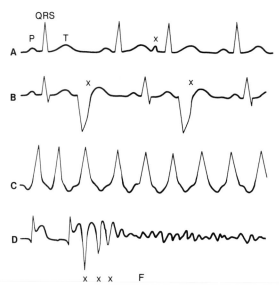

Figure 5.6. Electrocardiographic examples of arrhythmias. **A,** atrial extrasystole (X) after two normal beats, followed by a compensatory pause. **B,** ventricular extrasystoles (X), coupled regularly with normal beats (bigeminy). **C,** ventricular tachycardia; note wide QRS complexes, slightly irregular rhythm. **D,** two regular beats (with abnormal ST segment elevation) followed by three ventricular extrasystoles (X) and then ventricular fibrillation (F).

tation is spreading in a cephalad direction, the opposite of its normal progression. The QRS duration and waveform are normal in extrasystoles that originate above the bifurcation of the His bundle, but they may be anomalous in beats caused by ectopic foci in the bundle branches.

Ventricular extrasystoles, which are produced by an ectopic site in the distal Purkinje system or in injured ventricular muscle, can be identified by the broad, distinctly abnormal QRS complex and the absence of a preceding P wave (Figure 5.6B). The overall duration of ventricular depolarization, and hence of the QRS complex, is prolonged because excitation spreads directly through the muscle, without the benefit of the relatively fast, specialized conducting system. For example, an ectopic site in a terminal Purkinje fiber in the free wall of the left ventricle first excites adjacent muscle cells, whose action potentials activate neighboring cells. The wave of excitation travels through the left ventricular wall to its basal and apical regions, and eventually to the right ventricle. The QRS complex is not only longer than normal in duration but also large in amplitude because excitation advances more or less in one direction, rather than activating both ventricular free walls simultaneously and generating wave fronts that tend to cancel partially in the surface electrocardiogram. In many cases, the location of the ectopic site can be determined by vector analysis of the leads. Ventricular extrasystoles have been observed occasionally in some individuals who have no other cardiac dysfunction.

Ventricular extrasystoles are often systematically coupled to normally driven contractions, which is to say that each normal beat is followed by a beat of ventricular origin (Figure 5.6B). More often than not, the normal contraction and the extrasystole both produce a detectable pulse in peripheral arteries, and continued coupling of this kind produces what is called *bigeminal rhythm*. Less frequently, two extrasystoles may follow each normal excitation, a phenomenon called (with regrettable disregard for the Latin root) *trigeminy*. Regular coupling of normal beats and ventricular extrasystoles is probably an example of triggered activity (see above) in a Purkinje fiber.

Supraventricular tachycardias

Fast heart rates driven by an ectopic focus in the atria, atrioventricular junction, or His bundle are referred to as *supraventricular*. Such tachycardias usually range from 120 to 200 beats/min and are quite regular. The ectopic impulses are transmitted down the conduction system in the normal way, and the shape and duration of the QRS complex are the same as if the normal sinoatrial pacemaker were in control, unless there is in addition some abnormality of conduction through the ventricular muscle. Atrial tachycardias frequently originate from cells at the inferior caval border of the right atrium, the coronary sinus, or the muscle at the roots of the atrioventricular valves. External pressure over the carotid artery, which tends to stimulate the carotid sinus and elicit efferent vagal impulses, often causes an atrial tachycardia to cease abruptly. The maneuver has no effect on tachycardias of ventricular origin and is consequently used as a diagnostic test.

When the atrial rate is much above 150 beats/min, the refractory period of the atrioventricular conducting paths blocks transmission of some of the impulses, usually in a repetitive pattern. Frequently, one impulse arriving at the atrioventricular junction will be transmitted and the next one blocked, giving the electrocardiographic picture of 2 : 1 atrioventricular block. Atrial tachycardias faster than 250 beats/min produce a "sawtooth" pattern in the electrocardiogram, and the disturbance is then labeled *atrial flutter.* In place of distinct individual P waves, the electrocardiogram shows a continuous, regular oscillation, systematically related to normal QRS complexes in accordance with the degree of block. This electrocardiographic pattern suggests that a reentrant circuit may be the basis of atrial flutter, but that conclusion is not universally accepted.

Ventricular tachycardia

Rapid heart rates driven by foci below the bifurcation of the His bundle are classified as ventricular tachycardias. The usual range is 120 to 180 beats/min, much faster than that seen when a ventricular pacemaker takes over because of the failure of higher centers of impulse formation. Unlike atrial tachycardias, the rhythm is usually not perfectly regular. As with ventricular extrasystoles, no regular P wave precedes the QRS complexes, which are wide, large in amplitude, and often blend indistinguishably into the T wave (Figure 5.6C). At the highest rates, no clear interval between one QRS-T complex and the next can be discerned, and the arrhythmia is then called *ventricular flutter.* Ventricular tachycardias can continue for long periods of time, but they occasionally occur in bursts of 10 to 20 beats followed by a return to normal rhythm.

Fibrillation

Under certain conditions, the normal sequence of cardiac excitation disappears and is replaced by a chaotic electrical and mechanical activity referred to as *fibrillation.* The muscle of the affected chamber trembles instead of contracting regularly, and there is no orderly spread of the contraction wave. Small areas of muscle twitch irregularly, with no relation to others. The process is self-perpetuating and usually continues indefinitely unless therapeutic measures are undertaken. It may occur independently in the atria or the ventricles, but it involves both right and left chambers in either case.

The *sine qua non* for the onset of fibrillation is a chamber populated by cells in which various states of refractoriness exist in an irregular pattern.

Given that setting, a single ectopic stimulus is enough to disrupt the orderly sequence of systole and diastole, making it impossible for the normal pacemaker to regain control. Excitation spreads from the ectopic site to whatever adjacent cells it finds responsive, and continues to advance over narrow pathways that become available as the refractory period ends in one cell after another, eventually returning to the site of origin. If the pathway has been sufficiently long and the conduction velocity just right, the initial site is now ready to respond to arriving excitation, and a continuous process has been established. No further ectopic stimulation is required. Fibrillation thus appears to be founded on circus movements and reentry, but current hypotheses envision a complex pattern of serpentine pathways rather than an unbranching circle. Multiple circuitous routes probably operate independently and in no constant pattern. Some investigators maintain that the process is not regenerative but is sustained by repeated firing of ectopic foci.

Atrial fibrillation is a common clinical condition and is well tolerated in most cases. The electrocardiographic sign of atrial fibrillation is a continuous series of small, irregular waves at rates of approximately 500 to 600 impulses/min. These waves reflect uncoordinated atrial electrical activity at rates much higher than the atrioventricular node can transmit, and most of the atrial impulses that impinge on the atrioventricular node find it refractory. Those that are successfully conducted produce irregular ventricular responses at rates ranging from 120 to 180 contractions/min. Careful experimental measurements show that absence of the atrial contraction that usually precedes ventricular systole causes a modest decrease in cardiac output, but this effect is of little practical importance. The response to exercise is limited, however, by inability to control the ventricular rate.

Ventricular fibrillation, unlike the atrial variety, is a life-threatening disturbance. Blood flow ceases immediately, and irreversible brain damage develops in a few minutes. The arrhythmia often begins with several ventricular extrasystoles, after which the electrocardiogram loses all semblance of normality, displaying waves that are roughly sinusoidal for a few minutes before becoming quite irregular (Figure 5.6D). The record is unmistakable, and electrocardiographic monitors are commonly installed in clinical wards where there is a high risk of such events in order to detect them immediately.

The ventricles are most susceptible to fibrillation in one specific part of the cardiac cycle, a 20- to 30-msec period near the peak of the T wave called the *vulnerable* or *supernormal period* (Chapter 3), during which an external stimulus or a spontaneous extrasystole can precipitate ventricular fibrillation. This empiric observation is consistent with the notion that variable refractoriness is the essential prerequisite. Repolarization, unlike depolarization, is not forced into an orderly sequence by a conducting system, and the duration of the action potential is not the same in all myocardial cells. As a result, cell recovery develops in a pattern less regular than that of the activation wave front, and a mixture of responsive and refractory cells exists during the vulnerable period.

Although ventricular fibrillation was once almost uniformly fatal, that prognosis changed with the discovery that an electrical stimulus of the proper kind can interrupt the arrhythmia and that its cessation is often followed by a return to normal rhythm.[7,23] What is required is a current through the heart that is sufficient to stimulate all responsive cells and lasts long enough to affect the remaining cells as they emerge from their refractive periods. Instruments that provide such a stimulus through large electrodes placed on the body surface are now readily available. Nothing reveals the nature of fibrillation as a functional, reversible discoordination more dramatically than the sudden reawakening of a patient successfully treated by this method. Apparatus has recently been devised to defibrillate the heart through electrodes on an intracardiac catheter, monitoring the electrocardiogram to detect fibrillation and applying the stimulus automatically, when needed, in appropriate patients.

Myocardial injury and arrhythmias

The localized ischemia produced in a ventricle by coronary thrombosis or other disease states is often accompanied by arrhythmias. These disturbances take the form of ventricular extrasystoles and tachycardias, which often turn suddenly into ventricular fibrillation. That injured cells might come to act as ectopic pacemakers seems reasonable and the literature abounds in theories of how that happens, but rigorous proof has been elusive. One or more of the mechanisms already discussed is presumably involved, and reentrant circuits seem the most likely choice.

Inhomogeneity with respect to excitability and conduction velocity is characteristic of ischemic areas, setting the stage for reentry. Injured cells suffer a net loss of potassium, and extracellular K^+ rises within an ischemic region, at the same time that lactate accumulates and pH falls. High $[K^+]_o$, especially when combined with hypoxia, slows the upstroke of the action potential, depressing conduction. The concentrations of $[K^+]_o$ vary widely within a damaged region, and a sharp gradient can exist between the border of the lesion and the normal cells outside it. Conduction is slowed inhomogeneously by these changes, and small areas of block appear. Impairment of intercellular coupling in the injured cells offers a further impediment to conduction. Adjacent cells may depolarize to different degrees in such a way that their resting as well as active voltages differ.[19] As a result, local injury currents develop, not unlike those between excited and resting cells in normal conduction. A single stimulus, even the arrival of a normally propagated impulse, can trigger an ectopic focus or start a reentrant process under these conditions. Either one can serve as a source of ventricular extrasystoles, and the setting is conducive to fibrillation.

Drugs and arrhythmias

The mechanisms responsible for arrhythmias suggest the actions required of drugs used to treat them. It is not always possible to identify the mechanism in a given case, but the physiological principles that have been discussed provide a rational approach to therapy. The appropriate goals in combatting specific mechanisms are as follows:

1. To inhibit automaticity, hyperpolarize the cell membranes or slow the phase 4 depolarization in the ectopic focus.
2. To discourage reentry, interrupt the circuit by prolonging the refractory period, slowing conduction, or applying a suitable electrical stimulus.

The factors that inhibit triggered activity are less clear, but they are probably the same as those that discourage automaticity. Catecholamines, compounds related to digitalis, and myocardial injury enhance the probability of afterpotentials that can act as triggers,[3] just as they do for ectopic beats.

Most of the drugs used to treat arrhythmias have multiple actions, but with relatively low, therapeutic concentrations, one effect is usually dominant. Antiarrhythmic agents can be divided into several classes: (1) membrane-stabilizing agents, (2) inhibitors of Ca^{2+} influx, (3) beta-adrenergic antagonists, and (4) parasympathetic stimulators. The effects of digitalis and related compounds merit separate consideration, as does the relatively new technique of suppressing arrhythmias by appropriate electrical stimuli.

Membrane-stabilizing drugs

Quinidine, a typical member of this group, slows the upstroke velocity (phase 0) and prolongs the duration of the action potential. The first of these actions, brought about by inhibition of sodium channel activation and the fast sodium current, is predictably accompanied by slowing of conduction. The second action extends the refractory period, producing a long QT interval in the electrocardiogram, and the combined effects account for the suppression of reentrant arrhythmias by this drug. The clinical observation that atrial fibrillation, presumably a reentrant abnormality, often ceases under the influence of quinidine is well documented. Drugs in this class also slow the rate of firing in ectopic foci and in the sinoatrial node.

Reduction of sodium conductance (g_{Na}) is a central factor in the action of such agents, a conclusion based largely on measurements of the rate of rise of action potentials and the assumption that the maximum dV/dt is an index of sodium conductance. The validity of this approach has been questioned by some investigators, but the results appear to be consistent with more direct measurements now becoming available from isolated myocytes and from sodium channels studied individually by patch clamping.[4] The effects depend in part on the frequency with which the controlling focus is firing. Therapeutic concentrations of quinidine and local anesthetics reduce g_{Na} and the rate of rise of the action potential when ventricular muscle is being stimulated at rapid rates, but not as slow rates. Blockade of sodium conductance is thus frequency dependent, tending to suppress beats occurring in quick succession during an arrhythmia but not those developing at slower, physiological rates. This phenomenon fits with the clinical observation that low doses of these drugs have little effect on the normal heart but suppress ectopic foci when they exist. The basic action on g_{Na} is the same in both cases, but normal heart rates allow sufficient time between beats for complete recovery of the sodium channels, and full expression of the fast sodium influx appears in the next action potential, along with a rapid phase 0 and normal conduction. Other factors also influence the phenomenon. The restoration of maximum phase 0 dV/dt is modulated by the transmembrane voltage and by extracellular K^+, Ca^{2+}, and pH. Slowing of recovery is directly correlated with the physical size of the drug molecule, its lipid solubility, and the channel–drug affinity.

Some drugs classified as membrane-stabilizing agents are local anesthetics. Lidocaine, procaine amide, and other drugs in this subset produce many of the same effects as quinidine and are used in a similar way in the treatment of arrhythmias. Subtle differences between the groups have been pointed out, but they remain controversial. Quinidine, for example, is said to obliterate the voltage dependence but not the time dependence of the action potential upstroke, whereas the reverse is the case with lidocaine. Lidocaine has been reported to shorten rather than lengthen the action potential under some conditions.

The effect of quinidine and related drugs on conduction is not an unmixed blessing, because it carries with it the possibility that conduction may fail at some points in the myocardium but not at others, creating the conditions for reentry. Such a sequence of events is probably the source of the serious arrhythmias, both atrial and ventricular, that can be caused by toxic doses of quinidine.

Calcium-flux inhibitors

The *calcium blockers* are a relatively recent addition to the list of antiarrhythmic agents. These drugs inhibit the passage of calcium ions through selective channels in the cell membrane but do not affect the sodium–calcium exchange mechanism.[22] As would be expected, they have profound effects on muscle contraction through their influence on the availability of calcium within the cells. The antiarrhythmic action is derived from inhibition of the slow inward calcium current that sustains the plateau of the action potential. In the sinoatrial and atrioventricular nodes, where the calcium current contributes significantly to the rise as well as the plateau of potential, calcium blockers presumably also act on that phase of the response.

The receptor for these agents is unknown. It has even been suggested that it may lie on the inner, not the outer, layer of the plasma membrane. Alternatively, the calcium blockers may act within the membrane itself. Verapamil in high concentrations, for example, appears to enter the lipid bilayer and modify its properties, thus altering the activity of the calcium channel proteins.[29] This mechanism can be regarded as nonspecific in the sense that it is shared by many local anesthetics. In addition, calcium blockers interact in an unexplained way with some neurotransmitter receptors. Verapamil competes with muscarinic antagonists for binding sites, but with a low affinity that may be nonspecific.[22] The same is true for alpha-adrenergic receptors, and some suggest that the site in question is the calcium channel itself.[16]

Beta-adrenergic antagonists

The activation of beta-adrenergic cardiac receptors by high levels of norepinephrine or epinephrine predisposes to the formation of automatic or triggered ectopic foci, hence the use of beta-adrenergic antagonists like propranolol in the treatment of ectopic rhythms. The alpha-adrenergic receptors of cardiac tissues apparently have a less prominent role. High concentrations of most beta-blocking agents have membrane-stabilizing effects like those of local anesthetics.

Norepinephrine and epinephrine speed up and increase the amplitude of phase 0 depolarization and hence increase firing rates. The source of the arrhythmias they can produce is not entirely clear, but it is probably related to the shortening of action potentials, a response attributable to an accelerated closure of channels bearing the outward potassium current, and consequently a more rapid repolarization back to the resting level. Given a constant (or increased) rate of slow phase 4 depolarization from that resting level, the result is a faster rate. These transmitters actually cause a slight hyperpolarization at the end of the repolarization period, which would tend to slow the rate, but that effect is small and the overall outcome is a shorter beat-to-beat interval.

In the sinoatrial node, at least, the increase of the inward calcium current caused by catecholamines helps to speed repolarization.

Catecholamines can increase the rate of any ectopic region that is inclined to become a controlling pacemaker, encouraging the development of extrasystoles or ectopic tachycardia. Such events are rare in the normal heart under resting conditions, but they occasionally develop when catecholamine concentrations are elevated by emotional or physical stress. High concentrations can also lead to an inhomogeneous distribution of refractory periods and thus to reentrant tachycardias or fibrillation. The likelihood of serious dysrhythmias is higher in patients who already have myocardial disease.

Parasympathetic stimulation

External pressure over the carotid sinus is a maneuver that has long been employed in treating paroxysmal tachycardias. The effect is like that of stimulating the vagus nerve, and this procedure often succeeds in arresting an ectopic atrial tachycardia, although it has no effect on ventricular tachycardia. Acetylcholine and its more stable analogues tend to suppress automatic foci by hyperpolarization and slowing of phase 4 depolarization. Both actions tend to extend the time required for spontaneous depolarization to reach threshold, and they consequently slow the firing rate. The simultaneous slowing of the normal pacemaker is an undesirable effect, however, because it reduces the ability of the higher pacemaker to take over from the slowing ectopic focus. Because of the concomitant slowing of atrioventricular conduction and a number of unwanted side effects, parasympathetic drugs are now used much less frequently than in the past for the treatment of arrhythmias.

Digitalis and related drugs

The cardiac glycosides (Chapter 3) are best known for their remarkable therapeutic effect in heart failure, but they have some specific uses in the treatment of atrial disturbances of rhythm. In high concentrations, however, they can *cause* serious arrhythmias. The first action of digitalis to be considered is an indirect one: It causes a reflex increase in the frequency of vagal impulses to the heart. This response can be greatly reduced by section of the carotid sinus nerves,[17] suggesting that the drug has a direct action on the arterial baroreceptors. As a result of this rather curious effect on noncardiac tissues, digitalis causes, among other things, slowing of conduction in the atrioventricular node and slowing of the heart rate. Postganglionic parasympathetic fibers carry the reflex signals to the heart, and the effects on the nodal cells are those of acetylcholine: hyperpolarization and slowing of the upstroke of the action potential.[2]

These actions are the basis for the use of digitalis in cases of atrial fibrillation, where the effects of therapeutic doses on atrioventricular conduction reduce the number of impulses that reach the ventricles, slowing the irregular ventricular responses from the untreated level of 120 to 180 beats/min to a more tolerable rate. Slowing of the ventricular rate with atrial flutter or tachycardia can be accomplished in the same way. The fibrillation of the atria in such cases is occasionally suppressed by digitalis and replaced by a normal rhythm.

The propensity of the cardiac glycosides to produce arrhythmias is observed all too frequently. Disturbances of rhythm or conduction of virtually any type can result from toxic concentrations, but the abnormalities often take the form of ventricular extrasystoles, tachycardia, or fibrillation. Bigeminy arising from regularly coupled premature beats of ventricular origin is especially common, an example of triggered activity (see above) in Purkinje fibers. The cellular mechanism responsible for these abnormal conditions is probably the same as the one that provides the desirable inotropic effects of digitalis, namely, an increase in the intracellular availability of Ca^{2+}. At the cellular level, the difference between therapeutic and toxic effects is only one of degree.

Elevation of $[Ca^{2+}]_i$ by cardiac glycosides is well documented,[13,30] and this response is generally accepted as an adequate explanation of the enhancement of contractility. Arrhythmogenic conditions can appear along with the effects on calcium and inotropy, as indicated by small, spontaneous depolarizations and contractions after a stimulated action potential.[27] The mechanism for the increase of $[Ca^{2+}]_i$ has been intensively studied, but some aspects of it remain unclear. Inhibition of the Na^+,K^+-activated ATPase of the myocardial cell membrane (the enzymatic equivalent of the sodium pump) is one element in the response to these glycosides, along with a net loss of intracellular K^+ and a gain of Na^+. Just how this phenomenon leads to an increment in $[Ca^{2+}]_i$ is uncertain, but many investigators now believe that the $Na^+–Ca^{2+}$ exchange mechanism by which intracellular Na^+ is exchanged for extracellular Ca^{2+} is the key[21] (Chapter 3). Other alternatives or contributing factors have been suggested, including the possibility that the glycosides act directly on the release of intracellular stores of Ca^{2+} or on the channel of the slow inward Ca^{2+} current. Some evidence suggests that arrhythmias produced by toxic doses of digitalis and related drugs arise from afterdepolarizations that increase $[Ca^{2+}]_i$ and induce automaticity in Purkinje fibers. These afterpotentials are accompanied by release of prostaglandins and inhibited by indomethacin.[26]

Electrical stimulation

The use of an electrical stimulus to arrest arrhythmias, a technique first applied to ventricular fibrillation (see above), has been extended to supraventricular tachycardias, atrial fibrillation, and ventricular tachycardias.[7] The method is now known as *cardioversion* in recognition of its effectiveness in causing the heart to revert to normal rhythm. The electrical shock, typically amounting to an energy of 25 to 50 J, is delivered through electrodes positioned on the body surface so as to send current through the heart. The object is to create a suprathreshold stimulus for all cells more or less simultaneously. In many cases, the normal pacemaker will regain control when the effects of abnormal foci are interrupted. The same technique has recently been adapted for use with catheter-mounted electrodes. Specialized equipment and careful selection of patients are obviously required. Many instruments specially designed to provide appropriate waveforms and timing are now available for cardioversion.

References

Reviews

1. Burch, G.E., DePasquale, N.P. (1964). *A History of Electrocardiography.* Chicago, Year Book Medical Publishers.

2. Cranefield, P.F. (1975). *The Conduction of the Cardiac Impulse: The Slow Response and the Cardiac Arrhythmias.* Mt. Kisco, N.Y., Futura.

3. Cranefield, P.F. (1977). Action potentials, afterpotentials, and arrhythmias. *Circ. Res.* 41:415–423.

4. Grant, A.O., Starmer, C.F., Strauss, H.C. (1984). Antiarrhythmic drug action blockade of the inward sodium current. *Circ. Res.* 55:427–439.

5. Katz, L.N. (1946). *Electrocardiography,* 2nd ed. Philadelphia, Lea & Febiger.

6. Lipman, B.S., Massie, E., Kleiger, R.E. (1972). *Clinical Scalar Electrocardiography,* 6th ed. Chicago, Year Book Medical Publishers.

7. Mandel, W.J. (1987). *Cardiac Arrhythmias,* 2nd ed. Philadelphia, J.B. Lippincott.

8. Marriott, H.J.L. (1983). *Practical Electrocardiography.* Baltimore, Williams & Wilkins.

9. Milnor, W.R. (1980). The electrocardiogram. In: *Medical Physiology,* V.B. Mountcastle, ed. St. Louis, C.V. Mosby, pp. 1007–1016.

10. Pipberger, H.V., Dunn, R.A., Berson, A.S. (1975). Computer methods in electrocardiography. *Ann. Rev. Biophys. Bioeng.* 4:15–42.

11. Scher, A.M., Spach, M.S. (1979). Cardiac depolarization and repolarization and the electrocardiogram. In: *Handbook of Physiology, Section 2: The Cardiovascular System. Vol. I, The Heart,* R.M. Berne, ed. Bethesda, Md. American Physiological Society, pp. 357–392.

12. Simonson, E. (1961). *Differentiation between Normal and Abnormal in Electrocardiography.* St. Louis, C.V. Mosby.

13. Smith, T.W., Antman, E.A., Friedman, P.L., Blatt, C.M., Marsh, J.D. (1984).

Digitalis glycosides: Mechanisms and manifestations of toxicity. *Prog. Cardiovasc. Dis.* 26:413–441.

14. Webster, J.G. (ed.) (1978). *Medical Instrumentation.* Boston, Houghton, Mifflin.

Research Reports

15. Allessie, M.A., Bonke, F.I.M., Schopman, F.J.G. (1977). Circus movement in rabbit atrial muscle as a mechanism of tachycardia. III. The "leading circle" concept: A new model of circus movement in cardiac tissue without the involvement of an anatomical obstacle. *Circ. Res.* 41:9–18.

16. Atlas, D., Adler, M. (1981). Alpha-adrenergic antagonists as possible calcium channel inhibitors. *Proc. Natl. Acad. Sci. USA* 78:1237–1241.

17. Chai, C.Y., Wang, H.H., Hoffman, B.F., Wang, S.C. (1967). Mechanisms of bradycardia induced by digitalis substances. *Am. J. Physiol.* 212:26–34.

18. Corbin, L.V., II, Scher, A.M. (1977). The canine heart as an electrocardiographic generator: Dependence on cardiac cell orientation. *Circ. Res.* 41:58–67.

19. Downar, E., Janse, M.J., Durrer, D. (1977). The effect of acute coronary artery occlusion on subepicardial transmembrane potentials in the intact porcine heart. *Circulation* 56:217–224.

20. Einthoven, W. (1903). Die galvanometrische Registrierung des menschlichen Elektrokardiogramms, zugleich eine Beurtheilung der Anwendung des Capillar-Elektrometers in der Physiologie. *Arch. Gesamte Physiol.* 99:472.

21. Glitsch, H.G., Reuter, H., Scholz, H. (1970). The effect of the internal sodium concentration on calcium fluxes in isolated guinea pig auricles. *J. Physiol.* 209:25–43.

22. Katz, A.M., Hager, W.D., Messineo, F.C., Pappano, A.J. (1984). Cellular actions and pharmacology of the calcium channel blocking drugs. *Am. J. Med.* 77:2–10.

23. Kouwenhoven, W.B., Milnor, W.R., Knickerbocker, G.G., Chesnut, W.R. (1957). Closed chest defibrillation of the heart. *Surgery* 42:550–561.

24. Milnor, W.R., Talbot, S.A., and Newman, E.V. (1953). A study of the relationship between unipolar leads and spatial vectorcardiograms, using the panoramic vectorcardiograph. *Circulation* 7:545–557.

25. Mines, G.R. (1913). On dynamic equilibrium in the heart. *J. Physiol.* 46:349–382.

26. Moffat, M.P., Ferrier, G.R., Karmazyn, M. (1986). A possible role for endogenous prostaglandins in the electrophysiological effects of acetylstrophanthidin on isolated canine ventricular tissues. *Circ. Res.* 58:486–494.

27. Orchard, C.H., Eisner, D.A., Allen, D.G. (1983). Oscillations of intracellular Ca^{2+} in mammalian cardiac muscle. *Nature* 304:735–738.

28. Scherlag, B.J., Lau, S.H., Helfant, R.H. (1969). Catheter technique for recording His bundle activity in man. *Circulation* 39:13–18.

29. Singh, B.N., Vaughan Williams, E.M. (1972). A fourth class of antidysrhythmic action? Effect of verapamil on ouabain toxicity, on atrial and ventricular intracellular potentials, and on other features of cardiac function. *Cardiovasc. Res.* 6:109–119.

30. Weir, W.G., Hess, P. (1984). Excitation–contraction coupling in cardiac Purkinje fibers. Effect of cardiotonic steroids on the intracellular $[Ca^{2+}]$ transient, membrane potential, and contraction. *J. Gen. Physiol.* 83:395–415.

PRINCIPLES OF HEMODYNAMICS

Physical principles are used extensively in analyzing cardiovascular function because the heart and blood vessels are a mechanical pumping system. Hemodynamics applies these principles to the circulation in order to relate the movement of blood and the strength of cardiac contraction to the physical properties of the structures involved. The tools employed are mainly the classical laws of force and motion described by Newton and Galileo, expressed in forms appropriate to the unusual nature of the pump, the circulating fluid, and the tubular conducting system.

The origins of hemodynamics can be traced to William Harvey's seventeenth-century estimates of the stroke volume of the heart from casts of the ventricular chambers and to the first measurements of arterial pressure in mammals a century later by Stephen Hales (see Chapter 1 for references). An equal place of honor belongs to J.L.B. Poiseuille, a French physiologist and physician, who not only introduced the mercury manometer for measuring blood pressure, but also studied the flow of liquids through tubes with a precision that has scarcely been matched since his classical report[42] in 1846.

Poiseuille measured the flow of water through long, straight glass tubes of small bore and presented his results in the form of an equation that described the relationships among pressure, flow, and the dimensions of the tube.[42] For a given volumetric rate of flow, Q, through a tube of length L and inner diameter D, he discovered that the difference between pressure at the entrance and exit to the tube (P_1 and P_2, respectively) fitted the equation

$$Q = \frac{kD^4(P_1 - P_2)}{L} \tag{6.1}$$

We will refer hereafter to the difference $(P_1 - P_2)$ as the *driving pressure*. This formulation was based entirely on Poiseuille's empiric observations, although theoretic equations for the motion of fluids in tubes had been published a few years earlier. The coefficient k, he found, was independent of the length and diameter of the conduit and did not vary with flow rate under the conditions of his experiments.

In the light of later developments, it is now clear that k depends on the nature of the fluid employed, specifically on a fluid property called *viscosity*, and on the kind of motion that exists within the flowing stream. Both of these variables appear in general theories of fluid dynamics, and they must be defined before considering their application in the present context. With that as a foundation, we can move on to the principles that govern pressure and flow in the cardiovascular system.

To adopt a systematic approach, we will begin by describing steady, non-pulsatile flow in a rigid tube and then advance, step by step, to distensible tubes, pulsating flow, and branching assemblies that resemble the arterial tree. The final complications to be dealt with are the interactions within a closed circular system where fluid returns to its starting point after passing through a peripheral network. Fortunately, although new phenomena must be considered at each step in this progress from a very simple model to a more or less realistic picture of the circulation *in vivo*, the hemodynamic principles involved are simply an enlargement or a slight modification of those in the preceding stages. The microcirculation is a special case, and none of the analyses in this chapter apply to the tiny vessels in that region. Capillary pressure and flow are considered in Chapter 10 and the deformability of red cells, which plays a major hemodynamic role in those vessels, in Chapter 13.

Steady Flow

Fluid dynamics

Fluids have no fixed shape; any part of a homogeneous body of liquid can slide over adjoining parts. One need look no further than a familiar river for an example. The middle of the stream tends to move more rapidly than the water adjacent to it, which in turn slides past the relatively slow-moving water nearer the banks. In other words, fluids can move in layers, or *laminae*, of different velocity. In this example, the differences arise in part from a frictional "drag" imposed by the banks and the river bed, but fluids themselves differ in the ease with which laminar flow can be induced. The energy required to move one lamina over another is greater for some liquids than for others. This property of a fluid is called its *viscosity*, which Isaac Newton aptly described as "a lack of slipperiness" between layers. Viscosity is the property referred to when tar is described as a "thick" fluid or kerosene as "thin," and blood falls somewhere in between.

The physical definition of viscosity is illustrated by the diagram in Figure 6.1, which represents two hypothetical fluid laminae of thickness dx, in contact over an area A, moving at velocities that differ by dv. The stress (S), or force per unit area (F/A), required to produce that differential movement is directly proportional to the velocity gradient between the layers, and the viscosity of the fluid is the proportionality constant, η:

$$S = \frac{F}{A} = \eta \frac{dv}{dx} \qquad (6.2)$$

The standard unit of viscosity is the *poise*, named in recognition of the scientific contributions made by Poiseuille. One poise equals 1 dyn sec/cm². The viscosity of water is 0.010 poise at 20° C; viscosity rises as temperature falls in most fluids. The gradient dv/dx, which has the dimension $(\text{sec})^{-1}$, is called the *shear rate*. Note that stress is not related to absolute velocity but to the relative velocity of different laminae. Water and other liquids that behave in this way are called *Newtonian fluids*; their viscosity is not influenced by absolute velocity. The viscosity of non-Newtonian liquids is said to be *anomalous* because it changes with the forward velocity and shear rates in the stream.[4,8]

Shear rate is among the factors that determine whether fluid laminae move smoothly or irregularly (see below). It is highest near the vessel wall, where it

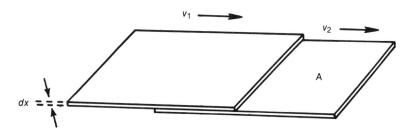

Figure 6.1. The concept of fluid viscosity. Two infinitely thin layers of fluid are shown (dx = thickness), each moving at a different velocity (v_1, v_2). The "friction as one layer slides across the other is expressed as the force required to produce the motion, divided by the area of contact (A). In a Newtonian fluid, this force per unit area, or stress, is proportional to velocity gradient dv/dx, and the proportionality constant is the viscosity of the fluid (see equation 6.2).

averages about 50/sec in the human aorta and 150/sec in the femoral artery. The movement of blood along the wall exerts a shearing force on the endothelium, and high stresses of this kind may play some part in the formation of atherosclerotic vascular lesions. Experiments have shown, for example, that prolonged wall shear stresses above a critical level can alter the flux of proteins and lipids into the wall.[23] Equations for calculating shear rate and stress can be found in other textbooks.[4,8]

Blood is not a perfectly Newtonian fluid; its apparent viscosity varies with cell concentration and rises at very low shear rates (Chapter 13). Within the normal range of hematocrits and blood flows, however, the viscosity of human and canine blood is virtually constant, with a value[7] between 0.030 and 0.040 poise at 37° C. The relevance to hemodynamics is that blood viscosity contributes to the term k in equation 6.1, a fact that became clear when later investigators arrived at a theoretic solution to Poiseuille's problem in which viscosity (η) appeared explicitly[8] and the tube lumen was described in terms of its radius, r:

$$Q = \frac{\pi r^4 (P_1 - P_2)}{8 \eta L} \qquad (6.3)$$

This equation, which was derived from the physical definition of viscosity just given and from certain assumptions about the conditions of flow (see below), indicates that Poiseuille's empiric constant k is equal to $\pi/128\eta$.

The relationship expressed in equation 6.3 is now referred to as *Poiseuille's law,* and its validity has been firmly established for the special conditions of steady laminar flow in cylindrical tubes. *Steady* flow denotes an absence of pulsations, a continuous stream moving at a constant rate. Other equations that describe pulsatile flow are considered later in this chapter, but even under pulsatile conditions, equation 6.3 approximates the relationships for *mean* pressure and flow averaged over an integral number of cardiac cycles.

Laminar flow, in this context, means that the fluid layers all move in a longitudinal direction, with no eddies or other radial deviations. Laminar flow in a straight tube of circular cross section can be regarded as a set of concentric, cylindrical shells. The most rapid motion is in the central axis of the stream, and velocity falls progressively from the axis out to the wall of the tube. The distribution of velocities across the lumen has the form of a parabola (Figure 6.2), a mathematical result of the circular shape and the nature of fluid viscosity. (The quantity $\pi/8$ in equation 6.3 comes from integration of the parabolically distributed velocities to derive a volumetric rate of flow.[8]) The plot of velocities shown in Figure 6.2 is called a *velocity profile,* and motion of this kind is termed *Newtonian* or *parabolic flow.*

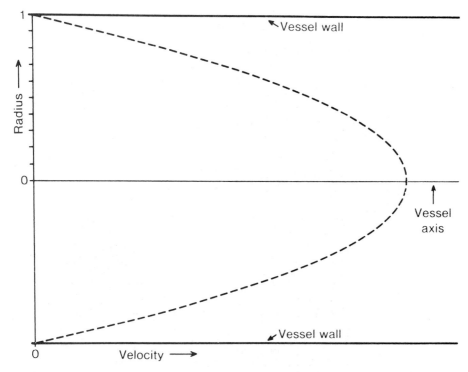

Figure 6.2.   Parabolic velocity profile in steady laminar flow in a tube. *Abscissa*, velocity. *Ordinate*, radial distance from central axis. (Reproduced from Milnor,[8] with permission of Williams & Wilkins)

The velocity profile of a laminar flow is not invariably parabolic. At the entrance of a tube supplied by a large reservoir (and in the ascending aorta just beyond the aortic valve), all lamina move with about the same velocity (Figure 6.3). The layers nearest the wall are immediately slowed by viscous "drag," however, while the central core continues to advance with a flat profile. As the fluid moves further, the blunt central portion becomes smaller and smaller, and eventually a complete parabolic profile develops. The distance required for complete development of parabolic flow is referred to as the *entrance length* and the progressive stages prior to its development as *entrance effects*.[4,8] Blood flow in the mammalian circulation is parabolic in virtually all parts of the vascular tree beyond the aortic arch.

The smooth flow of fluid laminae can be disturbed under certain conditions, producing eddies and vortices; such flow is described as *turbulent*. Sharp bends in the tube or obstructions in the stream can have this effect, but flow can become turbulent even in the absence of such complications. The hemodynamic significance of turbulence is that it dissipates energy; Poiseuille's law no longer applies, and the pressure drop is much greater than equation 6.3

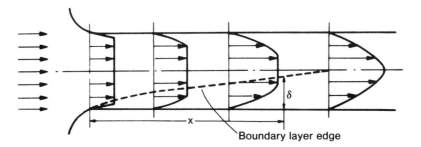

Figure 6.3. Velocity profiles in steady laminar flow at the entrance to a tube, showing width of boundary layer (δ) and change from initially flat profile to fully developed parabolic profile. (Reproduced with modifications from Caro et al.,[4] with permission of Oxford University Press)

would predict. The critical factors have been combined in a dimensionless term called the *Reynolds number* (N_R), which is a function of tube radius (r), fluid density (ρ), viscosity (η) and mean velocity ($\bar{v}$).

The Reynolds number expresses the tendency of flow to become turbulent under specific conditions, and in a cylindrical tube it takes the form

$$N_R = \frac{2r\bar{v}\rho}{\eta} \tag{6.4}$$

The higher the Reynolds number, the greater the likelihood of turbulence, an interpretation that follows from the definition of N_R as a ratio of inertial to viscous factors. The critical value at which turbulence can be expected is approximately 2,300, but that number is based on empiric observations and varies with the experimental conditions. Inasmuch as blood density is relatively constant, the important fact is that the possibility of turbulence is increased by high blood velocity, large vessel radius, and low viscosity.

Reynolds numbers in the mammalian circulation rarely come anywhere near the turbulence-producing level, and laminar flow is the rule. The Reynolds numbers in the human aorta and main pulmonary artery are about 1,600 under resting conditions, although they may reach much higher values transiently at the peak of flow. Disturbance of the laminar pattern when flow is pulsatile depends in part on the rate of pulsation and the peak velocity (rather than the average in equation 6.4), and parameters that take these factors into account have been described.[8,14] Turbulence can produce audible vibrations, which take the form of *murmurs* in the heart or blood vessels, and are caused at times by unusually high rates of flow but more often pathological conditions that partially obstruct blood flow.

Vascular resistance

Poiseuille's law states that the ratio of driving pressure to blood flow is a function of the physical properties of the vascular system. The motion of blood through a tube depends not only on the force applied to move it but also on the length and radius of the tube and the viscosity of the fluid. In a sense, the system opposes the flow of blood to an extent determined by the dimensions of the conduit, the source of the resistance being a kind of friction at the walls of the tube and between laminae of blood.

This physical opposition to flow has been named *vascular resistance* (**R**), a parameter defined as the ratio of driving pressure to flow

$$\mathbf{R} = \frac{(P_1 - P_2)}{Q} \tag{6.5}$$

Mean pressures are used in this equation because Poiseuille's law applies to steady flow, not pulsations (see below). The relationship resembles the definition given by Ohm's law for electrical resistance, the ratio of driving voltage to electrical current. If pressure is expressed in dyn/cm^2 and flow in cm^3/sec, equation 6.5 gives vascular resistance in $dyn\ sec/cm^5$. Alternatively, pressure can be expressed in mm Hg and flow in liters/min, in which case the resistance unit becomes (mm Hg)/(liter/min).

If conditions are such that Poiseuille's law is applicable, the relation between resistance and the physical properties of the system can be derived by rearranging equation 6.3 to give

$$\mathbf{R} = \frac{8\eta L}{\pi r^4} \tag{6.6}$$

In other words, the pressure difference required to pump a selected number of liters of blood per minute through a tube is directly proportional to the viscosity of the blood and the length of the tube and inversely proportional to the fourth power of the tube radius.

For Poiseuille's law to be a valid description of the phenomena, flow must be laminar and a number of other conditions must be met.[8] First, the conduit must be cylindrical in shape, not elliptical or flattened. Second, flow must be steady, not pulsatile. Third, the fluid must have Newtonian viscosity. If the system meets these requirements, its vascular resistance will be a constant, independent of the driving pressure and defined precisely by equation 6.6. Strictly speaking, none of the conditions is satisfied perfectly in blood vessels, yet in arteries the relationships among pressure, flow, vascular dimensions, and blood viscosity depart only moderately from Poiseuille's law. There are small anomalies, but they are significant only in careful investigations of hemodynamic theory.[8,30,46] For instance, although most arteries are approximately cylindrical they taper slightly, and this convergence has a detectable effect on pressure–flow relationships.[30] The Poiseuille equation is not just an accurate description of steady flow but also a fair approximation of the ratio of the *mean* pressure and flow components of pulsatile flow. The *pulsations* around those means fit a different equation, which includes terms for the distensibility of the vessel, as discussed in a later section.

The concept of vascular resistance has been most useful in its application to whole vascular beds, however, not single vessels. The basic principles are the same, but the goal is to detect constriction or dilatation of vessels. The resistance of the pulmonary vascular bed, for example, can be determined from equation 6.5, substituting the cardiac output for Q, and mean pressures in the pulmonary artery and left atrium for P_1 and P_2, respectively. Similarly, resistance of the entire systemic circulation can be calculated by using systemic arterial pressure for P_1 and right atrial (or large vein) pressure for P_2. Renal vascular resistance can be calculated from measurements of renal blood flow and pressure in a systemic artery and vein.

The utility of such resistance estimates is implied by equation 6.6, although a vascular bed consists of a sequence of numerous segments of different lengths and radii. If we assume that each segment is subject to Poiseuille's law, certain conclusions can be drawn from changes in the resistance of a bed. Segment length is essentially constant, but physiological alterations of vessel diameter are common, especially in the arterioles and venules (Chapter 8). Therefore, when an increase in the resistance of some region is observed, it is usually safe to conclude that the lumen of vessels somewhere in the bed has decreased, and vice versa. More often than not, the cause is constriction or dilatation of arterioles.

Such conclusions must be only tentative, and the principles involved in overall resistance measurements should be kept in mind. The most important limitations are as follows:

1. Changes in resistance do not indicate their cause, which may be neural stimuli, transmural pressure, the action of local metabolites, or a blood clot.
2. They do not reveal where in the pathway from P_1 to P_2 the vessels responsible for the change are situated.
3. They represent the net effect of changes throughout the bed; these changes may be the result of constriction in some vessels and dilatation in others, for example.

4. They do not distinguish between dilatation of vessels and the addition of new channels by opening of vessels previously closed (*recruitment*).
5. They do not include changes in gravitational or kinetic energy within the bed (see below).
6. They may be the result of changes in blood viscosity (which can be measured independently).

Provided that these limitations are recognized, measurements of vascular resistance can be extremely useful in research and clinical medicine. The hemodynamic disturbance in the disease called *essential hypertension,* for example, is an increased resistance of the systemic bed; *primary pulmonary hypertension* is an analogous condition in the vessels of the lungs. The increased resistance is the result of arteriolar constriction. Research on these disorders has therefore concentrated on possible mechanisms for the constriction, thus far without success. Increased cardiac output can produce high blood pressure in a vascular bed with normal resistance, as equations 6.5 and 6.6 imply, but that is not the situation in essential hypertension.

Vascular resistance is often employed in research as an indicator of vasomotor responses. When a substance or experimental maneuver produces an increase in resistance in some region, the intervention may have caused arteriolar constriction, although the other possibilities already mentioned must be kept in mind. Normal values for the resistance of several vascular beds are given in Table 6.1. A related parameter, *input resistance* (R_{in}), is calculated by omitting P_2 from equation 6.5. Input resistance at any point in the circulation is related to the total pressure energy that must be supplied per unit flow to move blood on.

Vascular resistance of the systemic or pulmonary bed in various animals is *inversely* correlated with body size (Table 6.1), a relationship that arises from the architecture of the circulation and the effects of parallel, in contrast with

Table 6.1. Typical Vascular Resistances Under Basal Conditions[a]

VASCULAR BED	DOG (20 KG)	MAN (70 KG)
Pulmonic	320	80
Systemic	4,200	1,150
Splanchnic	11,700	4,650
Renal (both kidneys)	14,600	5,800
Cerebral	23,400	9,300

[a]Dyn sec/cm^5, calculated by equation 6.5 from regional blood flows and pressures given in Table 2.1, Table 2.4, and Chapter 12.

series, connections of resistances. If three tubes are connected in sequence, the total resistance of the combination, R_T, is the sum of the individual resistances, as with electrical components:

$$\text{In series:} \quad R_T = R_1 + R_2 + R_3 \tag{6.7}$$

When the same resistances are in parallel (i.e., all with the same pressure, P_1 at their inlets, P_2 at their outlets, and a total flow, Q, throughout the whole assembly), a reciprocal relationship defines the overall resistance:

$$\text{In parallel:} \quad \frac{1}{R_T} = \frac{1}{R_1} + \frac{1}{R_2} + \frac{1}{R_3} \tag{6.8}$$

The greater the number of similar resistances in parallel, the lower the total resistance of the array.

All mammals have essentially the same number of large arteries and veins, one aorta, two renal arteries, and so on. They differ, however, in the periphery, where the number of small vessels in parallel increases with the size of the animal. Equation 6.8, not 6.7, thus dominates comparative resistances in the vascular beds of different animals. The relatively long overall vascular pathways in large animals might be expected to increase resistance, and their relatively large aortic diameter to reduce it, but those factors have relatively little influence; resistance is concentrated in the microcirculation because of its relation to the fourth power of the vessel radius (equation 6.6). The diameters and lengths of arterioles, capillaries, and venules are only slightly size dependent. Pulmonary vascular resistance in the mouse is consequently much higher than it is in man, a situation that can be pictured dramatically by imagining the enormous pressure that would be required to push 6 liters of blood per minute through the lungs of the smaller animal. The same structural and hemodynamic principles apply within species as an animal develops from infancy to adulthood.[21]

Hydraulic energy

Poiseuille's law defines the fall in hydraulic pressure along a tube under certain conditions of flow, a fall that is related to the energy being dissipated as the fluid advances. The heart supplies that energy, and the motion of viscous fluid through the system dissipates it. In addition, the inertia of the fluid must be overcome, and the heart must at times move blood against the force of gravity to reach the head or other regions. The Poiseuille equation thus includes only one of the three kinds of energy associated with blood flow. Energy is the product of force and distance (dyn cm), and hemodynamics is concerned with three different kinds: pressure, kinetic, and gravitational.[8]

Pressure energy

Pressure is defined as force per unit area (dyn/cm²), but in the present context it can also be regarded as an expression of energy per unit volume of fluid (dyn cm/cm³). This is a kind of potential energy, transferred to blood by contractions of the heart and stored in the elastic walls of blood vessels. Pressure energy, W_P, is the product of a volume of blood, V, and the pressure, P, associated with it:

$$W_P = PV \tag{6.9}$$

This energy component is the only one included in the Poiseuille equation, but it is the largest of the three kinds of hydraulic energy in the circulation.

Atmospheric pressure is taken as the zero reference point in this calculation, as it almost always is in hemodynamics. If ambient pressure happens to be 760 mm Hg, for example, then a blood pressure reported as 100 mm Hg means that the *absolute* pressure is 860 mm Hg. Calibration and measurements are all carried out in relative terms, so atmospheric pressure rarely needs to be considered.

Kinetic energy

Like all moving bodies, circulating blood possesses a kinetic energy (W_K) that is related to its mass (m) and the square of its velocity (v). Mass is the product of volume (V) and density (ρ, g(mass)/cm³), so that

$$W_K = \frac{\rho V v^2}{2} \tag{6.10}$$

The relative magnitudes of blood pressure and velocity *in vivo* are such that the kinetic energy associated with blood flow is always much smaller than the pressure energy.

Gravitational energy

Energy must be exerted to lift an object vertically in the earth's gravitational field. The object can then be said to be endowed with a *gravitational energy* that could cause it to fall back to its original position. This fact is relevant when blood must be pumped to a level higher than the heart, a situation that exists for the head in the erect posture. Gravitational energy (W_G) can be calculated from the volume (V) of blood involved, its height (h) above a reference level, the gravitational acceleration constant (g), and the density (ρ) of blood:

$$W_G = \rho g h V \qquad (6.11)$$

The reference level is usually an imaginary plane passing through the heart. Gravitational energy is the source of what are called *hydrostatic pressures,* which are discussed in a later section. It is of particular importance in the return of blood from dependent regions like the feet, and in the pulmonary circulation, where the pressure energy delivered by the right ventricle is of about the same order of magnitude as the gravitational energy needed to move blood to the apices of the lungs (Chapter 11).

The physiological significance of these categories of hydraulic energy is that all three are involved in the motion of fluids through conduits. Blood moves down a gradient of hydraulic energy, not pressure energy alone, and to that extent Poiseuille's equation is incomplete. Total hydraulic energy (W_T) at any point in the circulation is

$$W_T = PV + \frac{1}{2}\rho V v^2 + \rho g h V \qquad (6.12)$$

and blood always flows toward regions of lower hydraulic energy.

Poiseuille could safely neglect kinetic and gravitational energies in his experiments because velocities were low and the tubes horizontal. Similar conditions often exist *in vivo,* and pressure energy in the circulation is usually much larger than the kinetic or gravitational components. When those components are absent, pressure falls in a linear way along the length of a tube (Figure 6.4A), in accordance with Poiseuille's law (equation 6.3). If the cross section of the flowing stream changes abruptly, however, kinetic energy can be converted into pressure, or vice versa, a phenomenon exhibited in what is called the *Bernoulli principle,* and in the difference between the *end pressure* and the *lateral pressure* measured by a catheter.

Bernoulli's law

Flow through a tube that suddenly widens at one point, as in Figure 6.4B, illustrates the significance of total hydraulic energy. If flow is steady and laminar, the volumetric rate of flow (Q) is the same at all cross sections of the tube. Velocity (v), however, is related to flow and cross-sectional area (A): $v = Q/A$. Therefore, velocity is lower at point 2 in the figure, where the area has increased, than at point 1. If the distance between the two points is very small the total energy does not change, but kinetic energy decreases at the cross

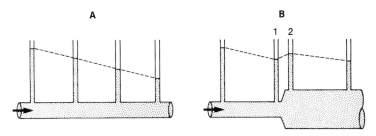

Figure 6.4. Pressure–flow relationships described by Poiseuille's law and Bernoulli's principle. Pressure is indicated at several points by the height of fluid in small side tubes. **A**, Poiseuille relationship: Constant laminar flow through cylindrical tube is associated with linear fall in pressure (see equation 6.3). **B**, Bernoulli effect: Abrupt change in cross section of tube modifies the fall in pressure. Volumetric rate of flow is the same just after the expansion of the tube (*2*) as before it (*1*), and velocity equals flow divided by cross-sectional area. For that reason, velocity decreases abruptly between *1* and *2*; the kinetic energy corresponding to that loss of velocity is converted into pressure; and the lateral pressure rises slightly.

section between points 1 and 2. The difference is made up by an increase in pressure at point 2 through conversion of kinetic energy into pressure.

Gravitational energy is zero in this example because the system is horizontal, and the last term in equation 6.12 can be ignored for that reason. The increase in pressure between points 1 and 2 ($P_2 - P_1$) equals the loss of kinetic energy between the two points, therefore, in terms of volumetric flow (which is the same at both places) and the two cross-sectional areas (A_1, A_2):

$$P_2 - P_1 = \frac{\rho Q^2}{2}\left\{\frac{1}{A_2^2} - \frac{1}{A_1^2}\right\} \tag{6.13}$$

The right-hand side of equation 6.13 represents the kinetic energy converted into pressure under these conditions. At any sudden downstream narrowing the effect would be reversed, and pressure would be converted into kinetic energy.

Bernoulli's law has little application in the normal circulation, for changes in cross section are gradual and viscous losses far outweigh any small interconversions of energy. On the other hand, pathological conditions like partial stenosis of an artery by disease or a local aneurysm (dilatation) of the aorta can produce prominent Bernoulli effects. Such abnormalities often produce turbulence as well, which tends to dissipate both kinetic and pressure energy.

Lateral and end pressures

Another situation in which kinetic energy must be taken into account is in the measurement of blood pressure through a catheter or needle in a vessel. Such probes obstruct flow in some tiny part of the stream, bringing blood that impinges on them to almost zero velocity, so that its previous kinetic energy is converted into local pressure. If the opening of the catheter (or a sensor at the tip) faces laterally (i.e., in a radial direction), this phenomenon has no effect on the pressure that is recorded (*lateral pressure*), but if it faces upstream, the *end pressure* so detected is higher than the lateral pressure by an amount equivalent to the kinetic energy. The effect is reversed when the opening faces downstream, making end pressure lower than lateral pressure. The difference is less than 1 mm Hg in normal arteries, but it can amount to more than 10 mm Hg in the jet that issues through a pinpoint opening in a stenosed aortic or pulmonic valve. Lateral pressure is the one to be measured for most purposes and the one referred to throughout this volume.

Vascular Distensibility

Blood vessels are elastic, which means that they can be distended by raising intravascular pressure or diminished in radius by lowering it. This fact does not alter any of the principles already discussed; the ratio of driving pressure to flow still depends on length, radius, and other variables, as indicated in equation 6.3. The one new phenomenon in distensible tubes is that *transmural pressure*, the difference between the pressures inside and outside the vessel, is now one of the factors that *control* the radius. Extravascular, or interstitial space, pressure is 0 to 3 mm Hg under most conditions, much lower than intravascular pressure. The elasticity of the blood vessel walls plays a large role in hemodynamics for two reasons. First, the contraction or relaxation of vascular smooth muscle alters vessel diameter by changing the elasticity of the wall. Second, the elasticity of a vascular bed determines how much of the blood volume is accommodated within that region at the existing local pressure.

Elasticity of materials[8,11]

Elasticity is a physical property of materials, and it is necessary to be clear about its definition. A body is said to be *elastic* if it can be elongated (or otherwise deformed) by application of a stress and completely recovers its original dimensions when the stress is removed. The degree of deformation is expressed as a *strain,* the ratio of the observed change to the original dimension. In stretching, for example, strain is the change in length divided by the initial length ($\Delta L/L_0$). *Extensibility* refers to the degree of elongation produced by a given stress. Rubber is very extensible and steel is not, although both are elastic materials to the physicist. In a purely elastic body, the strain produced by a sudden stress occurs instantaneously. Materials in which the strain changes with time are called *viscous* or *viscoelastic*.

Circumferential stress in a vascular wall can be calculated from the dimensions of the vessel and the transmural pressure. Equations for this purpose are derived from what is usually called *Laplace's law,* which states that the tension (*T,* force per unit length) in the wall of a very thin cylindrical shell is related to transmural pressure (P_t) and radius (*r*): $T = P_t r$. The circumferential stress (force/area) on the wall also depends on wall thickness, however. The longitudinal area on which distending stress acts along each centimeter of length is numerically equal to the wall thickness, *h,* so the circumferential stress (*S*) is

$$S = \frac{P_t \mathrm{r}}{h} \tag{6.14}$$

(The word *tension* is rarely used elsewhere in this volume because it has been given many different meanings in the literature on muscle physiology, where it has been variously employed to denote force per unit length [dyn/cm, as in surface tension], force per unit area [dyn/cm^2], or simply as a synonym for *force* [dyn]).

The elasticity of any material is expressed by an *elastic modulus (E),* the relevant one here being Young's modulus of elasticity by stretching. This parameter is defined as the ratio of applied stress, or force per unit area ($\Delta F/A$), to resulting strain ($\Delta L/L_0$)

$$E = \frac{\Delta F/A}{\Delta L/L_0} \tag{6.15}$$

The elastic modulus is thus expressed in units of stress (e.g., dyn/cm^2 or g/cm^2); its value is equivalent to the stress required to double the length of the specimen, although in practice the strain is kept very small. The length and stress involved in applications to blood vessels are principally those in a circumferential direction, although longitudinal stretching also occurs *in vivo* and has been studied in detail.[8] Circumferential strain can be expressed by the quantity ($\Delta r/r$), where *r* is the initial radius.

The assumption of a thin wall makes equation 6.14 an *inexact* description of conditions in blood vessels, although the qualitative implications of the expression are correct. More rigorous equations must take into account variations of stress in different parts of the wall.[2,8,15] Accurate calculation of the elastic modulus of the wall of a blood vessel should take into account the thickness of the wall, which generally ranges from 7 to 15% of the external radius in arteries and reaches larger proportions in arterioles. Under such conditions, circumferential stress and strain are more complicated than stated in equation 6.15. One of the many equations[8] that have been derived to overcome this problem has the form[15]

$$E = \frac{3r_o^2}{2(r_o^2 - r_i^2)} \cdot \frac{\Delta P}{(\Delta r_i/r_i)} \qquad (6.16)$$

where r_o represents outer radius and r_i inner radius. This equation assumes that the material of the wall is incompressible;[8] wall thickness enters into it through the appearance of both the inner and outer radii.

Just as the elastic modulus is an expression employed to characterize material properties, so *compliance* is a term used to describe the elastic behavior of a hollow vessel or chamber. It refers to changes in the capacity, or volume, of the structure (ΔV) in relation to changes in transmural pressure (ΔP). The parameter most often used is *relative compliance* (C), in which the volumetric change is expressed as a fraction of the initial volume, V_1:

$$C = \frac{\Delta V}{V_1 \Delta P} \qquad (6.17)$$

Note that compliance and elastic modulus are related in a reciprocal way; a tube with a large elastic modulus has a low compliance. *Distensibility* and *compliance* are virtually synonymous terms, but *distensibility* is generally used in a broad sense and is not employed in quantitative statements. The compliance of a whole vascular bed can be measured by appropriate experimental techniques,[31] and such observations are used in studying shifts of blood from one part of the circulation to another (Chapter 13).

Elastic behavior of blood vessels[2]

The elasticity of the blood vessel wall depends on the properties of its constituents, and the wall is not homogeneous but made up of a mixture of tissues arranged in a distinctive architectural pattern. Three layers can be identified in the walls of most arteries and veins. The inner lining, the part of the wall in direct contact with circulating blood, is a single layer of flat endothelial cells called the *intima* or *endothelium*. The outermost layer, or *adventitia*, consists of connective tissue that merges almost indistinguishably into the surrounding tissues. Between these two lies a broad *media,* which is made up largely of smooth muscle but also contains a complex arrangement of collagen and elastin fibers.[22] The proportions of various components of canine arterial walls are listed in Table 6.2. Water (intra- and extracellular) makes up 70 to 80% of wall weight.[7,19]

Elastic fibers consist of a rubber-like, highly extensible protein, *elastin.* *Collagen* fibers, which are also found in skeletal muscle tendons, are very inextensible and have a high tensile strength. Both kinds of fibers are embedded in

Table 6.2. Chemical Composition of Canine Arterial Walls[a]

COMPONENT	PERCENT WET WALL WEIGHT	
	ASCENDING AORTA	FEMORAL ARTERY
Smooth muscle	65	63
Interstitial fluid	19	19
Elastin	8	5
Collagen	4	9
Fat	1	1
Other	3	3

[a]Estimated from data in Fischer and Llaurado[22] and Milnor.[8]

an amorphous, mucopolysaccharide *ground substance*. Elastin fibers are dispersed within the media, and in arteries of medium size there are also two thin concentric layers of elastic tissue at the inner and outer limits of the media. Collagen fibers, in contrast, form a loose circumferential mesh. The smooth muscle consists of elongated cells 20 to 100 μm in length and 5 to 10 μm in diameter, attached end to end and side to side in bundles about 100 μm in diameter. Some of these bundles parallel the longitudinal axis of the vessel, but the majority travel around the circumference in a circular or helical fashion. Contraction of smooth muscle in these circumferential strings tends to shorten them and thus reduces the diameter of the vascular lumen.

The aorta and the proximal portion of its major branches are classified as *elastic arteries* because of their high elastin content, whereas the more distal parts of the tree are called *muscular arteries* because of the high proportion of smooth muscle in their walls. No sharp dividing line exists, but the relative amount of muscle increases continuously toward the periphery in the arterial tree, and the ratio of collagen to elastin decreases (Figure 1.2). The media of arterioles and venules consists almost entirely of one or two layers of muscle cells.

In simple elastic substances, stress and strain are directly proportional in accordance with Hooke's law, but that is *not* the case in blood vessels because the various components of the vascular wall differ markedly in their elasticity. The relative stiffness of collagen is indicated by its elastic modulus of about 50×10^6 dyn/cm^2, as contrasted with 5×10^6 dyn/cm^2 for elastin and 1×10^6 dyn/cm^2 for relaxed smooth muscle.[3] The endothelium is very compliant and makes little physical contribution to vascular distensibility. The mechanical behavior of the wall as a whole is also influenced by the way these elements are interconnected. Information on this point is incomplete, but there appear to be connections between muscle and elastin at some points, and attachments of muscle and elastin to collagen fibers have been described. The end result is that the vessel wall becomes *stiffer* (i.e., the elastic modulus increases) as the vessel is distended and the wall is stretched.[2,15,24,26]

Figure 6.5 illustrates the nonlinear nature of stress–strain relationships in arteries. The data in this figure were obtained from a vessel that was first allowed to relax completely in physiological saline; pressure within it was then raised in a series of steps. Each step was maintained for 2 min to allow the resulting distention to reach an equilibrium, after which the radius was measured. This procedure is called an *incremental* method of measuring elasticity because it is based on small increments in stress and strain. Because initial transient effects are ignored and strain is measured only after a steady state has been reached, the parameters calculated by equation 6.16 in such an experiment are called *static elastic moduli*.

Figure 6.5 shows that the vessel is readily distended when the radius is relatively small; a small increase in stress is accompanied by a large increase in radius (and circumference). At large radii, however, the vessel is stiff; small increments in stress produce only small increments in radius. Obviously, the elasticity of the wall cannot be described by a single number because it varies with the degree of stress and strain, but it can be defined at any point on the curve by an *incremental elastic modulus*. For the curve shown in Figure 6.5, the static modulus calculated by equation 6.16 is 1.05×10^6 dyn/cm^2 at a radius of 1.7 mm and 11.2×10^6 dyn/cm^2 at a radius of 2.1 mm. (These values were calculated from *incremental* strain, the difference between two radii divided by their average, and are hence equivalent to the slope of a line tangential to the curve at the average radius.)

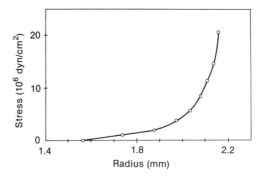

Figure 6.5.   Nonlinear relation between circumferential stress (*ordinate*, 10^6 dyn/cm^2) and outer radius (*abscissa*, mm) in a canine femoral artery. Vessel was distended by increments in transmural pressure and radius was measured after a 2-min equilibration period. Highest point was obtained at transmural pressure of 180 mm Hg.

The nonlinear stress–strain relationship is thought to be created by the mixture of materials being stretched. According to a widely accepted theory, the steepness of the right-hand portion of the curve develops as the stiff collagen network of the wall bears more and more of the strain. Little or none of the stress is borne by collagen until the vessel has been distended to a certain degree, but its stiffness begins to dominate the relationship as the wall is stretched farther, as if the collagenous fibers were disposed in a sort of loose basketwork, in which slack is not taken up until vessel diameter increases to a critical level. The curvilinearity may also to some extent be an inherent property of smooth muscle, however, for passive stress–strain curves of single cells have roughly the same shape.[18]

The effect of smooth muscle contraction on the elastic behavior of arteries[20] is shown in Figure 6.6, where the data are plotted in the more familiar terms of transmural pressure and radius. The control curve when the smooth muscle was inactive resembles that in Figure 6.5, exhibiting the "passive" elasticity attributable to relaxed muscle and nonmuscular elements of the wall. When contraction of the smooth muscle was induced by exposing the vessel to norepinephrine, the vessel constricted, reducing the radius at any given pressure and moving the curve upward and to the left. Stimulation of the muscle constricted the vessel even at a transmural pressure of zero, and stiffness increased with radius in both states. The curves also show that muscle stimulation combined with an increase in transmural pressure could leave the radius unchanged or even enlarge it.

Activation of vascular smooth muscle increases the elastic modulus of the vessel wall under most conditions, and consequently alters the relationship be-

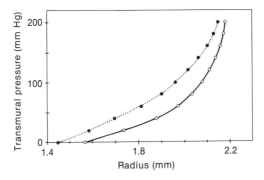

Figure 6.6. Effect of smooth muscle stimulation on stress–strain relationships in canine femoral artery (same vessel as in Figure 6.5). *Abscissa*, radius (mm); *ordinate*, transmural pressure (mm Hg). *Solid line*, relaxed state. *Dashed line*, observations after external application of 1-norepinephrine (10^{-6} M) to vessel wall. At any given transmural pressure, the contraction of vascular smooth muscle elicited by norepinephrine reduces radius.

tween distending pressure and the volume of the segment involved. In small vessels, such changes in distensibility are the source of constriction or dilatation, but in large vessels the change in diameter is small and has no significant effect on local resistance, which is low in any case. Nevertheless, any change in sympathetic constrictor impulses to the large veins has important hemodynamic results because of their large volume (Chapter 13). The effectiveness of venomotor activity in shifting blood from one region to another is discussed in a later section.

The blood volume of large arteries, unlike that of veins, changes relatively little under physiological conditions because of their relatively small total arterial capacity and distensibility. Arterial elasticity is subject to autonomic control, however, and it is the principal determinant of ventricular afterload and the transmission of pulsatile pressure and flow (Chapter 4). These factors are particularly important in the pulmonary circulation, where a large part of the right ventricular work is devoted to overcoming input impedance, and reflex alterations of elasticity in the major arteries are sometimes as great as those in small-vessel resistance.[28]

Hysteresis

Purely elastic bodies respond to a sudden stretching force by elongating instantaneously to an appropriate new length that remains constant until the stress is removed (Figure 6.7A), whereupon they return to their original dimensions. The vascular wall does *not* behave in this way, but requires a finite time to reach a new equilibrium between stress and strain. Such behavior is called *hysteresis,* from the Greek word for delay or lagging behind, and materials that exhibit hysteresis are said to be *viscous.* Blood vessels are *viscoelastic,* meaning that they appear to contain a mixture of elastic and viscous materials.

The viscoelasticity of vessel walls becomes evident in a variety of ways in different experiments and *in vivo.* The imposition of a constant strain causes an initial sharp increment followed by a gradual decline in wall stress, called *stress relaxation* or *delayed compliance*[47] (Figure 6.7B). Conversely, vessels exposed suddenly to a constant force—an increase in transmural pressure, for example—distend promptly to a certain degree and then continue to stretch gradually over a period of seconds or minutes, a response referred to as *creep* (Figure 6.7C). Stress relaxation and creep appear to be two manifestations of the same underlying process, the former occurring when the circumference is kept constant, the latter when wall stress is the controlled variable. Both phenomena are observed in the smooth muscle of other organs. They presumably originate in detachment and reattachment of muscle cross-bridges, as well as in the properties of other wall components. Another kind of behavior, the *myo-*

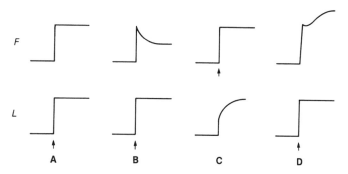

Figure 6.7. Typical relations between force and length in viscoelastic materials and smooth muscle. *Arrows* indicate which variable is experimentally controlled (step-function of length in **A**, **B**, **D**; force in **C**). **A**, purely elastic response; force increases instantly when material is stretched. **B**, *stress relaxation*; length-step produces immediate increment in force, which decays with time as length is held constant. **C**, *creep*; force-step produces an immediate stretch, but material continues to lengthen with time. **D**, *myogenic response* in vascular smooth muscle; force increases after length-step.

genic response, occurs in some blood vessels when they are stretched quickly. A sudden elongation elicits first an immediate step and then a slow increase in force (Figure 6.7D), as if the stretch had stimulated contraction of smooth muscle (Chapter 9). Myogenic responses can be demonstrated *in vitro* and hence do not involve neural reflex arcs.

All of these types of time-dependent behavior occur *in vivo* and are of physiological significance. Stress relaxation and creep are part of the response when blood is displaced into the venous bed from other regions (see below), allowing the venous compartment to accommodate a greater volume at lower pressure. The myogenic response may be a factor in vascular autoregulation (Chapter 12). Vessel walls can also be overstretched, although it is not clear whether this ever happens in living animals. Very large strains *in vitro* (distending a systemic artery with a pressure greater than 250 mm Hg, for example) usually diminish the subsequent responsiveness of the vessel, probably because of structural damage to the cells.

Blood flow in distensible vessels

One consequence of the distensibility of blood vessels is that the relation between perfusing pressure and blood flow in a vascular bed is nonlinear. Poiseuille's law implies a straight-line relationship (equation 6.3 and Figure 6.4), but only if rigid vessels are assumed. In a rigid system, where the radius of each segment would be constant, a driving pressure of 50 mm Hg would produce the same flow whether $(P_1 - P_2)$ were $(100 - 50)$ or $(60 - 10)$. In a distensible system, however, the first pair of entrance and exit pressures would be accompanied by higher transmural pressures than the second, making the radii larger and thus the flow greater. The Poiseuille equation still applies, but the correct radii must be inserted.

The pressure–flow relationship in a real vascular bed is shown in Figure 6.8, the result of an experiment on the perfused vascular bed of a rabbit ear as arterial pressure was raised in a series of steps. Venous outflow pressure was atmospheric. The changes were characteristic of a distensible bed, with no evidence of autoregulation (Chapter 12). The increment in flow that followed each increase in pressure became greater with each step because transmural as well as driving pressure was increased, distending the bed to a slightly greater degree at each stage. As a result, the plot is curvilinear, with a convexity toward the pressure axis. This relationship is characteristic of distensible beds and is often seen *in vivo*. The curvilinearity does not arise from the nonlinear elasticity of vessel walls shown in Figure 6.5, but occurs even in the absence of nonlinearity. In regional beds that exhibit autoregulation the curve is quite different, flattening out to a constant flow at all but the lowest perfusion pressures.

Figure 6.8 also shows two other general features of vascular beds in live animals. First, the curve intercepts the horizontal axis at a finite pressure. As arterial pressure is raised from zero, no flow occurs until a critical level is reached. The obstruction to flow comes from the closure of very small vessels

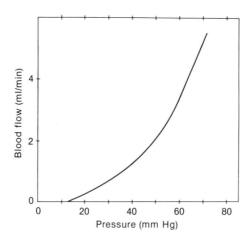

Figure 6.8. Passive pressure–flow relations in vascular bed of rabbit ear. *Ordinate*, blood flow (ml/min). *Abscissa*, arterial perfusion pressure (mm Hg), identical with driving pressure because terminal venous pressure was zero. Slight convexity of curve toward pressure axis is result of progressive distention of elastic vessels by transmural pressure (see text). Straight line at higher pressures indicates relative rigidity of vessels at maximum distention. Note that no flow occurs unless perfusion pressure is greater than about 12 mm Hg (critical closing pressure).

at low transmural pressure, and in this example they did not open until the pressure was raised to 12 mm Hg. The same phenomenon appears when pressure is allowed to fall gradually from an initially high level, and the point at which flow ceases in that case is called the *critical closing pressure*. In the presence of normal vascular tone the critical level is between 10 and 25 mm Hg, but it is made higher by stimuli that cause contraction of vascular smooth muscle, suggesting that the active stress generated by muscle can close some microvessels completely unless transmural pressure is high enough to balance it.[3] With a few exceptions, such as vessels at the apex of the lung and those within ventricular walls, critical closing probably does not occur under physiological conditions. The other point illustrated in Figure 6.8 is the tightening of the collagen net around large vessels distended by relatively high transmural pressures. The pressure–flow relationship became approximately linear above 50 mm Hg in this experiment, indicating that the vessels had become effectively rigid.

Pulse wave velocity

Pulse waves are transmitted very rapidly through the arterial tree, and their velocity should not be confused with the much slower speed with which blood moves through the system. A pressure wave originating in the left ventricle reaches the radial artery in about 0.1 sec, whereas a drop of blood takes at least 8 sec to make the same journey. The contrast is analogous to that between the speed of sound in water and the actual motion of a stream.

Pulse wave velocity depends in part on the elasticity of the vessel wall. The stiffer the wall, the greater the speed; wave velocities in the circulation range from 1 m/sec in the main pulmonary artery to more than 15 m/sec in small systemic arteries. The relation between wave transmission and vascular distensibility can be derived from basic physical principles, and details are given in specialized textbooks.[4,8] The fundamental concept is that pressure and flow waves traveling in a distensible tube are slowed to the extent that they move in radial as well as longitudinal directions with each pulsation. If vessels were completely rigid, the waves would travel at an almost infinitely high speed, since the extremely small compressibility of blood would then be the only limiting factor.

Pulse wave velocity was long regarded as a matter of more theoretic than practical interest, but it is now recognized as a reliable and clinically useful index of vascular elasticity. Abnormal or premature stiffening of the arteries may be a feature of some disease states. The transcutaneous ultrasonic flowmeter provides a noninvasive method of measurement by making it possible to compare the arrival times of waves at two different sites; that procedure has been used in a number of human studies (Chapters 2, 14). It is difficult at present to identify the functional significance of wave velocities, but some possibilities have been suggested. The normal transmission time through the lungs, for instance, delivers blood into the left atrium at exactly the time of rapid ventricular filling, a temporal arrangement that may contribute to ventricular performance (Chapter 11).

Collapsible vessels

The elastic nature of blood vessels allows them not only to be distended but also to collapse and lose their circular cross section under some conditions. Arteries rarely behave this way because their shape is maintained by the structure and thickness of the walls. Large peripheral veins, however, with their thin walls and low transmural pressures, are often in a collapsed state. Veins on the back of the hand can be seen to collapse as the arm is raised above heart level, and the external jugular vein, which is usually visible in supine subjects, virtually disappears in the erect posture. Blood continues to flow through such vessels, but the lumen is slit-like or dumbbell shaped. Small coronary vessels deep within the ventricular walls furnish examples of partial or complete occlusion by external systolic pressure.[13]

Hemodynamic conditions in vessels that collapse or are forced into an elliptical or flat configuration are different from those in the more or less cylindrical tubes that have been discussed in preceding sections. One is not surprised that a sufficiently high extravascular force can occlude a vessel completely, but an unexpected finding is that relatively small external and internal pressures can establish a balance that keeps collapsible vessels barely open and at the same time makes flow independent of downstream pressure.[41] Poiseuille's law clearly does not apply, but appropriate equations have been developed[29] and flow through a bed in this state is *lower* than would be expected from the arteriovenous pressure difference.

Partially collapsed vessels dissipate more hydraulic energy than normally rounded ones do, producing a discrepancy between apparent driving pressure and blood flow. That generalization suffices to explain qualitatively a number of physiological observations in regions where vessels can collapse, but a detailed examination of exactly what happens in the affected vessels is a lengthy and somewhat speculative exercise. Although the phenomena can be duplicated in rubber tubes, direct experimental measurements that would identify the mechanism involved in live animals are almost impossible to obtain. Nevertheless, the probable physical source of such behavior can be reasoned out, and the explanation that follows is given for readers who may wish to pursue it.

Transmural pressure is a major factor in determining the shape and dimensions of collapsible vessels, and the hydrostatic contributions to distending force can be significant (see above). In some situations, the extravascular and intravascular pressures may be of the same order of magnitude. The interaction between the two is illustrated in Figure 6.9, which shows a collapsible tube fed by a reservoir and draining through a tube with a controlled distal pressure. The collapsible segment is surrounded by a box representing the source of extravascular pressure. Energy is supplied hydrostatically by the height of the water in the reservoir, and distal pressure is controlled by the vertical position of a beaker at the outflow. The collapsible segment in this model is sometimes called a *Starling resistor.*

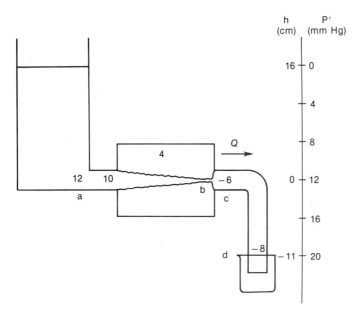

Figure 6.9.   Pressure and flow in a tubular, water-filled system containing a collapsible segment. Pressure supplied by reservoir on left. Scale at right: *h*, height above bottom of reservoir in cm; *P′*, hydrostatic pressure in mm Hg. Collapsible portion lies within a sealed compartment in which pressure is 4 mm Hg, the "extravascular" pressure. Exit of system is 11 cm below collapsible segment and bottom of reservoir. Under these conditions, the tube within the box is almost but not quite completely closed at its distal end, and a steady flow (*Q*) is maintained. Pressures inside the tubing are shown in mm Hg. Changes of pressure in the box will alter flow, but raising the level of the outflow beaker will not, unless the beaker is raised high enough to counteract the box pressure (see text). The collapsible tube surrounded by a controllable external pressure is called a Starling resistor, and a situation in which flow is independent of the pressure far downstream is sometimes referred to as a vascular waterfall.[41] (Reproduced from Milnor,[8] with permission of Williams & Wilkins)

For purposes of this example, the fluid level in the beaker is 11 cm *below* the midline of the horizontal tubing, and the level in the reservoir is 16 cm *above* it. The driving pressure is thus the difference between 12 mm Hg at the bottom of the reservoir and − 8 mm Hg in the beaker. If extravascular pressure were zero (not positive, as in the diagram), then the collapsible tube would remain fully open and flow would proceed through the system in accordance with the driving pressure and the dimensions and distensibility of the conduits.

Raising the pressure in the box to 4 mm Hg partially collapses the tubing within it, leaving it barely open at its distal end and greatly reducing flow through the system. (The elasticity of the collapsible segment has been defined so that it is fully open at transmural pressures above 0.2 mm Hg and collapses progressively at lower pressures until it closes completely at P_t = 0 mm Hg.). As water flows through the tubing there is a drop in pressure, described by the Poiseuille equation, between the reservoir exit and the beginning of the collapsible tube, and between the end of the box and the distal beaker. The resulting pressure in the collapsible segment is 10 mm Hg at its entrance, which viscous flow reduces to slightly over 4.0 mm Hg at point b.

Now, at long last, we arrive at the point of this demonstration. Increasing the pressure within the box will decrease the flow, and vice versa, as might be expected. Contrary to any expectations derived from rigid systems, however, raising or lowering the beaker to change the distal pressure will *not* affect the flow as long as it is not raised high enough to bring the pressure at point c to more than +4.0 mm Hg (Figure 6.10).

The size of the opening (if any) at the terminus of the collapsible tube is controlled by the difference between pressures in the box and at point b. The critical factor in our example is thus the intravascular pressure at point b; if it is greater than +4.0 mm Hg, it will hold the terminal part of the segment open; otherwise, it will not. The pressure at point b is self-adjusting in a sense, however. The smaller the opening, the lower the flow, the less the viscous drop along the segment, and the closer the pressure at b approaches 12 mm Hg, the pressure that would exist were the terminus closed. Provided that the pressure at point c is lower than +4.1 mm Hg, what the system does is to achieve an equilibrium in which the rate of flow is such that pressure b barely keeps the end of the collapsing segment open. A large pressure gradient exists from b to c, and flow in that region may be turbulent, but the pressure at c has no effect on the flow rate.

In short, if the distal component of the driving pressure (P_2 in our terminology, d in Figure 6.9) is *lower* than the extravascular pressure, flow through a collapsible system is controlled by the inflow and *extravascular* pressures, not by the inflow and outflow pressures that determine flow in a noncollapsible system. Strictly speaking, the intravascular pressure gradients from a to b, b

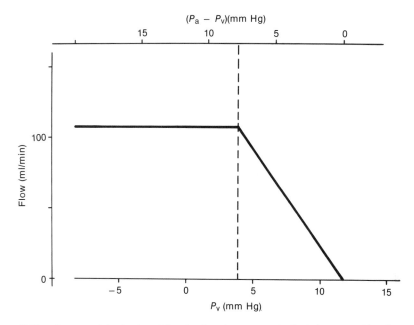

Figure 6.10. Pressure (*abscissa*) and flow (*ordinate*) in a vascular bed that resembles the system in Figure 6.9. Arterial pressure, P_a, is constant, like that in the reservoir. Venous pressure (P_v, *bottom scale*) is analogous to that at point *c* in Figure 6.9. When $P_v = P_a$ (12 mm Hg), there is no flow. When P_v is then gradually lowered, flow begins and increases. If P_v falls below the external pressure on collapsible vessels (4 mm Hg), however, further lowering of P_v has no effect on flow even though the arteriovenous gradient ($P_a - P_v$, *top scale*) continues to get larger.[41] (Reproduced from Milnor,[8] with permission of Williams & Wilkins)

to c, and c to d, together with the size of the vessel lumen at all locations, still govern the flow rate. The pressure at c automatically remains close to the extravascular value, however, and most of the resistance is concentrated at that point.

The relevance of this phenomenon to the circulation *in vivo* is that the pressure outside collapsible vessels in certain regions *can* become greater than the intravascular pressure; the pulmonary circulation provides a striking example. The principal force acting externally on pulmonary capillaries is the pressure within the alveoli of the lung. Although it seems unlikely, on first thought, that alveolar pressure, which is usually close to zero, could be higher than intravascular pressures, hydrostatic effects and the negative intrapleural force can make vascular pressures subatmospheric at the apex of the lung (Chapter 11). Capillaries or venules then act like the collapsible segment in Figure 6.9, and pressure in the terminal pulmonary veins or left atrium has no effect on flow. In zones of the lung where pressure is lower in the veins than in the alveoli, flow appears to depend on the difference between arterial and *alveolar* (not venous) pressures, although this is true only because intravascular pressure at the ends of partially collapsed vessels becomes almost identical to that in the alveoli.

Pressure–flow relationships in the regions where such conditions exist are like those shown in Figure 6.10, where arterial pressure (P_a) is analogous to that at point a in Figure 6.9 and venous pressure (P_v) to that at point c. Pressure within the alveoli corresponds to that in the extravascular box. Arterial pressure in Figure 6.10 is assumed to remain constant at 12 mm Hg, and if venous pressure is also 12 mm Hg there will be no flow, although the vessels remain open. Lowering the venous pressure creates an arteriovenous pressure gradient and produces flow. As venous pressure is lowered, this gradient becomes larger and flow increases, until venous pressure reaches the extravascular level (+4 mm Hg). As P_v is lowered further, the $P_a - P_v$ difference continues to increase, but flow remains *constant* because collapsible vessels are behaving in the fashion described above. The collapsing segments act like a sluice gate, permitting a certain flow regardless of the difference between upstream and downstream pressures. This hemodynamic state has been called a "vascular waterfall,"[41] by analogy with another situation in which flow is unrelated to downstream pressure.

Pulsatile Pressure and Flow

The principles that govern steady flow are the foundation for those that apply to the pulsatile flow seen in mammalian circulations. The heart pumps by repeated contraction, injecting a certain volume of blood at the origin of the vascular system at more or less regular intervals. The resulting rise and fall of blood pressure and flow in the ascending aorta and main pulmonary artery with each heartbeat were described in Chapter 2, and the cessation of flow in these vessels during diastole is shown in Figure 2.7. The velocity profile also oscillates with pulsatile flow, becoming parabolic when flow is near its peak and less so during the diastolic period, when velocity near the wall may even reverse its direction briefly.

As pulsations move on through the vascular system, the properties of the arterial tree transform the shape and timing of the waves.[8,12] The general features of this transformation and the reasons for it are important parts of cardiovascular physiology, but the quantitative details are of interest only to those engaged in specialized research. The mathematical analysis of pulsatile pressure and flow has reached a high level of sophistication.[8,10,39]

The elastic nature of arteries allows their diameter to follow the cyclic variations in pressure with each heartbeat, as shown in Figure 6.11. With nor-

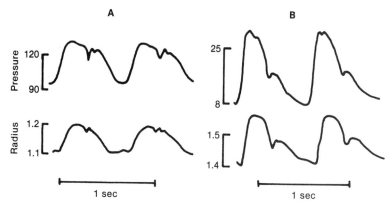

Figure 6.11.   Pressure (*above,* cm H$_2$O) and radius (*below,* cm) in ascending aorta (**A**) and main pulmonary artery (**B**) as functions of time, in human subject. (Reproduced with modifications from Patel et al.,[39] with permission of McGraw-Hill Book Co.)

mal pulse pressures, the diameter of the human and canine ascending aorta undergoes a pulsatile excursion that amounts to about ±2% of the mean diameter. Large distal branches like the common iliac artery are stiffer, and their radial pulsation is smaller for that reason.[8,40] The main pulmonary artery is the most compliant of the large arteries, and its distention with each heartbeat is about ±8%. Elastic modulus and pulsatile distention are thus correlated inversely, as shown in Table 6.3

The elastic parameters in Table 6.3 describe pressure–radius relationships for sinusoidal waves of a particular frequency, and represent *dynamic* measurements rather than the static moduli described earlier. They are expressed by what are known in mathematics as *complex numbers,* which consist of an amplitude and a phase angle.[5,8] The amplitude is the ratio of sinusoidal pressure to flow amplitudes, and the phase represents the relative timing of the two waves. Arterial distention lags slightly behind pressure, and this delay appears in Table 6.3 as a positive phase angle of the *complex viscoelastic modulus, E_c.* The equation for E_c is the same as equation 6.16, except that Δr and ΔP are complex numbers.

Although the word *stiffness* is often used in its everyday sense in discussions of elasticity, that term is applied to a specific variable in some experimental work and used instead of the viscoelastic modulus. *Stiffness* in that case is defined as the ratio $\Delta F/\Delta L$, which differs from the conventional elastic modulus by omitting the cross-sectional area and initial length (compare equation 6.15) and neglecting phase angles. This variable is a convenient way of expressing responses to experimental interventions in any given vascular strip if the phase shift between force and length is small. The cross-sectional area may

Table 6.3. Viscoelasticity of Canine Arterial Walls

ARTERY	PULSATION[a]	E_c (F = 1–3 HZ)[b] AMPLITUDE (10^6 DYN/CM^2)	PHASE (RAD)
Pulmonary (main)	7.8%	0.1	—
Aorta (thoracic)	1.5%	3.0	+0.09
Aorta (abdominal)	1.0%	9.9	+0.12
Iliac	0.2%	11.2	+0.20

[a]Percent of mean radius; from Patel et al.[40]

[b]E_c = complex viscoelastic modulus; pulmonary artery data from Patel et al.,[40] others from Gow and Taylor.[26]

change as the specimen is stretched, but the number of muscle fibers per unit area does not, making it appropriate to consider force rather than stress.

Pulse pressures

Part of each stroke volume moves through the aortic arch and into the thoracic aorta during systole, but another part distends the ascending aorta and is temporarily stored there, so to speak, until diastole begins. A portion of the right ventricular stroke volume is similarly stored in the main pulmonary artery. This storage takes on physiological significance because it determines the difference between systolic and diastolic pressures (i.e., the *pulse pressure*; Chapter 2).

Arterial pulse pressure depends on the size of the stroke volume and the elastic modulus of the vessel. The stiffer the vessel, the larger the pulse pressure for a given stroke volume. This relationship is consistently observed at the origins of the systemic and pulmonic circulations, and to some extent it persists into the large arteries. The distensibility of arteries is consequently the basis for the hemodynamic interpretation of systolic and diastolic pressures. Mean arterial pressure is also involved in this process, but equations 6.5 and 6.17 make it clear that mean pressure and pulse pressure are not determined by the same factors. Mean arterial pressure depends on mean flow, or cardiac output, and peripheral resistance. Cardiac output is the product of stroke volume and heart rate, to be sure, but mean pressure is not influenced by stroke volume per se.

Figure 6.12 illustrates these points, presenting diagrammatically the influence of resistance and stroke on mean and pulse pressures if there is no change in venous pressure or aortic elastic modulus. A control state is shown in Figure

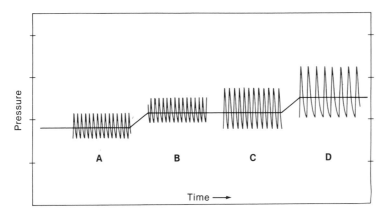

Figure 6.12. Effects of vascular resistance and stroke volume on arterial blood pressure, assuming constant venous pressure and arterial elasticity. Under such conditions, mean arterial pressure varies with cardiac output and resistance (equation 6.3), whereas pulse pressure varies with stroke volume. **A**, control state. **B**, increased vascular resistance, while stroke and heart rate (hence cardiac output) remain constant; mean pressure increases, but pulse pressure does not change. **C**, slower rate and proportionately increased stroke volume (giving same cardiac output as in **B**); mean pressure does not change because there has been no alteration of resistance or total blood flow, but pulse pressure increases because of elevated stroke. **D**, further slowing of rate and increase in stroke (still keeping output unchanged), plus increased resistance; both mean pressure and pulse pressure increase.

6.12A. Raising peripheral resistance while keeping cardiac output constant (i.e., no change in stroke volume or heart rate) causes an elevation in mean pressure but no change in pulse pressure, so that systolic and diastolic pressures necessarily rise (Figure 6.12B). If, starting from this new state and keeping the same peripheral resistance, stroke volume is increased and heart rate is reduced proportionately so that cardiac output remains the same, mean pressure will not change. Pulse pressure will increase, however, and this change, superimposed on a constant mean, raises systolic pressure and lowers diastolic pressure (Figure 6.12C). Next, a combination of these two maneuvers, further increasing resistance and stroke (but not output), raises both the mean and the pulse pressure, with the result that systolic pressure inevitably rises (Figure 6.12D). There is usually also an increase in diastolic pressure, but it may show no change or may even fall if the stroke volume increment dominates the response.

These simple rules are all that is needed to explain physiological changes in pulsatile blood pressure under most conditions. The principle is straightforward: Resistance and cardiac output themselves do not affect systolic or diastolic pressure, but the mean pressure they determine carries those oscillations up or down with it. This fact is a useful practical guide, although it does not provide quantitative interpretations because vascular elasticity is both frequency dependent and nonlinear. Quantitative analysis of each of the frequency components contained in pressure, flow, and radial pulsations is possible (see below) but is required only in certain kinds of research.

Note that the effects of a given hemodynamic change on diastolic pressure cannot always be predicted, a fact that is not widely appreciated. An impression once prevailed that diastolic pressure is directly related to peripheral resistance, but that is true only in special cases. Although raising peripheral resistance in the examples of Figure 6.12 did, indeed, raise diastolic pressure, exceptions can easily be imagined. A greater increase in stroke volume in Figure 6.12D, for instance, could have lowered diastolic pressure in spite of the increase in resistance.

Quantitative descriptions of pulsations

Any attempt to relate time-varying pulsations of blood pressure and flow to the properties of the cardiovascular system in a precise way requires that some specific model be adopted. An appropriate one should be translatable into mathematical equations in which properties like vascular resistance and viscoelasticity appear; given those properties, the equations should predict pulsatile waves like those found in the circulation. The best-known model of this kind was devised by Stephen Hales early in the eighteenth century. Perceiving that elastic arteries transform the discontinuous outflow from the heart into a relatively steady motion of blood in the peripheral vessels, he compared the arteries to an essential component of old-fashioned fire engines: the air compression chamber, where the repeated strokes of the water pump were smoothed into an almost continuous stream. This chamber, in the German translation *Windkessel,* is an enlightening metaphor that still permeates thinking about arterial function.

The *Windkessel* model, illustrated in Figure 6.13, has characteristics that are easily expressed in equations. Flow from a pump enters an elastic chamber through a one-way valve, entering more rapidly than it can leave by way of a narrow exit tube, or resistance, that impedes outflow. At the end of one pump stroke, pressure within the now distended chamber has been raised to P_0. The valve prevents backward flow, and fluid is driven through the resistance ($\mathbf{R}$) by the pressure within the chamber as the elastic wall begins to recoil. The outflow rate, Q, is then the decrease in chamber volume, V, per unit time, and $Q = dV/dt$. Resistance is defined in the usual way as the ratio of pressure to flow ($\mathbf{R} = P/Q$), and the absolute volumetric compliance of the chamber, dV/dP, is denoted by C. The quantity $\mathbf{R}C$ is then

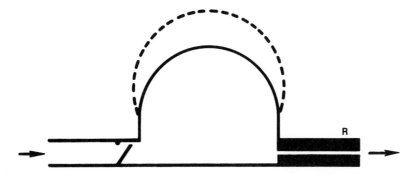

Figure 6.13.   Standard *Windkessel* model of the aorta and major arteries. Flow enters chamber through one-way valve on the left faster than it can leave through the exit on the right, raising the pressure and distending the elastic wall to position shown by *dashed line*. When inflow stops, valve closes and fluid leaves the chamber through the narrow resistance (**R**) on the right.

$$\frac{1}{RC} = \frac{dP}{PdV} \cdot \frac{dV}{dt} \qquad\qquad (6.18)$$

Integration of equation 6.18 with respect to time shows that pressure in the chamber declines exponentially from its initial value, P_0, during the period of outflow:

$$P(t) = P_0 \exp\left[\frac{-t}{RC}\right] \qquad\qquad (6.19)$$

One method of measuring arterial compliance, C, is to apply this equation to the declining diastolic portion of a pressure pulsation (which is approximately exponential in most cases), the resistance having been determined from mean pressure and flow.[44]

The simplicity of the *Windkessel* concept has made it popular, and countless modifications have been proposed to make it more suitable for various parts of the circulation.[8,39,45] Treating the whole arterial tree as a single compartment is unrealistic, of course, but that simplification is acceptable for many purposes.[45] In theory, equations derived from the *Windkessel* could be used to calculate stroke volume from measured pulse pressure, and many variations on this theme have been reported, but the accuracy of such calculations leaves much to be desired.[7] The *Windkessel* model is a vivid and instructive analogue for the behavior of elastic arteries, but its use as a source of quantitative physiological data is limited.

A quite different model of the circulation, with an equally long history, describes the movement of blood at every point in a tubular system by standard differential equations of force and motion. The classical foundations of this approach are the Navier-Stokes equations, which define, in cylindrical coordinates, the balance among forces associated with pressure, inertia, and viscosity.[8,9] These equations are nonlinear and general solutions are not available, but linear abbreviations of them are the basis for most theoretic work today. The versions most widely accepted as a basis for experimental work, which were developed by Womersley[46] and extended by McDonald and his associates,[7,43] take into account the viscoelasticity of blood and the vessel wall, and also the "tethering" of blood vessels to surrounding tissues. Each of these factors has small but significant effects on the relationships among the pressure, flow, and physical properties of the system. Equations that retain many of the appropriate nonlinear terms have also been derived.[30] A detailed account of these theories would be inappropriate here, but they have been reviewed elsewhere.[8,9]

Most analyses of this kind treat the blood vessel as a string of identical units, chained together so that pressure and flow waves pass through each one in sequence. The mathematical expression of such an arrangement has been extensively developed in the design of cables that transmit electricity over long distances, and for that reason such constructs are called *transmission-line models*.[8,32,43,46] Distributed systems avoid many of the limitations of simpler models, and the more intricate computations they entail can be readily performed by a digital computer.

Single-compartment, or *lumped,* models neglect all the variations in dimensions and physical properties within the arterial tree, and cannot be used to study pulse wave velocity or the transformation of pulse waves as they travel through the system. The *Windkessel* theory, for example, assumes that pressure is transmitted instantaneously to all parts of the chamber, that is, all arteries. Attempts to circumvent that problem by picturing the aorta as a series of *Windkessels* merely moves a few steps in the direction of transmission-line models.

The behavior of models of the circulation can often be duplicated in electrical networks, representing pressure by voltages and flow by electrical currents (or vice versa). Such models can be physical analogues made up of resistors, capacitors, and inductances, but more often the appropriate circuits are used as a kind of shorthand for the corresponding equations. A circuit that roughly imitates the *Windkessel* model is shown in Figure 6.14A. The network shown in Figure 6.14B is one of the repeated units in a mathematical transmission-line model designed by Taylor[43] to simulate the effects of viscoelasticity in the walls of blood vessels.

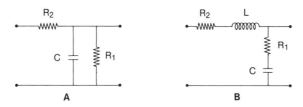

Figure 6.14.   Some electrical models of arteries. Resistor R_1 is the electrical analogue of longitudinal, steady-flow resistance. Capacitor C imitates the behavior of an elastic wall. Resistor R_2, coupled with C, represents wall viscoelasticity or leakage through side branches. Inductance L corresponds to inertia of the blood. **A**, *Windkessel* model. **B**, repeated element in transmission-line model of Taylor.[43]

Frequency analysis

Many theories of pulsatile hemodynamics are concerned with sinusoidal waves of pressure and flow oscillating around some positive average value. This approach, far from restricting the application of such theories, gives them unmatched power and versatility because of the array of mathematical techniques developed in the physical sciences for analysis of sinusoidal waveforms. The waves that occur in the circulation are not sinusoidal in shape, but they are equivalent to the sum of sinusoids of different amplitude and frequency, each of which can be defined quantitatively by numerical calculations. This principle holds for pulses of any shape as long as they are periodic, repeating at regular intervals.

Frequency analysis by Fourier or other methods has found many applications, ranging from astronomy to the molecular structure of DNA. It provides a complete quantitative expression of pressure and flow pulses when that is required, but it is well to remember that such precision is not always needed. The marked changes in the contour of pressure waves sometimes caused by reflections, for instance, is easily recognized in oscillographic records (Figure 2.6), and the slow rise of the arterial pulse in certain types of valvular disease can be detected clinically by palpation.

Frequency analysis techniques dissect a waveform into a series of sinusoids, as shown in Figure 6.15. The observed wave in this example consisted of a single flow pulsation from a canine pulmonary artery, indicated by the dotted line in the topmost record. The four sinusoidal waves below were calculated by the Fourier method (see below) after the observed wave was first converted into a string of digits equivalent to readings of flow every 0.01 sec (analogue-to-digital conversion; Chapter 14). The continuous line in the top

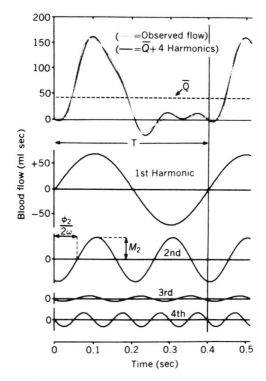

Figure 6.15. Fourier series derived from an experimentally recorded flow pulsation. *Abscissa*, time; *ordinates*, blood flow. *Dotted line* in uppermost panel is a record of flow in the canine pulmonary artery. This record was converted to digital form and subjected to harmonic analysis, producing a Fourier-series representation of the original data. The Fourier series consists of a mean flow ($\bar{Q}$) and a set of sinusoidal waves, or harmonics. The first harmonic is at the frequency of the heartbeat; the second harmonic, at twice that frequency; and so on. Four harmonics are shown here, and their sum equals the *solid line* superimposed on the record in the upper panel. The amplitude (M_2) and phase (ϕ_2) of the second harmonic are indicated. Phase angles specify the timing of each sinusoidal wave in relation to the others.

panel is the sum of those four waves at each instant of time, plus mean flow, and the result is almost identical to the original pulsation.

The four computed sinusoidal waves in Figure 6.15 are an example of a *Fourier series,* one of the most common methods of examining the frequency content of a periodic function. An alternative technique called *spectral analysis,* based on correlation functions,[6,8] is preferred in some applications. The description and equations that follow are intended to convey the general nature of the Fourier approach; other text books should be consulted for many details that are important in theory and in practice.[1,5,6,8] The calculation of Fourier terms from experimental data is usually carried out in the laboratory by a digital computer and commercially available programs, but it is unwise to delegate any computational task to a machine without understanding, at least in principle, the processes involved.

Fourier's theorem states that any periodic function, $g(t)$, is equal to the sum of an infinite series of terms:

$$g(t) = \frac{A_0}{2} + \sum_{n=1}^{n=\infty} \cdot (A_n \cos n\omega t + B_n \sin n\omega t) \qquad (6.20)$$

The mean value of the function is $A_0/2$, and for each value of n the corresponding cosine–sine pair defines a sinusoidal wave of frequency $n\omega$, the nth harmonic. Each harmonic is a complex number equivalent to $M \cos (n\omega t - \phi)$, where the amplitude $M = (A^2 + B^2)^{1/2}$, and the phase angle ϕ is arctan (B/A). The theory is based on integration, but the finite summation in equation 6.20 is the form used in practice. The sum cannot include an infinite number of terms, of course, but it is carried to a number consonant with the frequencies contained in the original data, within limits set by the analogue-to-digital conversion interval.[6,8]

By definition, a periodic function of time, $g(t)$, equals $g(t + T)$ for all t; the interval between repetitions is thus T. The fundamental frequency, f, is $1/T$ pulses/sec (the same as the heart rate in cardiovascular applications). The sinusoidal wave calculated at that frequency is called the *first harmonic* of the original pulsation. The second harmonic is a wave at twice that frequency, and further harmonics can be calculated at integral multiples of the fundamental frequency. In Figure 6.15, the sum of the first four harmonics comes very close to reproducing the waveform from which they were derived, but in other cases more harmonics are required to achieve that result.

The first, or fundamental, harmonic is always the largest in amplitude, and the size of the subsequent terms decreases rapidly with frequency. The first five harmonics contain 95% of the energy in most pressure and flow waves *in vivo*, but harmonics up to the 20th may be required to include all the sharp details. As heart rate increases, the second and higher harmonics diminish in size, and at very fast rates the arterial pressure comes to resemble an almost pure sinusoidal oscillation at the fundamental frequency.

Frequencies can be expressed in cycles per second (hertz) or radians per second. Radians, like degrees, measure angles; $90° = 1.57 \ldots$ radians. Sinusoids can be represented graphically as projections of the rotating radius of a circle, and angular units are useful in describing time relationships between sinusoidal waves because one revolution (i.e., one complete cycle) equals 360°, or 2π radians. The customary symbol for circular frequency is ω ($= 2\pi f$).

The Fourier coefficients A and B are calculated from the following equations:

$$A_n = \frac{2}{T} \int_{-T/2}^{T/2} g(t) \cos n\omega t \cdot dt \qquad \text{(for } n = 0, 1, 2, \ldots\text{)} \qquad (6.21)$$

$$B_n = \frac{2}{T} \int_{-T/2}^{T/2} g(t) \sin n\omega t \cdot dt \qquad \text{(for } n = 0, 1, 2, \ldots\text{)} \qquad (6.22)$$

Linear systems

From one point of view, a vascular bed can be regarded as a system in which a given driving pressure (input) produces a certain blood flow (output). Like other waveforms, this input and output can be expressed as the sum of a set of sinusoidal waves. Furthermore, in what are called *linear systems*, each of those sinusoidal components seems to preserve an independent existence, unaffected by others that may accompany it. A blood vessel can thus be treated as a "black box" that transforms waveforms at its input into waves of different size and timing at its output. The interior of the box is the most fascinating part for the physiologist; defining the relation between input and output is one step toward discovering the mechanisms concealed there.

By applying sinusoidal pressures generated by a pump, the relation of output to input can be determined at a number of different frequencies, taking into account any time delays as well as the relative amplitudes. If the system is linear with respect to pressure–flow relations—which has been found to be approximately true for the pulmonic and systemic beds as a whole—several consequences follow. First, the output will be sinusoidal, and its frequency will be the same as that at the input. Second, the output/input amplitude ratio and time shift will be constant at any one frequency, regardless of the absolute size of the input. Third, the output/input characteristics at any one frequency will remain unchanged when other frequencies are added to them at the input, which is the case with waves of physiological shape. The behavior at 1 Hz, for example, will be the same whether the 1-Hz wave is present in isolation or accompanied by harmonics at other frequencies.

It is this last property that opens the door to a number of physiological applications. Any linear, frequency-dependent phenomenon can be studied with the pulsations that exist *in vivo*, and the conclusions reached will apply to pulses of other shapes. Vascular impedance,[8] a ratio of pressure to flow pulsations, falls in this category (see below), as do some modes of calculating external cardiac work (Chapter 4). The approach cannot be used with all cardiovascular relationships, however, as the nonlinear correlation between transmural pressure and vessel diameter demonstrates (Figure 6.5). Indeed, no system in the real world is perfectly linear; the questions to be asked are how far it departs from linearity and what errors are introduced by treating it as if it were linear.

Vascular impedance

The effect of vascular dimensions and viscoelasticity on the relation between pulses of pressure and flow is defined as an impedance. In contrast to vascular resistance, which is *mean* pressure divided by *mean* flow (equation 6.5), *vascular impedance* is the ratio of pressure to flow *pulsations,* or, to be exact, the ratios of their sinusoidal components at each harmonic frequency. Impedance thus expresses the opposition offered by vessels or vascular beds to pulsatile flow, just as resistance expresses the opposition to steady flow. Both must be overcome by energy that the heart supplies to move blood in a pulsatile fashion.

Vascular impedance of any part of the circulation can be calculated by frequency analysis of pressure and flow pulsations that have been recorded simultaneously.[8,16,34-36] The impedance amplitude at each harmonic frequency is the ratio of pressure to flow amplitudes, and the phase difference between pressure and flow sinusoids is the impedance phase angle. The result is a complex impedance spectrum like that shown in Figure 6.16, which was constructed from measurements in the ascending aortas of a group of normal human subjects.[36] Impedance at this site, the origin of the systemic circulation, has a fundamental significance: The spectrum represents the energy-dissipating properties of the systemic vascular tree, the opposition faced by the left ventricle as it ejects blood. In effect, aortic impedance expresses the afterload on the ventricle and determines how much work the ventricle must do to produce a given pulsatile flow (Chapter 4).

The frequency of the first harmonic in Figure 6.16 is 1.1 Hz, the heart rate, and nine harmonics are shown. The ratio of mean arterial pressure to mean flow (cardiac output) is plotted at $f = 0$. This term can be regarded as the impedance at a "frequency" of zero, but it is usually referred to as the *input resistance* (see above), and it is considerably higher than the impedance to pulsatile waves. The impedance observed in any artery is called the *input impedance* of the vascular bed it supplies. The amplitude of the aortic input impedance, $|Z_x|$, falls sharply from 0 to about 2 Hz, decreases less steeply to a minimum in the neighborhood of 3 Hz, and rises to a secondary peak in the 6- to 8-Hz region. Phase angles are negative between 0 and about 3 Hz, indicating that flow leads pressure. The spectrum of impedance in the main pulmonary artery is similar, but the amplitudes are smaller. Normal values of impedance and input resistance in some vessels are given in Table 6.4

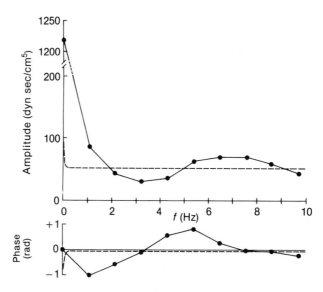

Figure 6.16. Impedance in ascending aorta as a function of frequency (*abscissa*) in normal adult human subjects. *Ordinates*, impedance amplitude above, phase angle below. *Solid line*, observed (input) impedance; *dashed line*, theoretical characteristic impedance in the absence of reflections, calculated from equation 6.23. (From data reported by Nichols et al.[36])

The frequency-dependent swings of impedance amplitude and phase are the result of reflected waves that are always present in the arterial system (see below). Peripheral vasoconstriction increases the reflections and thus changes the spectrum, making the impedance amplitudes larger at some frequencies and smaller at others. Arteriolar vasodilatation has the opposite effect, minimizing the impedance oscillations. Reflections do not affect mean pressure and flow or resistance. If reflections were absent, the spectrum would depend only on

Table 6.4. Impedance and Input Resistance in Canine and Human Blood Vessels[a]

	DOG		MAN	
	R_{in}[b]	Z_0[c]	R_{in}[b]	Z_0[c]
Ascending aorta	4,700	250	1,200	50
Pulmonary	580	180	190	22
Femoral	110,000	16,000	42,000	7,400

[a]Units, dyn sec/cm[5]; from data reported on canine vessels by Attinger,[12] Bergel and Milnor,[16] Milnor and Nichols,[34]; human vessels, Nichols et al.,[36] Patel et al.,[39] Murgo and Westerhof.[35]

[b]R_{in} = input resistance, based on input pressure alone (see text) and hence higher than the conventional resistances in Table 6.1.

[c]Characteristic impedance amplitude at 2 Hz.

the properties of the vessel where the measurements were made, the *characteristic impedance* (Z_0). In large vessels Z_0 is almost independent of frequency, as indicated by the dashed line in Figure 6.16, and it is the baseline around which the swings generated by reflections occur.

The properties of a vessel that determine its impedance can be formulated in the same way that the factors involved in resistance are expressed in equation 6.6, but in this case a number of different equations have been proposed. One of the most widely used mathematical models, devised by Womersley,[46] describes characteristic impedance at a frequency f as follows:

$$Z_0(f) = \frac{P(f)}{Q(f)} = \frac{\rho}{\pi r^2} \cdot \Phi \tag{6.23}$$

where all terms except the radius, r, are complex (i.e., expressed by an amplitude and a phase angle), and Φ is a function of frequency, viscosity, the ratio of wall thickness to radius, and the elastic modulus of the vessel.

The resemblance to the Poiseuille relationship is evident (equation 6.3), but the function Φ contains several new variables that are now relevant, notably elasticity. Descriptions of the other relationships symbolized here by the complex function Φ can be found elsewhere.[8,43,46] The most important consequence is that impedance amplitude is directly related to elastic modulus. Other factors being equal, the stiffer the vessel, the higher the impedance, a theoretic prediction that has been confirmed experimentally.[37] Stimulation of the sympathetic constrictor nerves of pulmonary vessels, which activates and stiffens the vascular smooth muscle, raises the characteristic impedance of that bed.[28,38] The system described by equation 6.23 is a linear one, but experimental tests show that this linear model comes very close to predicting hemodynamic conditions *in vivo*. Numerous small nonlinearities have been detected,[30] each of them capable of producing discrepancies of 2 or 3%, but the cumulative error appears to be about $\pm 10\%$ in practice.

The concept of impedance can also be applied in ways that do not require quantitative analysis. It implies, for example, that the higher the impedance amplitude, the greater the pulse pressure for a given pulsatile flow. This rule is usually a reliable guide, although the mixture of waves of different frequency and phase in physiological pulsations sometimes invalidates it. The spectra of aortic and pulmonary impedance also suggest an important relation between cardiac work and heart rate. The rate determines the frequency of the fundamental harmonic, which is associated with most of the energy involved in moving blood, and the impedance minimum found at approximately 2 to 3 Hz in man (Figure 6.16) corresponds to heart rates during exercise. The relation between rate and the impedance spectrum thus seems to be optimal, minimizing the pulsatile work of the heart. (The distinction between steady and pulsatile cardiac work is discussed in Chapter 4.) This conclusion must be regarded as no more than a tempting hypothesis at present, but it is supported by observations on species that have faster heart rates, where the impedance spectrum is displaced to the right and the early minimum falls at higher frequencies.[33]

Branching Systems

The tree-like branching of the arterial system is one of its most obvious features, and from a hemodynamic point of view it can be treated as an assembly of elastic tubes, each of them conducting pulsatile flow according to the principles already considered. The one new phenomenon that appears in branching systems arises from the changing dimensions and elasticity of arteries from origin to periphery. The sites of branching, in particular, represent abrupt modifications of local vascular properties, and wherever there is such a change, the oncoming waves of pressure and flow are partially reflected.[8,9]

As a result, the pulsation observed at any point in the arterial tree is the sum of a forward-moving and a retrograde wave. There is no hint of this mixture in ordinary records, but with appropriate experimental procedures it can be shown that about 20% of the pressure wave arriving at the origin of the femoral artery is reflected back, while the remaining 80% travels on.[25] In a tube that contains pulses traveling in both directions, the waves will be exactly in phase at some points but 180° out of phase at others. The pulsation observed at any point will be the algebraic sum of the antegrade and retrograde waves, which will partly cancel each other at out-of-phase sites and add together to produce a relatively large pulse at points where they are in phase. The situation is much like that in the string of a musical instrument, which vibrates with a large amplitude at some places and scarcely moves at others.

The effects can be illustrated by comparing the transmission of pressure waves in a uniform tube with that in a branching system that generates reflections. In the first case (Figure 6.17A), where no reflected waves are present, the pulsations are simply attenuated by viscous effects as they move down the tube. This dissipation of pulsatile pressure is analogous to the fall in mean pressure along the length of the tube in accordance with Poiseuille's law (equation 6.3 and Figure 6.4A). In the presence of reflections, however, the alternate reinforcement and cancellation of forward- and backward-moving waves causes the pressure amplitude to oscillate regularly (Figure 6.17B).

The same phenomena appear in the circulation, although the aorta is the only place where they are readily apparent. Pulse pressure is greater in the distal than in the ascending aorta in most subjects (Figure 6.18), and it would be difficult to explain that observation without assuming the presence of reflected waves. In terms of wavelength, which is the relevant parameter, the

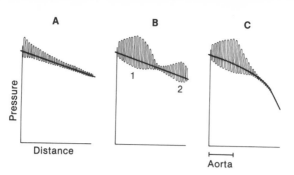

Figure 6.17. Transmission of pulsatile pressure waves (*ordinate*, showing mean, systolic, and diastolic) as a function of distance (*abscissa*). **A**, attenuation of pulse pressure by viscous effects in an infinitely long tube of constant diameter and elasticity (no reflections). **B**, waxing and waning of pulse pressure in a similar tube terminated by an impedance that generates reflected waves; incident and reflected waves are in phase at some points and produce large pulse pressure (*1, 2*) but are out of phase at others, yielding small pulses; mean pressure falls as in **A**, and viscous attenuation makes the second maximum smaller than the first. **C**, pressures in mammalian systemic arterial tree; reflections cause pulse pressure to rise to a maximum near the end of aorta; in more distal vessels, viscosity reduces pulse (and mean) pressures so that a second maximum does not appear.

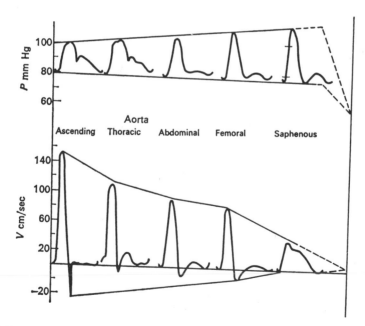

Figure 6.18. Pressure (*above*) and blood velocity (*below*) in canine aorta and distal branches, showing amplification of pressure pulses by reflected waves. (Reproduced from McDonald,[7] with permission of Edward Arnold, Ltd)

aorta is not long enough to exhibit repeated waxing and waning of pressure pulsations, but it clearly shows a gradual enlargement of pulse pressure from its origin to its distal portion. Beyond that, viscous attenuation dominates the picture, and pulse pressure diminishes steadily as the vessel radii become smaller and smaller (Figure 6.17C). The reflected waves originate mainly from small peripheral arteries, but also from the progressively changing diameter and elasticity of the aorta itself.

Circular Systems

One last group of facts about the mammalian cardiovascular system must be considered to complete this discussion of the hemodynamic principles that operate as blood moves in a pulsating fashion through a branching, viscoelastic array of vessels. To begin with, the system is one that literally *circulates* the blood, moving it continuously out to the periphery and back to the heart again. It is also a *closed* system except for transfers through capillary walls, where any small net loss of fluid is balanced by lymph returned to the central veins (Chapter 10). The closed nature of the circulation ensures that pressures and volumes in different parts of the system are interdependent. Finally, it is an *elastic* system that has been filled with a volume of blood sufficient to distend it.

The distended state signifies an underlying pressure that depends on total blood volume and vascular compliance. The pressures generated by cardiac contraction are not part of this baseline level but are superimposed on it. Evidence for the existence of such a noncardiac pressure comes from experiments in which the action of the heart is temporarily interrupted, usually by causing ventricular fibrillation (Chapter 5). Arterial pressure falls rapidly to a low level, but venous pressures rise as blood redistributes itself within the vascular system, running from the previously high-pressure arteries into the veins.

The volume of the venous compartment thus rises at the expense of the arteries, and in about 30 sec an equilibrium has been established, with a uniform pressure in all parts of the vascular system, the MCFP.[27] When the heart is restarted, pressures return to their former levels after a few heartbeats. The fact that arterial pressures fall and venous pressures rise to reach an equilibrium while the heart is inactive suggests that some point in the microcirculation is at the MCFP level when the heart is beating normally, and this point appears to be in the venules.

The usual MCFP is between 7 and 12 mm Hg, but it becomes higher when total blood volume is increased by transfusion of blood or lower after a hemorrhage. Alterations in vascular compliance can have a similar effect, as can be demonstrated by infusing drugs that cause venoconstriction while total blood volume remains constant. The MCFP rises because activation of venous smooth muscle alters pressure–volume relationships in the venous compartment, displacing a certain amount of blood from veins to arteries and raising the overall equilibrium pressure. Vasomotor stimuli or changes in blood volume produce similar changes in mean pressures when the heart is beating normally, but reflex actions are often mixed with the effects of MCFP under those conditions.

The potency of venomotor stimuli was measured in experiments on dogs by substituting a pump for the heart and connecting an external reservoir connected to the venous circulation.[17] When reflex venodilatation was induced by raising pressure in the isolated carotid sinuses, blood moved from the reservoir into the animal's vascular system unless the "cardiac output" of the pump was lowered by 20 to 30%, demonstrating the large circulatory effect of the change in venomotor tone.

Similar experiments have shown that venoconstriction can displace at least 10% of the total blood volume from veins into other parts of the circulation. The influence of regional compliances on such shifts is discussed in Chapter 13. Increased venous tone not only redistributes the blood volume but also often raises venous pressure, an effect that acts on cardiac output by raising ventricular filling pressure (Chapter 4). Evidence of this nature shows the hemodynamic importance of venous distensibility and the significant role played by vasomotor control of capacitance vessels, which might not be guessed from the relatively small changes in venous and arterial pressure that occur. It also demonstrates the interaction among different segments of a circular system.

Hemodynamic Effects of Vasomotor Activity

The hemodynamic effects to be expected from neural or other vasomotor stimuli can, as a rule, be predicted from the principles outlined in this chapter. Localized events cannot be interpreted in isolation, however, and the interdependence of different parts of the circulation makes it necessary to view the system as a whole. For instance, when the resistance of arterioles or venules is altered by small changes in the caliber of those vessels, such vasomotor activity causes a change in local blood flow *provided* that pressure in the main perfusing artery remains constant. The latter proviso must be added because simultaneous cardiac and vascular responses can interact. A combination of regional arteriolar constriction and enhanced cardiac performance could raise prearteriolar pressure, and local blood flow might then remain constant or even increase in spite of the new, higher resistance. Another instance of interdependence can be found in the effects of parallel resistances; if cardiac output is constant, vasodilatation in one organ necessarily reduces flow to others.

The influence of transmural pressure on diameter must also be kept in mind, and it is desirable to adopt a terminology that distinguishes between the effects of transmural pressure and those of smooth muscle activity. The terms *vasoconstriction* and *vasodilatation* should be reserved for changes in vascular caliber produced by smooth muscle activity. Changes in active smooth muscle force can be described in terms of *tone,* whether or not accompanied by changes in vessel diameter (increased tone and increased transmural pressure together might leave the diameter unchanged). Passive responses to transmural pressure alone can appropriately be referred to as *distention* or *collapse.*

References

Reviews

1. Bendat, J.S., Piersol, A.G. (1971). *Random Data: Analysis and Measurement Procedures.* New York, Wiley Interscience.
2. Bergel, D.H., Schultz, D.L. (1971). Arterial elasticity and fluid dynamics. *Prog. Biophys. Mol. Biol.* 22:1–36.
3. Burton, A.C. (1954). Relation of structure to function of the tissues of the walls of blood vessels. *Physiol. Rev.* 34:619–642.
4. Caro, C.G., Pedley, J.G., Schroter, R.C., Seed, W.A. (1978). *The Mechanics of the Circulation.* Oxford, Oxford University Press.
5. Franklin, P. (1949). *An Introduction to Fourier Methods and the Laplace Transformation.* New York, Dover.
6. Lee, Y.W. (1960). *Statistical Theory of Communication.* New York, Wiley.
7. McDonald, D.A. (1974). *Blood Flow in Arteries.* London, Edward Arnold.
8. Milnor, W.R. (1989). *Hemodynamics,* 2nd ed. Baltimore, Williams & Wilkins.
9. Noordergraaf, A. (1969). Hemodynamics. In: *Bio-Engineering,* H. Schwann, ed. New York, McGraw-Hill, pp. 391–545.
10. Wetterer, E., Kenner, T. (1978). *Die Dynamik des Arterien-pulses.* Berlin, Springer-Verlag.
11. Whitmore, R.L. (1968). *Rheology of the Circulation.* Oxford, Pergamon Press.

Research Papers

12. Attinger, E.O., Sugawara, H., Navarro, A., Mikami, T., Martin, R. (1967). Flow patterns in the peripheral circulation of the anesthetized dog. *Angiologica* 4:1–27.
13. Bellamy, F.F. (1978). Diastolic coronary artery pressure–flow relations in the dog. *Circ. Res.* 43:92–101.
14. Bellhouse, B.J., Bellhouse, F.H. (1968). Mechanism of closure of the aortic valve. *Nature* 217:86–87.

15. Bergel, D.H. (1961). The dynamic elastic properties of the arterial wall. *J. Physiol.* 156:458–469.

16. Bergel, D.H., Milnor, W.R. (1965). Pulmonary vascular impedance in the dog. *Circ. Res.* 16:401–415.

17. Braunwald, E., Ross, J., Jr., Kamler, R.L., Gaffney, T.E., Goldblatt, A., Mason, D.T. (1963). Reflex control of the systemic venous bed. *Circ. Res.* 12:539–549.

18. Cooke, P.H., Fay, F.S. (1972). Correlation between fiber length, ultrastructure, and the length–tension relationship of mammalian smooth muscle. *Cell Biol.* 52: 105–116.

19. Cox, R.H. 1984). Viscoelastic properties of canine pulmonary arteries. *Am. J. Physiol.* 246. (*Heart Circ. Physiol.* 15):H90–H96.

20. Dobrin, P.B., Rovick, A.A. (1969). Influence of vascular smooth muscle on contractile mechanics and elasticity of arteries. *Am. J. Physiol.* 217:1644–1651.

21. Ferencz, C. (1969). Pulmonary arterial design in mammals. Morphologic variation and physiologic constancy. *Johns Hopkins Med. J.* 125:207–224.

22. Fischer, G.M., Liaurado, J.G. (1966). Collagen and elastin content in canine arteries selected from functionally different vascular beds. *Circ. Res.* 19:394–399.

23. Fry, D.L. (1973). Responses of the arterial wall to certain physical factors. In: *Atherosclerosis: Initiating Factors.* Ciba Foundation Symposium 12 (N.S.). Amsterdam, Association of Scientific Publishers, pp. 93–125.

24. Gentile, B.J., Gross, D.R. (1985). Viscoelastic behavior of the thoracic aorta of dogs and rabbits. *Circ. Res.* 56:690–695.

25. Gessner, U., Bergel, D.H. (1966). Methods of determining the distensibility of blood vessels. *IEEE Trans. Biomed. Eng.* BME-13:2–10.

26. Gow, B.S., Taylor, M.G. (1968). Measurement of viscoelastic properties of arteries in the living dog. *Circ. Res.* 23:111–122.

27. Guyton, A.C., Polizo, D., Armstrong, G.G. (1954). Mean circulatory filling pressure measured immediately after cessation of heart pumping. *Am. J. Physiol.* 179:261–272.

28. Ingram, R.H., Szidon, J.O., Skalak, R., Fishman, A.P. (1968). Effects of sympathetic nerve stimulation on the pulmonary arterial tree of the isolated lobe perfused in situ. *Circ. Res.* 22:801–815.

29. Katz, A.I., Chen, Y., Moreno, A.L. (1969). Flow through a collapsible tube. Experimental analysis and mathematical model. *Biophys. J.* 9:1261–1279.

30. Ling, S.C., Atabek, H.B., Letzing, W.G., Patel, D.J. (1973). Nonlinear analysis of aortic flow in living dogs. *Circ. Res.* 33:198–212.

31. Liu, Z., Brin, K.P., Yin, F.C.P. (1986). Estimation of total arterial compliance: An improved method and evaluation of current methods. *Am. J. Physiol.* 251 (*Heart Circ. Physiol*) 20:H588–H600.

32. McIlroy, M.B., Seitz, W.S., Targett, R.C. (1986). A transmission line model of the normal aorta and its branches. *Cardiovasc. Res.* 20:581–587.

33. Milnor, W.R. (1979). Aortic wavelength as a determinant of the relation between heart rate and body size in mammals. *Am. J. Physiol.* 237 (*Reg. Integr. Comp. Physiol.* 6):R3–R6.

34. Milnor, W.R., Nichols, W.W. (1975). A new method of measuring propagation coefficients and characteristic impedance in blood vessels. *Circ. Res.* 36:631–639.

35. Murgo, J.P., Westerhof, N. (1984). Input impedance of the pulmonary arterial system in normal man. Effects of respiration and comparison to systemic impedance. *Circ. Res.* 54:666–673.

36. Nichols, W.W., Conti, C.R., Walker, W.E., Milnor, W.R. (1977). Input impedance of the systemic circulation in man. *Circ. Res.* 40:451–458.

37. O'Rourke, M.F. (1967). Steady and pulsatile energy losses in the systemic circulation under normal conditions and in simulated arterial disease. *Cardiovasc. Res.* 1:312–326.

38. Pace, J.B., Cox, R.H., Alvarez-Vara, F., Karreman, G. (1972). Influence of sympathetic nerve stimulation on pulmonary hydraulic input power. *Am. J. Physiol.* 222:196–201.

39. Patel, D.J., Greenfield, J.C., Jr., Auten, W.G., Morrow, A.G., Fry, D.L. (1965). Pressure–flow relationships in the ascending aorta and femoral artery of man. *J. Appl. Physiol.* 20:459–463.

40. Patel, D.J., Greenfield, J.C., Jr., Fry, D.L. (1964). In vivo pressure–length–radius relationship of certain blood vessels in man and dog. In: *Pulsatile Blood Flow*, E.O. Attinger, ed. New York, McGraw-Hill, pp. 293–305.

41. Permutt, S., Riley, R.L. (1963). Hemodynamics of collapsible vessels with tone: The vascular waterfall. *J. Appl. Physiol.* 17:893–898.

42. Poiseuille, J.L.M. (1846). Recherches experimentales sur le mouvement des liquides dans les tubes de tres-petits diametres. *Memoires presentes par divers savants a l'Acad. Sci. de l'Institut de France* 9:433.

43. Taylor, M.G. (1959). An experimental determination of the propagation of fluid oscillations in a tube with a visco-elastic wall; together with an analysis of the characteristics required in an electrical analogue. *Phys. Med. Biol.* 4:63–82.

44. Toorop, G.P., Westerhof, N., Elzinga, G. (1987). Beat-to-beat estimation of peripheral resistance and arterial compliance during pressure transients. *Am. J. Physiol.* 252 (*Heart Circ. Physiol.* 21):H1275–H1283.

45. Westerhof, N., Elzinga, G., Sipkema, P. (1971). An artificial system for pumping hearts. *J. Appl. Physiol.* 31:776–781.

46. Womersley, J.R. (1957). Oscillatory flow in arteries: The constrained elastic tube as a model of arterial flow and pulse transmission. *Phys. Med. Biol.* 2:178–187.

47. Zatzman, M., Stacy, R.W., Randall, J., Eberstein, A. (1954). Time course of stress relaxation in isolated arterial segments. *Am. J. Physiol.* 197:299–302.

7

THE CARDIOVASCULAR CONTROL SYSTEM

A highly organized control system ensures adequate circulation of blood to all parts of the body under a wide variety of external conditions. During physical exertion, for example, cardiac output increases and vascular adjustments direct most of the increment to the exercising muscles. This continuous adaptation of function to physiological needs depends on a communication and control network that may be divided into four parts for purposes of discussion:

1. Central nervous system.
2. Sensors and afferent nerves.
3. Autonomic (efferent) nerves.
4. Humoral agents (blood-borne or local).

The first three of these divisions, which are agents of what might be called *central* control, are covered in this chapter. The fourth category, which represents mechanisms of *peripheral* regulation that do not necessarily involve the central nervous system, is described in Chapter 8. Central and peripheral mechanisms are equally important in cardiovascular regulation.

The state of the circulation is monitored at critical points by structures that act as *sensors,* which send information back to the brain over *afferent* neural pathways. Stretch sensors in arterial walls (baroreceptors) are the classical example, but other kinds exist in various regions. The brain integrates the information received from all sources and generates outgoing (*efferent*) signals to the active tissues of the cardiovascular system, namely, the myocardium,

219

the pacemaking and conducting cells of the heart, and the smooth muscle of blood vessels. Data from all parts of the body are taken into account.

The efferent impulses are carried in branches of the autonomic nervous system, which innervate the heart and blood vessels as well as many other organs. Autonomic nerves are classified as either *sympathetic* or *parasympathetic,* a distinction based primarily on the anatomical location of the fibers. The peripheral outflow of parasympathetic nerves is limited to the cranial and sacral regions, whereas that of sympathetic nerves extends along the spinal cord. Postganglionic sympathetic fibers originate from the lateral chain of ganglia adjacent to the cord and travel relatively long distances to the tissue they supply. Parasympathetic ganglia lie near, or even within, the structures they innervate. Norepinephrine is the characteristic postganglionic neurotransmitter for most sympathetic nerves, and acetylcholine is the neurotransmitter for parasympathetic terminals.

This neural system is not the only means by which cardiovascular function is regulated. Hormones and other active substances are carried by the bloodstream to all tissues, the catecholamines secreted by the adrenal medulla being a prominent example. In addition, the cells of the heart and vessels are affected by the locally modulated concentrations of metabolites and a host of other compounds. All the parts of this complex regulatory system interact, and the operation of each separate part contributes to the net effect.

Central Nervous System

Early students of cardiovascular control observed the effects of transection of the brain stem at various levels, or of stimulation of selected points in the central nervous system. The results of such experiments suggested that vasoconstriction and vasodilatation are controlled by two "centers" in the medulla and pons (Figure 7.1). Subsequent research showed this view to be an oversimplification, for regulation of the heart and blood vessels is by no means restricted to the medulla. The so-called vasomotor centers do indeed contain many neurons involved with cardiovascular control, but their function is modulated by signals from other areas.

Modern technology has provided many new tools for the investigation of neural control, including autoradiography, immunohistology, axonally transported labels, and compounds that mark the degree of activity of cell bodies. The picture that has emerged is one of complex circuits that connect different levels, rather than specialized centers.[19] Neurons in the spinal cord, medulla, hypothalamus, and limbic and other forebrain structures are involved, and communication among them is an inherent part of the process that leads to the final output signal. Pathways concerned with a particular physiological re-

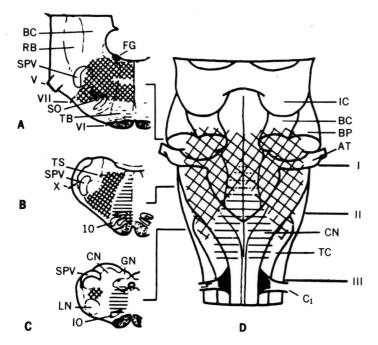

Figure 7.1.   Localization of pressor (*crosshatched*) and depressor (*horizontal lines*) "centers" in feline brain stem. **A, B, C,** cross sections through medulla at levels indicated. **D,** projection of pressor and depressor regions onto dorsal surface of brain stem (cerebral penduncles cut and cerebellum removed). *AT,* auditory tubercle; *BC,* brachium conjunctiva; *BP,* brachium pontis; C_1, first cervical nerve; *CN,* cuneate nucleus; *FG,* facial genu; *GN,* gracile nucleus; *IC,* inferior colliculus; *IO,* inferior olivary nucleus; *LN,* lateral reticular nucleus; *RB,* restiform body; *SO,* superior olivary nucleus; *SPV,* spinal trigeminal tract; *TB,* trapezoidal body; *TC,* tuberculum cinereum; *TS,* tractus solitarius; *V* to *VII,* cranial nerves; *I* to *III,* levels of transection discussed in text. (Reproduced from Alexander,[26] with permission of *J. Neurophysiol.*)

sponse often come together in circumscribed medullary or hypothalamic regions, but such areas are only part of a widely distributed network. Any combination of afferent signals, sometimes described as an *input profile,*[14,62] is converted by the central processing system into a set of efferent impulses that triggers an appropriate peripheral response. The regulatory network is capable of producing general or localized peripheral responses. Autonomic signals can be limited to effects on heart rate, contractile force, or the blood vessels of one particular region, as the situation requires. The regions in the nervous system that receive input from peripheral sensors, the interconnections within the system, and the eventual sources of outgoing signals are gradually being identified, but the map is far from complete.

The basal pattern of sympathetic efferent impulses is set by one or more groups of central nervous system neurons that act as oscillators, firing two to six impulses per second (Chapter 8). These oscillators maintain a more or less constant rate even after baroreceptor denervation and decerebration at the mid-collicular level. In the intact animal, they are modulated by inputs from baroreceptors, so that the sympathetic output is synchronized with the arterial pulse. Parasympathetic efferent signals are less regular, but some are entrained by cyclic inputs from pulmonary stretch receptors. Parasympathetic neurons in the nucleus ambiguus, for example, fire only during expiration.[54] The ultimate rate and pattern of autonomic efferent impulses are thus determined by oscillator outputs modified by central processing.[10]

Spinal cord

The spinal cord was long regarded as no more than a relay station for signals to the cardiovascular system, but that view has been revised. Newer evidence shows that both excitatory and inhibitory messages from medullary and higher levels are integrated in the cord.[5] The spinal cord and its associated ganglia can maintain a certain amount of vascular regulation even in the absence of higher centers.

Transection of the spinal cord in the cervical region produces an abrupt fall in blood pressure that has been called *spinal shock*. If the phrenic nerve and sympathetic preganglionic outflow are preserved, as is the case for sections between C6 and T1, the animal survives and after a few days exhibits a normal blood pressure. Such chronic spinal animals can compensate almost as well as normal specimens for moderate losses of blood up to about 20% of total blood volume. This adaptation is difficult to account for in the absence of a baroreceptor feedback loop, but it may arise from hypoxia and spontaneous firing of sympathetic neurons. The animals also respond to stimulation of the central end of a cut sensory nerve with tachycardia and an elevation of pressure, showing that neurons within the cord can receive input signals and produce an output.

Medulla and pons

The so-called vasomotor centers of the medulla are only one part of the vascular regulatory system, as indicated above, but the experiments by which they were discovered laid the foundation for modern knowledge. The critical observations were made at Carl Ludwig's laboratory in Leipzig in the early 1870s by two of his students, Owsjannikow and Dittmar. Their evidence for circumscribed centers was twofold. First, they found that, in rabbits and cats, separation of the higher levels of the brain from the medulla oblongata did not prevent the normal reflex rise in arterial pressure when the central end of the sciatic nerve was stimulated. Second, they showed that successive transections of the brain stem from above down did not alter blood pressure or reflexes until the cut was made at the lower end of the pons. Transections below that point produced marked hypotension and blunting of reflexes, and a level was eventually reached where pressure fell to the levels seen on acute cervical cord section and pressure reflexes disappeared. They concluded, and subsequent investigations confirmed, that a region of major importance in the maintenance of normal blood pressure and reflex activity lies between the calamus scriptorius and the fovea superior.

The location and nature of this region were later clarified by localized stimulation. Exploration of the floor of the fourth ventricle revealed one area where stimulation produced a rise in arterial pressure and another area where a decrease in pressure was elicited. These observations have been confirmed repeatedly, although the *depressor* region has been found to be less sharply defined than the *pressor* area. Their approximate location is shown in Figure 7.1, but both regions are now believed to be more limited in extent than is shown in that diagram (see below). Transection at the level labeled *II* in the figure leads to a fall in arterial pressure and blunting of reflex responses to stimulation of somatic nerves. The frequency of impulses in sympathetic nerves to the heart is also reduced, but it can be partially restored by section below the depressor center. Neurons of the depressor region deliver inhibition directly to efferent sympathetic fibers, not by way of the pressor area. Clearly, these two regions are involved in the maintenance of normal blood pressure, and are at least partly responsible for the tonic levels of sympathetic signals to the heart and blood vessels.

Subsequent investigation showed that the ventrolateral portions of the medulla are the ones involved in cardiovascular regulation; destruction of the dorsal and ventromedial parts has little effect on blood pressure. Moreover, the ventrolateral region in the reticular formation of the medulla has been found to contain a number of functionally identifiable concentrations of neurons connected with higher and lower levels and concerned with autonomic function.[15] For example, one cluster in the ventrolateral medulla consists mainly of catecholamine-containing cells, which communicate with the intermediolateral cell column of the cord and the intercalated spinal nucleus through a dense assembly of noradrenergic nerve fibers. Projections from this group also extend to specific supraspinal areas, including the nucleus tractus solitarius, parabrachial nucleus, central nucleus of the amygdala, paraventricular hypothalamic nucleus, and dorsal motor nucleus of the vagus nerve. These nuclei, in turn, are connected with each other in virtually every possible combination.

Other ventromedullary cell groups contain serotonin, acetylcholine, or neuropeptides. The excitation and inhibition of parasympathetic cholinergic fibers that innervate the heart and some blood vessels are largely controlled by the nucleus ambiguus and the dorsal motor nucleus of the vagus nerve,[43] but the existence of connections between the dorsal nucleus and the ventrolateral medulla suggests that the latter may also influence peripheral cholinergic responses. The concept of a simple vasomotor center has thus expanded into an array of multiple pathways that combine information from various levels and lead eventually to preganglionic efferents.

The terms *pressor* and *depressor* in this context are slightly misleading, as they are in the case of vasomotor nerves. They were adopted because the experimentally induced changes in *pressure* were easy to measure and large in magnitude, but we now know that the responses include actions on all effectors that respond to autonomic nerve impulses. Stimulation of the pressor area increases the heart rate, the force of cardiac contraction, the resistance of arterioles, the wall tension in veins, and the adrenal secretion of catecholamines. All of these responses tend to raise blood pressure, and stimulation of a depressor region has the opposite effects. It is obvious now, as it was not when the study of cardiovascular reflexes began, that changes in blood pressure are not always the most sensitive indicators of reflex activity. Changes in ventricular function or in the distribution of blood flow to the various organ systems can occur without significant alteration of arterial pressure.

Hypothalamus

Exploration of the hypothalamus with a stimulating electrode can evoke such a variety of cardiovascular responses that this region could be a competitor for the title of *vasomotor center*. Separate locations that influence the renal, muscular, or splanchnic beds can be identified,[40] as well as others that affect heart rate or adrenal medullary secretion. None of these functions is regulated exclusively by the hypothalamus, however.

The hypothalamus is crucial in responses that require the integrated action of several organ systems. Thermoregulation in a hot environment, for example, involves cutaneous vasodilatation, visceral vasoconstriction, sweating, and panting in some animals. All of these reactions are mediated through one particular part of the hypothalamus. The same region is essential for cutaneous vasoconstriction and muscular shivering on exposure to cold. Stimulation of other diencephalic areas, the fields of Forel, produces changes in cardiac rate, volume, and work that are similar to those that occur with exercise.[20] Responses like those in the defense reaction (Chapter 8) follow stimulation in still another location.[41] Although the hypothalamus is essential for the complete expression of these overall patterns of response, it is worth emphasizing again that other parts of the central nervous system also influence them.

The hypothalamus plays a significant role in the arterial chemoreceptor reflex, being essential to the bradycardia and increased peripheral resistance that are part of the response. The same thing is true to a lesser degree of the baroreceptor reflex, which is reduced by damage to the hypothalamus. These reflexes are normally modulated by the hypothalamus, but they operate to some extent in the decerebrate animal if the medulla is left intact.

Cerebral cortex

The highest levels of the brain have some influence on cardiovascular performance, as is apparent in the tachycardia of emotional stress or the now archaic response known as *blushing*. The importance of the mental state can be seen in studies of animals that have been trained to run on a treadmill. Many of the characteristic cardiovascular responses to exercise begin when the investigator is seen to reach for the switch, anticipating by a few seconds the actual muscular exertion.[20]

Relatively little is known about pathways from the cerebral cortex to neurons at lower levels that influence cardiovascular function, but electrical stimulation of the motor, temporal, or fronto-orbital cortex can alter heart rate and blood pressure.[14] At least three cortical systems appear to affect autonomic function: one originating in the sensory-motor cortex, another in the temporal-cingulate region, and a third in the orbital-cingulate area.[63] Only the last of these connects to neurons in the hypothalamus. Some pathways from the motor cortex elicit sympathetic cholinergic vasodilatation, relaying first in the hypothalamus and mesencephalon, and then passing directly to neurons of the preganglionic spinal outflow. At least two specific functional consequences of cortical lesions have been demonstrated. First, removal of the sensory-motor area of one hemisphere leads to vasodilatation in the contralateral limbs and reduced cutaneous vasoconstriction on exposure to cold. The cortex thus has a significant, although not indispensable, effect on temperature regulation. Second, some parts of the cortex and diencephalon are critical in the lung inflation reflex,[14,62] again demonstrating the close connection between autonomic activity and respiratory performance (Chapter 11).

Cardiovascular Sensors

Sensors that are activated by mechanical deformation and others that respond to certain chemicals exist in many parts of the cardiovascular system, as well as in other organs. These structures are called *receptors,* but they should be referred to specifically as *mechanoreceptors* (baroreceptors, stretch receptors) or *chemoreceptors* to avoid confusion with the more recently discovered receptor proteins of the cell membrane and interior (Chapter 1). The axons for many of these sensors are C fibers, unmyelinated, slow-conducting axons $1\mu m$

Table 7.1.   Classification of Cardiovascular Sensors

STIMULUS	LOCATION	AFFERENT NERVES[a]
Mechanoreceptors		
Stretch, broad range	Carotid sinuses	Vagal
Stretch, broad range	Aortic arch	Vagal
Stretch, low threshold	Atria, ventricles, pulmonary artery	Vagal
Stretch, high threshold	Heart and great vessels	Sympathetic
Chemoreceptors		
pO_2, pCO_2	Carotid bodies, aortic body	Vagal, IX
Bradykinin, other[b]	Heart and great vessels	Vagal
Bradykinin, other[b]	Heart and great vessels	Sympathetic

[a]Sympathetic afferent fibers travel in branches of sympathetic nerves and have cell bodies in dorsal root ganglia (see text). Afferents of carotid bodies and sinuses are located in cranial nerve IX.

[b]For example, veratrum, prostaglandins, and lactic acid.

or less in diameter, while others are typical A fibers, myelinated and of somewhat larger cross section.

The baroreceptors and chemoreceptors of the carotid arteries and aortic arch, which were the first to be discovered, have their afferent fibers in cranial nerves IX and X. An additional system of sensors is now known to exist in the form of nerve endings that are sensitive to mechanical deformation or chemical stimuli; these are widely distributed in the heart and great vessels. Many of the afferent fibers associated with them follow vagal pathways, but a significant number lie in branches of sympathetic nerves.[8,32] Fibers of the latter group are called *sympathetic afferents,* a name appropriate only in the sense that they travel in peripheral branches of sympathetic nerve trunks. Their cell bodies are in the dorsal spinal ganglia, *not* in the paravertebral chains of sympathetic ganglia. A summary of the known cardiovascular mechanical and chemoreceptors is given in Table 7.1

Carotid and aortic baroreceptors

Structure and innervation

The carotid sinuses and aortic arch contain specialized nerve terminals that are sensitive to mechanical deformation.[9,18,21] These structures, which are called *baroreceptors* because stretching of the vascular wall by intravascular pressure is the stress they normally experience, generate afferent nerve impulses when they are deformed. Immobilizing the vessel wall with a plaster cast in experimental animals makes the baroreceptors immune to changes of distending pressure. Lowering the pressure in a box surrounding the neck produces a typical baroreflex effect in humans.[29] These receptors can be activated by deformation in any direction, including longitudinal stretching or collapse of the sinus wall at extremely low pressures, but such events rarely occur under physiological conditions,[12] and distention in a radial direction is the normal stimulus.

The carotid sinus is a dilatation at the origin of the internal carotid artery. The arterial wall is slightly thinner there than in the more distal parts of the vessel, and it contains more elastin and less muscle. Separate *carotid sinus nerves,* which are anatomical branches of the glossopharyngeal nerve, transmit signals from the baroreceptors back to the central nervous system and also carry at least a few efferent sympathetic fibers.[8,58] The aortic baroreceptor area is innervated by the left aortic nerve. The right aortic nerve supplies a group of baroreceptors at the bifurcation of the right subclavian and common carotid arteries, and both aortic nerves receive fibers from the *aortic body,* a chemoreceptor structure (see below).

The deformation-sensitive structures are part of a diffuse arborization of nerve terminals in the adventitia and outermost medial layer of the arterial wall (Figure 7.2). They are of several morphological types, ranging from bare nerve endings to more organized globular networks.[1] The afferent nerve fibers are generally of intermediate size, 3 to 5 μm in diameter. A few are much larger and are said to correspond to receptors of relatively high sensitivity.[11] Some are myelinated, others not. Although all the sensing elements are qualitatively similar in that mechanical deformation is their effective stimulus, they vary quantitatively in threshold and in the amplitude of the impulses they generate.

Although the most important systemic arterial baroreceptors are those in the carotid sinuses and the arch of the aorta, others are scattered more sparsely in segments of the common carotid arteries (Figure 7.3). Under normal circumstances, the mean pressure is almost the same in all of these regions. The multiplicity of baroreceptor sites provides a redundant system in which selective stimulation of a single region can be counteracted by the activity of the others. Experimental distention of one carotid sinus has only transient effects unless the aortic region and the other carotid sinus have been denervated. Carotid baroreceptors operate over a wide range of arterial pressures above and below the normal level. In contrast, most of those in the aorta have a higher threshold and function only at high pressures. Afferent signals appear in the sinus nerve of the dog whenever arterial pressure is above about 60 mm Hg (Figure 7.4), but the threshold for aortic baroreceptors is closer to 100 mm Hg.[57] The sinuses

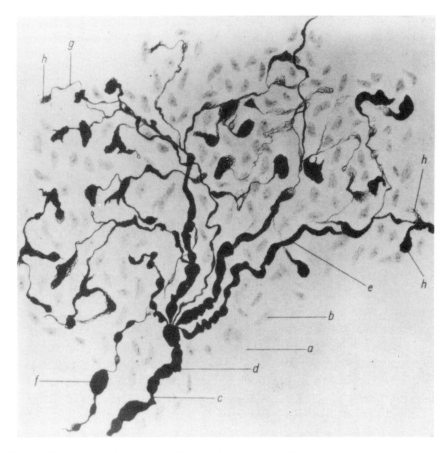

Figure 7.2.   Baroreceptors in adventitia of canine aortic arch. The following structures are labeled: *a*, connective tissue; *b*, nucleus of connective tissue cell; *c*, axon; *d*, main branch; *e*, lateral branch; *f*, widening or "varicosity" of fiber; *g*, terminal fiber; *h*, terminal network, sometimes called end plate but not to be confused with structure of that name in motor nerves. × 400. (Reproduced from Abraham,[1] with permission of Pergamon Press)

also contain some low-threshold receptors, which return relatively low-amplitude spikes through unmedullated afferents. Differences between carotid and aortic systems vary with the species studied; in the rabbit, for instance, the two regions have approximately the same threshold.[24]

The specific reflex responses initiated by the baroreceptors are described in detail in a later section. In brief, elevation of pressure in the carotid and aortic baroreceptive areas leads to a reflex slowing of the heart, arteriolar dilatation in many vascular beds, decreased venomotor tone, and a lowering of myocardial contractility. The efferent arm of the reflex for arteriolar and venous responses is a reduction in the frequency of sympathetic constrictor im-

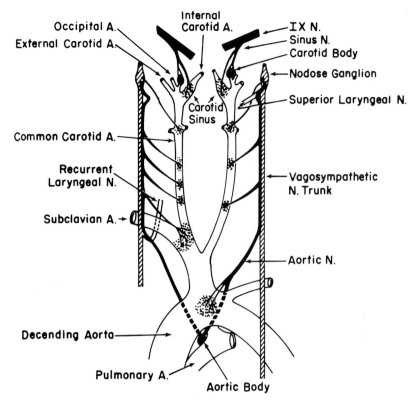

Figure 7.3. Location and innervation of aortic and carotid baroreceptors and chemoreceptors in cat and dog. *N*, nerve; *A*, artery. Baroreceptor areas indicated by *stippling*. Chemoreceptors are located in aortic and carotid bodies. (Based on data reported by Heymans and Neil[11] and Kejdi[12])

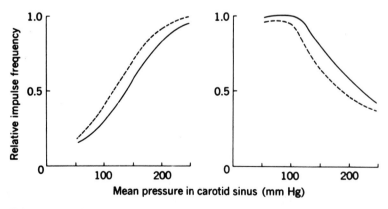

Figure 7.4. Impulse frequency in carotid sinus nerve (*left*) and in postganglionic sympathetic nerve (*right*) as functions of pressure in canine carotid sinus. *Solid line* represents response to steady pressure; *dashed line* to pulsatile pressure. Raising pressure in sinus increases average frequency of afferent impulses from baroreceptors, and reflex response is a decrease in frequency of efferent impulses in sympathetic constrictor fibers. (Based on experimental observations by Spickler[60])

pulses. The cardiac response involves parasympathetic as well as sympathetic efferents.

Baroreceptor afferent nerve fibers terminate in the dorsal medulla, in the nucleus tractus solitarius. The sympathetic efferent signals elicited by the baroreceptor reflex travel down to the spinal intermediolateral cell column, and the parasympathetic components issue from the dorsal vagal motor nucleus and nucleus ambiguus. Between these inputs and outputs, the nature of the reflex response is determined by neural processes that have not been completely identified but include information from other sensors, other parts of the brain stem and the forebrain, as well as the neurons that generate a basic 2/sec to 6/sec sympathetic oscillation.[10,13] Systems as disparate as the pulmonary stretch receptors and the cerebral cortex influence the final autonomic discharge. Conversely, activation of baroreceptors has effects on cortical activity, respiratory function, and somatomotor reflexes. As far as the cardiovascular system is concerned, the baroreceptor reflex tends to maintain arterial pressure at its normal level but is sometimes outvoted by other physiological demands.

Afferent signals

A train of afferent impulses appears in the baroreceptor nerves under normal conditions, and distention of the mechanosensitive regions increases their frequency. The overall relation between distention and signal frequency is sigmoid, but it is approximately linear for pressures from 100 to 180 mm Hg (Figure 7.4). With normal pulsatile distending pressures the baroreceptors do not transmit afferent impulses at a steady rate, but fire rapidly during the rising phase of pressure and less rapidly as pressure declines from its peak; in diastole they may be silent (Figure 7.5). The average firing rate over a whole cycle is higher with pulsatile pressure than with a constant pressure of the same mean value (Figure 7.4).

Baroreceptors consequently respond in two ways, one directly related to the instantaneous pressure, the other to its rate of change. The records in Figure 7.5 demonstrate that instantaneous pressure is not the only monitored variable, for firing sometimes ceases on the downstroke of the pulsation at a pressure that was accompanied by firing on the upstroke. On this time scale the baroreceptor sensitivity is asymmetric, being greater for rising than for falling pressures. Over longer time periods, however, baroreceptors behave like slowly adapting sensory transducers.[11] If carotid sinus pressure is gradually increased to a new level and held there, the afferent impulse rate will rise proportionately and then remain constant for as much as an hour, exhibiting no adaptation. A sudden increase in pressure, on the other hand, produces a short, transient burst of rapid firing.

The average firing rate measured in single afferent fibers at normal pres-

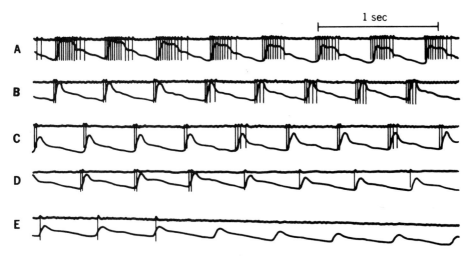

Figure 7.5. Impulses in single fiber of left aortic nerve, and blood pressure recorded simultaneously from left common carotid artery, as pressure was lowered. **A–E**, Mean pressures: 125, 80, 62, 55, and 42 mm Hg. (Reproduced from Neil,[56] with permission of the Middlesex Hospital)

sures is between 10 and 30 impulses per second.[11,12] The traffic in the nerve as a whole comes from a large population of receptors that differ in threshold and fire asynchronously, producing a continuous, patterned stream of signals. These afferent impulses impinge on the brain stem, where they contribute their share to the formulation of efferent signal patterns that regulate the performance of the heart and the resistance of vascular beds. The reflex effect of an increase in the afferent impulse rate is ordinarily manifested in a decrease in the sympathetic efferent firing rate (Figure 7.4).

The resulting vasomotor tone and cardiac output, in their turn, influence arterial pressure, so that the baroreceptor system is part of a feedback loop. A rise in arterial pressure, for example, elicits through the baroreceptors a set of responses that tends to return the pressure to normal, which in turn is sensed and acknowledged by the baroreceptors. This system operates so effectively that it is difficult to study the reflex in the intact animal, and investigators often resort to *open-loop* experiments in which the feedback pathways are interrupted[27] (see below).

Reflex responses

Although the baroreceptors are only one of many elements in the system that regulates the heart and blood vessels, certain stereotyped responses to baroreceptor activation are observed unless other inputs to the central nervous system override them. The cardiovascular responses elicited when an increase in pressure distends the carotid sinuses and aortic arch, for example, are as follows:

1. Slowing of the heart rate, owing to a prominent increase in efferent vagal parasympathetic impulses, and a small decrease in sympathetic discharge, to the sinoatrial node.
2. Slowing of conduction in myocardium and conducting tissues, mediated in the same way.
3. Decreased contractility of the heart, produced mainly by a reduction of sympathetic discharge to myocardial cells. Diminished vagal tone also contributes to a small degree.[53]
4. Decreased cardiac output, in which the slowed heart rate plays a greater part than the depressed ventricular performance.
5. Systemic arteriolar vasodilatation, brought about by a lessening of sympathetic constrictor tone. All vascular beds share in this response to some extent and total peripheral resistance falls, but the dilatation in skeletal muscle exceeds that elsewhere. There is little or no change in cerebral vascular resistance. Because of these regional differences in the effects on resistance there is a redistribution of cardiac output, so that skeletal muscle receives an increased fraction of the total blood flow.
6. Decreased mean systemic arterial pressure, mainly attributable to the fall in total vascular resistance. A small decrease in cardiac output is also a contributing factor.[29,34]
7. Relaxation of tone in systemic veins as a result of diminished sympathetic adrenergic impulses. This change tends to lower atrial filling pressure and is thus another cause of diminished cardiac output.

The effects of *decreased* pressure are the reverse of those listed above, plus a sympathetic stimulation of adrenal catecholamine secretion.

Set point and gain

Quantitative studies of baroreceptor function are often carried out by "opening" the feedback loop, as mentioned earlier. In the case of the carotid baroreceptors, this can be accomplished by isolating the carotid sinuses from the rest of the circulation while preserving their innervation and perfusing them at controlled pressures. The results can then be analyzed in accordance with *control theory,* a set of concepts and equations devised to study the inanimate control systems designed by engineers.[21] (see below). This approach treats the regulating system as a unit that reacts to certain input signals by generating specific outputs.

In the present context, the transmural pressure distending the isolated sinus may be regarded as the *input* and the reflex alteration of systemic arterial pressure as the *output*. The baroreceptors are a *negative feedback* system, meaning that an increase in input tends to cause a decrease in output. A rise in carotid sinus pressure triggers a reflex response that tends to lower arterial pressure. The slope of the relation between input and output (Δ output/Δ input) is called the *gain* of the system. The relationship is a sigmoidal curve, however, not a straight line, and gain reaches a maximum near the midpoint of the curve. The maximum static open-loop gain of isolated carotid sinus baroreceptors in anesthetized animals is typically close to unity; lowering the sinus pressure from 125 to 75 mm Hg produces an increase in systemic arterial pressure of about the same amount, 50 mm Hg.[21]

The equilibrium point under closed-loop conditions—in other words, the steady-state blood pressure level maintained by reflex action of the carotid and aortic stretch receptors—is called the baroreceptor *set point*. The set point may or may not coincide with the point of maximum gain. Although hypertension and some other pathological states have been attributed to *resetting* of the baroreceptor reflex, it is important to recognize that the set point varies considerably under normal conditions. Increased blood pressure during exercise does not lead to reflex slowing of the heart, for example.[55] The afferent impulses that report deformation of baroreceptors are only part of the information considered by the central nervous system as it chooses an appropriate pattern of sympathetic outflow, albeit an important part.

The host of nonbaroreceptor inputs that enters into the formulation of the efferent sympathetic discharge includes signals from chemoreceptors, pulmonary stretch receptors, and many other peripheral sensors, but inputs from central nervous system neurons that reflect higher functions of the brain are even more important. The response to changes in the baroreceptor input is not the same when an animal perceives some threat to its well-being, for instance, as it is in a relaxed, nonalert state. Sleep, to cite another example, induces a fall in blood pressure, but there is no reflex attempt to compensate for that change. In fact, the heart rate slows, peripheral resistance falls, and cardiac output decreases slightly, as if the baroreceptor system were inactive.[50] Nevertheless, any sudden increment in arterial pressure elicits a marked bradycardia, showing a heightened sensitivity of the baroreceptor system to that stimulus in the sleeping state.[59]

Physiological resetting can occur, in other words, but it usually represents a change in the weighting of various inputs by the central nervous system, not in the properties of the mechanical receptors. The earlier concept of the baroreceptor reflex as a single, invariant input–output relation has now been replaced by a picture of the baroreceptors as just one of a constellation of inputs. The essential feature of processing by the central nervous system is that it makes use of all the information available to it, whether from peripheral sensors or the highest levels of the brain. The interneuronal connections of these inputs and the basal sympathetic oscillators already mentioned have yet to be defined in detail, but in effect they converge at some point in the efferent sympathetic pathways. As a result, virtually all central nervous system reflexes in the intact animal are responses to multiple inputs.

Chronic systemic hypertension, a pathological elevation of arterial pressure, is accompanied by a resetting of the baroreceptor system to a higher threshold and lower sensitivity. Afferent impulse frequency is lower at any given pressure in hypertensive than in normal animals, and the sensitivity of the reflex at all levels is diminished.[12] The mechanism of this resetting remains unknown at present, and it is not even possible to say whether it is a cause or an effect of the persistently high pressure.

Arteries in general become less distensible in hypertension,[24] and the lowered sensitivity of the baroreceptors may be the result of stiffening of the carotids and aorta (see below). Impairment or loss of some of the sensing units is suggested by a lowering of the maximum afferent rate that can be evoked by very high pressure.[12] The effects of eliminating the baroreceptor mechanism experimentally are not the same as those of hypertensive disease. Denervation of the major baroreceptors does lead to a mild degree of hypertension, but the principal result is a marked lability of the pressure,[35] with inappropriately high elevations in response to minor environmental stimuli. In pathological hypertension, the baroreceptors apparently act to maintain high blood pressure once it has developed.

The baroreceptor as transducer

The location of the carotid and aortic baroreceptors subjects them to changes in the diameter of the carotid sinus or aortic arch; it is accepted as axiomatic that the receptors are stretched along with the wall, and to about the same degree, when these regions are distended. Other kinds of mechanical deformation can also activate the receptors, as we have seen, but radial distention is the physiological mode of deformation. Any decrease in the diameter of the carotid sinus, for example, reduces strain on the mechanoreceptors and hence leads to a reduction of afferent impulses.[13] The afferent rate in a baroreceptive region increases when pressure and diameter rise,[25] but not when pressure is raised while diameter is held constant. The transducing function of carotid baroreceptors thus seems to be the generation of afferent impulses with a frequency directly related to the diameter of the sinus.

The baroreceptor system serves to monitor arterial *pressure,* however, and sensing the diameter of the carotid sinus or aortic arch is no more than a means to an end. For that reason, the relation between transmural pressure and diameter is a potentially important factor in the operation of the system. The baroreceptive sites are supplied with functioning sympathetic motor fibers that can alter the compliance of the wall, so that local activity of smooth muscle can alter the pressure–diameter relationship. The extent to which such activity influences normal baroreceptor function is a mystery, but it seems safe to say that afferent baroreceptor signals depend not only on the pressure in the sensing vessel but also on the viscoelasticity of its wall. The definitive experiments that would allow a more exact statement have yet to be done, for what is required is simultaneous measurement of sinus diameter, sinus pressure, efferent nerve impulses, and afferent signals, all in conscious animals—a technical *tour de force*.

In spite of the theoretic significance of the elasticity of the vascular walls that contain stretch receptors, that variable does not seem to interfere greatly with the normal operation of baroreceptors. Virtually all work in which changes of arterial pressure are imposed experimentally show a direct correlation between sinus pressure and afferent frequency in the sinus nerve, although the relationship is nonlinear and limited to a certain range. Consequently, the function of baroreceptors as transducers can be expressed as a curve relating afferent signal rate to pressure (Figure 7.4). The slope of such a curve, the change in afferent frequency per unit change in pressure, describes the *sensitivity* of the transduction process. Note that the sensitivity so defined refers to afferent frequency as the output, because we are considering here the transducing properties of the receptors, not the overall performance of the reflex. Deviations from the normal relationship can be due to impairment of the receptors themselves or to altered distensibility of the vessels that contain the receptors.

With this background in mind, what effects would be expected from stimulating sympathetic nerve fibers that supply the carotid sinus or aortic arch? As far as the *sensitivity* of the receptor is concerned, the results are in accord with the known elastic behavior of blood vessels. Smooth muscle activation usually raises the elastic modulus of the vascular wall, meaning that the increase in diameter for a given pressure increment becomes smaller (Chapter 6). This fact suggests that stimulation of efferent sympathetic constrictor fibers to the carotid sinus should diminish the sensitivity of the baroreceptor reflex, and exactly that effect has been observed.[64]

The effects on the steady-state level of afferent signals are puzzling, however, and difficult to reconcile with the idea that stretching of the wall is the only source of receptor activation. Inasmuch as activation of smooth muscle makes a vascular wall less distensible, sympathetic constrictor impulses under conditions of constant transmural pressure should reduce the stretching of the receptors and lower the output signal level, but the results of experimental work are *not* consistent with this expectation. External application of norepinephrine to the carotid sinus or stimulation of its sympathetic innervation does, indeed, raise the pressure/diameter ratio,[28] but it *increases* the impulse rate in the sinus nerve and produces reflex hypotension, effects similar to those of *raising* intrasinus pressure. The diameter of the sinus usually becomes smaller, yet the increased afferent traffic suggests that the mechanoreceptors are being stretched. Tension in the wall as a whole is not involved, because the same response occurs even when the sinus has been opened so that it is under no tension.[49]

The explanation most frequently offered is that the contraction of smooth muscle stretches the receptors, regardless of changes in the circumference of the vascular segment in which they are located. The implication is that muscle and receptors are connected in series. An alternative explanation postulates a direct action of norepinephrine on the mechanical sensors, causing them to fire as if stretched. Perhaps the baroreceptors that are accessible and responsive to norepinephrine per se are a subset of the total population.

To complicate the picture further, the action of Na^+–K^+ pumps in the chemosensitive cells may also be involved in baroreceptor activity, for most mechanoreceptors are sensitive to the concentrations of those ions. Even a small reduction of $[Na^+]$ in the fluid perfusing a carotid sinus causes an appreciable rise in arterial pressure,[8,51] but the physiological significance of this reaction is uncertain because the plasma sodium concentration is essentially constant under normal conditions.

Pulmonary arterial baroreceptors

Mechanoreceptors similar to those in the carotids and aorta also exist at the bifurcation of the main pulmonary artery and in the right and left main branches.[33] Their function is essentially the same as that of the systemic baroreceptors, which is to say that a rise in pulmonary arterial pressure leads to a reflex decrease in systemic arterial pressure. A fall in pulmonary arterial pressure has the opposite effect, and in addition produces an increase in the rate and depth of respiration. These responses occur with variations of pressure in the physiological range, but gross distention of the arteries by pressures above 50 mm Hg elicits systemic vasoconstriction, the mechanism of which is not known. Some experiments suggest that baroreceptors of the large pulmonary arteries also mediate reflex vasomotion in smaller vessels downstream, but more experimental evidence on that point is needed.[11]

Cardiovascular mechanoreceptors

Bare nerve endings that act as mechanoreceptors are widely distributed in the heart and great vessels, specifically in atria, ventricles, thoracic aorta, venae cavae, pulmonary vessels, and pericardium. With the exception of those in the atria, they have a relatively high threshold and fire infrequently under normal conditions, often without relation to the cardiac cycle.

Atria

In effect, the atria act as sensors of intravascular volume, because atrial pressure generally rises and falls along with total blood volume. They not only contain stretch-sensitive nerve endings that generate reflex arcs, but also produce a hormone that contributes to regulation of fluid volume (see below). Mechanosensitive nerve endings are found just under the endocardium in both atria, mainly in the region of the venoatrial junctions. Two different types can be distinguished (Figure 7.6). One fires during atrial contraction (type A), the other late in ventricular systole near the peak of the atrial v wave (type B). The two kinds exist in approximately equal numbers,[17] and both can be activated by stretching the atrial wall. The rate of receptor firing is raised by increased atrial filling and by increased blood volume. Type B receptors are slower to adapt and perhaps less sensitive to rate of stretch than type A. The afferents of most atrial mechanoreceptors are in sympathetic nerves, but some are vagal.

The reflex responses to activation of type B receptors are qualitatively similar to those elicited from arterial baroreceptors, but the atrial type is sensitive to much smaller changes in pressure, as is appropriate in this low-pressure part of the circulation. One puzzling feature of the reflex initiated by atrial stretch receptors is that sympathetic discharge is stimulated by activation of

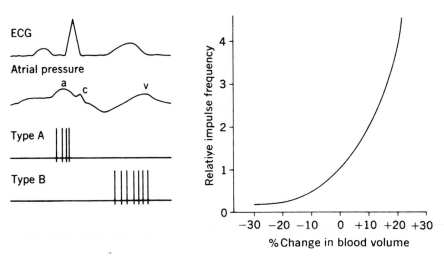

Figure 7.6. Atrial mechanoreceptor activity. *Left*, electrocardiogram (ECG), atrial pressure, impulses in afferent vagal fibers from type A and type B atrial receptors. *Right*, relative frequency of impulses (*ordinate*) in afferent from type B receptor when total blood volume (*abscissa*) was changed from its normal level. Change in atrial pressure was approximately 5 cm H_2O for 20% change in blood volume. (Based on data given by Paintal[17] and Gupta[45])

type A but inhibited by type B. The resulting reflex response may be a function of the A/B impulse ratio.[46] The *Bainbridge reflex,* an increased heart rate produced by large intravenous infusions of saline or blood,[52] originates in atrial type A stretch receptors, and the afferent fibers travel in the vagus nerve. High atrial pressures are required to elicit the reflex; its physiological significance is uncertain.

Stretching the atrial walls affects not only cardiovascular function but also the renal excretion of water and sodium. A connection between atrial distention and the flow of urine was discovered by early investigators who found that inflation of a balloon in the right atrium produced marked diuresis, whereas acute increases in blood volume had no effect on urinary output if atrial distention was prevented. Such phenomena are now known to depend in part on a group of *atrial natriuretic peptides* (*ANP*) produced in the atrial walls. The detailed structure of these hormones has been identified and their genetic relationships have been described.[4,16]

The production of ANP by the atria is a function of the degree of stretch experienced by atrial muscle cells, and a measurable level of the peptides appears in the blood under physiological conditions. Congestive heart failure, renal damage, and disturbances of atrial rhythm are accompanied by higher levels. Experimental injections of ANP cause increased excretion of sodium and water through mechanisms that include inhibition of renin release, changes in glomerular filtration rate, and perhaps suppression of aldosterone. The possibility of direct action on renal tubules is also under active investigation.[4] Specific cellular receptors for ANP have been detected in vascular smooth muscle as well as in kidney tissues, and ANP is a potent inhibitor of vasoconstriction, especially in the renal vascular bed. It does not necessarily alter total renal blood flow, but it changes the local resistance in afferent and efferent arterioles. Although these responses to infused ANP are now well established, recent evidence shows that the alterations of renal function that follow atrial distention are, at least in part, neurally mediated reflex actions generated by stretching the atrium, quite apart from (and presumably in addition to) an increase in circulating ANP.[44]

Ventricles

Both ventricles contain mechanoreceptor nerve endings, the left ventricle more than the right. Most of those with vagal afferents are unmyelinated and have a relatively high threshold. About half of them are silent under normal conditions, and the remainder tend to fire only in systole. Those with sympathetic afferents not only have a high threshold but also adapt rapidly to steady deformation, returning to their normal pattern of discharge in seconds. The physiological function of these sensors is not clear, but they evidently provide for detection of changing conditions rather than continuous monitoring.

Chemoreceptors

Cardiovascular chemoreceptors are of two kinds. One group, which is limited to specific regions at the carotid bifurcations and in the aortic arch, is sensitive to the O_2 and CO_2 tensions in arterial blood. Its afferent pathways run in cranial nerves IX and X. The other, which consists of chemosensitive nerve endings widely distributed in the heart and great vessels, responds to bradykinin and other endogenous substances. The sensory innervation of chemoreceptor endings in this second group is vagal in some cases and by way of fibers in sympathetic branches in others. In general, the vagal afferents evoke depressor responses like vasodilatation, bradycardia, and reduced myocardial contractility, whereas the sympathetic afferents produce the opposite effects.[32]

Carotid and aortic chemoreceptors

The location of the carotid and aortic "bodies" that contain chemoreceptors is shown in Figure 7.3. These specialized tissues sense the partial pressure of O_2 and CO_2 in arterial blood, but under normal conditions they send relatively few impulses to the central nervous system. Moderate deviations of blood gases from their normal levels produce marked respiratory responses but only slight changes in cardiovascular function. Extreme deviations, however, have definite effects on both systems. These chemoreceptors thus constitute a kind of emergency system for the circulation, unlike baroreceptors, which provide a more continuous tonic regulatory function. Respiration is subject to more or less constant fine tuning by chemoreceptor reflex control.[6,18,23]

The carotid and aortic bodies are highly vascular, an appropriate arrangement for organs that monitor chemical contents of the blood. Although the total blood flow to these structures is very small, their local blood flow per gram of tissue is on the order of 20 ml/g min, by far the highest in the body. The microcirculation in these organs consists of wide sinusoids lined with chemosensitive cells. The fact that the critical variable is the partial pressure, not the absolute amount, of respiratory gases in the blood has been demonstrated by observations made in CO poisoning. By competing with O_2 for the hemoglobin binding sites, CO lowers the amount of O_2 carried by the blood without altering its partial pressure. In such experiments chemoreceptor discharge is related to arterial pO_2, not content.

Receptor firing depends on the partial pressure of both O_2 and CO_2, with an interaction that makes the reflex response greatest when the two gases change in opposite directions (Figure 7.7). Elevation of pCO_2, for example, has less effect at normal than at low O_2 tensions. Individual receptors differ widely in threshold, and at least some afferent fibers respond to both O_2 and CO_2 tensions. The chemoreceptors are also sensitive to hydrogen ion concentration, and the effects of CO_2 may in part be attributable to concomitant changes in

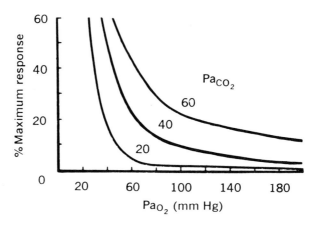

Figure 7.7. Average afferent chemoreceptor impulse frequency from multifiber preparation, expressed as percentage of maximum response (*ordinate*), in relation to changes in arterial pO_2 (*abscissa*) and pCO_2 (numbers beside curves). (Reproduced from Korner,[14] with permission of the American Physiological Society)

pH. Drugs that stimulate these receptors include cyanide, nicotine, and lobeline, which are often used as experimental tools.

The straightforward response to gas tensions is only one aspect of chemoreceptor function.[2] The picture is more complex because the aortic and carotid body sensors also seem to be sensitive to the rate of blood *flow*. Decreased flow increases chemoreceptor discharge and increased blood flow has the opposite effect, even when arterial pO_2 is kept constant.[39] Activation of chemoreceptors in moderate arterial hypotension, or during vasoconstriction of the arterioles that supply the chemosensitive areas,[30] is apparently the result of decreased flow.

Inasmuch as pO_2 falls steadily along the length of capillaries in most tissues, one could argue that decreased flow causes a widening of the arteriovenous pO_2 difference, and hence a lowering of pO_2 at the venous end of the sinusoids, which would be sensed by at least some chemoreceptor cells. This explanation is contradicted, however, by the experimental evidence. The arteriovenous O_2 difference in the carotid body, measured directly, is in fact quite small, perhaps 0.5 ml O_2/100 ml blood at normal blood pressures. Evidently, the amount of O_2 carried in simple solution in the plasma is more than sufficient for the metabolic and sensory needs of the chemoreceptors. Moreover, the chemoreceptor discharge elicited by a constant degree of anoxia can be almost completely abolished by raising the blood pressure. Observations of this kind have given rise to the hypothesis that blood flow influences the chemoreceptor response by carrying away some locally produced substance, thus reducing the action of that substance on the chemoreceptor nerve endings.[23] The validity of this hypothesis and the nature of the "transmitter" are still in question, but serotonin, which stimulates chemoreceptors (Chapter 8), is one possibility being considered.

The cardiovascular response to activation of the carotid chemoreceptors consists of bradycardia, arteriolar constriction in all the principal vascular beds, and increased adrenal secretion of catecholamines. The cardiac effect is brought about by increased parasympathetic and decreased sympathetic activity, whereas the vasoconstriction results from an increase in the rate of efferent sympathetic constrictor impulses.[37] The cardiac output falls, but the total peripheral resistance increases to such an extent that arterial pressure may become higher.

These *primary* effects are seen in pure form only in experiments where respiration is artificially kept constant, however, for chemoreceptor activation causes a marked increase in the rate and depth of breathing. Under normal conditions, the respiratory effects are not only more striking than the effects on heart and blood vessels, but they also modify the circulatory response, resulting in an *increase* in heart rate and output (especially if hypercapnia occurs). The secondary effects of respiratory effort thus outweigh the primary reflex action on the heart and blood vessels. In addition, the dilatation of systemic arterioles that is a direct local response to hypoxia partially counteracts the reflex vasoconstriction, with results that differ in different regions. Cerebral blood flow usually increases slightly, whereas gastrointestinal and renal flows often fall.

Cardiac and other chemoreceptors

The carotid and aortic bodies are what might be called the *classical* chemoreceptors, but it has gradually become clear that nerve endings in the heart and other blood vessels also serve as important chemical sensors. These terminals are not sensitive to hypoxia or hypercapnia, but they can be activated by bradykinin, some of the prostaglandins, and a number of other substances. The chemicals that activate this second chemoreceptor system are metabolized rapidly, so that these receptors monitor local conditions, not the bloodstream in general.

The heart, for example, contains chemosensitive *vagal* nerve endings that induce reflex vasodilatation, particularly in the coronary arteries. These sensors are most numerous in the left ventricle, but they also appear in the right ventricle, atria, great veins, pulmonary artery, and aorta.[7] They are sensitive to bradykinin, 5-hydroxytryptamine, and prostaglandins $PGF_{2\alpha}$ and PGE_2, but are often studied experimentally by stimulation with veratrum alkaloids or other foreign substances.

The terminals of *sympathetic afferent* fibers in the ventricles can be stimulated by epicardial application of bradykinin or lactic acid;[61] in this case, the resulting reflex response is constriction of blood vessels. Prostaglandins play some role in the response of sympathetic afferent endings to bradykinin, for PGE_1 potentiates such effects. Interest has centered on chemoreceptors of this kind in the myocardium and its arteries, because they elicit reflex coronary constriction and possibly the pain associated with myocardial ischemia.

Injured tissues in general generate some pain-producing substance locally,[31] and much evidence points to bradykinin as the culprit. Damaged cells apparently release proteolytic enzymes into the interstitial space, where they convert an already existing substrate into bradykinin, which is an effective stimulus to unmyelinated sensory afferents. *Angina pectoris*, the deep pain associated with severe reduction of blood flow to the myocardium, may arise in this way. At the same time, one would expect prostaglandins produced by ischemic myocardium to stimulate vagal afferent chemosensors. The final reflex response is difficult to predict because of the completely opposite vasomotor effects mediated by vagal as contrasted with sympathetic afferent fiber endings, and the physiological significance of these two opposing chemosensitive systems, both activated by bradykinin, is by no means clear. To complicate the picture further, bradykinin also exerts a direct local action on vascular smooth muscle, causing vasodilatation (Chapter 8).

Cerebral chemoreceptors

Reduction of blood flow to the brain leads to acute general vasoconstriction, tachycardia, and an elevation in systemic arterial pressure. A fall in cerebral perfusion pressure can produce this response, but it does not appear in experiments where blood O_2 tension is maintained at a high level.[38] The reaction does not depend on pressure per se, in other words, but instead has the appearance of a chemoreflex. It does not arise from chemosensitive nerve endings in cerebral vessels, however, but from local hypoxia and hypercapnia of neurons somewhere in the central nervous system. The cerebral vessels themselves are dilated by hypercapnia, to which their smooth muscle is exquisitely sensitive (Chapter 12).

Except for the tachycardia elicited by the reflex, the overall effects are similar to those mediated by the chemoreceptors of the carotid sinuses and aorta. In generalized anoxia, the primary bradycardia that the arterial baroreceptors would otherwise produce (see above) is often suppressed by the tachycardia caused by the cerebral component of the responses and by hyperventilation. Constant autoregulation is prominent in the circulation of the brain. The cerebral chemoreflex is an additional emergency system, called into play only in extreme hypotension or when local vasomotor mechanisms can no longer cope with arterial hypoxia or hypercapnia. Brain tumors or other lesions that raise intracranial pressure enough to reduce cerebral blood flow often fall in this category. In addition, tissue in some part of the brain acts as a sensor of hydrogen ion concentration and generates reflex responses in the respiratory and cardiovascular systems. The location of these cells is not known, but one theory places them in the ventral surface of the medulla.[22]

Extrinsic Sources of Afferent Signals

In many situations, afferent signals arising from organs other than the heart and blood vessels evoke reflex changes in the circulation. The principal extrinsic sources of such signals are the lungs, somatic sensory nerves, and skeletal muscle.

Pulmonary mechanoreceptors

The parenchymal, nonvascular tissue of the lung contains stretch-sensitive nerve endings that are activated by pulmonary inflation, and a large number of the afferent fibers in the vagi originate in these receptors. A second group exists in the narrow interstitial space between the capillaries and pulmonary alveoli, where they monitor pressure and hence local fluid volume. Unmyelinated C vagal afferents appear to carry signals from these sensors, providing a system that can monitor any increase in interstitial fluid volume even before the development of frank pulmonary edema.[6] The reflexes associated with both classes are described in Chapter 11.

Somatic and visceral sensory inputs

Experimental stimulation of the central stump of a cut somatic or visceral nerve may produce either a rise or fall in blood pressure, depending on the experimental conditions. The pressor response follows relatively strong stimuli and includes tachycardia and vasoconstriction. It probably arises from activation of small, myelinated fibers involved in the sensation of pain. The depressor response can be initiated by rapid stimulation of high-threshold C fibers or by low-frequency stimulation of small, myelinated fibers. The latter are responsible for the deep pain associated with manipulation of viscera or blood vessels, maneuvers that are often accompanied by bradycardia, sweating, and a sudden fall in blood pressure. Stimulation of afferent nerves from skeletal muscle can also elicit either vasoconstriction or dilatation, again depending on the particular fibers stimulated. The response is generalized, and its extent in different vascular beds depends on their initial tone.[48] Fibers from thermoreceptors may also be activated by stimulation of cutaneous sensory nerves.

Although the extraordinary vasodilatation in exercising muscle is due largely to the direct action of metabolites on vascular smooth muscle, the influence of some metabolic products that excite chemosensitive vascular nerve endings may contribute in a small way to the cardiovascular reflex response.

Evidence pointing in this direction comes from experiments in which the muscles of one limb are exercised while the circulation to that extremity is occluded (Chapter 8). Tachycardia and elevation of blood pressure result, even with levels of exertion far below those that produce pain under such conditions, and these effects persist after exercise until the occlusion is released.

Submersion and diving

The diving response consists of apnea, bradycardia, and peripheral vasoconstriction, reflexly triggered by somatic sensory inputs through the trigeminal nerve.[3,36] The phenomenon is most prominent in diving animals, although the same reflex occurs in humans. In the duck, for example, submersion of the head or just the nostrils produces an immediate bradycardia and intense peripheral vasoconstriction everywhere except in the heart and brain. Cardiac output is greatly reduced, in part because of the bradycardia and in part through negative inotropic stimuli. Arterial pressure remains essentially constant, and increased venomotor tone raises venous pressure slightly. This is not a response to asphyxia, because it develops instantaneously and cannot be duplicated by simple occlusion of the trachea. The presence of noxious gases or foreign bodies in the upper airways elicits a similar reflex response.

The breath holding is not merely voluntary but is maintained by reflex inhibition of respiration through the central nervous system. Continued apnea leads to arterial hypoxemia and hypercapnia, stimulating the carotid and aortic chemoreceptors, which reinforce the cardiovascular effects. The reflex stimulus to respiratory activity that the chemoreceptors would otherwise evoke is suppressed by sensory facial or airway input. In effect, the diving response conserves oxygen while protecting the brain and myocardium, minimizing oxygen usage by all but the most essential tissues. During prolonged submersion, the energy needed for muscular activity is obtained largely by anaerobic metabolism.

References

Reviews

1. Abraham, A. (1969). *Microscopic Innervation of the Heart and Blood Vessels in Vertebrates Including Man*. Oxford, Pergamon.
2. Acker, H. (1989). pO$_2$ Chemoreception in arterial chemoreceptors. *Annu. Rev. Physiol.* 51:835–844.

3. Andersen, H.T. (1966). Physiological adaptations in diving vertebrates. *Physiol. Rev.* 46:212–243.

4. Ballerman, B.J., Brenner, B.M. (1986). Role of atrial peptides in body fluid homeostasis. *Circ. Res.* 58:619–630.

5. Barman, S.M. (1984). Spinal cord control of the cardiovascular system. In: *Nervous Control of Cardiovascular Function*, W.C. Randall, ed. New York, Oxford University Press, pp. 321–345.

6. Coleridge, H.M., Coleridge, J.C.G. (1986). Reflexes from the tracheobronchial tree and lungs. In: *The Handbook of Physiology; The Respiratory System, Vol. 2, Control of Breathing, Part I*, N. Cherniak and J.G. Widdicombe, eds. Washington, D.C., American Physiological Society, pp. 395–429.

7. Coleridge, J.C.G., Coleridge, H.M. (1979). Chemoreflex regulation of the heart. In: *Handbook of Physiology, Section 2, Vol. 1, Circulation*, R.M. Berne, ed. Washington, D.C., American Physiological Society, pp. 653–676.

8. Donald, D.E., Shepherd, J.T. (1980). Autonomic regulation of the peripheral circulation. *Annu. Rev. Physiol.* 42:429–439.

9. Downing, S.E. (1979). Baroreceptor regulation of the heart. In: *Handbook of Physiology, Section 2: The Cardiovascular System. Vol. I, The Heart*. R.M. Berne, N. Sperelakis, and S.R. Geiger, eds. Bethesda, Md., American Physiological Society, pp. 621–652.

10. Gebber, G.L. (1984). Brainstem systems involved in cardiovascular regulation. In: *Nervous Control of Cardiosvascular Function*, W.C. Randall, ed. New York, Oxford University Press, pp. 346–368.

11. Heymans, C., Neil, E. (1958). *Reflexogenic Areas of the Cardiovascular System*. Boston, Little, Brown.

12. Kejdi, P. (ed.) (1967). *Baroreceptors and Hypertension*. Oxford, Pergamon Press.

13. Kirchheim, H.R. (1976). Systemic arterial baroreceptor reflexes. *Physiol. Rev.* 56:100–176.

14. Korner, P.I. (1971). Integrative neural cardiovascular control. *Physiol. Rev.* 51:312–367.

15. Loewy, A.D., McKellar, S. (1980). The neuroanatomical basis of central cardiovascular control. *Fed. Proc.* 39:2495–2503.

16. Needleman, P., Blaine, E.H., Greenwald, J.E., Michener, M.L., Saper, C.B., Stickman, P.T., Tolunay, E.H. (1989). The biochemical pharmacology of atrial peptides. *Ann. Rev. Pharmacol. Toxicol.* 29:23–54.

17. Paintal, A.S. (1973). Vagal sensory receptors and their reflex effects. *Physiol. Rev.* 53:159–227.

18. Pallot, D.J. (ed.) (1984). *The Peripheral Arterial Chemoreceptors*. New York, Oxford University Press.

19. Randall, W.C. (1984). *Nervous Control of Cardiovascular Function*. New York, Oxford University Press.

20. Rushmer, R.F., Smith, A.O., Jr., Lasher, E.P. (1960). Neural mechanisms of cardiac control during exertion. *Physiol. Rev.* 40(Suppl. 4):27–34.

21. Sagawa, K. (1983). Baroreflex control of systemic arterial pressure and vascular bed. In: *Handbook of Physiology, Section 2: The Cardiovascular System. Vol. 3, Peripheral circulation and organ blood flow, Part 2*. J.T. Shepherd and F.M. Abboud, eds. Bethesda, Md., American Physiological Society, pp. 453–496.

22. Schlaefky, M.E. (1981). Central chemosensitivity: A respiratory drive. *Rev. Physiol. Biochem. Pharmacol.* 90:171–244.

23. Torrance, R.W. (ed.) (1968). *Arterial Chemoreceptors*. Oxford, Blackwell Scientific.

Research Reports

24. Aars, H. (1968). Aortic baroreceptor activity in normal and hypertensive rabbits. *Acta Physiol. Scand.* 72:298–309.
25. Aars, H. (1971). Effect of noradrenaline on activity in single aortic baroreceptor fibers. *Acta Physiol. Scand.* 83:335–343.
26. Alexander, R.S. (1946). Tonic and reflex functions of medullary sympathetic cardiovascular centers. *J. Neurophysiol.* 9:205–217.
27. Allison, J.L., Sagawa, K., Kumada, M. (1969). Open-loop analysis of the aortic arch barostatic reflex. *Am. J. Physiol.* 217:1576–1584.
28. Bagshaw, R.J., Peterson, L.H. (1972). Sympathetic control of the mechanical properties of the canine carotid sinus. *Am. J. Physiol.* 222:1462–1468.
29. Bevegard, B.S., Shepherd, J.T. (1966). Circulatory effects of stimulating the carotid arterial stretch receptors in man at rest and during exercise. *J. Clin. Invest.* 45:132–142.
30. Biscoe, T.J., Purves, M.J. (1967). Observations on carotid body chemoreceptor activity and cervical sympathetic discharge in the cat. *J. Physiol.* 190:413–424.
31. Chapman, L.F., Ramos, A.O., Goodell, H., Wolff, H.G. (1961). Neurohumoral features of afferent fibers in man. Their role in vasodilatation, inflammation, and pain. *Arch Neurol.* 4:617–650.
32. Coleridge, H.M., Coleridge, J.C.G., Kidd, C. (1978). Afferent innervation of the heart and great vessels: A comparison of the vagal and sympathetic components. *Acta Physiol. Pol.* 29(Suppl. 17):55–79.
33. Coleridge, J.C.G., Kidd, C., Sharp, J.A. (1961). The distribution, connexions, and histology of baroreceptors in the pulmonary artery, with some observations on the sensory innervation of the ductus arteriosus. *J. Physiol.* 156:591–602.
34. Corcondilas, A., Donald, D.E., Shepherd, J.T. (1964). Assessment by two independent methods of the role of cardiac output in the pressor response to carotid occlusion. *J. Physiol.* 170:250–262.
35. Cowley, A.W., Liard, J.F., Guyton, A.C. (1973). Role of the baroreceptor reflex in daily control of arterial blood pressure and other variables in dogs. *Circ. Res.* 32:564–576.
36. Daly, M. de B., Angell-James, J.E. (1979). The "diving response" and its possible clinical implications. *Int. Med.* 1:12–19.
37. Daly, M. de B., Scott, M.J. (1963). The cardiovascular responses to stimulation of the carotid body chemoreceptors in the dog. *J. Physiol.* 165:179–197.
38. Downing, S.E., Mitchel, J.H., Wallace, A.G. (1963). Cardiovascular responses to ischemia, hypoxia, and hypercapnia of the central nervous system. *Am. J. Physiol.* 204:881–887.
39. Eyzaguirre, C., Lewin, C. (1961). Effect of different oxygen tensions on the carotid body in vitro. *J. Physiol.* 159:238–250.
40. Feigl, E.O. (1964). Vasoconstriction resulting from diencephalic stimulation. *Acta Physiol. Scand.* 60:372–380.
41. Folkow, B., Lisander, B., Tuttle, R.S., Wang, S.C. (1968). Changes in cardiac

output upon stimulation of the hypothalamic defense area and the medullary depressor area in the cat. *Acta Physiol. Scand.* 72:220–233.

42. Gebber, G.L. (1980). Central oscillators responsible for sympathetic nerve discharge. *Am. J. Physiol.* 239 (*Heart Circ. Physiol.* 8):H143–H155.

43. Geis, G.S., Kozelka, R.D., Wurster, R.D. (1981). Organization and reflex control of vagal cardio-motor neurons. *J. Autonomic Nerv. Sys.* 3:437–450.

44. Goetz, K.L., Wang, B.C., Bie, P., Leadley, R.J., Jr., Geer, P.G. (1988). Natriuresis during atrial distention and a concurrent decline in plasma atriopeptin. *Am. J. Physiol.* 255 (*Reg. Integrative Comp. Physiol.* 24):R259–R267.

45. Gupta, P.D., Henry, J.P., Sinclair, R., Von Baumgarten, R. (1966). Responses of atrial and aortic baroreceptors to nonhypotensive hemorrhage and to transfusion. *Am. J. Physiol.* 211:1429–1437.

46. Hakumaki, M.O.K. (1970). Function of the left atrial receptors. *Acta Physiol. Scand.* 79(Suppl. 344):1–54.

47. Hornbein, T.F., Griffo, Z.J., Roos, A. (1961). Quantitation of chemoreceptor activity: Interrelation of hypoxia and hypercapnia. *J. Neurophysiol.* 24:561–568.

48. Johannson, B. (1962). Circulatory responses to stimulation of somatic afferents. *Acta Physiol. Scand.* 57(Suppl. 198):1–91.

49. Kalkoff, W. (1959). Die Reflexbeeinflussung des blutdruckes wahrend Adrelalineinwirkung am Karotissinus. Ausserung einer spezifischen von der Pressorezeption unterscheidbaren Funktion. *Verh. Dtsch. Ges. Kreislaufforsch.* 25:173–178.

50. Kumazawa, T., Baccelli, G., Guazzi, M. Mancia, G., Zanchetti, A. (1969). Hemodynamic patterns during desynchronized sleep in intact cats and in cats with sinoaortic deafferentiation. *Circ. Res.* 34:923–937.

51. Kunze, D.L., Saum, W.R., Brown, A.M. (1977). Sodium sensitivity of baroreceptors mediates reflex changes of blood pressure and urine flow. *Nature* 267:75–78.

52. Ledsome, J.R., Linden, R.J. (1967). The effect of distending a pouch of the left atrium on the heart rate. *J. Physiol.* 193:121–129.

53. Levy, M.N., Ng, M., Lipman, R.I., Zieske, H. (1966). Vagus nerves and baroreceptor control of ventricular performance. *Circ. Res.* 18:101–106.

54. McAllen, R.M., Spyer, K.M. (1978). The baroreceptor input to cardiac vagal motoneurones. *J. Physiol.* 282:365–374.

55. McRitchie, R.J., Vatner, S.F., Boettcher, D., Heyndrickx, G.R., Patrick, T.A., Braunwald, E. (1976). Role of arterial baroreceptors in mediating cardiovascular response to exercise. *Am. J. Physiol.* 230:85–89.

56. Neil, E. (1954). Reflexogenic areas of the circulation. *Arch. Middlesex Hosp.* 4:16.

57. Pelletier, C.L., Clement, D.L., Shepherd, J.T. (1972). Comparison of afferent activity of canine aortic and sinus nerves. *Circ. Res.* 31:557–568.

58. Rees, P.M. (1967). The distribution of biogenic amines in the carotid bifurcation region. *J. Physiol.* 193:245–253.

59. Smyth, H.S., Sleight, P., Pickering, G.W. (1969). The reflex regulation of arterial pressure during sleep in man; a quantitative method of assessing baroreflex sensitivity. *Circ. Res.* 24:109–121.

60. Spickler, J.W., Kezdi, P., Geller, E. (1967). Transfer characteristics of the carotid sinus pressure control system. In: *Baroreceptors and Hypertension,* P. Kezdi, ed. Oxford, Pergamon Press, pp. 31–40.

61. Staszewski-Barczak, J., Ferriera, S.H., Vane, J.R. (1976). An excitatory no-

ciceptive cardiac reflex elicited by bradykinin and potentiated by prostaglandins and myocardial ischemia. *Cardiovasc. Res.* 10:314–327.

62. Uther, J.B., Hunyor, S.N., Shaw, J., Korner, P.I. (1970). Bulbar and supra-bulbar control of the cardiovascular autonomic effects during arterial hypoxia in the rabbit. *Circ. Res.* 26:491–506.

63. Wall, P.D., Davis, G.D. (1951). Three cerebral cortical systems affecting auto-nomic function. *J. Neurophysiol.* 14:507–517.

64. Wurster, R.D., Trobiani, S. (1973). Effects of cervical sympathetic stimulation on carotid occlusion reflexes in cats. *J. Physiol.* 225:978–981.

AUTONOMIC AND PERIPHERAL CONTROL MECHANISMS

The role of the central nervous system in regulating the heart and circulation was described in Chapter 7, along with an account of the peripheral sensors that provide the brain with relevant information. Here we move on to the neural and other mechanisms that send controlling signals to the cardiovascular tissues. These commands reach the cells of the heart and blood vessels in the form of specific substances, which may be delivered as neurotransmitters, hormones, or paracrine agents. In recent years, it has become apparent that some substances serve in all three capacities. Neural signals are carried through transmitters released at nerve terminals; endocrine control, by hormones that travel in the bloodstream. Paracrine regulation acts through locally produced materials that affect cells in the immediate vicinity. In each case, the active agent affects its target cells by binding to specific membrane-bound receptors (Chapter 1). These three modes of control will be considered separately in this section, although they interact under physiological conditions; the chapter concludes with a description of the integrated cardiovascular adaptations to hypoxia and other forms of stress.

Autonomic Nervous System

The peripheral nervous system contains two classes of nerves, somatic and autonomic. The heart and blood vessels, like other viscera, are innervated by the autonomic nervous system. The autonomic system, in turn, can be subdivided into two parts, sympathetic and parasympathetic. Although autonomic nerves were originally thought to be exclusively motor in function, certain sensory fibers are now also considered to be part of the system. The autonomic nervous system in general is covered in textbooks of general physiology, and the description that follows here is merely a brief recapitulation. Additional information can be found in a comprehensive monograph by Pick.[19]

Motor fibers of the sympathetic and parasympathetic systems follow pathways that originate in central nervous system neurons, synapse in peripheral ganglia, and then travel through postganglionic axons to the effector tissues. Sympathetic motor preganglionic nerves emerge along the length of the spinal cord and make synaptic contact with cell bodies in the paravertebral sympathetic chains or prevertebral ganglia. The parasympathetic outflow travels in cranial and sacral nerves to synapse with cell bodies in more distal ganglia, which sometimes lie within the tissue of the effector itself. In both systems, the postganglionic fibers destined for blood vessels usually lie in large peripheral nerve trunks and eventually in perivascular networks. Preganglionic autonomic neurons are cholinergic, meaning that their natural neurotransmitter is acetylcholine. Postganglionic parasympathetic terminals are also cholinergic. Sympathetic postganglionic neurons are adrenergic, releasing norepinephrine.

The peripheral nerve plexuses associated with the gastrointestinal tract were treated by some early investigators as a separate enteric nervous system, and recent studies give new justification for this view.[12] Although the enteric autonomic nerves and ganglia are usually considered part of the parasympathetic system, they are the site of a host of vasoactive substances that may be transmitters for nonadrenergic, noncholinergic nerves. In addition, this system apparently endows the gut with some reflexes that operate independently of the brain or spinal cord.

Neural control of the heart

Sympathetic and parasympathetic divisions of the autonomic system innervate the heart through a maze of cardiac nerves,[19,20] some of which are shown diagrammatically in Figure 8.1. Sympathetic preganglionic axons have their cell bodies in the interomediolateral columns of the upper thoracic cord (T1–T8). In mammals, virtually all postganglionic sympathetic fibers originate in the superior cervical, middle cervical, and stellate ganglia or cognate structures, although considerable variation appears among species. The preganglionic parasympathetic neurons that supply the heart issue predominantly from the dorsal motor nucleus and the nucleus ambiguous and travel in the vagus nerves. Neurons that represent parasympathetic ganglia exist in the atrial and ventricular walls. In the dog and a few other species, sympathetic axons join the vagi in the cervical and upper thoracic regions to form a common vagosympathetic trunk, which also includes some afferent fibers. The proximal

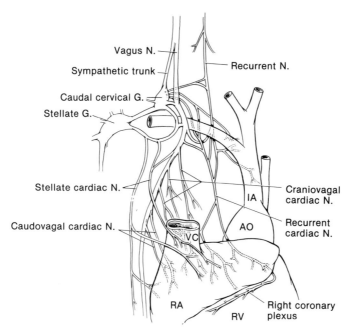

Figure 8.1. Principal right-sided cardiac nerves near base of the heart (dog). *VC,* superior vena cava; *RA,* right atrium; *RV,* right ventricle; *Ao,* aorta; *IA,* innominate artery; *G,* ganglion; *N,* nerve. (Semidiagrammatic and not to scale. Pulmonary artery and its innervation not shown.)

portion of this trunk contains nerves destined for noncardiac structures of the thorax and abdomen, as well as others that travel to the heart. Within the pericardium, it becomes possible to distinguish groups of fibers that extend to specific regions of the heart.[20]

   The cardiac sympathetic and parasympathetic fibers innervate atrial muscle, ventricular muscle, the sinoatrial node, the atrioventricular node, and the intraventricular conducting fibers. The density of nerve endings is high in both nodes; the typical distribution in the atrioventricular node is shown in Figure 8.2, a drawing derived from serial histological sections.[13] Neural density is greater in atrial than in ventricular muscle, and Purkinje fibers are only sparsely innervated. The microscopic structure of neuromyal junctions in the heart is a subject of debate, but adrenergic and cholinergic nerve terminals lie in close proximity to muscle cells at some sites.[39,46] Right and left vagosympathetic trunks both contain fibers that affect all cardiac tissues, but there is a marked quantitative difference in their action on the nodes. Stimulation of the right vagus causes a marked slowing of the heart rate and a much smaller inhibition of atrioventricular conduction, whereas slowing of atrioventricular conduction is the most prominent effect of left vagal stimulation.[20] The difference is quan-

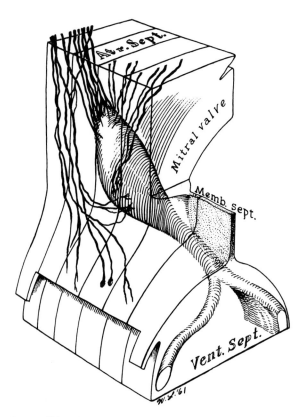

Figure 8.2.   The human AV node and His bundle, showing relation to mitral valve and septa. *Atr. Sept.*, interatrial septum; *Vent. Sept.*, interventricular septum; *Memb. Sept.*, membranous portion of septum. Bundle gives rise to a single right branch but multiple left branches, which form virtually a sheet of fibers down the left septal endocardium. (Reproduced from James,[13] with permission of McGraw-Hill Book Co.)

titative rather than absolute, and the contrast is more obvious in some subjects than in others. These *chronotropic* effects are mediated by a combination of parasympathetic and sympathetic neurons, the parasympathetic impulses acting to slow conduction velocity and the sinoatrial firing rate, while the sympathetic components have the opposite effect. Conduction velocity in muscle as well as in the specialized conducting system (Chapter 4) is affected.

Vagal stimulation affects the heart very quickly, within one or two heartbeats, whereas sympathetic actions develop more slowly. The refractory period of the atria, but not the ventricles, is reduced by parasympathetic stimulation, a response consistent with the effect of acetylcholine on atrial membrane potentials (Chapter 3). The quantitative effect of incoming vagal impulses depends not only on their frequency but also on the part of the cardiac cycle in which they arrive, yielding a complex input–output relationship.[15] Myocardial contractility is increased by sympathetic impulses (a positive *inotropic* effect), raising the ventricular work done from any given end-diastolic volume. Contractility of the heart is mildly depressed by parasympathetic impulses, although this response is so subtle that it went undetected for many years.

Cardiac performance is consequently regulated by signals from both divisions of the autonomic nervous system. In the resting state, the heart rate is dominated by parasympathetic impulses, and the rate increases when the vagi are cut. Increased sympathetic nerve activity produces enhanced contractility, but again, there is interaction between sympathetic and parasympathetic systems. The negative inotropic effect of vagal impulses seems to vary directly with the level of sympathetic activity.[15,63] This phenomenon, which investigators have named *accentuated antagonism,* probably arises from the presynaptic cholinergic inhibition of adrenergic nerves (see below). Any nerve-mediated increase in the work of the heart is usually accompanied by changes in coronary blood flow (Chapter 12).

Adrenergic control of the heart was once thought to act only through beta adrenoceptors, but more recent studies show that alpha receptors are also involved.[2] The intracellular messengers activated by these receptors are discussed in Chapter 1. Beta$_1$-, beta$_2$-, and alpha$_1$-adrenoceptor subtypes have been identified in myocardium by functional and radioligand methods. All mediate positive inotropic effects, but beta-adrenoceptor activation shortens the duration of the action potential and mechanical contraction, whereas alpha-adrenoceptor stimulation does not. Beta-adrenergic agonists increase the heart rate as well as the force of contraction. Changes in the numbers of beta receptors in the myocardium have been demonstrated in a number of situations. A decrease in the number of beta receptors (*down regulation*) follows prolonged administration of the natural transmitter norepinephrine or the synthetic agonist isoproterenol; it also occurs in some forms of experimental hypertension.[25] Thyroid hormone causes up regulation, which is also seen in myocardial hypertrophy. Receptor affinities are probably not altered in these responses. An alpha$_1$-adrenergic mechanism may play some part in the generation of a specific substance that mediates hypertrophy of cardiac muscle in hypertension and some other disease states.[65]

Neural control of blood vessels

Vasomotor activity

The walls of all blood vessels except capillaries contain smooth muscle, and activity of that tissue is the mechanism of vascular regulation. The physiological characteristics of vascular smooth muscle are described in Chapter 9;

here we will be concerned primarily with nervous control of those cells. The degree of force developed by vascular smooth muscle influences the diameter of the lumen of small vessels and the viscoelasticity of large vessel walls. Sympathetic adrenergic nerve fibers supply vascular smooth muscle in virtually all parts of the circulation, whereas sympathetic and parasympathetic cholinergic innervation is restricted to certain tissues or specific regions. Small arteries in the vascular bed of skeletal muscles have sympathetic cholinergic as well as adrenergic innervation, and a few vessels elsewhere receive cholinergic stimuli from the cranial or sacral divisions of the parasympathetic system (see below).

The magnitude of an adrenergic or cholinergic response is directly correlated with the amount of transmitter released from postganglionic terminals, which in turn is a function of the frequency of incoming nerve impulses. The adrenergic receptors of vascular smooth muscle include both alpha and beta types in most vessels, although their relative densities vary from one vascular region to another. The nature of the vascular smooth muscle response varies with the transmitter and the receptors that bind it: contraction in the case of norepinephrine and alpha-adrenergic receptors, relaxation by norepinephrine and beta-adrenergic receptors. The cholinergic receptors are of the muscarinic class, blocked by atropine; their vasomotor actions are discussed later in this chapter.

Although norepinephrine is an agonist for both alpha- and beta-adrenoceptors, the contraction mediated by the former dominates the response in almost all blood vessels. The fibers involved are often called *constrictor nerves* for that reason, but it would be more accurate to say that they control the degree of force exerted by vascular smooth muscle. The diameter of a vessel depends on the transmural pressure that tends to distend it, as well as the muscle activity that tends to constrict it. Moreover, any reduction in the frequency of sympathetic constrictor impulses diminishes muscle contraction and leads to relative vasodilatation. This flexibility is exploited in most reflex adjustments of the circulation, which utilize changes in the sympathetic adrenergic impulse rate to increase or decrease the caliber of arterioles.

The release of norepinephrine from sympathetic adrenergic terminals is the most widespread mode of neural vascular control, but the density of this innervation varies widely. Small arteries and arterioles in the skin, skeletal muscle, and splanchnic bed have a profuse network of such fibers at the adventitial–medial border, for example, whereas cerebral vessels have a relatively sparse innervation. Nerve terminals containing norepinephrine are scarcer in veins than in arteries, as can be demonstrated by fluorescent labeling of that neurotransmitter (Figure 8.3). Some evidence suggests that veins also contain fewer alpha-adrenergic receptors.

Central nervous system cardiovascular control usually operates by regu-

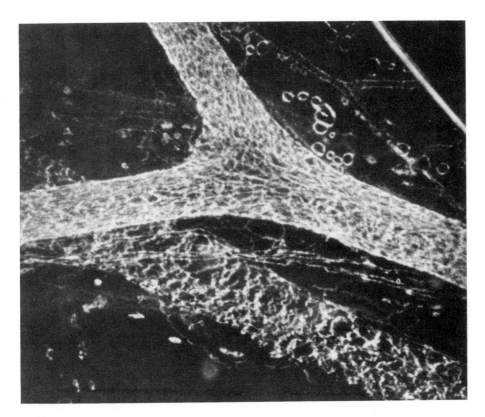

Figure 8.3. Plexus of adrenergic nerve fibers around small artery (*above*) and vein (*below*) in rat mesentery, demonstrated by fluorescence method. (Reproduced from Falck,[40] with permission of *Acta Physiol. Scand.*)

lating several hemodynamic variables simultaneously, but a few general statements about the effectors can be made. As a rule, moderate reflex augmentations of cardiac output owe more to tachycardia than to increased myocardial contractility. This principle is evident in responses to baroreceptors and in mild exercise, where stroke volume is little affected. More strenuous demands on the circulation raise contractility and stroke volume, as well as heart rate. A second generalization applies to reflex elevations of arterial pressure, which are accomplished principally by increasing vascular resistance rather than cardiac output, although this depends in part on the starting point.

VASOMOTOR TONE. In addition to the passive tension induced in blood vessel walls by transmural pressure, a certain degree of active force is exerted at all times by vascular smooth muscle, although not to the same extent in all vessels. This muscle activity arises in part from a small but constant release of neurotransmitters, in part from vasoactive chemicals in the local environment of the muscle cells, and in some cases from smooth muscle cells that act as pacemakers. The result is a characteristic basal *tone* in each part of the vascular tree, establishing a level on which dilatation or further constriction can be imposed. The amount of resting tone varies with the type and number of receptors in the smooth muscle cells, as well as the amount of muscle, the density of its innervation, and the frequency of nerve impulses. The full range of contraction is elicited by frequencies between 0 and 15 impulses/sec (Figure 8.4).

Vasomotor control in skeletal muscle is illustrated in Figure 8.4. The data were obtained in experiments on the leg muscles of the cat,[34] and vascular resistance was used as the measure of response to changing levels of nerve stimulation. Constrictor and dilator fibers were both present in the sympathetic nerve trunk stimulated, and their separate effects were observed by the use of appropriate blocking agents. A certain *intrinsic tone* and finite resistance are present even in the absence of vasomotor impulses (frequency = zero). Stimulation of constrictor fibers alone causes an increase in resistance above the basal level (rising curve) and stimulation of dilator fibers decreases it (falling curve), with a clear correlation between stimulus frequency and the magnitude of the effect in both cases.

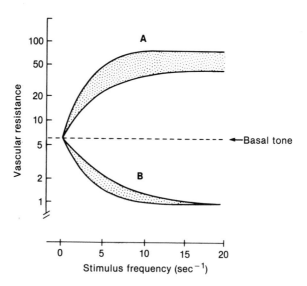

Figure 8.4.   Range of vasomotor control in feline leg muscles, showing relation of vascular resistance (*ordinate*, relative units, logarithmic scale) to frequency of stimulation applied to distal end of cut abdominal sympathetic chains (*abscissa*). *Stippled areas* indicate range of results observed in one series of experiments. **A**, effects of adrenergic constrictor fibers (sympathetic dilator fibers blocked by atropine). **B**, dilatation by sympathetic cholinergic neurons (adrenergic fibers blocked by dihydroergotamine). (Based on data from Celander[34])

Basal tone in each vascular bed determines the basal level of blood flow in that region, but the maximum blood flow in any bed when all its vessels are fully dilated depends on the vascularity of the tissue, that is, the number of small parallel vessels per unit weight or volume. As might be expected, this maximum is high in vascular structures like the salivary gland and low in avascular fatty tissue. Starting from the basal level and given a constant driving pressure, maximum regional vasodilation alone can increase flow through the kidney by less than 20%, but it can raise cerebral flow by a factor of about 2 and myocardial, splanchnic, or cutaneous flow by a factor of 6 to 24 (Figure 8.5).

FUNCTIONAL CLASSIFICATION OF VESSELS. Vasomotor control is exercised on vascular smooth muscle in all parts of the circulation, but the hemodynamic consequences vary with the size and location of the vessels affected. The resistance changes are produced by constriction or dilatation of arterioles and venules, which are consequently referred to as *resistance vessels*. Large arteries and veins also have a finite resistance, but it is extremely small because of their large diameter, as Poiseuille's law predicts (Chapter 6). The drop in mean pressure per millimeter of length is quite steep in an arteriole but very small in the aorta.

Veins of large and medium size offer relatively little resistance to flow, but the volume of the venous system as a whole is quite large, amounting to about two-thirds of the total blood volume. Because of this large capacity, veins are

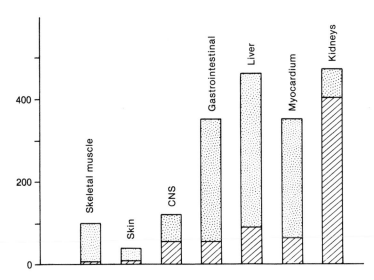

Figure 8.5. Regional blood flows in basal state (*diagonal lines*) and in maximum vasodilatation (*stipple*). *Ordinate*, ml blood flow/min per 100 g tissue, showing relative vascular resistance of each organ system.

classified as *capacitance vessels.*[16] An increase in venous tone can displace significant amounts of blood to other parts of the system, or raise venous pressure, by relatively small changes in the distensibility of veins. Large and intermediate arteries are sometimes called *conduit vessels,* as if they merely conveyed blood to the periphery, but that designation ignores the influence of these vessels on the impedance of the arterial system and on the transmission of pulsations of pressure and flow (Chapter 6). Increased smooth muscle tension in the aortic wall, for example, raises aortic input impedance and in that way places a greater burden on the left ventricle. The special place of capillaries in the circulation is recognized by their designation as *exchange vessels,* because they provide the delivery site for which all the rest is a transport system. To some extent, particularly in the pulmonary circulation, the arteriolar and venular segments at the entrance and exit of the capillary share in the transfer of solutes between vascular and interstitial compartments.

Resistance vessels also have an indirect effect on capillary function. Although the capillary wall contains no smooth muscle and is consequently not subject to direct vasomotor control, arteriolar constriction tends to lower intracapillary pressure and venular constriction to raise it. In this way, neural stimuli and local vasoactive substances can control indirectly the opening or closing of capillaries. Such changes not only alter local blood flow but also influence the net transfer of water and solutes across the capillary membrane, because the ratio of precapillary to postcapillary resistance influences capillary pressure. This ratio is among the variables affected by the atrial stretch receptor reflex, providing one element in the regulation of plasma volume (Chapter 10).

This functional classification is a useful way of thinking about the circulation for many purposes. In a broad sense, small-vessel resistance and large-vein distensibility are the main vascular properties controlled by neural and humoral stimuli. Resistance vessels determine the distribution of cardiac output among the various organs, and hence regional blood flow. Capacitance vessels influence the blood pressure and the filling pressure of the heart. This relatively simple picture of the circulation is sufficient in many cases to explain changes in *mean* blood pressure and flow.

Vasoconstriction

Constrictor nerves, meaning those in which an increase of impulse frequency causes smooth muscle contraction, all belong anatomically to the sympathetic division of the autonomic nervous system and release norepinephrine at their terminals. Adrenergic regulation of cardiac and smooth muscle cells by receptors is discussed in Chapters 3 and 9. Recent immunohistochemical and other studies show that many adrenergic nerves release a second transmitter along with norepinephrine; ATP is one example (Chapter 9), neuropeptide Y (NPY) another.[67] Exogenous NPY constricts peripheral systemic and cerebral arteries; this vasoconstriction is not affected by blockade of adrenergic receptors.

The *co-release* of NPY and norepinephrine from nerve terminals presumably has a more potent constrictor effect than would be evoked by either transmitter alone. NPY is distributed widely in the perivascular nerves of systemic vessels but appears in only about half of the cells of sympathetic ganglia, suggesting that adrenergic postganglionic fibers consist of two subpopulations. One releases NPY along with norepinephrine; this group includes the vasomotor axons. The other does not contain NPY and does not innervate blood vessels, but supplies exocrine glands, adipose tissue, and other cells.[18]

The physical effect of vasoconstriction is an increase in the pressure drop per unit length of the vessel (Chapter 6). If the constriction is widespread, the result *in vivo* is usually a rise in pressure upstream (i.e., in the arteries), with little change in the venous pressure downstream. This phenomenon is known by virtue of experimental observations. It could not have been predicted from physical laws like the Poiseuille equation, which defines the *ratio* of driving pressure to flow. The elevation of pressure comes about because the heart in such situations usually increases its external work enough to keep blood flow at about the previous level. This example illustrates the general principle that the net hemodynamic results of vasomotor activity depend partly on cardiac performance and partly on changes in the vascular tree.

EFFECTS OF DENERVATION. The observation that cutting of sympathetic nerves causes distal vasodilatation was the beginning of vasomotor physiology, and that effect is now known to result from withdrawal of normal sympathetic vasoconstrictor tone. Of equal importance, however, is the fact that the vasodilatation is only temporary. After sympathetic denervation of the hand, for example, vascular tone begins to return in a few days, and blood flow may be back to normal in a few weeks.[1] This recovery is not due to regeneration of the nerves, and the full explanation is not known. Spontaneous generation of action potentials in some smooth muscle cells, followed by cell-to-cell conduction throughout the wall, may account for partial recovery of tone.

Another aspect of this same phenomenon is the hypersensitivity of blood vessels to catecholamines after denervation. Exposure of a sympathectomized hand to cold or other stimuli that provoke increased secretion by the adrenal medulla produces very intense vasoconstriction, for example. This increased responsiveness probably comes about because local catecholamine concentrations regulate the properties of the smooth muscle alpha-adrenergic receptors. A decreased norepinephrine level in the wall of denervated vessels causes an increase in the number of these receptors, raising the response of the muscle cells to catecholamines available from the blood stream. Conversely, chronic elevation of circulating epinephrine leads to a decrease in the number of alpha-adrenergic receptors.[35]

Vasodilatation

CHOLINERGIC MECHANISMS. True vasodilator nerves in which stimulation evokes a relaxation of vascular smooth muscle are more restricted in their distribution than are the constrictor nerves. Sympathetic dilator fibers are limited to skeletal muscle vascular beds. Parasympathetic dilator nerves supply the external genitalia and some intracranial arteries (see below). Both kinds are cholinergic. The conclusion that the terminals of these sympathetic and parasympathetic nerves release acetylcholine is supported by several lines of evidence, including the fact that atropine tends to block the dilator response. Like other vasomotor nerves, they do not penetrate beyond the outer media, and one would expect rapid inactivation of the transmitter by acetylcholinesterase, yet it apparently diffuses far enough to reach significant numbers of muscle cells.

The mechanism by which vasodilator fibers act has been called into question by recent investigations, however. The blockade by atropine is often incomplete,and recognition of a number of noncholinergic dilator substances has prompted reexamination of the experimental evidence for cholinergic activity. Of equal importance is the finding that muscarinic cholinergic receptors activated by acetylcholine exist not only in smooth muscle but also in endothelial cells and at presynaptic sites in adrenergic nerves. Furthermore, at least one of the mechanisms of active sympathetic vasodilatation seems to act through atropine-blockable cholinergic receptors in peripheral ganglion cells.[55]

The discovery that endothelial cells release substances that cause vasodilatation under physiological conditions is a relatively recent advance of major proportions. The binding of acetylcholine to muscarinic cholinergic receptors of endothelium causes release of *endothelial relaxing factors*, which in turn act directly on vascular smooth muscle cells. The number of such factors is not yet known; nitric oxide is one of them (Chapter 9). The nature of the phenomenon has been demonstrated by a variety of experimental methods. In vessels that are relaxed by acetylcholine *in vitro,* for example, relaxation no longer occurs after removal of the endothelial layer from the vascular wall.[11] Moreover, the factor that is released when the endothelium is intact can be recovered and applied to an unstimulated vessel, where it causes relaxation. This form of cholinergic vasodilatation is thus indirect in the sense that it is mediated by endothelial cells.

Nevertheless, the role of endothelial cells in vasomotor regulation under physiological conditions is far from clear, in part because of uncertainty about the source of acetylcholine that might stimulate them. The distribution of parasympathetic cholinergic terminals is limited, and the circulating blood does not contain significant levels of acetylcholine because of the rapid enzymatic mechanisms for degrading that transmitter. The fact that substances other than acetylcholine—namely, ATP, histamine, bradykinin, substance P,[17] and vasopressin[11]—can also stimulate endothelial release of relaxing factor may well be relevant.

The vascular muscle cells themselves possess muscarinic cholinergic receptors, but their activation by acetylcholine causes contraction, or vasoconstriction, a response that can be demonstrated *in vitro* in some vessels.[53] The reaction of a particular artery or vein to acetylcholine apparently depends on the relative magnitude of these two opposing responses, an indirect relaxation via endothelium and a direct contractile effect on muscle. In most instances, relaxation appears with low concentrations of the transmitter, and some degree of contraction occurs with higher concentrations.

Another effect of acetylcholine arises from its inhibition of norepinephrine release by adrenergic nerves, an action mediated by presynaptic muscarinic receptors near the vascular nerve terminals and blocked by muscarinic antagonists. In this way, acetylcholine reduces the amount of norepinephrine released and the resulting vasoconstriction caused by adrenergic nerve stimulation. In vessels where adrenergic and cholinergic fibers both innervate the adventitial–medial border, this interaction provides an axoaxonal form of adrenergic regulation.[39]

Because of these multiple sites of action and the recognition of other natural dilator substances, the extent and mechanism of dilatation mediated through autonomic cholinergic nerves are controversial at present. As far as sympathetic cholinergic fibers are concerned, the consensus is that they are responsible for muscle vasodilatation in the *defense reaction* and in anticipation of exercise, but not during muscle exertion or in the dilatation that persists for a short time afterward.[4] The marked dilatation that occurs with exercise is to some extent the product of local metabolites, but it also has a neural component that may be mediated by sympathetic purinergic nerves (see below).

SYMPATHETIC VASODILATORS. Vascular beds in the skeletal musculature are supplied with sympathetic cholinergic dilator as well as adrenergic constrictor nerves. These fibers are silent at rest but transmit impulses in circumstances that evoke the defense reaction (see below) and in response to various forms of psychological stress, causing a vasodilatation that can be blocked by atropine. The fibers act to relax the smooth muscle of some arterioles, but in spite of this microcirculatory reaction, oxygen uptake tends to fall slightly (Chapter 12). Since there is no change in the number of functioning capillaries,[61] nonnutritive shunt pathways have apparently opened, a response that might be interpreted as a preparation for muscular activity before any increase in oxygen uptake is actually required. The same sympathetic vasodilator nerves were once thought to mediate the dilatation that accompanies physical exercise, but that response appears to be neither cholinergic nor adrenergic because it is not completely blocked by atropine or sympathectomy.[4]

The external genitalia are supplied with both sympathetic and parasympathetic cholinergic vasodilator nerves, which mediate penile engorgement and erection. These sympathetic erector fibers originate in lumbar spinal segments L2–L4 and reach the pelvis by way of the hypogastric nerves. Abdominal sympathectomy interrupts these pathways and eliminates the emission of seminal fluid because it inactivates the sympathetic motor fibers to the seminal vesicles, but it does not otherwise alter overt sexual behavior.

The existence of sympathetic vasodilator nerves in other mammalian organs is dubious. Vasodilatation in the skin, gastrointestinal tract, pulmonary vessels, and salivary glands is probably attributable to other mechanisms, either parasympathetic dilators, withdrawal of sympathetic constriction, purinergic stimuli, or local paracrine effects (Chapters 11 and 12). Sympathetic cholinergic fibers innervate sweat glands, and in some species they may also supply some cutaneous blood vessels, but the cutaneous circulation is controlled mainly by changes in sympathetic constrictor tone, locally generated peptides, and purinergic mechanisms.

PARASYMPATHETIC DILATOR NERVES. Cerebral and genital blood vessels are the two principal groups known to be supplied with parasympathetic cholinergic vasodilator fibers. Acetylcholine-containing nerve endings have been demonstrated in many cerebral vessels, including prominent cholinergic plexuses on the circle of Willis and terminals on the pial, anterior and middle cerebral, basilar, and internal carotid arteries. Adrenergic terminals of sympathetic fibers are also present to a lesser degree. Atropine-sensitive dilatation can be demonstrated by the increased cerebral blood flow caused by infusion of cholinergic agonists and by the dilatation of pial arteries to which carbamylcholine has been applied.[48] Pial arteries receive parasympathetic dilator fibers from the medulla by way of a plexus on the internal carotid artery and the facial nerve. In the cat and monkey, stimulation of the geniculate ganglion or the facial nerve hear the medulla causes an ipsilateral dilatation of arterial vessels of the parietal cortex.

Small coronary vessels and arterioles are supplied with cholinergic dilator nerves, but it is not clear whether they should be classed as sympathetic or parasympathetic.[4] Acetylcholine-containing fibers have been identified histologically in small coronary arteries, but they are unaffected by complete cardiac denervation and presumably arise from ganglia within the heart.[36] This peripheral location argues that they are parasympathetic. The presence of parasympathetic vasodilatation in other organ systems is even less certain, but it probably exists to some extent in the gastrointestinal tract, salivary glands, uterus, and pulmonary vascular bed. Pulmonary vessels are dilated by acetylcholine, for example, although that can be demonstrated only if a significant level of constrictor tone has first been established. There are marked species differences in each case, and the cholinergic mechanism is not the only one that contributes to vasodilatation.

INHIBITION OF ADRENERGIC NERVES. Many adrenergic nerves possess presynaptic receptors that inhibit the release of norephinephrine at the nerve terminals. Specific receptors of this kind exist for a number of naturally occurring substances. The alpha$_2$-adrenoceptors of nerves, for example, have a high affinity for norepinephrine itself, and binding of that transmitter to presynaptic alpha$_2$ adrenoceptors inhibits norepinephrine release at the synaptic terminals, creating a negative feedback loop. (These nerve cell receptors should not be confused with the postsynaptic alpha$_2$-receptors of smooth muscle cells described in Chapter 9.)

Other compounds that mediate similar presynaptic inhibition include acetylcholine, purine nucleotides, serotonin (5-hydroxytryptamine, 5-HT) dopamine, histamine, and prostaglandins. Some of these agents may be important in cardiovascular regulation, but the evidence for such a conclusion is still far from complete. To the extent that these materials are released by nonadrenergic nerves (see below), an axoaxonal interaction could be established. In the case of *adenosine* and *ATP*, the co-release of those transmitters with norepinephrine in certain nerves provides another example of feedback control (Chapter 9). Prejunctional *angiotensin* receptors of adrenergic nerves have exactly the opposite effect, namely, an enhancement of nerve-stimulated responses, and the same may be true of beta-adrenoceptors in some situations.[14]

Serotonin receptors of vascular smooth muscle cells mediate vasoconstriction directly, but in addition, there are presynaptic 5-HT receptors on adrenergic nerve fibers in some blood vessels. The latter are responsible for the inhibition of nerve-stimulated release of norepinephrine and for the dilator response to 5-HT observed in canine limbs, a response that is blocked by specific 5-HT antagonists.[57] *Dopamine* acts in a similar way,[5] but the results are extraordinarily variable in different species. Blockade of prejunctional dopamine receptors potentiates the responses to constrictor nerve stimulation in the rabbit ear artery, for example, but not in the dog hind limb. Multiple receptor subtypes have been described, but the physiological role of endogenous dopamine remains uncertain. *Prostaglandins* E1 and E2 (but not I2) produce the same kind of presynaptic adrenergic nerve inhibition, a response that can be demonstrated by exogenous administration of these prostaglandins or arachidonic acid. Stimulation of sympathetic nerves leads to release of prostaglandins of the E series,[41] but they probably come from postjunctional tissues, not from the nerve terminals. *Histamine* has an inhibitory effect on adrenergic neuro-transmission via presynaptic H_2 receptors. Although this agent is present in high concentrations in sympathetic nerves, blood vessel walls and the heart, the physiological consequences of such inhibition are dubious because the histamine antagonists currently available do not alter the response to sympathetic nerve stimulation.

SECRETOMOTOR NERVES. Local vasodilatation occurs on stimulation of the parasympathetic nerves to the salivary glands, but these are not true vasodilator nerves. The dilatation is caused by a substance secreted by the glandular cells, not by a conventional neurotransmitter. The secretomotor fibers that evoke secretion in these glands thus influence the vascular smooth muscle of the region only indirectly.

This phenomenon has been under investigation for more than a century, and the gradual clarification of the mechanism is a good example of the way physiological knowledge grows through research. Claude Bernard found in 1858 that stimulation of the cervical sympathetic trunk reduced blood flow through the submandibular salivary gland, suggesting vasoconstriction. Stimulation of the chorda tympani nerve had the opposite effect, causing the venous outflow from the gland to increase, become pulsatile, and change to a more nearly arterial color. The vasodilatation these signs suggested was confirmed repeatedly in later years, and the chorda tympani came to be regarded as the classical example of a nerve containing vasodilator fibers. In 1872 Heidenhain discovered that the vasodilatation was not abolished by doses of atropine that prevented salivary secretion, and concluded that separate secretomotor and vasodilator fibers exist in the chorda tympani nerve. Joseph Barcroft disputed that conclusion some years later (1914), rejecting the idea of separate vasodilator fibers. Noting that stimulation of the chorda increased oxygen consumption of the salivary gland even when secretion was blocked by atropine, he suggested that metabolic activity of the gland released some substance that caused vasodilatation. This view, which was not widely accepted for a long time, is now known to be correct in principle.

Subsequent investigation confirmed and extended the theory that activation of the salivary glands produces a substance that causes vasodilatation.[45] Physiological salt solutions perfused through the gland during chorda stimulation acquire vasodilating properties, which can be demonstrated by injecting the solution into a normal blood-perfused gland. Botulinus toxin, which selectively inactivates cholinergic fibers, abolishes both secretory and vasodilating effects of chorda stimulation, indicating that some cholinergic link is an integral part of the response. The vasoactive material is released after arterial injection of acetylcholine, as well as by stimulation of the chorda tympani, yet the dilatation is not antagonized by atropine.

Eventually, the sequence of events became clearer. Stimulation of the chorda causes the glandular cells to release an enzyme (*kallikrein*) into the local extracellular space (Figure 8.6). This enzyme acts with a normal endogenous globulin (*kininogen*) to produce a polypeptide, *kallidin,* which is rapidly transformed to *bradykinin.* The last two products are both potent vasodilators, and they are least one source of the vasodilatation that follows stimulation of the nerves to the salivary glands and tongue. This response, brought about by locally produced agents, is now recognized as one of several types of paracrine vasomotor regulation (see below). Later investigations brought the story full circle by showing that vasodilatation by nerve stimulation can occur in salivary glands perfused with kininogen-free solutions, suggesting that some dilator nerve fibers may, after all, function in addition to the bradykinin mechanism.[44] Bradykinin is involved in a number of different physiological responses, and may be the pain-producing agent that is liberated by myocardial ischemia and other kinds of tissue injury (Chapter 7).

Cutaneous vasodilatation has also been ascribed to bradykinin, sweat glands being the source in this case, but increasing evidence makes that conclusion unlikely. Active, atropine-resistant vasodilatation unquestionably occurs in the skin and is indeed the principal component of indirect responses to heat or cold. The direct, local response to applied heat is predominantly a physical effect of the temperature itself. Warming of one part of the body causes reflex vasodilatation in other parts, however, and it is such indirect vasomotor effects that concern us here. In experiments of this kind, sweating occurs and blood flow increases, but bradykinin has not been found in the venous effluent

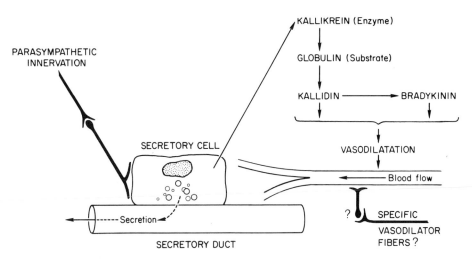

Figure 8.6. Mechanisms of vasodilatation in salivary gland on stimulation of parasympathetic nerve supply. See text for discussion. (After Gautvik,[44] Hilton and Lewis,[45] and others)

from the affected limbs. Nevertheless, active vasodilatation in the skin does not occur in subjects with congenital absence of sweat glands,[22,32] pointing to the secretion of some other vasoactive substance not yet identified. Adenosine, ATP, and prostaglandins are among the candidates. Purinergic nerves have been suggested as the source of cutaneous vasodilatation in some species, but they have not been found in man.

AXON REFLEXES. Localized vasodilatation can be generated by the terminal branches of some sensory nerves in the skin and mucous membranes. Mechanical or chemical irritation of the skin generates action potentials in such sensory fibers, and these impulses not only travel in the normal direction toward the spinal cord but also enter other branches nearby, where they travel back out to local cutaneous blood vessels (*antidromic conduction*) and cause dilatation. True afferent nerves are involved, for their cell bodies lie in somatic sensory ganglia. Stimulating the distal end of a cut dorsal spinal root brings on the same response, and a similar local reflex causes hyperemia in the intestinal mucosa upon mechanical stimulation.

This *axon reflex* underlies one part of the "triple response" of the skin to sharply localized pressure, stroking firmly with a needle, for example. The skin around the affected area reddens because of arteriolar dilatation. The reaction can be elicited for a short time after nerves to the region are cut, but not after the somatic sensory fibers have degenerated. The transmitter is not known but it may be histamine, because the other components of the response (reddening of the traumatized spot and formation of an edematous wheal in the region) are caused by local release of that substance (see below). Intense, localized cooling can evoke the same kind of vasodilatation.

At the level of the central nervous system, the mediation of painful sensations in general may involve serotonergic neurons. Drugs that inhibit the uptake of 5-HT potentiate the action of morphine, for example, and tryptophan, a precursor of 5-HT, has been said to have antinociceptive effects. The current literature on this subject is extensive and the evidence is mixed,[21] but some investigators postulate the existence of an antinociceptive system of neurons that projects from the periaqueductal gray to the nucleus raphe magnus and then to the dorsal horn via cells containing 5-HT. This hypothesis raises the possibility that a pain-relieving 5-HT antagonist may be discovered.

Nonadrenergic, noncholinergic nerves

Nerves that contain neither norepinephrine nor acetylcholine have been found in a number of regions, and in some cases stimulation of these nerves has vasomotor effects. The neurotransmitters involved are the subject of intense investigation, and the list of substances that might serve this function continues to lengthen. Vasoactive intestinal peptide (VIP), serotonin, ATP, substance P, somatostatin, enkephalins, and prostaglandins have been found in the enteric plexuses and some of their axons.[12]

Purinergic nerves, in which ATP or adenosine acts as the neurotransmitter, are perhaps the class most clearly identified so far. Their terminals can be identified histologically by the presence of large, opaque vesicles, as contrasted with the small, agranular vesicles characteristic of acetylcholine storage sites and the small, granular vesicles typical of adrenergic fibers.[4] Adenosine and ATP are both effective vasodilators in most blood vessels, ATP being the more potent of the two; their general vascular effects are treated in a later section. Purinergic nerves have been identified in the gastrointestinal tract and a number of other organ systems, as well as in the portal vein and in vessels of the intestine and mesentery. Whether other blood vessels possess such innervation is still a matter for conjecture, as is its physiological significance. Elevated levels of adenyl compounds have been found in the venous effluent from the heart and in a number of other vascular beds during hypoxia, although it is not yet possible to say whether they come from nerve terminals or tissue metabolism. Some of the ganglia from which purinergic nerves arise lie peripherally, in the organ itself, like those of the parasympathetic system.

Serotonergic nerves, which release serotonin, exist in the brain and in the myenteric plexus of the gut. They affect the muscle of the stomach and intestines in much the same way as vagal stimulation, but their physiological functions with respect to blood vessels are unknown. The effects of serotonin on the circulation, and its action as a presynaptic modulator of adrenergic nerves, are discussed elsewhere in this chapter.

Endocrine Control

Catecholamines from the adrenal medulla

The adrenal medulla is in many ways analogous to a postganglionic sympathetic neuron, secreting transmitters when stimulated through preganglionic sympathetic fibers. It releases both epinephrine and norepinephrine (in their physiologically active levo-rotatory forms) into the bloodstream, although the proportions vary in different species. Quantitative changes in the amounts secreted are reflected in plasma levels and are one of the mechanisms of cardiovascular control. These catecholamines are thus hormones in the conventional sense, and norepinephrine is in addition a neural transmitter. Adrenergic receptors mediate the action of blood-borne catecholamines on the heart and blood vessels, just as they do when these same substances are neurally released. In many circulatory response, catecholamines released by nerve terminals and the adrenal medulla act in concert as a sympathoadrenal system, as illustrated by the response to hypoxia (see below).

The plasma level of norepinephrine is approximately 200 picograms/ml in supine human subjects at rest and about twice that during quiet standing.[7] Intravenous infusions show that levels greater than 1500 pg/ml must be reached to produce hemodynamic effects, indicating that blood-borne norepinephrine plays little part in circulatory control under basal conditions.[64] During strenuous exercise, however, adrenal secretion increases sufficiently to establish norepinephrine plasma concentrations well above the cardiovascular threshold. In contrast, the circulating plasma level of epinephrine averages about 30 pg/ml in man at rest, and only moderate elevations (50 to 100 pg/ml) cause an increase in heart rate and arterial pressure. Epinephrine thus acts as a cardiovascular-regulating hormone under almost all conditions. Other effects, such as those of glycolysis and suppression of insulin secretion, appear only at higher epinephrine concentrations.

The effects of administering these catecholamines to intact animals are well known because of their use in experimental studies and in some clinical situations. Intravenous administration of epinephrine in humans increases heart rate, myocardial contractility, and venomotor tone. The positive inotropic effects on the heart, added to the effects of venoconstriction on filling pressure, raise cardiac output, stroke volume, and left ventricular work. Epinephrine speeds the slow repolarization phase in pacemaker cells, returning their potential to the resting level more rapidly and increasing their firing rate. This effect is not seen in atrial or ventricular muscle cells, although ectopic atrial or ventricular arrhythmias occasionally appear. The refractory period of atrial and ventricular muscle becomes shorter, along with that of the atrioventricular node, and atrioventricular conduction becomes faster.

The vasomotor effects of epinephrine arise from its affinity for both alpha- and beta-adrenergic receptors. The response in each vascular bed is the net result of smooth muscle activation by the former and relaxation by the latter. The arterioles in cutaneous and renal beds constrict, but those in skeletal muscle and the splanchnic region dilate and total peripheral resistance falls. In spite of the fall in resistance, the increase in cardiac output is great enough to raise arterial blood pressure. The elevation of pressure is usually only moderate, however, because it is curbed by a prompt baroreceptor response. Pulse pressure enlarges because of the increased stroke volume, and that change, together with the rise in mean pressure, pushes the systolic pressure higher. If the increase in pulse amplitude is large and the rise in mean pressure is relatively small, diastolic pressure tends to fall (Chapter 6). One probable cause of these regional differences is that alpha- and beta-adrenoceptors are not present in the same proportions in all vessels.

Norepinephrine has similar effects, but its affinity for beta-adrenergic receptors is lower than that of epinephrine, whereas both catecholamines have roughly the same affinity for alpha-adrenergic receptors. Consequently, norepinephrine causes more vasoconstriction and less excitation of the heart than does epinephrine. Virtually all vascular beds constrict, and peripheral resistance increases. Mean and systolic systemic arterial pressures tend to rise to a greater extent than with epinephrine, and diastolic pressure often increases.

Renin and angiotensin

Renin is secreted by the *juxtaglomerular cells* of the kidney, epithelioid types that lie in the wall of the afferent arteriole at its entrance to Bowman's capsule. In the same region, cells in an adjacent loop of the distal convoluted tubule form a histologically identifiable structure called the *macula densa*. The specialized cells of the arteriolar wall and those of the macula densa together are referred to as the *juxtaglomerular apparatus*. The amount of renin released under various circumstances by the juxtaglomerular cells is directly correlated with the concentration of intracellular granules they contain, which provides one method of estimating secretory activity. Granularity is reduced by high renal perfusion pressure and increased by a sodium-free diet. According to one widely held theory, the cells of the macula densa are sensitive to the sodium content or osmolality of distal tubular fluid, and control release of renin by the juxtaglomerular cells.

The biologically active peptide and vasoconstrictor, angiotensin II, is the end result of a series of substrates and enzymes that have come to be known as the *renin-angiotensin system*. The enzyme renin acts on a substrate manufactured by the liver to produce *angiotensin-I,* which is rapidly converted to *angiotensin-II*. Elevation of the levels of angiotensin-II stimulates secretion of *aldosterone* by the adrenal gland, leading to reduction of the output of sodium in the urine.

Renin is released from the kidney into the bloodstream and into the local interstitial spaces, whence it finds its way into the renal lymphatic drainage. Renin-like materials, probably isoenzymes of kidney renin, have been found in other organs, but their physiological significance is not known. Renin is inactivated by the liver, and its half-life in the bloodstream is 15 to 20 min. The angiotensin-I generated from renin substrate by renin is converted into angiotension-II, principally by a single passage through the pulmonary circulation. A similar conversion may take place to some extent in the juxtaglomerular apparatus itself, permitting direct local effects of angiotensin-II on the kidney. Angiotensin-II is rapidly degraded by nonspecific peptidases, and its effects are consequently of short duration. The vasoconstricting action of injected angiotensin-II disappears in a few minutes.

Any decrease in renal arterial pressure stimulates renin release, and thus a rise in the circulating level of angiotensin-II, implying that juxtaglomerular cells sense, and are activated by, distention of the walls of the afferent arterioles. The effective stimulus is apparently the local transmural pressure, not decreased blood flow. The same response follows partial clamping of the renal artery, which is consistent with the finding of high circulating renin levels in clinical cases of hypertension associated with pathological stenosis of that vessel. Other pathological forms of hypertension have been carefully studied in this respect because of the marked pressor action of angiotensin-II, but abnormal levels of renin have not been found consistently. Plasma renin is increased in congestive heart failure, however, and in subjects whose dietary intake of salt has been greatly reduced. Renin release is affected by pressure in the atria as well as in the distal renal arterial tree, and the elevated levels of ANP produced by atrial distention (Chapter 7) inhibit renin release. The renin-angiotensin-aldosterone system is thus a central element in the regulation of body fluids, blood volume, and arterial pressure. It serves both homeostatic and protective functions, reacting not only to severe hemorrhage but also to hemodynamic stresses as mild as a change of posture.

Blood pressure is not the only physiological stimulus for renin release, for it appears to be controlled in part by neural pathways. Stimulation of sympathetic nerves to the kidney elicits not only renal vasoconstriction but also secretion of renin. Both responses can be duplicated by norepinephrine infusion and blocked by beta-adrenoceptor antagonists,[28] but such observations do not make clear whether the renin release is caused by nerve impulses or by the vasoconstriction they elicit. Stronger evidence for neural control is the fact that the reflex effects of mild hemorrhage increase renin release even when the blood loss is too small to alter blood pressure. The possibility that the supply of renin may be influenced by the composition of renal tubular fluid has also been raised.

The vasoconstrictor effect of angiotensin-II is greatest in arterioles of the skin, splanchnic region, and kidney. Vascular beds of skeletal muscle, heart, brain, and lungs are affected to a much smaller degree. An increase in myocardial contractility can be demonstrated experimentally, but the cardiac effects are small compared to the elevation of blood pressure. With extreme peripheral vasoconstriction, ventricular end-diastolic pressure may rise to some extent. Angiotensin-II acts directly on receptors in vascular smooth muscle and the myocardium.[29] The action on myocardial cells, unlike that mediated by beta-adrenoceptors, does not employ cyclic AMP as the intracellular messenger. Prejunctional angiotensin receptors exist on some adrenergic nerves, and angiotensin is one of the few substances to enhance, rather than diminish, the release of norepinephrine by this mechanism.[69] Increases in the plasma level of angiotensin-II stimulate production of vasopressin and are suspected of modifying baroreceptor reflex function.[33] The influence of the renin-angiotensin system on arterial blood pressure has naturally made it a suspect in human hypertension, and it is known to play a part in some but not all forms of that disorder.[9]

Posterior pituitary hormones

Vasopressin (antidiuretic hormone, ADH) contracts vascular smooth muscle in most of the arterial tree, including the coronaries, and in venules. Apart from coronary vasoconstriction, its effects on the heart are slowing of atrioventricular conduction and a transient tachycardia followed by a baroreceptor-induced decrease in heart rate. The renal effect of ADH—reduced volume and increased osmolarity of the urine—are not the result of vasomotor changes but of altered permeability of tubular cells to water. *Oxytocin* is another posterior pituitary hormone that acts on blood vessels, but with an opposite and more transient effect, namely, relaxation of vascular smooth muscle and increased blood flow to the limbs. Oxytocin is best known for its potent contraction of uterine smooth muscle. ADH and oxytocin are similar in structure, and the vasodilator action of oxytocin is blocked by ADH. It seems unlikely that either ADH or oxytocin is involved in the physiological regulation of resting tone in blood vessels, but their cardiovascular effects must be taken into account whenever they are administered for therapeutic purposes.

Paracrine Control

Some vasoactive materials are synthesized by nonneural cells and released into the local extracellular space, where they act on other cells nearby. Bradykinin is one example of this *paracrine* mode of action that has already been discussed, but there are many others. In some instances, a substance has both paracrine and endocrine functions, as in the case of renin and angiotensin-II. In others, the same agent serves as a neurotransmitter and a paracrine agent.

Prostaglandins

Prostaglandins (PG) are a class of lipids derived from arachidonic acid and grouped with the family of *eicosanoids,* a term applied to oxygenated 20-carbon fatty acids, which also include leukotrienes and thromboxanes. A number of different prostaglandins are synthesized from arachidonic acid by vascular smooth muscle and endothelial cells, as well as by other cell types, in virtually all organs. Prostacyclin (PGI_2) is the principal variety produced by large vessels, and arteries have a much greater capacity to produce it than do veins. Microvessels tend to produce types other than PGI_2. The kidney, especially its medullary portion, generates a mixture of prostaglandins that stimulate renin release by direct action on juxtoglomerular cells.[43]

The transformation of arachidonic acid into the intermediate metabolites that lead to these prostaglandins is controlled by an enzyme system, endoperoxide synthetase, which is inhibited by indomethacin and other aspirin-like drugs. The parent compound, arachidonic acid, has no effect on blood vessels, but PGE_2 and PGI_2 cause vasodilatation, and $PGF_{2\alpha}$ constriction, in some vascular beds.[10] The cellular mechanism of action of prostaglandins is unknown. Prostaglandin production is regulated not only by signals that involve phosphoinositides, as might be expected from its relation to arachidonic acid, but also by non-specific stimuli such as thrombin. Mechanical shear stress is another interesting but little explored stimulus for prostaglandin synthesis.[42]

The physiological functions of prostaglandins have yet to be unraveled, but these substances can produce many different effects.[52] PGI_2 and PGE_2 are vasodilators and can modulate constrictor stimuli from other sources. Systemic arterial blood pressure falls when PGE_2 or PGI_2 is given intravenously, and there is marked vasodilatation in the kidney, intestines, and mesentery. This dilatation is not endothelium dependent. Regional differences exist in the action of these two prostaglandins, however. In pulmonary arteries and veins, PGI_2 causes dilatation but PGE_2 produces constriction. In mesenteric vessels, PGE_2 elicits a transient increase in resistance, quickly followed by a return to the control state.

$PGF_{2\alpha}$ is predominantly a vasoconstrictor in the dog and rat, but not in all other species and not in all organs. Intravenous infusion of $PGF_{2\alpha}$ leads to mesenteric and pulmonary vasoconstriction, but renal vascular resistance is not affected. The net result is usually a rise in systemic arterial pressure. Prostaglandins of the E type also inhibit the release of norepinephrine by adrenergic nerves. As a result, indomethacin reduces the effect of stimulating sympathetic constrictor fibers.

Prostaglandins are not stored in tissues but are synthesized as needed. Moreover, they are *local hormones* in the sense that they act almost entirely on the cells that produce them and on others nearby. PGE_2 and $PGF_{2\alpha}$, but not PGI_2, are removed from the bloodstream by a single passage through the pulmonary circulation. The substances are also taken up by the liver and kidney, and circulating blood levels are extremely low. Prostaglandin production takes place in the vicinity of the cell membrane,[23] and endothelial cells probably release eicosanoids in two directions: from the luminal surface, where they can reach blood platelets, and from the abluminal side, where they act on the adjacent smooth muscle.

Other arachidonic metabolites

Prostaglandins as a class also include the *leukotrienes*[58] and *thromboxanes,* Leukotrienes are produced by many large vessels, but their physiological role in circulatory regulation is still uncertain. The production of leukotrienes from arachidonic acid does not follow the enzyme pathway of the prostaglandins described above, and they are consequently not influenced by indomethacin. They act on vascular smooth muscle and some are vasoconstrictors, at least for the coronary and mesenteric beds, whereas others relax the smooth muscle of blood vessels, at least *in vitro*.[30] The dominant function of leukotrienes is as mediators of immunological and inflammatory reactions through effects on leukocyte activity and vascular permeability. They are among the slow-acting substances of anaphylaxis.

Thromboxanes synthesized by platelets and other tissues are potent vasoconstrictors. Thromboxane TXA_2 is found in blood platelets and acts to promote their aggregation, which can lead to thrombosis. PGI_2 has an antiaggregatory effect, and the balance between these two prostaglandins probably regulates platelet aggregation in man. The lung can generate thromboxanes (and prostaglandin 6-keto-$PGF_{1\alpha}$) actively; the specific tissue source is unknown, but it could be smooth muscle, endothelium, or parenchymal cells. The pulmonary hypertension that develops when plasma complement is activated by contact with artificial membranes, an occasional complication of cardiopulmonary bypass, is apparently caused by this process.

Purine nucleotides

It has become increasingly evident that adenosine and ATP have major physiological roles in vascular regulation, although their function as neurotransmitters, as contrasted with that of locally produced paracrine agents, is still unclear. Myocardial hypoxia or ischemia causes a marked increase in ATP and adenosine in the coronary venous effluent, and a similar increase occurs with functional hyperemia of the heart, skeletal muscle, and brain. Adenosine has consequently been proposed as the principal agent in the muscle vasodilatation that accompanies exercise, but that hypothesis is still controversial.

ATP is a powerful dilator of most vascular beds, including those of the heart, kidney, salivary glands, and gastrointestinal tract. ATP and ADP are the most potent dilators of coronary arteries, whereas AMP and adenosine are less effective. Vasodilatation in the intestine can be produced by doses of adenyl compounds lower than those required to produce relaxation of the gut. The effects on pulmonary vessels are confusing, both constriction and dilatation having been observed in various experiments.

In many instances, vasodilatation is produced not only by ATP receptors of the vascular smooth muscle cells, but also by inhibition of adrenergic norepinephrine release via presynaptic ATP receptors on adrenergic terminals (see above). Similar modulation of adrenergic function by a negative feedback loop is an attribute of adenosine, acetylcholine, dopamine, and the prostaglandins of the E series. This fact suggests still another potential adenylic source of vasodilatation inasmuch as ATP promotes prostaglandin synthesis.[4]

Histamine

Histamine, which is released from cells of almost all tissues by injury and by antigen–antibody reactions, is one of the most potent dilators of arterioles and venules in the dog, monkey, and human. This response is highly species dependent, and constriction is the rule in cats and rodents. Direct effects on the myocardium are minimal, but histamine initially increases the venous tone and filling pressure, leading to a transient rise in cardiac output. As a result of species differences in the magnitude and interaction of these variables, histamine usually decreases blood pressure in the dog but raises it in the rabbit.

Increased permeability of the microcirculation is another effect of histamine, leading to extravasation of plasma protein and fluid into interstitial spaces. This response accounts for the regional edema of allergic reactions. The capillary wall plays some part in this phenomenon, but the gaps that develop between endothelial cells in venules are probably the principal sites of increased permeability.[51] Toxic doses of histamine in the dog produce marked hypotension that resembles traumatic shock, the result of peripheral pooling of blood as well as of an actual decrease in blood volume. The vascular actions are mediated by H_1 and H_2 histamine receptors of vascular smooth muscle cells.[24,60] The inhibitory action of histamine on adrenergic neurotransmission is mediated by H_2 receptors.

Effects on other organs include strong stimulation of secretion by gastric glands and constriction of bronchioles in most species, the latter being an important factor in bronchial asthma. Local intracutaneous injection of histamine in humans produces the so-called triple response, consisting of a red spot immediately around the site of injection, edema that forms a wheal in that same small area, and a more intense flush (*flare*) extending about 1 cm from the site. The first two elements of the response illustrate the vasodilatation and increased vascular permeability, but the wider dilatation in the third component involves a local axon reflex (see above).

Physical trauma is not the only stimulus that can cause cells to release histamine granules. Mast cells do so upon interaction of specific antigens and a cell-fixed antibody; this is the basis for allergic responses and anphylaxis.

The precise mechanism by which antigen acts on mast cells is not known, but it involves promotion of calcium influx. Histamine release does not account for all the features of hypersensitivity; a number of other substances appear in such reactions, including 5-HT, various kinins, and the *slowly reacting substance* that is now believed to be a leukotriene.

Serotonin

Serotonin is a naturally occurring substance that has a wide variety of effects, especially on the cardiovascular, respiratory, and gastrointestinal systems. In addition to its direct actions on various effector tissues, it serves as a neurotransmitter in some neurons of the central and enteric nervous systems (see above). Vasoconstriction is the most prominent vascular effect of serotonin. Pulmonary and renal arterioles are particularly sensitive to it, and large systemic veins are strongly constricted. In the hind limb of the dog, however, low doses of serotonin cause dilatation and increase blood flow, probably by way of serotonin's presynaptic inhibition of sympathetic adrenergic tone (see above). Species differences are marked, as illustrated by the observation that serotonin, like histamine, increases capillary permeability in rodents, but not in humans. As for its cardiac effects, a positive inotropic action of serotonin is evident in isolated papillary muscles, and the heart rate and cardiac output are increased in intact animals.

These responses are largely due to direct actions on vascular smooth muscle and myocardium, but in addition, serotonin, like acetylcholine, may act on endothelial cells to release their *relaxing factor.* One observation that points in this direction is that coronary vasoconstriction by serotonin is potentiated by removal of the endothelium.[49] The picture is further complicated by reflex effects by way of chemosensitive afferent nerve endings that are activated by serotonin (Chapter 7). In the heart, for example, serotonin is one of the substances that can stimulate vagal afferent nerve endings in the left ventricle to produce the *coronary chemoreflex,* leading to marked hypotension and bradycardia (Bezold-Jarisch reflex). Serotonin also stimulates chemoreceptors of the carotid and aortic bodies, provoking a brief increase in the depth, and sometimes the rate, of respiration. Actions on other organs include contraction of intestinal smooth muscle and increased motility in the gut. Bronchial smooth muscle is contracted by serotonin *in vitro,* but bronchoconstriction is not consistently observed *in vivo.*

Serotonin acts through specific serotonin receptors to exert its effects, which can be blocked by selective antagonists. The excitatory effect on smooth muscle is presumably brought about by increased calcium influx. On nerves, however, the action of serotonin is usually inhibitory and appears to operate through potassium channels (for references, see Chapter 3). The endogenous source of serotonin is synthesis by neurons, chromaffin cells of the gut, and the pineal gland. Platelets do not synthesize the substance but acquire high concentrations by uptake from the blood. Production and degradation proceed at a fairly rapid pace. This fact, combined with the wide distribution and multiple effects of the material, make it likely that serotonin has an important, although not yet clearly defined, place in physiological regulations.

Dopamine

Dopamine (DOPA), a precursor of norepinephrine, has a positive inotropic effect on the heart, raising cardiac output and thereby increasing arterial pressure in man even though peripheral resistance is not altered. It causes renal vasodilatation, however, and increases sodium excretion. The direct effect on blood vessels apparently operates through specific DOPA receptors of vascular smooth muscle cells. Other DOPA receptors located presynaptically on adrenergic nerve fibers mediate the inhibition of norepinephrine release already mentioned. Although dopaminergic neurons have been found in the brain, there is no clear evidence of their existence in the cardiovascular system.

Vasoactive intestinal peptide

Vasoactive intestinal peptide (VIP) was originally found in the gastrointestinal tract, where it is located in neurons of stomach muscle, intestinal mucosa, and in blood vessel walls.[62] VIP dilates small vessels of the intestinal vascular bed, and reflex hyperemia provoked by mechanical stimulation is followed by a marked rise of VIP in the venous outflow from that bed. The vascular responses are inhibited when local nerve conduction is blocked by tetrodotoxin, supporting the hypothesis that this peptide is a neurotransmitter. VIP also appears in the walls of other peripheral vessels, although the concentrations vary greatly among species. Vasodilator fibers in cerebral arteries of the cat contain both acetylcholine and VIP, suggesting neural co-release of these two substances.[8] VIP levels in cerebral arteries of the rabbit, on the other hand, are very low, a contrast that matches the active cerebral vasodilator mechanism observed in the cat and its absence in the rabbit.[8] Neural vasodilatation in the salivary and other exocrine glands may be another example of cholinergic–VIP co-release.[50]

Other peptides

That many peptides are biologically active has been known for years, but knowledge in this field is now advancing at a dizzying pace.[50,62,67] The precise structure of substance P, angiotensin-II, vasopressin, oxytocin, thyrotropin-releasing hormone, enkephalins, somatostatin, and neurotensin, to name just a few of these peptides, is now known. Many of these substances may be neurally released, and the distinction between endocrine, paracrine, and neural transmitters is becoming hazy.

Substance P[17] has been identified by immunocytochemical methods in enteric nervous system neurons[12] and in chromaffin cells of the gastrointestinal mucosa, as well as the dental pulp. In addition to being a potent vasodilator, it has been implicated in antidromic nerve stimulation in the teeth and skin, and may be one of the pain-producing substances released by injured cells.

Integrated Reactions to Stress

Reactions of the body to stress range from relatively simple reflexes initiated by specific peripheral sensors to complex adaptations in which higher centers of consciousness play an important part. The chemoreceptor-triggered response to hypoxia is among the less complicated reactions, whereas the physiological adjustments to exercise and hemorrhage call on a great variety of peripheral sensors. Reflex adjustments to the erect posture modify the properties of the circulation to counteract the effects of gravity (Chapter 13). The so-called defense reaction, to which visual perceptions and the emotional state make significant contributions, is an example of involvement of higher levels of the brain. In each case, changes occur in several organ systems, and it is evident that the central nervous system does not merely alter a single variable like heart rate, but deploys a wide range of effectors to achieve a particular goal.

Specific centers in the hypothalamus are associated with some of the more highly integrated responses, including exercise, temperature regulation, and the defense reaction. Stimulating such a region evokes most of the components of the reaction, and damaging it blunts the normal response, but these areas are simply concentrations of neurons that process information from various parts of the brain and transmit the results to lower levels (Chapter 7).

Hypoxia

The reflex responses to hypoxia involve neural, adrenal, and local mechanisms.[47] The consequences of two different types of hypoxia provide an instructive contrast, revealed by comparing the effects of two respiratory gas mixtures, one containing 8% O_2, the other containing 0.2% CO and the normal 21% O_2. The former produces a low arterial pO_2 (*arterial hypoxia*) and therefore stimulates the chemoreceptors, which sense the partial pressure of oxygen, not the amount of oxygen in each unit of blood. The CO mixture does not activate them because it does not alter the normal arterial pO_2, but it lowers the amount of O_2 carried to the periphery because of the affinity of CO for hemoglobin and thus causes *tissue hypoxia*. In both cases the supply of O_2 to peripheral tissues declines, and the local vascular response is vasodilatation. The autonomic responses and the part played by adrenal secretion of catecholamines differ in the two situations, however.

Arterial hypoxia causes a transient drop in cardiac output and heart rate, together with an abrupt rise in total peripheral resistance, but all of these variables return toward control values in a few minutes. The heart tends to stabilize at a higher rate, and the vascular system at a slightly lower resistance, than before. The consequences for arterial pressure are a brief rise followed by a return to the control level, which is generally maintained without further deviations. Tests comparing adrenalectomized and sympathectomized animals show that the autonomic nervous system is the principal efferent path for the whole response, although adrenal release of catecholamines also contributes. Both divisions of the autonomic efferent system join in the response. The initial bradycardia, for example, involves an increase in parasympathetic and a reduction in sympathetic impulses to the pacemaker.

Although arterial hypoxia of this degree causes only a small decrease in total peripheral resistance in the steady state, the effects are not uniform in all organs. Vascular resistance falls in skin and muscle of the limbs, but resistance increases sharply in the splanchnic vascular bed and moderately in the kidneys. This regional difference has been attributed to corresponding variations in the distribution of beta-adrenoceptors, which are activated by epinephrine from the adrenal medulla and cause relaxation of vascular smooth muscle. This explanation implies that the discharge of sympathetic constrictor impulses under these conditions is diffuse, not regionally selective, and there is no evidence that contradicts this assumption. The particularly high sensitivity of the portal bed to dilatation by low pO_2 also plays a part. Cholinergic sympathetic vasodilatation is not involved. The cardiovascular reactions are accompanied by a marked respiratory hyperventilation, and signals from lung inflation receptors become part of the afferent information that contributes to the overall response.

Tissue hypoxia induced by CO has somewhat different consequences. Respiration is not affected, cardiac output rises and remains elevated, and heart rate increases slightly. There is a marked fall in total peripheral resistance, with no early transient increase, and systemic arterial pressure declines in parallel with the resistance, in spite of the increased cardiac output. Again, the regional vascular changes are not uniform, but in this case the splanchnic resistance falls, a response just opposite to that in arterial hypoxia. A slight vasoconstriction occurs in skeletal muscle in some instances; renal vascular resistance undergoes little change.

Plasma catecholamines rise considerably during the response in intact animals, and the hypotensive reaction is accentuated after adrenalectomy or sympathectomy. The two elements of sympathoadrenal control, neural and secretory, thus appear to play more equal roles than they do in arterial hypoxia. A smaller sympathetic constrictor discharge and a greater epinephrine release in tissue hypoxia could account for the striking drop in pressure.

Although tissues are adversely affected by hypoxia of any kind and cells begin to deteriorate quickly when their blood supply is interrupted, additional cell damage often occurs when blood flow is restored. This paradoxical *reperfusion effect* is a serious clinical complication of attempts to relieve coronary artery occlusions. Current evidence points to free radicals like superoxide (two oxygen atoms with an extra free electron, O_2^-) and other reactive O_2 species as the deleterious agents.[31] Normal aerobic metabolism operates predominantly through divalent O_2 pathways, and the small amounts of O_2^- that are produced are eliminated by the action of superoxide dismutase, an enzyme present in most tissues. Upon reperfusion of cells that have been deprived of O_2 for a critical period, however, superoxide may be produced in amounts that overwhelm the natural scavenging mechanisms. O_2-derived free radicals also appear to be the source of damage in pulmonary O_2 poisoning, a disorder caused by high environmental O_2 tensions and characterized by pulmonary edema and alveolar hemorrhage.

Hemorrhage

Acute loss of blood triggers the compensatory responses summarized in Figure 8.7. The reduction in total blood volume lowers the MCFP (Chapter 6), and hence pressures throughout the circulation, a change sensed by the atrial stretch receptors and baroreceptors. The resulting reflex causes a sympathetic adrenergic discharge that increases the heart rate, raises myocardial contractility, constricts arterioles and veins, and increases adrenal secretion of catecholamines. The tachycardia, pallor of the skin, sweating, and rapid breathing that are characteristic clinical signs of acute hemorrhage reflect this sympathetic response. The magnitude of the reflexes and their net effect depend on the amount of blood lost. Systemic arterial pressure usually remains normal with losses of up to 10% of the total blood volume, but it falls if the hemorrhage is rapid and exceeds that amount. Slow bleeding may produce no hypotension until one-third of the blood volume has been lost.

Arteriolar constriction is most marked in skin, muscle, and splanchnic beds, and less prominent in the renal blood vessels, probably because of the high degree of autoregulation in the kidney. No constriction occurs in the cerebral and coronary vascular beds, so blood flow to the brain and heart is main-

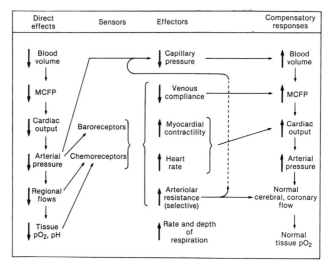

Figure 8.7. Schematic summary of responses to hemorrhage. MCFP, mean circulatory filling pressure. *Heavy upward arrows* denote an increase; *downward*, a decrease. Compensatory responses tend to counteract direct effects of hemorrhage.

tained at the expense of flow to other organs. Venous constriction tends to reduce the capacity of the circulatory system to match the new blood volume, thus returning MCFP toward normal values. Increased venomotor tone is one of the most important compensatory mechanisms in this situation, because relatively large amounts of blood can be displaced from the venous tree with little effect on venous pressure. The venous beds of the liver and splanchnic region in particular are, in a sense, emergency "reservoirs" of blood (Chapter 13).

Sympathetic nervous activity is not the only compensatory response that acts to sustain blood pressure by vasoconstriction. Large amounts of epinephrine and norepinephrine are released by the adrenal medulla, and the plasma concentration of these catecholamines rises sharply. In addition, the posterior pituitary increases the amount of vasopressin (ADH) released into the bloodstream. This hormone provides a powerful vasoconstrictor and acts on the kidney to reduce water excretion. If hypotension develops and renal perfusion falls, the renin-angiotensin system comes into play, adding angiotensin to the repertoire of constrictors and at the same time stimulating increasing aldosterone production by the adrenal cortex, which promotes retention of sodium and water. A variety of mechanisms thus combine to raise peripheral vascular resistance and maintain total body fluids at a tolerable level.

The responses that tend to maintain intravascular volume include a passive effect at the capillary level. As arteriolar constriction lowers capillary pressure, the balance of forces across the capillary wall changes to favor net transfer into the vascular compartment. By this means, plasma volume is increased at the expense of the extracellular fluid, diluting the blood, lowering the hematocrit, and reducing osmotic pressure of the plasma. The baroreceptor reflex itself stimulates adrenal secretion of cortisol, which in concert with other unidentified factors causes a shift of fluid from the intracellular to the interstitial space.

Powerful as these compensatory mechanisms are, severe hemorrhage can lead to marked hypotension and inadequate blood flow to the tissues. At arterial pressures below about 60 mm Hg the arterial baroreceptor reflex has reached its maximum, and no further constriction can be generated by that route. Some evidence suggests that sympathetic efferent impulses actually decrease in frequency at very low pressures. The brain is likely to be underperfused in this extreme situation, however, and cerebral ischemia becomes a source of constrictor impulses and tachycardia (Chapter 12). Local blood flow through the carotid and aortic bodies may also fall to such an extent that the chemoreceptors are activated, in which case the heart rate slows and bradycardia develops. If blood loss has not been too great or prolonged, transfusion often restores circulatory conditions to normal, but reduction of blood volume by more than one-third for longer than an hour frequently leads to irreversible hypotension and death.

Extreme hypotension that is resistant to therapeutic measures is called *circulatory shock*; its cause is not definitely known. Hemorrhage evokes many effects other than the protective mechanisms discussed above, and some of them tend to be self-perpetuating. Reduced coronary blood flow as arterial pressure falls is an obvious example, because the consequent depression of cardiac output leads to further hypotension. Similarly, local hypoxia and hypercapnia cause relaxation of vascular smooth muscle, tending to counteract reflex vasoconstriction, and in time these abnormalities tend to reduce vascular responsiveness to any stimulus. Metabolic acidosis is another deleterious effect of severe blood loss. If blood flow decreases to such an extent that the O_2 delivered directly to the tissues is insufficient for their needs, the deficiency is met by anaerobic metabolism, producing lactic acid and other metabolites that lower blood pH. The resulting acidosis has a negative inotropic effect on the myocardium and tends to cause vasodilatation. It also stimulates the chemoreceptors, producing hyperventilation. Clearly, there is no lack of factors that might make hypotensive hemorrhage irreversible, but it is not yet clear which ones are of critical importance.

Cardiac failure is a frequent complication of severe hemorrhage and shock. Reduced coronary perfusion and acidosis are doubtless major sources of the impairment of myocardial function, but some recent evidence suggests that amino acids and peptides released by ischemic tissues may be additional factors. In other organs, severe ischemia in an underperfused region can lead to tissue necrosis and bleeding, a complication to which the intestines are particularly susceptible. Even if treatment is successful and pressure is eventually restored to normal levels, significant damage to the kidney, intestine, or brain may already have occurred.

Exercise

The hemodynamic changes that accompany muscular exertion have been extensively studied in dogs trained to run on a treadmill and in human subjects. The responses begin immediately at the onset of exercise, although a steady state is not reached for several minutes. Heart rate and cardiac output increase abruptly, and total peripheral resistance falls. The increase in cardiac output to meet the needs of exercise is the most marked hemodynamic effect. Blood flow increases as a function of the intensity of the exercise, primarily in the exercising muscles. Mean systemic arterial pressure tends to remain constant with mild exertion, the increased output balancing the fall in peripheral resistance, but at higher levels of exercise and output the pressure rises moderately. The double burden imposed by exercise in high environmental temperatures is considered in Chapter 12.

The cardiac responses to exercise were confusing in early studies until the effects of posture alone on cardiac output were recognized. Stroke volume at rest is lower in the erect than in the supine position, and at any given level of cardiac output during exercise, there is a tendency for heart rate to be higher and stroke volume smaller in the upright than in the supine posture. In addition, small and inconsistent changes in ventricular volumes were observed in dogs, leading to the erroneous conclusion that the Starling mechanism played no part in the circulatory adaptations to exercise.

More recent investigations with improved techniques for measuring volumes have resolved the uncertainties, at least in man. Ventricular end-diastolic and stroke volumes increase at virtually all levels of muscular exertion.[59] Stroke volume increases only a little with mild exercise, so that tachycardia accounts for most of the increment in cardiac output. With higher degrees of effort, stroke and end-diastolic volumes both increase. Conflicting reports on ventricular filling pressure have appeared,[38,66] but it seems wise to assume that the observed increase in end-diastolic volume implies increased end-diastolic transmural pressure in the absence of evidence to the contrary. Most investigators now agree that the Starling mechanism does operate during exercise, but the increase in cardiac output is mostly the result of a sympathetically stimulated enhancement of myocardial contractility. End-systolic ventricular volume decreases, especially in the upright posture, and the left ventricular ejection fraction rises from the resting level of about 0.60 to as much as 0.85.

The cardiac effects result from sympathetic adrenergic discharge, which also increases vasomotor tone. The muscular and abdominal pump mechanisms also come into play immediately. Marked vasodilatation in the exercising muscles is caused mainly by local metabolic changes, including a falling pO_2 and a rising pCO_2. Because of this vasodilatation, and because the renal and splanchnic beds constrict just enough to maintain their blood flow at the preexercise level, most of the increased cardiac output goes to skeletal muscle. The contribution of neural impulses delivered through sympathetic cholinergic fibers to the reduced vascular resistance in muscle is debatable (see above). In any event, the combined mechanisms for dilatation in the muscle bed during exercise are so effective that stimulation of sympathetic constrictor nerves scarcely changes the resistance.

The rise in cardiac output is directly correlated with oxygen consumption and workload (Figure 8.8A). The mechanism for this close matching of blood flow to metabolic needs is not entirely clear. Conventional baroreceptors apparently play no part, for adequate output is achieved even though mean pressure does not change. Furthermore, the major chemoreceptors are not involved. Systemic arterial O_2 saturation does not change in normal subjects, but the arteriovenous O_2 difference widens as more O_2 is taken up by the muscles, and venous O_2 saturation typically falls with heavy exercise from the normal 80% to about 50%. Given normal pulmonary function, the arterial pCO_2 does not change. Blood lactate rises in proportion to the severity of the exertion. When exercise stops, the heart rate and ventilation remain elevated for several

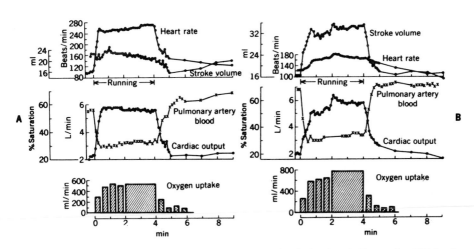

Figure 8.8. Cardiovascular responses and oxygen uptake during treadmill exercise (5.5 km/hr, 21% grade). **A**, normal dog. **B**, dog with chronic cardiac denervation. (Reproduced from Donald and Shepherd,[37] with permission of the American Physiological Society)

minutes. The arteriovenous O_2 difference falls rapidly, reaching control levels in 2 to 5 min, indicating that an oxygen "debt" has been repaid.

The source of afferent signals that dictate just how much increase in total cardiac output is required is not obvious. This adjustment has the characteristics of a central reflex, and it may be regulated by signals from the mechanoreceptors of the atria, lungs, skeletal muscles, and joints. However mediated, the result is an appropriate increase in output, even in the absence of cardiac nerves. After denervation the heart develops tachycardia more slowly and to a lesser extent, but it increases the stroke volume so as to reach the required cardiac output (Figure 8.8B). This phenomenon suggests that the reflex element of control is exerted through the vascular system, possibly through an increase in venomotor tone.

Stimulation of a circumscribed hypothalamic region dorsolateral to the mammillary bodies produces cardiovascular responses very similar to those observed during exercise.[66] The same changes in stroke and end-diastolic volumes appear, together with approximately the same patterns of regional vasodilatation and constriction. As we have already said, the identification of such a center does not mean that it is the sole source of adaptation to the needs of exercise, but only that some of the important elements in the control path are located there.

Physical training

The effectiveness of physical training in improving athletic performance in situations that call for enhanced cardiovascular function is well known. Most of the readjustments that come into play have been identified, and although the physiological mechanisms that generate them remain obscure, the end result is that training increases the maximum O_2 uptake and cardiac output that an individual can attain during exercise.[6] Cardiac output at rest is similar in trained and untrained persons, but physical training tends to lower the resting heart rate and increase the stroke volume.

Studies of college students before and after a 2-month training period have shown an average increase in maximum O_2 uptake from a pretraining control value of 3.30 liters/min to 3.91 liters/min and a small but significant elevation of maximum cardiac output from 20.0 to 22.8 liters/min. Stroke volume increased with training from 104 to 120 ml, but exercising heart rates were unchanged. Olympic athletes were found to be literally in a class by themselves,[3] with stroke volumes of about 170 ml, maximum O_2 uptakes of 5.4 liters/min, and cardiac outputs of 30 liters/min. The high level of O_2 uptake that trained individuals can attain is directly correlated with the maximum cardiac output they can achieve. The principal effect of training, in other words, is to increase the maximum ability of the cardiovascular transport system to deliver oxygen to the tissues. No major changes develop in pulmonary function or the ability to ventilate, except at the most extreme levels of performance.

One of the cardiac effects of training is an increase in ventricular end-diastolic volume, and hence preload, both at rest and during exercise. There is also a modest hypertrophy of the left ventricular wall in some cases,[54] although the degree of enlargement is nothing like that seen in valvular heart disease. These are the only cardiac changes that have been documented convincingly. Myocardial contractility, the inherent ability of the cardiac muscle cells to contract, seems to undergo no change. The vascular tree makes things easier for the heart, however, by a training-induced lowering of afterload. The decrease in the resistance of the arterioles of skeletal muscle during exercise is even more marked in trained than in untrained individuals, reducing the amount of work required of the heart for any given cardiac output.

All of these alterations improve the capacity of the system to deliver O_2 but in addition, there may be changes in the ability of the peripheral tissues to utilize it. The arteriovenous O_2 difference during exercise is widened by training (although arterial O_2 saturation is not altered), showing an increased efficiency of skeletal muscle in taking up O_2 from the blood supplied to it. Furthermore, there is enlargement of mitochondrial volume in the muscle cells and increased levels of oxidative enzymes.[3] The mechanism of these peripheral changes remains unknown.

Defense reaction

An animal confronted by a threatening situation exhibits a more or less stereotyped complex of physiological responses, which has come to be known as the *defense reaction*.[26,68] The cardiovascular changes consist of an increase in cardiac output, heart rate, and systemic arterial pressure, together with vasoconstriction in cutaneous, intestinal, and renal vascular beds and vasodilatation in skeletal muscle. These responses are mediated by an increased sympathetic adrenergic discharge except in skeletal muscle, where the vascular resistance is decreased by a combination of reduced sympathetic constrictor tone and dilatation by sympathetic cholinergic nerves.

The responses are thus similar to those in exercise, but in this case there is little or no muscular exertion, and the initial input must involve the visual cortex and other sensory centers, not to mention memory. The reaction is evoked by the animal's perception of something potentially harmful, and the reaction varies to some degree with the behavior it adopts. The muscle vasodilatation occurs only with hind limb movements, which may presage an effort to attack or escape; in the absence of such movements, the heart rate is not greatly elevated or may even fall. The same set of physiological responses can be produced by stimulation of a specific part of the hypothalamus, and the full reaction requires integrity of a region that extends longitudinally from the hypothalamus through the midbrain and pons to the medulla.

References

Reviews

1. Barcroft, H., Swan, H.J.C. (1953). *Sympathetic Control of Human Blood Vessels*. London, Edward Arnold.

2. Benfey, B.G. (1980). Cardiac alpha-adrenoceptors. *Can. J. Physiol. Pharmacol.* 58:1145–1157.

3. Blomqvist, C.G., Saltin, B. (1983). Cardiovascular adaptations to physical training. *Annu. Rev. Physiol.* 45:169–189.

4. Burnstock, G. (1980). Cholinergic and purinergic regulation of blood vessels. In: *Handbook of Physiology, Section 2: The Cardiovascular System. Vol. II, Vascular Smooth Muscle*, D.F. Bohr, A.P. Somlyo, and H.V. Sparks, Jr., eds. Bethesda, MD., American Physiological Society, pp. 567–612.

5. Buylaert, W.A., Willems, J.L., Bogaert, M.G. (1981). Peripheral prejunctional dopamine receptors. In: *Vasodilatation*, P.M. Vanhoutte and I. Leusen, eds. New York, Raven Press, pp. 125–130.

6. Clausen, J.P. (1977). Effect of physical training on cardiovascular adjustments to exercise in man. *Physiol. Rev.* 57:779–815.

7. Cryer, P.E. (1980). Physiology and pathophysiology of the human sympathoadrenal neuroendocrine system. *N. Engl. J. Med.* 303:436–444.

8. Duckles, S. (1981). Vasodilator innervation of cerebral blood vessels. In: *Vasodilatation*, P. M. Vanhoutte and I. Leusen, eds. New York, Raven Press, p. 27–37.

9. Dzau, V.J., Gibbons, G., Levin, D. (1983). Renovascular hypertension. An update on pathophysiology, diagnosis, and management. *Am. J. Nephrol.* 3:172–184.

10. Feigen, L.P., Hyman, A.L. (1981). Vascular influences of prostaglandins. *Fed. Proc.* 40:1985–1990.

11. Furchgott, R.F. (1984). The role of endothelium in the responses of vascular smooth muscle to drugs. *Annu. Rev. Pharmacol. Toxicol.* 24:175–197.

12. Gershon, M.D. (1981). The enteric nervous system: Multiplicity of neurotransmitters outside the brain. In: *Smooth Muscle*, E. Bulbring et al., ed. Austin, University of Texas Press, pp. 263–284.

13. James, T.N. (1974). Anatomy of the conduction system of the heart. In: *The Heart, Arteries and Veins*, 3rd ed., J.W. Hurst, R.B. Logue, R.C. Schlant, and N.K. Wenger, eds. New York, McGraw-Hill, pp. 52–62.

14. Langer, S.Z. (1981). Presynaptic regulation of the release of catecholamines. *Pharmacol. Rev.* 32:337–362.

15. Levy, M.N., Martin, P.J. (1979). Neural control of the heart. In: *Handbook of*

Physiology, Section 2, Vol. I, The Heart, R.M. Berne, N. Sperelakis, and S.R. Geiger, eds. Bethesda, Md., American Physiological Society, pp. 581–620.

16. Mellander, S., Johansson, B. (1968). Control of resistance, exchange and capacitance functions in the peripheral circulation. *Pharmacol. Rev.* 20:177–196.

17. Payan, D.G. (1989). Neuropeptides and inflammation: The role of Substance P. *Ann. Rev. Med.* 40:341–352.

18. Pernow, J. (1988). Co-release and functional interactions of neuropeptide Y and noradrenaline in peripheral sympathetic vascular control. *Acta Physiol. Scand.* 133(Suppl. 568):1–56.

19. Pick, J. (1970). *The Autonomic Nervous System.* Philadelphia, J.B. Lippincott.

20. Randall, W.C. (1984). *Nervous Control of Cardiovascular Function.* New York, Oxford University Press.

21. Roberts, M.H.T. (1984). 5-Hydroxytryptamine and antinociception. *Neuropharmacology* 23:1529–1536.

22. Rowell, L.B. (1981). Active neurogenic vasodilatation in man. In: *Vasodilatation,* P.M. Vanhoutte and I. Leusen, eds. New York, Raven Press, pp. 1–17.

23. Smith, W.L. (1986). Prostaglandin biosynthesis and its compartmentation in vascular smooth muscle and endothelial cells. *Annu. Rev. Physiol.* 48:251–262.

24. Westfall, T.C. (1980). Neuroeffector mechanisms. *Annu. Rev. Physiol.* 42:383–397.

25. Wikberg, J.E.S., Lefkowitz, R.J. (1984). Adrenergic receptors in the heart: Pre- and postsynaptic mechanisms. In: *Nervous Control of Cardiovascular Function,* W.C. Randall, New York, Oxford University Press, pp. 95–129.

Research Reports

26. Abrahams, V.C., Hilton, S.M., Zbrozyna, A.W. (1964). The role of active muscle vasodilatation in the altering stage of the defence reaction. *J. Physiol.* 171:189–202.

27. Armour, J.A., Hopkins, D.A. (1984). Anatomy of the extrinsic efferent autonomic nerves and ganglia innervating the mammalian heart. In: *Nervous Control of Cardiovascular Function,* W.C. Randall, ed. New York, Oxford University Press, pp. 20–45.

28. Assaykeen, T.A., Clayton, A., Goldfien, A. (1970). Effect of alpha- and beta-adrenergic blocking agents on the renin response to hypoglycemia and epinephrine in the dog. *Endocrinology* 87:1318–1322.

29. Baker, K.M., Capanile, C.P., Trachte, G.J., Peach, M.J. (1984). Identification and characterization of the rabbit angiotensin II myocardial receptor. *Circ. Res.* 54:286–293.

30. Berkowitz, B.A., Zabko-Potapovich, B., Valocik, R., Gleason, J.R. (1984). Effects of leukotrienes on the vasculature and blood pressure of different species. *J. Pharmacol. Exp. Ther.* 229:105–112.

31. Bernier, M., Hearse, D.J., Manning, A.S. (1986). Reperfusion-induced arrhythmias and oxygen-derived free radicals. Studies with "anti-free radical" interventions and a free-radical generating system in the isolated perfused rat heart. *Circ. Res.* 58:331–340.

32. Brengelmann, G.L., Freund, P.R., Rowell, L.B., Olerud, J.E., Kraning, K.K.

(1981). Absence of active cutaneous vasodilation associated with congenital absence of sweat glands in man. *Am. J. Physiol.* 240 (*Heart Circ. Physiol.*) 9):H571–H575.

33. Brooks, V.L., Keil, L.C., Reid, I.A. (1986). Role of the renin-angiotensin system in the control of vasopressin secretion in conscious dogs. *Circ. Res.* 58:829–838.

34. Celander, O. (1954). The range of control exercised by the "sympatheticoadrenal system." *Acta Phsyiol. Scand.* 32 (Suppl. 116):1–132.

35. Colucci, W.S., Gimbrone, M.A., Jr., Alexander, R.W. (1981). Regulation of the postsynaptic α-adrenergic receptor in rat mesenteric artery. Effects of chemical sympathectomy and epinephrine treatment. *Circ. Res.* 48:104–111.

36. Denn, M.J., Stone, H.L. (1976). Autonomic innervation of dog coronary arteries. *J. Appl. Physiol.* 41:30–35.

37. Donald, D.E., Shepherd, J.T. (1964). Initial cardiovascular adjustment to exercise in dogs with chronic cardiac denervation. *Am. J. Physiol.* 207:1325–1329.

38. Ekelund, L.-G., Holmgren, A. (1967). Central hemodynamics during exercise. *Circ. Res.* 21(Suppl. I):I33–I43.

39. Ehinger, B., Falck, B., Sporrong, B. (1970). Possible axoaxonal synapses between peripheral adrenergic and cholinergic nerve terminals. *Z. Zellforsch. Mikroskop. Anat.* 107:508–521.

40. Falck, B. (1962). Observations on the possibilities of the cellular localization of monoamines by a fluorescence method. *Acta Physiol. Scand.* 56(Suppl. 197):1–25.

41. Frame, M.H., Hedqvist, P. (1975). Evidence for prostaglandin mediated prejunctional control of renal sympathetic transmitter release and vascular tone. *Br. J. Pharmacol.* 54:189–196.

42. Francos, J.A., Eskin, S.G., McIntire, L.V., Ives, C.L. (1985). Flow effects on prostacyclin production by cultured human endothelial cells. *Science* 227:1477–1479.

43. Freeman, R.H., Davis, J.O., Villarreal, D. (1984). Role of renal prostaglandins in the control of renin release. *Circ. Res.* 54:1–9.

44. Gautvik, K. (1970). The interaction of two different vasodilator mechanisms in the chorda tympani–activated submandibular salivary gland. *Acta Physiol. Scand.* 79:188–203.

45. Hilton, S.M., Lewis, G.P. (1956). The relationship between glandular activity, bradykinin formation and functional vasodilatation in the submandibular salivary gland. *J. Physiol.* 134:471–483.

46. Hirsch, E.F., Nigh, C.A., Kaye, M.P., Cooper, T. (1964). Terminal innervation of the heart. II. Studies of the perimysial innervation apparatus and of the sensory receptors in the rabbit and in the dog with the technics of total extrinsic denervation, bilateral cervical vagotomy, and bilateral thoracic sympathectomy. *Arch. Pathol.* 77:172–187.

47. Korner, P.I., Chalmers, J.P., White, S.W. (1967). Some mechanisms of reflex control of the circulation by the sympatho-adrenal system. *Circ. Res.* 20–21(Suppl. III):157–172.

48. Kuschinsky, W., Wahl, M., Neiss, A. (1974). Evidence for cholinergic dilatory receptors in pial arteries of cats. *Pfluegers Arch.* 347:199–208.

49. Lamping, K.G., Marcus, M.L., Dole, W.P. (1985). Removal of the endothelium potentiates canine large coronary artery constrictor responses to 5-hydroxytryptamine in vivo. *Circ. Res.* 57:46–54.

50. Lundberg, J.M. (1981). Evidence for coexistence of vasoactive intestinal peptide (VIP) and acetylcholine in neurones of cat exocrine glands. Morphological, biochemical and functional studies. *Acta Physiol. Scand.* 496(Suppl):1–57.

51. Majno, G., Gilmore, V., Leventhal, M. (1967). On the mechanism of vascular leakage caused by histamine-type mediators. *Circ. Res.* 21:833–847.

52. Messina, E.J., Weiner, R., Kaley, G. (1976). Prostaglandins and local circulatory control. *Fed. Proc.* 35:2367–2375.

53. Milnor, W.R., Sastre, A. (1988). Cholinergic receptors and contraction of smooth muscle in canine portal vein. *J. Pharmacol. Exp. Ther.* 245:244–249.

54. Morganroth, J. Maron, B.J., Henry, W.L., Epstein, S.E. (1975). Comparative left ventricular dimensions in trained athletes. *Ann. Intern. Med.* 82:521–524.

55. Myers, H.A., Schenk, E.A., Honig, C.R. (1975). Ganglion cells in arterioles of skeletal muscle: Role in sympathetic vasodilatation. *Am. J. Physiol.* 229:126–138.

56. Palmer, R.M.J., Ferrige, A.G., Moncada, S. (1987). Nitric oxide release accounts for the biological activity of endothelium-derived relaxing factor. *Nature* 327:524–526.

57. Phillips, C.A., Mylecharane, E.J., Shaw, J. (1985). Mechanisms involved in the vasodilator action of 5-hydroxytryptamine in the dog femoral arterial circulation in vivo. *Eur. J. Pharmacol.* 113:325–334.

58. Piper, P.J. (1984). Formation and actions of leucotrienes. *Physiol. Rev.* 64:744–761.

59. Poliner, L.R., Dehmer, G.J., Lewis, S.E., Parkey, R.W., Blomqvist, C.G., Willerson, J.T. (1980). Left ventricular performance in normal subjects: A comparison of the responses to exercise in the upright and supine positions. *Circulation* 62:528–534.

60. Powell, J.R., Brody, M.J. (1976). Identification and specific blockade of two receptors for histamine in the cardiovascular system. *J. Pharmacol. Exp. Ther.* 196:1–14.

61. Renkin, E.M., Rosell, S. (1962). Effects of different types of vasodilator mechanisms on vascular tone and on transcapillary exchange of diffusible material in skeletal muscle. *Acta Physiol. Scand.* 45:241–251.

62. Said, S.I., Mutt, V. (1970). Polypeptide with broad biological activity: Isolation from small intestine. *Science* 169:1217–1218.

63. Schwegler, M. (1974). Sympathetic-parasympathetic interactions on the ventricular myocardium: Possible role of cyclic nucleotides, *Basic Res. Cardiol.* 3:215–221.

64. Silverberg, A.B., Shah, S.D., Haymond, M.W., Cryer, P.E. (1978). Norepinephrine: Hormone and neurotransmitter in man. *Am. J. Physiol.* 234 (*Endocrinol. Physiol.* 3):E252–E256.

65. Simpson, P. (1983). Norepinephrine-stimulated hypertrophy of cultured myocardial cells in an alpha$_1$ adrenergic response. *J. Clin. Invest.* 72:732–738.

66. Smith, O.A., Jr., Rushmer, R.F., Lasher, E.P. (1960). Similarity of cardiovascular responses to exercise and to diencephalic stimulation. *Am. J. Physiol.* 198:1139–1142.

67. Tatemoto, K., Carlquist, C., Mutt, V. (1982). Neuropeptide Y—a novel brain peptide with structural similarities to peptide YY and pancreatic polypeptide. *Nature* 296:659–660.

68. Zanchetti, A., Baccelli, G., Mancia, G. (1976). Fighting, emotions and exercise: Cardiovascular effects in the cat. In: *Regulation of Blood Pressure by the Central Nervous System.* G. Onesti et al., eds. New York, Grune & Stratton, pp. 87–103.

69. Zimmerman, B.G. (1983). Peripheral neurogenic factors in acute and chronic alterations of arterial pressure. *Circ. Res.* 53:121–130.

VASCULAR SMOOTH MUSCLE AND ITS REGULATION

Smooth muscle is the mechanically active tissue in blood vessels, the *effector* of control in the vascular tree. All blood vessels except capillaries contain smooth muscle cells, and their contraction or relaxation changes the distensibility of the vascular wall. Vasoconstriction and vasodilatation are consequently brought about by the activity of vascular smooth muscle. Although nerve signals are an important element in controlling this muscle,[2,40] a variety of blood-borne or locally produced substances also act directly on vascular smooth muscle cells.

In the smallest arteries and veins, regulation of diameter is equivalent to control of vascular resistance, in accordance with the principles of hemodynamics already discussed (Chapter 6). Vasoconstriction can reduce the lumen of an arteriole to a fraction of its normal size, greatly increasing its hydraulic resistance. Activating vascular muscle in large arteries like the major branches of the aorta has a different hemodynamic effect, although the muscle response is qualitatively similar. The resistance in such vessels is extremely low to begin with, and smooth muscle activity rarely changes their diameters by more than 15%. What smooth muscle contraction does in large arteries, however, is to increase their stiffness, raising their impedance and increasing the energy that must be expended to move blood through them. In a similar way, vasomotor activity controls the compliance of large veins, and consequently their function as blood reservoirs. Vascular smooth muscle has an exclusively autonomic motor innervation. It maintains some degree of contractile force, or *tone,* at all times, and can sustain a steady state of contraction with the expenditure of relatively little energy.

Blood vessels in different parts of the vascular tree, and in different species, do not all react the same way to a given stimulus. An increased frequency of impulses in the sympathetic fibers that innervate a blood vessel usually produces vasoconstriction, for example, but a few vessels respond by dilating. Moreover, the contraction is accompanied by muscle action potentials in some cases, but not in others. The facts discussed in this chapter help to explain why such diversity exists. For one thing, the smooth muscle cells can be excited by a variety of physiological mechanisms. Furthermore, the specific cell membrane receptors that mediate the contractile response in smooth muscle cells differ in kind and number from one blood vessel to another. Finally, vasomotor regulation in the intact animal involves local as well as central nervous control, and inhibitory as well as excitatory stimuli.

Structure and Function

Vascular muscle cells are similar in structure to those of smooth muscle in the gastrointestinal tract, uterus, and other regions, although responses to neurotransmitters vary considerably in different organs. The contractile apparatus of smooth muscle cells is not arranged in sarcomeres like those of skeletal and cardiac muscles, and the absence of regular microscopic striations is what gives *smooth* muscle its name. Smooth muscle cells do, however, contain actin and myosin, and cross sections demonstrate about 15 actin filaments disposed around each thick myosin filament in a kind of rosette pattern.

Individual smooth muscle cells are elongated structures 20 to 100 μm in length and 5 to 10 μm in diameter. Although often described as spindle-shaped, they do not always taper at the ends and may have an uneven contour. Structures analogous to the cross-bridges of striated muscle have not been observed, but contractile filaments are present, aligned at an angle of 5° to 45° with the long axis of the cell and inserted at each end on *dense bodies* in the cell wall. Stimulation of single, isolated smooth muscle cells demonstrates this arrangement clearly; the cell wall invaginates at the sites of dense bodies, and the cell contracts in a helical fashion along its length.[27,50] In spite of this orientation of the contractile apparatus, the main contraction is longitudinal. The dense bodies are often in contact with those of neighboring cells and apparently attached to them, providing a mechanical continuum that enables the cells to act as a contractile sheet.

Smooth muscle cells make up 40 to 60% of the medial portion of blood vessel walls.[5,13,38] The remainder consists of elastic tissue, collagen, and connective tissue, all embedded in an amorphous mucopolysaccharide ground substance (Table 6.2). The muscle cells are arranged in strings and sheets that travel helically around the vessel. The pitch of the helix varies, and both circular and longitudinal strands are found in some regions. Although the majority of muscle cells are attached to each other end to end or side to side, some insert on collagen fibers and others on elastin. The collagen forms a relatively loose network when blood pressure is normal and vessels are functioning at their normal diameter. Vascular distention, however, places a strain on this relatively stiff material, and the vessel becomes much less distensible as the diameter is increased.

The behavior of smooth muscle resembles in many ways that of striated muscle, where the cross-bridge mechanism is well established,[12] yet the way actin and myosin filaments interact in smooth muscle is not known. Troponins, which play an important role in striated muscle, are absent from smooth muscle. The physicochemical properties of actin are essentially the same in both types of muscle, and the same is true for myosin, although some differences in amino acid content have been noted.[38] Vascular muscle contains more actin and less myosin than striated muscle does per unit weight of tissue.[38] Maximum force per cell is much greater in vascular than in skeletal or cardiac muscle, even though the cross-bridge arrangement in the latter types would lead one to expect that force would be directly correlated with the amount of myosin. The difference may arise from a spatial organization of filaments that favors high force in smooth muscle, but that is no more than speculation at present. Recent information suggests that actin–myosin interaction may not be the only force-generating mechanism in smooth muscle. Intermediate strands of the protein *filamin* may bind to actin and regulate cell length without the intervention of cross-bridges.[43]

Virtually all arteries and veins are innervated by branches of the autonomic system called *vasomotor nerves,* but the density of innervation varies greatly in different vessels. The anatomy of this neural system has been described in detail by Pick.[6] The sympathetic postganglionic axons originate in the paravertebral chains of sympathetic ganglia, often at a great distance from the vessel they eventually supply. Parasympathetic pathways are restricted to a cranial and a sacral outflow and their ganglia lie more peripherally, sometimes in the walls of blood vessels.

Most autonomic axons reach the periphery through large nerve tracts that contain a mixture of fiber types, and they eventually travel in fine perivascular networks. The fibers penetrate the adventitia of the blood vessel and terminate as a plexus in the outermost layers of the media, extending into the outer half of the media in the largest arteries but not in smaller vessels. Many vascular smooth muscle cells thus lie in a considerable distance, physiologically speaking, from the nearest source of neuronally released transmitter. The separation is rarely less, and often greater, than 100 nm, so that diffusion from nerve to muscle cell becomes an important factor in the effects of neurotransmitters. In addition to the efferent fibers with which we are primarily concerned here, some afferent nerve fibers that serve a sensory function originate in the vascular wall[6] (Chapter 7).

The final *synapse* of vasomotor fibers consists of one or more swellings of the axon near its termination (Figure 9.1), a configuration quite different from the *motor end plate* of skeletal muscle. These varicosities contain granules of the transmitter, which are released into the extracellular space on arrival of a nerve action potential. Norepinephrine is the classical postganglionic transmitter for most sympathetic fibers and acetylcholine for parasympathetic nerves. Other neurally released substances include ATP and serotonin (Chapter 8).

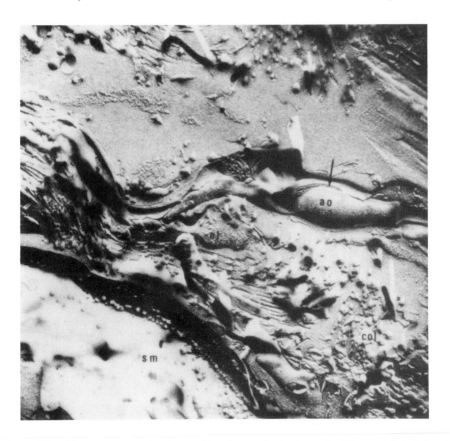

Figure 9.1.   Electronmicrograph of innervation of mesenteric artery of rat (freeze-etch technique). Portion of one smooth muscle cell (*sm*) apperars at lower left; *ao, arrow,* axon bundle and varicosity; *col,* collagen; *el,* elastic tissue. × 11,000 (Reproduced from Devine et al.,[22] with permission of Cambridge University Press)

Vascular smooth muscle receptors

Vascular smooth muscle cells possess several different kinds of membrane-bound receptors; the general character of these regulatory proteins was described in Chapter 1. Alpha-adrenergic, beta-adrenergic, and muscarinic cholinergic receptors are major elements in vascular control. Receptors for histamine, serotonin, ATP, and other vasoactive substances are also present in many vessels.

Alpha-adrenergic receptors

The $alpha_1$ and $alpha_2$ subtypes are both found in vascular smooth muscle cells of many blood vessels, and their binding by agonists leads to muscle contraction. *Presynaptic* $alpha_2$-receptors also appear on some adrenergic nerve terminals, where their activation inhibits the release of norepinephrine from the nerve terminal, thus creating a feedback loop that modulates the extraneural concentration of the transmitter. The numbers and relative proportions of alpha-adrenoceptor subtypes vary widely in different parts of the vascular tree and in different species. In general, alpha adrenoceptors are found in greater numbers in arterial than in venous smooth muscle, and sensitivity to norepinephrine is greatest in arteries. Alpha-adrenergic receptors have approximately the same affinity for the adrenally released catecholamine epinephrine as for norepinephrine.

Cerebral arteries apparently differ from all other vessels in their adrenergic responses.[18,24] Pial arteries, for example, have very few $alpha_1$-adrenoceptors and respond only weakly to norepinephrine for that reason. The basilar artery apparently contains an adrenergic receptor that is unique in failing to distinguish between isomers of norepinephrine. Such observations raise the possibility of regional and species differences in the receptors themselves, but differences of innervation and perhaps receptor coupling seem a more likely explanation.

Beta-adrenergic receptors

These receptors are found in most blood vessels, where they inhibit contraction and thus relax the smooth muscle. Relaxation can be demonstrated only if some degree of contraction already exists, either spontaneously or as a result of contractile stimuli. The degree of relaxation is then directly (although nonlinearly) correlated with the initial level of active force. Alpha- and beta-adrenoceptors not only share the same neurotransmitter, norepinephrine, but often coexist in the same vessel. In such cases, the net effect depends on the relative affinity and numbers of the two classes of receptors. The alpha effect usually predominates and the muscle contracts, but there are exceptions. The facial vein of the rabbit, for example, dilates in response to norepinephrine, and so do small coronary vessels. Beta-adrenergic receptors have a greater affinity for epinephrine than for norepinephrine.

As in the case of alpha and other receptors, two types of beta-adrenoceptors, $beta_1$ and $beta_2$, have been identified by their ligand-binding properties and their responses to selective drugs. Both inhibit contraction of vascular smooth muscle, which is to say that they reduce preexisting active force, and both are coupled to the contractile apparatus by events that begin with activation of adenylate cyclase (Chapter 1). Beta receptors are also found in other tissues, including the heart, lung, gastrointestinal tract, uterus, and the erythrocytes of birds and frogs. Certain regulatory proteins play a part in their action, so that beta-receptor signals are based on the interaction of three membrane-bound proteins: the receptor itself, a stimulatory guanine nucleotide regulatory protein (N_s), and the enzyme adenylate cyclase.

Desensitization is a prominent characteristic of beta adrenoceptors, meaning that their effects diminish with repeated or prolonged exposure to agonists. Receptor and postreceptor mechanisms have been implicated in this phenomenon, and no single explanation seems to account for all cases. In some instances it is accompanied by a decrease in the number of beta receptors (*down regulation*), the receptors being internalized and either destroyed or else later returned to the membrane. In other examples, the receptor is uncoupled from adenylate cyclase, probably by phosphorylation.

Muscarinic cholinergic receptors

Cholinergic receptors of the muscarinic type are found in many parts of the vascular tree. Their action is complicated by the fact that they appear in endothelial as well as smooth muscle cells. Binding of acetylcholine to such receptors in endothelial cells releases a substance that causes muscle relaxation. In contrast, binding to cholinergic receptors of smooth muscle cells causes contraction. The messenger system employed by cholinergic receptors to invoke contraction of smooth muscle is believed to involve phosphoinositides (see below).

The response observed is thus the net result of two opposite effects. Vasodilatation is dominant in most arteries,[21] whereas constriction occurs in mesenteric veins, portal veins, and the vena cava, as well as in human coronary arteries. Peripheral systemic veins tend to dilate with low doses of acetylcholine and constrict at higher concentrations. Although the nerves that provide acetylcholine for these responses are mainly parasympathetic, one specific group of postganglionic cholinergic fibers that are part of the sympathetic nervous system innervates and causes dilatation of vessels in skeletal muscle (Chapter 8).

The nature of the *relaxing factor* released by the endothelium was long a mystery, but it has recently been identified as nitric oxide,[39] a pleasant contrast to the chemically complex signals responsible for many other functions of vascular smooth muscle. Nitric oxide is one of the many activators of guanylate cyclase. Acetylcholine is not the only substance that can stimulate the release of relaxing factor by endothelial cells; ATP, histamine, bradykinin, and other agents have the same effect (Chapter 8). A few vessels exhibit neurogenic cholinergic vasodilatation that is not endothelium dependent. Examples include the posterior auricular and cerebral arteries of the cat.[18] VIP may be the neurotransmitter.

Vasomotor responses

Vascular smooth muscle exerts its effects on the circulation by modifying the compliance of blood vessel walls, but the hemodynamic results of changes in distensibility are not the same in all parts of the vascular tree. Vasomotor regulation affects principally the resistance of very small vessels, the transmission properties of large arteries, and the capacity of large veins.

The main result of activating the smooth muscle of arterioles and venules is a change in their diameter. The diameter of an intact vessel is a function of two variables, its distensibility and the transmural pressure (Chapter 6). Transmural pressure in a given vessel depends on the hydraulic energy initially supplied by the heart and its dissipation in the vascular bed upstream. Distensibility, on the other hand, is determined by the passive elastic elements in the vessel wall and the active force generated by smooth muscle. Contractile stimuli to the muscle consequently produce vasoconstriction provided that transmural pressure remains constant, which is often but not always the case.

The situation in large arteries is quite different, even though the behavior of the smooth muscle is basically the same. The structure of a vessel like the aorta is such that maximum activity of its smooth muscle reduces its diameter only slightly, increasing aortic resistance (which is not large to begin with) by a negligible amount. Nevertheless, the alteration of distensibility can lead to significant changes in impedance, wave velocity, and reflection (Chapter 6), which influence the arterial transmission of pulsatile pressure and flow waves. The distensibility of large veins like the venae cavae can also be modified by smooth muscle activity. Although these relatively thin-walled vessels also offer little resistance, they can undergo larger changes in diameter than most arteries, and the result is a modification of their capacity as blood reservoirs (Chapter 13).

Vascular Heterogeneity

The diversity of the mechanisms that can produce excitation is a prominent characteristic of vascular smooth muscle. Some cells that have access to neurally released neurotransmitters are excited by corresponding receptors. Others receive their effective stimulus electrotonically from neighboring cells, which may have been excited by receptors or by independent pacemakers. The electrical activity that accompanies excitation may consist of action potentials (*spikes*) that occur regularly or in bursts (Figure 9.4), graded depolarization without spikes, excitatory junction potentials (see below), or no evidence of depolarization at all. This multiplicity of excitation pathways explains to some extent the differences in behavior that are observed throughout the vascular tree. Such differences are both qualitative and quantitative; they are not limited to the smooth muscle of blood vessels but appear in other organs as well. Norepinephrine, for example, causes contraction of most (not all) blood vessels but relaxation of gastrointestinal smooth muscle.

The various modes of excitation are considered in later sections, but it is useful to characterize them briefly before going further. Smooth muscles in different vessels vary in two fundamental ways: the presence or absence of full action potentials as a trigger for contraction, and the means by which action potentials, if present, are initiated. The categories of excitation defined by these criteria, together with vessels in which they have been observed, are as follows:

1. Excitation mediated by muscle action potentials that are triggered by arrival of nerve-released transmitter at cell receptors; this is the mechanism seen in many large systemic arteries. An increase in nerve impulse frequency causes increased contraction.
2. Contractions excited by spontaneous action potentials, occurring regularly or in bursts, generated by smooth muscle cells that act as pacemakers (e.g., portal and mesenteric veins in many species). Excitation spreads by cell-to-cell conduction, and the frequency of firing can be increased by nerve stimulation.
3. Muscle contraction directly related to sustained depolarization caused by neurotransmitters or other vasoactive substances, a phenomenon observed in carotid arteries of dogs and sheep. Spontaneous action potentials may be superimposed on the steady level of depolarization.
4. Contractile response to nerve stimulation or norepinephrine with no change in membrane potential, exhibited by the pulmonary artery and ear arteries in the rabbit.

The connection between stimulus and response when partial depolarization or complete action potentials trigger muscle contraction is described as *electromechanical coupling,* whereas the mechanism for responses that do not involve changes of membrane potential (category 4 above) is called *pharmacomechanical coupling.*[3] Note that this distinction is between two modes of excitation–contraction coupling, and can depend on the vasoactive material as well as on the specific blood vessel. Bozler[17] suggested a division of smooth muscle into spontaneously firing "single-unit" types and nerve-regulated "multi-unit" varieties, thus emphasizing the degree of neural control. That classification is less useful in the vascular system than in other organs, however, because the rate of spontaneous firing can be influenced by neural stimuli, as indicated above.

Vessel tone

Almost all blood vessels continually maintain a certain degree of active force, or tone, *in vivo.* This force has its origin in the contraction of smooth muscle cells, and together with transmural pressure (Chapter 6), it determines the vessel diameter. Curiously enough, we do not yet know whether this sustained stress is the result of prolonged contractions of each muscle cell, or of repeated asynchronous individual contractions that blend into an apparently steady force in the wall as a whole.

The degree of tonic contraction varies widely in the vessels of different organs (Figure 8.5), and these regional variations probably arise from differences in the type of innervation, its density, and the mode of excitation. In addition, vessels do not all possess the same type or numbers of muscle cell receptors, which accounts for differences in the response to nerve stimulation or drugs. Finally, vessels differ in the number of low-resistance gap junctions between cells and in the population of ion channels. The opportunities that this repertoire of control mechanisms provides for subtle adjustments of the vascular tree are obvious, and regional differences have doubtless evolved to serve particular functions. Detailed correlation of receptor populations and excitation processes with particular local functions, however, lies in the future.

The normal resistance of a vascular bed depends on the resting tone of its arterioles and venules, which in turn depends on a host of factors, including the number of receptors of each class that the cells contain and the local concentrations of ions, hormones, neurotransmitters, and metabolites. Neural control is exerted through transmitter release in amounts determined by the frequency of impulses arriving at nerve terminals. Norepinephrine and epinephrine levels in the bloodstream are also neurally controlled, the adrenal medulla that releases them being analogous to a postganglionic adrenergic fiber. Ultimately, the total response of each muscle cell depends on the number of cross-bridges that become active, which is mainly a function of cytosolic Ca^{2+} (see below).

Neural Excitation

The various modes of excitation in vascular smooth muscle operate through one or both of two different but related mechanisms, the binding of agonists to cellular receptors or membrane depolarization. Receptor activation itself can lead to depolarization in some cases. Both increase the availability of calcium ions within the cell, initiating a series of reactions that culminate in activation of the contractile apparatus. The physiological agents that bind to receptors of blood vessels may be released from autonomic nerve terminals, transported by the bloodstream, or produced by cells in the vicinity of the receptor.

Neural excitation of vascular smooth muscle has been intensively studied, and a detailed account of the response to stimulation of a sympathetic adrenergic vasomotor nerve will serve as an introduction to the subject. For the moment, we will limit the description to events mediated by the alpha$_1$ type of adrenergic receptors and accompanied by full-scale action potentials. The excitatory role of partial depolarizations, transient or sustained, will be considered in a later section.

First, the arrival of an action potential at one of the varicosities near the termination of the nerve causes the release of some of the norepinephrine stored there. Diffusion then brings that transmitter, progressively diluted by extracellular fluid and diminished by uptake mechanisms, to the immediate environment of muscle cells. If the cell membrane contains receptors of the alpha$_1$-adrenergic class, which is the case in many blood vessels, then norepinephrine binds to them, the number bound being directly related to the affinity and total number of the receptors, as well as the local concentration of the transmitter.

By no means does all of the nerve-released norepinephrine reach smooth muscle cells, however. The neuronal membrane actively transports norepinephrine back into the nerve, and 30 to 70% of the released transmitter is taken up in this way. Catecholamines are also sequestered by other components of the vascular wall and metabolized by local enzymes (monoamine oxidase and catechol-O-methyltransferase), further reducing the amount of norepinephrine that can diffuse to the vicinity of smooth muscle cells. Many of the differences in the response of various blood vessels to nerve stimulation arise from quantitative differences in these uptake mechanisms, as well as anatomical variations in the distance from axon varicosity to muscle cells.

Norepinephrine that finds its way to smooth muscle binds to the adrenergic receptors. In the case of alpha-receptors, one effect is an opening of receptor-controlled calcium channels in the cell membrane, which results in calcium influx because the extracellular concentration of calcium is four orders of magnitude higher than that inside the resting cell (e.g., 4×10^{-3} M versus 2×10^{-7} M). The intracellular concentration of free Ca^{2+} rises and this increment makes the cell membrane potential less negative, a partial depolarization that opens voltage-gated channels in the membrane, thus adding to the inward calcium and sodium currents.

Calcium also enters the cell interior from the SR on alpha$_1$-adrenoceptor activation by a process that has yet to be identified but probably involves binding of inositol 1,4,5-triphosphate to a specific SR receptor. This entry appears to be modulated by the existing intracellular level of calcium ions, for increases of $[Ca^{2+}]_i$ that are too small to activate the myofilaments have been shown to be sufficient to induce calcium release from the SR.[26] Release of calcium from intracellular organelles also contributes to increased $[Ca^{2+}]_i$, but the mechanism of this release is unknown and its contribution is thought to be relatively small. When the intracellular Ca^{2+} from all these sources rises above a threshold level, about 0.2 M, it enters into a series of reactions that activate the contractile apparatus (see below) and the cell contracts.

In the excitation mode we are considering, these events are accompanied by an action potential, a rapid and complete depolarization of the cell, followed by a plateau of approximately zero potential difference and then repolarization to the initial state. Such action potentials, which are not unlike those of myocardial cells (Chapter 3), are described in more detail later in this chapter, together with the underlying redistribution of various ions across the cell membrane, in which movements of sodium, potassium, and calcium ions play an important part. The beginning of mechanical contraction ordinarily follows the onset of depolarization after a very short *latent period* and does not end until well after complete repolarization. (As already indicated, action potentials do not occur in all blood vessels or under all conditions; contraction of vascular smooth muscle can be elicited by depolarization to a new steady-state level or by other mechanisms.)

Excitation of vascular smooth muscle by sympathetic nerves thus invokes a variety of mechanisms. Voltage-gated as well as receptor-controlled ion channels are involved, and the membrane potential modulates some of the processes directly. Control is transmitted by the vasomotor nerve impulse frequency, which ranges in sympathetic fibers from <1 to 20/sec (Chapter 8). The higher the frequency, the greater the amount of norepinephrine liberated at the nerve terminals, the greater the number of adrenergic receptors activated, and the greater the force generated.

Although the description just given attributes the contraction produced by

adrenergic nerve stimulation to norepinephrine and alpha adrenoceptors, recent evidence indicates that some adrenergic sympathetic fibers release ATP
and others NPY, in addition to norepinephrine. ATP apparently activates P_2
purinergic receptors of muscle cells, which also open calcium channels and
thus lead to contraction. These ATP-receptor–activated channels can carry
either Ca^{2+} or Na^+ ions, with a relatively low (3:1) selectivity ratio.[15] Endothelial cells also contain P_2 receptors, but their activation causes release of
endothelium-derived relaxing factor and hence relaxation.[19] The vasodilatation
commonly produced by exogenous ATP and adenosine may well be mediated
in this way. Co-release of the constrictor peptide NPY and norepinephrine is
described in Chapter 8.

Other Modes of Excitation

Blood-borne transmitters

All the events entrained by neurally released transmitters can be initiated
by blood-borne delivery of the same agents if they reach the vicinity of appropriate cells and receptors. Epinephrine and norepinephrine both circulate in
the blood after secretion by the adrenal medulla. Diffusion occurs from the
bloodstream into the vessel wall, but the major effects are presumably limited
to the muscle layers nearest the lumen because of progressive dilution as the
substance travels through the interstitial space and because of transmitter uptake by nonmuscular tissue. The beta-adrenoceptors have a much higher affinity for epinephrine than for norepinephrine, whereas the alpha-adrenoceptors
bind to the two catecholamines with about equal affinity. Other neurotransmitters, such as acetylcholine, do not appear in the blood in significant amounts
because they are taken up in various organs or enzymatically degraded in the
blood.

The effect *in vivo* of active substances that reach vascular smooth muscle
by way of the bloodstream is the net result of changes that vary in intensity,
and sometimes even in direction, in different parts of the circulation. This vari-
ability makes it difficult to generalize, but as a rule norepinephrine, serotonin,
angiotensin II, and ADH (vasopressin) are vasoconstrictors, and ATP is a vasodilator. Epinephrine constricts the cutaneous and renal vascular beds by way
of alpha-adrenoceptors but dilates the vessels of skeletal muscle and the
splanchnic regions, where beta-adrenoceptor effects are dominant. Histamine
acts as a dilator on vessels of the microcirculation but causes contraction of
smooth muscle in large arteries of the pig. The overall effect of intravenous
histamine is species dependent; it lowers blood pressure in man and the dog

and raises it in the rabbit. These responses are considered in more detail in Chapter 8.

Metabolic agents

A number of substances involved in tissue metabolism affect smooth muscle contractility, the most important being O_2, CO_2, hydrogen ions, and potassium. These agents act directly on the muscle cells, and their concentration in the cellular environment determines the magnitude of the effect. In addition to this local action, some of them elicit reflexes in the intact animal, as in the chemoreceptor response to arterial pO_2 (Chapter 7).

Oxygen

The partial pressure of O_2 influences the contractile activity of vascular smooth muscle, and in most vessels of the systemic circulation a decrease in pO_2 causes vasodilatation. This effect is a local one, demonstrable *in vitro,* and it operates in the intact animal in addition to the reflexes generated by arterial hypoxia. Pulmonary vessels exhibit just the opposite response; they constrict when pO_2 falls. The response of the pulmonary vasculature to hypoxia, a subject in itself, is discussed in Chapter 11. Contraction caused by low pO_2 has also been reported in mesenteric and saphenous veins, but the smooth muscle of virtually all other systemic vessels relaxes when pO_2 is lowered.

Vasodilatation as a result of vascular smooth muscle relaxation is evident when the pO_2 of the perfusate is lowered in isolated limbs, skeletal muscle, kidneys, and intestine. This response usually appears when the pO_2 has fallen to about 40 mm Hg, but organs vary considerably in their sensitivity. A decrease in pO_2 from 100 to 70 mm Hg causes measurable relaxation of vascular strips of rabbit aorta *in vitro,* and further graded decrements in pO_2 are accompanied by stepwise decreases in isometric force.[8] Such experiments are carried out on muscle that is in a steady state of contraction induced by norepinephrine or another vasoactive agent, and the magnitude of the relaxation caused by hypoxia is roughly proportional to the initial degree of contraction. Increasing pO_2 above the normal level causes vasoconstriction in most systemic vessels.

The mechanism of these responses remains unknown in spite of many attempts to discover whether it is a direct or an indirect effect on smooth muscle cells. Low pO_2 may simply reduce the energy available to muscle by decreasing the generation of ATP required for contraction, or it may act indirectly by stimulating local production of some muscle-relaxing substance. Evidence to support both hypotheses has been reported, and both may be involved under physiological conditions. The arguments in favor of a direct effect are quite convincing, including the fact that inhibitors of oxidative metabolism diminish the influence of changes in pO_2. On the other hand, the decrease in contractile force with lowered pO_2 is not always closely correlated with reduced tissue ATP, and experiments on some vessels show that about two-thirds of the energy production during isometric contractions is supplied by *anaerobic* metabolism.[8]

In addition, the degree of relaxation induced by low pO_2 depends in part on the agent used to produce the initial contracted state. Contraction caused by high K^+ concentrations is less sensitive to hypoxia than is contraction stimulated by norepinephrine. Relaxation by low pO_2 is accompanied by a reduction in the frequency of spontaneous firing in some veins, suggesting that hypoxia acts on cell membrane activity, an effect that might be minimized by sustained depolarization. All of these observations suggest that oxygen tension per se is at least not the only stimulus.

The precapillary segments of systemic arterioles are particularly sensitive to low pO_2, and they are the major source of the decrease in vascular resistance. Local pO_2 in the microcirculation has been carefully examined, and the results indicate that pO_2 is about 1 mm Hg lower just outside an arteriole than in its lumen. A longitudinal gradient of pO_2 also exists along the small arteries, such that pO_2 in the walls of terminal arterioles can be about 20 mm Hg when that in large arteries is about 70 mm Hg and that in tissue a short distance away is 8 mm Hg.[25] These data confirm that O_2 diffuses out through arteriolar as well as capillary walls and suggests that pO_2 in the wall is close to that of arteriolar blood.

This is not to say that tissue pO_2 has no effect; on the contrary, perfusion experiments and *in vitro* studies show that it has a powerful influence on local vascular tone. The question that remains unanswered is whether smooth muscle cells are the O_2 sensors in local responses, or whether changes in tissue pO_2 release a vasoactive substance from nonvascular cells. If the muscle cell is the primary sensor, relaxation still need not necessarily be a direct effect, for the vasodilatation may be stimulated by agents produced by muscle or other cells in the vascular wall. Bovine coronary arteries, for example, increase their production of prostaglandins of the PGE type when bath pO_2 is lowered (Chapter 8), and the release of adenosine has been reported in hog carotid artery.[8]

Whatever the mechanism, there can be no doubt that local blood and tissue pO_2 have significant physiological effects on vasomotion, vascular resistance, and blood flow. The functional hyperemia of working cardiac and skeletal muscle, in which O_2 consumption, blood flow, and decreased vascular resistance are closely correlated, is an example, although here again, the problem of direct and indirect effects is unresolved.[8] Autoregulation of blood flow has also been attributed to O_2 tensions in the vascular wall, although that hypothesis is not now among the front runners (Chapter 12). The creation and harmful effects of

O_2-derived free radicals in situations where tissue is reperfused after a period of ischemia are discussed in Chapter 8.

Carbon dioxide and acidosis

Elevations of CO_2 tension cause relaxation of smooth muscle in systemic vessels as a rule, and the result is vasodilatation. Local elevations of pCO_2 thus tend to increase blood flow and return the CO_2 to normal, just as the vasomotor effect of low pO_2 tends to restore local O_2 levels. The cerebral vascular system is the one most sensitive to hypercapnia, but a significant degree of vasodilatation has also been demonstrated in the coronary, mesenteric, and femoral arteries and probably occurs in all systemic vascular beds. Muscle relaxation occurs even in nerve-free umbilical vessels, demonstrating the local tissue component of the response. Arterial hypercapnia in the intact animal moderates the direct local effects of elevated pCO_2 through the chemoreceptor reflex. This response enlists predominantly alpha-adrenergic actions that tend to counteract any locally generated vasodilatation, with results that vary in different organs and different species.

The mechanism of these vascular reactions appears to be the fall in blood pH that accompanies hypercapnia, not the pCO_2 itself. Lowering the pH from 7.4 to 7.1 by addition of acids causes vasodilatation in perfused organs and relaxation of contracted vascular strips *in vitro*. Acidosis of this degree also reduces the contractile effects of catecholamines and other constrictor agents. Vascular smooth muscle cells are hyperpolarized by acidosis,[42] and the resting potential increases (i.e., becomes more negative) almost linearly as the pH is lowered from 7.7 to 6.7. The isometric force developed in the vascular wall by alpha-adrenergic stimulation also falls linearly with pH in this range. The relation between contractile force and membrane potential during alterations of pH is virtually the same as that observed with changes in $[K^+]_o$ (see below).

Potassium

The effect of potassium ions on vascular smooth muscle depends on the extracellular K^+ concentration. Studies *in vitro* show that raising the concentration from zero up to the normal mammalian level of approximately 4 mM produces relaxation; concentrations greater than 10 to 30 mM cause contraction.[8,42] These reactions have been observed *in vitro* in human and canine cerebral arteries, as well as in the aorta, portal vein, and femoral artery of the rat. Increasing the $[K^+]$ to high levels in the organ bath of such preparations is a standard method of stimulating smooth muscle contraction, and graded responses can be produced by stepwise increments in concentration. The relation between $[K^+]_o$ and active force in smooth muscle is thus biphasic; as the concentration is raised from zero the muscle first relaxes, and then, at higher levels, contracts.

The explanation of this behavior lies in the relation between $[K^+]_o$ and membrane voltage, which does not follow the simple K^+ equilibrium potential[42] (Chapter 3) but exhibits a maximum polarization between 2.0 and 5.0 mM $[K^+]_o$. Studies of isolated carotid arteries have shown that the greatest degree of polarization (i.e., most negative potential) occurs when external K^+ is in that range;[42] lower (or higher) concentrations are accompanied by smaller membrane potentials (i.e., a lesser degree of polarization). Maximum relaxation thus corresponds to maximum hyperpolarization. In vessels that exhibit spontaneous action potentials, hyperpolarization also slows the frequency of firing and lowers the force. This inhibitory effect appears to be mediated by the Na^+–K^+ transport system of the cell, because relaxation and hyperpolarization are both blocked by oubain, which inhibits that system.

The membrane potential is a key factor in determining the active force of smooth muscle contraction because it regulates Ca^{2+} influx by voltage-controlled channels,[7] allowing greater Ca^{2+} influx when the membrane potential becomes less negative[34] (Figure 9.2C). Inasmuch as displacement of $[K^+]_o$ in *either* direction from the physiological range reduces the negative potential, this interaction accounts for the biphasic nature of responses to $[K^+]_o$. Isometric force is closely correlated with the changes in potential brought on by alterations of either pH or K^+ (Figure 9.2B), indicating a tight coupling between potential and $[Ca^{2+}]_i$ (Figure 9.2C).

The reactions to $[K^+]_o$ are thus typical of one mode of smooth muscle excitation, namely, the regulation of Ca^{2+} influx by voltage-controlled channels, leading to graded contraction related to steady membrane potentials rather than spikes. The connection between membrane potential and calcium influx explains the contraction that occurs when vascular smooth muscle is depolarized by high K^+ concentrations, and at the same time accounts for the

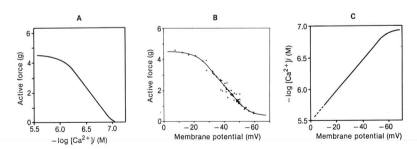

Figure 9.2. Membrane potential and intracellular free calcium concentration (expressed as $-\log$ molar $[Ca^{2+}]_i$) in relation to isometric force in vascular smooth muscle (isolated carotid artery segments). **A**, active force in relation to $[Ca^{2+}]_i$ (The lower the $[Ca^{2+}]_i$, the larger its negative logarithm.) **B**, active force when membrane potential was modified by altering K^+ (*circles*) or pH (*triangles*). **C**, relation between membrane potential and $[Ca^{2+}]_i$. (**B**, Reproduced from Siegel et al.,[42] with permission of Raven Press. **A** and **C**, from data published by Filo et al.[28])

fact that *reducing* potassium concentrations below the normal level also causes slight contraction. Responses in the intact animal are consistent with this interpretation and with the observations made on isolated vessels. Intravenous administration of potassium to intact animals also causes release of catecholamines from the adrenal medulla, producing the generalized effects of those agents.

The relation between intracellular calcium ions and active force is discussed in detail later in this chapter (and in Chapter 3). It has been demonstrated most clearly by *in vitro* experiments on "skinned" muscle fibers, in which cell membranes have been made freely permeable and the $[Ca^{2+}]$ available to the contractile apparatus can be controlled by adjusting the concentration in the tissue bath. The full range of contraction develops as $[Ca^{2+}]_i$ is raised from about 0.2 to 1.0 μM (Figure 9.2A), although the exact position of these boundaries varies to some extent in different reports.[28] The concentration of ionized calcium in intact muscle cells at rest is so low that it is difficult to measure accurately.

These observations, together with the Ca^{2+}/membrane potential relationship shown in Figure 9.2C, suggest that the normal mammalian $[K^+]_o$, 4.0 to 4.5 mM, may be accompanied by a $[Ca^{2+}]_i$ slightly above the contraction threshold in resting vascular smooth muscle,[42] which may account for the tone exhibited by blood vessels *in vivo* in the absence of neural stimuli. By the same token, vascular strips that are thought to be completely relaxed after bathing in physiological salt solution for 1 or 2 hr may actually be in a minimally contracted state.

Osmolarity

The infusion of hyperosmotic solutions usually reduces vascular resistance, a response that has been demonstrated in vascular beds of the forearm, myocardium, kidney, and pia mater.[8] The total solute concentration, or *osmolarity,* of human and canine body fluids is approximately 285 mOsmol/liter, and substances like NaCl, sucrose, and urea are commonly used to increase osmolarity in experimental studies. Plasma proteins contribute only about 1 mOsmol/liter of the total because of their low molar concentration. Increasing plasma osmolarity by 25 mOsmol/liter typically causes a marked but transient fall in resistance, followed by a slower vasodilatation to 20 to 50% of control resistance values, which tends to wane after 5 to 10 min. Dilatation of arterioles in hamster cremaster muscle has been observed with elevations of osmolarity above 330 mOsmol/liter. The effects on blood viscosity are much too small to account for these vascular responses.

A change of osmolarity in any one of the major fluid compartments—vascular, interstitial, or extracellular—is soon shared with the others because of the relatively free passage of water across cell membranes. Infusion of hypertonic solutions (or increased blood osmolarity) consequently pulls fluid from tissues, and the total weight of the organ involved decreases. The vasodilating effect can be attributed in part to loss of water from smooth muscle cells, which raises $[K^+]_i$ and thus causes a hyperpolarization that reduces contractile activity (see above). Increased ionic strength may also influence the contractile process by reducing actomyosin ATPase activity, as in the *rigor state* (see below).

Changes in the osmolarity of body fluids are not a mere laboratory curiosity, for they occur in many physiological adjustments. Exercise is a prominent example; the particles contributing to osmolarity in that case are inorganic phosphates generated from high-energy compounds and the lactate and pyruvate formed from glucose. The osmolarity of venous blood rises during contraction of skeletal muscles, and the fall of resistance in the muscle bed is roughly proportional to this increase. The vasodilatation produced by infusion of hyperosmotic solutions reaches a peak in about 1 min, however, and then declines, unlike that during muscular exertion. The degree of dilatation after 2 or 3 min of such infusions is much less than that found with comparable levels of osmolarity during exercise. Changes in osmolarity may, therefore, contribute to the rapid development of muscle hyperemia in exercise but cannot account for sustained vasodilatation over long periods. The alterations of osmolarity in the vascular response to exercise are not the same in all species; they are prominent in the cat, less so in man, and relatively minor in the dog.[8]

Myogenic contractions

Sudden stretching of the vascular wall is followed in some vessels by contraction of the smooth muscle, a response evoked directly by physical stretching of the muscle cells and therefore called *myogenic contraction*.[4,45] The phenomenon can be demonstrated in isolated vascular segments and does not involve neural reflex pathways. A quick stretch of any elastic structure to a new constant length is accompanied by an equally rapid increment in force, but the myogenic response consists of a later further development of force by an isometric muscle. In the case of the umbilical artery (a noninnervated vessel), contraction develops after a latency of about 9 sec, when the initial peak force has declined slightly (Figures 6.7 and 9.3), and continues for several minutes.

A similar response occurs in small mesenteric and cerebral vessels and in many nonvascular smooth muscles,[4] although these tissues differ in the speed and extent of the stretch required and in the duration of the contraction. The umbilical artery exhibits a myogenic response when stretched at least 25% of its initial length in 0.1 sec, but not with shorter or slower elongations (Figure 9.3). Smaller stretches are needed in smooth muscle of the intestine and blad-

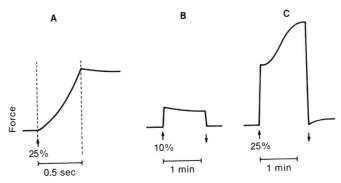

Figure 9.3.   Dependence of myogenic response on speed and magnitude of stretch (expressed as percentage of resting length) in human umbilical artery *in vitro. Arrows* indicate time of stretch and release. A slow 25% stretch over a period of 0.5 sec (**A**) does not elicit myogenic response, nor does a smaller, faster stretch (**B**, 10% in 0.04 sec). A large fast stretch (**C**, 25% in 0.04 sec) stimulates development of active force after a brief latency. (Reproduced with modifications from Sparks,[45] with permission of the American Heart Association)

der, and the latency is shorter. The reaction apparently does not occur in all vascular beds, and some vessels merely exhibit a gradual stress relaxation when stretched (Chapter 6). Even in vessels prone to the myogenic response, it is rarely elicited in every specimen tested.

The mechanism is unknown, but stretching of the muscle cell membrane appears to be the primary stimulus. In vessels that show spontaneous electrical activity of the muscle (see records from the guinea pig portal vein in Figure 9.4B), stretching increases the frequency of the spikes at the same time that it produces a mechanical response, suggesting that depolarization is the trigger for subsequent mechanical events.[33] The involvement of membrane potentials is supported by observations on other excitable tissues, for example, the increase in pacemaker rate that occurs when intracardiac pressure is raised in isolated hearts.[4]

Contraction of vascular smooth muscle on stretching occurs in live animals, as well as *in vitro*. Sudden elevation of transmural pressure in an arteriole has the same effect, and the vasoconstriction that results is the reason for attributing autoregulation of blood flow to a myogenic mechanism (Chapter 12 and Figure 12.1). The effects of stretch are not always transient, and some experiments have shown that a sustained elevation of intravascular pressure is accompanied by a steady state of increased smooth muscle force and electrical activity.[33] Moreover, shifting from steady to pulsatile perfusion pressure in a vascular bed causes resistance to rise,[4] as if the intermittent stretching were an additional stimulus to constriction.

Such observations make one wonder whether myogenic activity is a pervasive element in physiological regulation of blood vessels. They also bring to mind the superficial resemblance between the myogenic response to stretch and the force–length relationship described in an earlier section, even though the former is a direct reaction to a stimulus and the latter is a change in ability to generate force when the next stimulus comes along. Accumulating evidence makes it possible to imagine that the fundamental mechanism may be the same in both cases, because it appears that the force–length relationship in smooth and striated muscles arises not only from an increment in the number of sites available for cross-bridge attachment but also from a length-dependent enhancement of $[Ca^{2+}]_i$ (Chapter 3). The second of these factors may be the operative one in myogenic contractions.

Depolarization

The depolarization that is a key element in many forms of smooth muscle excitation is similar to that in striated muscle and nerve (Chapter 3), although it differs in some details. As in all excitable tissues, action potentials in vascular smooth muscle arise from specific ion movements across the cell membrane. These transfers take place passively through specific channels or with the aid of energy-expending "pumps" that usually exchange an intracellular ion for one or more of another kind in the external environment. The channels are integral membrane proteins that permit the passage of selected ions in accordance with the channel properties and the electrochemical gradients. Opening and closing (*gating*) of channels are controlled by receptor agonists in some cases and by the membrane potential in others, often both. Secondary modulation of the gating may be generated by such processes as phosphorylation of the channel protein.[40]

The membrane potential depends on the selective permeability of the cell wall and the relative ion concentrations on each side of it, the ions of most importance being Ca^{2+} Na^+, K^+, and Cl^- (Chapter 3). The distribution of K^+ is responsible for a large part of the resting potential, but K^+ is not the only ion involved. The equilibrium potential for K^+ under physiological conditions is about -100 mV, and that would be the resting potential if K^+ were the only effective species. The less negative potential observed in vascular smooth muscle cells indicates that permeability to the other ions mentioned above is a contributing factor. Nevertheless the potential is highly dependent on the external K^+ concentration; increasing $[K^+]_o$ is a common experimental way of producing depolarization.

Many different types of potassium channels have been described (Chapter 3). The repertoire available in vascular smooth muscle is not known with certainty, but it probably includes both fast and slow, delayed-rectification, and calcium-sensitive K^+ channels. All of these perform in effect as buffers, moderating the degree of depolarization that would otherwise result from the activity of other ion channels. Active, electrogenic transport mechanisms also contribute to the resting potential,[30] and the Na^+,K^+-ATPase pump helps to maintain normal intracellular concentrations of ions.

Typical membrane potentials recorded from vascular smooth muscle cells by an intracellular microelectrode are shown in Figure 9.4. Resting potentials are about -50 mV, much less negative than those observed in nerve and striated muscle. The slow action potentials in the aorta of the turtle follow a prolonged time course similar in shape to that of myocardial cells, but in warm-blooded species the duration of the potential is less than 0.5 sec and the plateau phase is very short. Depolarization to the neighborhood of the threshold (about -35 mV), however produced, usually initiates a full action potential, or *spike*. The rising phase of the signal is associated with rapid Ca^{2+} and Na^+ influx, but these two ions are involved in different degrees in different vessels. The action potentials of portal and mesenteric veins appear to be predominantly Ca^{2+} mediated, since they are not affected by reduction of $[Na^+]_o$ and are abolished by calcium-blocking drugs. Muscle in the carotid arteries of sheep, on the other hand, responds electrically in calcium-free solutions.[3]

The ionic basis for the action potential thus varies quantitatively in different parts of the vascular tree and in different species. In general, however, the upstroke of the action potential arises largely from calcium influx, in contrast to the inward sodium current responsible for rapid depolarization in nerve. This is not to say that sodium influx does not also occur in vascular smooth muscle, but only that calcium has a more prominent role. The height of the spike is

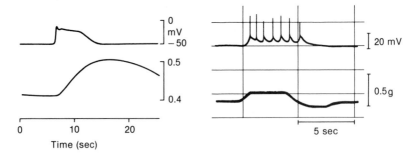

Figure 9.4. Action potentials (*above*) and simultaneous contractile force (*below*) in vascular smooth muscle. **A**, single action potential and resulting development of force in turtle aorta (Reproduced from Roddie,[41] with permission of S. Karger AG) **B**, repeated action potentials, and force, in guinea pig portal vein. (Reproduced from von Loh,[48] with permission of S. Karger AG)

limited by the fact that high $[Ca^{2+}]_i$ itself tends to reduce Ca^{2+} influx, possibly by accumulation of ions in the channel.

The voltage plateau is maintained by slow calcium influx, as it is in cardiac muscle, and by an outward potassium current. Intracellular Ca^{2+} does not remain elevated for long, however, in part because free intracellular Ca^{2+} is rapidly sequestered by the SR; the resulting fall in $[Ca^{2+}]_i$ contributes to the gradual repolarization of the membrane. The sodium–calcium exchange that has been demonstrated in myocardial cells (Chapter 3) may also exist in vascular smooth muscle, and its reversal to extrude calcium could play a part in late repolarization.

Cell-to-cell conduction

Regardless of whether an action potential is evoked by receptor-mediated excitation, by experimentally lowering the external K^+ to produce depolarization to threshold, or by other means, it can under certain circumstances produce depolarization in neighboring cells. The basis for such conduction is the existence of *tight junctions* of low electrical resistance, which allow currents to flow readily from one cell to another.[14] Under such conditions, excitation is transmitted consecutively through a series of cells (Chapter 3).

Local pacemakers

In some vessels a few muscle cells tend to fire spontaneously, like the pacemaker cells of the heart. Rhythmic contractions originating from such pacemakers often appear in veins *in vitro,* particularly mesenteric and portal veins, and occasionally in arteries. Spontaneous action potentials have also been recorded in many vessels, often recurring regularly for long periods of time. If a spontaneously firing cell is connected to its neighbors by tight junctions, the pacemaker may "drive" a small region of vascular muscle by cell-to-cell conduction. Spontaneous potentials sometimes occur in bursts separated by inactive periods (Figure 9.4), rather than continuing steadily at a fixed rate. Bursting has been attributed to the operation of calcium-sensitive K^+ channels.

Repeated individual action potentials can cause a relatively steady, prolonged tension because the contraction produced by each one does not relax completely before the next one begins, a phenomenon called *summation.* When the concentration of norepinephrine is varied *in vitro,* for example, the spike frequency increases along with the agonist concentration, and the force produced is directly related to the frequency of the individual contractions. The same phenomenon has been observed with sympathetic nerve stimulation.

Partial depolarization

Stimulation of perivascular nerves sometimes produces small, localized potential changes of short duration[8] called *excitatory junction potentials* (*EJPs*). Single EJPs are typically less than 15 mV in amplitude, decay exponentially with a time constant of a few hundred milliseconds, and do not evoke contraction. Pharmacological studies suggest that these responses are evoked through adrenergic nerve fibers, and there is some evidence that two kinds of norepinephrine receptors are involved: the conventional alpha type and a blockade-resistant gamma receptor.[31] Trains of stimuli cause successive EJPs that may summate, leading to a full action potential and contraction.

In carotid arteries and some other vessels, stimulation by low concentrations of norepinephrine depolarizes cells to a new membrane potential that is maintained steadily without spikes or decay. The change in potential is directly correlated with the agonist concentration, and the *graded depolarization* is accompanied by a similarly graded contraction. Even in vessels that normally exhibit action potentials, depolarization by high-K^+ solutions produces a steady voltage and tonic force, showing that action potentials per se are not necessary for contraction.

These observations show that either partial depolarization or complete action potentials can be associated with mechanical responses, but the range of possibilities is even wider, for contraction sometimes occurs in the absence of depolarization. Reports of this phenomenon were at first regarded as heresy, but it has now been demonstrated convincingly in a number of vessels, including pulmonary and ear arteries of the rabbit and arterioles of the rat.[3,20,49] Stimulation of the sympathetic nerves of such vessels produces constriction with no apparent change in membrane potential. At first, this was not regarded as strong evidence for contraction without action potentials because the cell in which the microelectrode was inserted might not be representative of the contracting population, but repeated confirmation in many laboratories finally ruled out that possibility. The conclusion is now accepted more readily because many other observations discussed in this chapter support the hypothesis that a rise in $[Ca^{2+}]_i$ is the *sine qua non* for contraction, whether or not depolarization occurs.

Excitation–Contraction Coupling

Excitation of the smooth muscle cell is only the first in a series of steps that lead eventually to a mechanical response. The chemical reactions involved in contraction have been studied intensively since Szent-Gyorgyi's[11] discovery that strands of actomyosin made from solutions of those proteins could be made to contract, but the story is still incomplete, particularly in smooth muscle. As we indicated in an earlier section, two different modes of excitation–contraction coupling are distinguished in discussions of vascular smooth muscle responses. *Electromechanical coupling* is a term applied to processes that induce contraction by way of depolarization, in contrast to *pharmacomechanical coupling* that is not accompanied by action potentials.[44] This distinction is useful as a description, but it can now be expanded to take into account the effects of partial depolarization (see above) and the various receptor–messenger combinations.

Among the reactions that couple excitation to the contractile apparatus, the intracellular concentration of Ca^{2+} is one crucial component and the level of cyclic AMP is another; the latter is involved in the function of beta-adrenergic receptors and in the relaxation of some vessels by nitro-compounds.[35] Within limits, raising $[Ca^{2+}]_i$ increases force in smooth muscle, and raising cyclic-AMP diminishes it. These are the two most firmly established of a host of *second messengers* now under active investigation. Phosphoinositides are probably also involved in the intracellular physiology of vascular smooth muscle cells (Chapter 1), but clear evidence for such activity has yet to be presented.

The role of calcium

Smooth muscle contraction is initiated by any process that elevates the cytosolic free $[Ca^{2+}]$ concentration above 0.2 μM, and active force increases along with Ca^{2+} up to a maximum at about 1 μM. Intra- and extracellular sources of calcium both contribute to the elevation in normal modes of excitation. In cardiac muscle, troponins on the actin filament prevent myosin–actin interaction at low (i.e., resting) calcium concentrations; that inhibition is removed when $[Ca^{2+}]_i$ rises (Chapter 3). Troponins are absent in smooth muscle, however, and the initial link in the chain that connects Ca^{2+} to contraction is not known unequivocally, although it clearly is not the same in smooth as in striated muscle.

The most widely accepted hypothesis is that the establishment of actomyosin bridges in smooth muscle first requires the formation of a complex of Ca^{2+} and calmodulin. The calmodulin molecule binds Ca^{2+} at several different sites and undergoes conformational changes as it does so, thus acting as a calcium sensor. The altered conformation increases the affinity of calmodulin for myosin light chain kinase, thus increasing the phosphorylation of regulatory myosin light chains. A non-calcium-sensitive dephosphorylating enzyme, myosin phosphatase, inhibits contraction at low concentrations of free Ca^{2+}.

Once the myosin light chain has been phosphorylated, the subsequent steps are probably the same in smooth as in striated muscle. Contact of a myosin head with an active site on the actin filament brings into play an actin-Mg^{2+}–activated myosin ATPase, resulting in splitting of ATP to ADP and phosphate (P_i) and binding of the head to the actin filament. ATP is promptly re-created from ADP and phosphocreatine, however, so that the net ATP concentration remains almost constant. The persistent presence of ATP then breaks the binding of myosin to actin, ending the energy "stroke" of the cross-bridge. Two consecutive actions thus occur when ATP is hydrolyzed by myosin ATPase. First, ATP acts as an energy-supplying substrate. Second, it dissociates actin from myosin, breaking the bridge attachment. Many of the intermediate steps and products of these reactions have been defined.[1] Under experimental conditions that provide no ATP, the bridge remains attached for long periods of time, creating the state called *rigor.*

Although the theory outlined above has been widely accepted, many investigators doubt that myosin phosphorylation is the only mechanism for coupling excitation to contraction in smooth muscle. Some evidence suggests that a complex of calmodulin with another thin-filament protein, caldesmon, exerts an inhibitory influence on actin–myosin interaction,[36] much as tropomyosin does in skeletal muscle.

Mechanical Behavior

Contraction

Vascular smooth muscle, like other types, responds to excitation by developing force and shortening. The amount of force and the extent of shortening depend on the strength of the stimulus, but they also depend on the mechanical constraints imposed on the contracting muscle. Isometric or isotonic conditions represent extreme degrees of constraint, and vascular smooth muscle normally functions somewhere between those two limits. The muscle is free to shorten, so that isometric conditions do not obtain, and transmural pressure may not be constant, so the state is not isotonic.

Contraction elicited by effective stimuli can be maintained at a steady level for long periods of time if the stimulus continues. The response to norepinephrine of a strip of vascular wall, held at constant length *in vitro,* is typical (Figure 9.5). To demonstrate such a response, a resting strip is first stretched to a suitable length, which requires a certain amount of force (compare Figure 3.9). In the absence of spontaneous pacemakers, this passive force arises only from elongation of the structural elements in the vessel wall, not from cross-bridge activity. When stimulation activates the cross-bridges, they generate an additional "active" force. The speed with which this force develops when the tissue

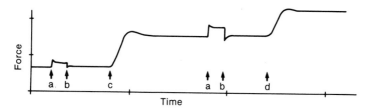

Figure 9.5. Development of isometric force in strip of blood vessel wall *in vitro* (rabbit aorta) stimulated by norepinephrine; *a*, quick stretch, and *b*, quick release, to measure control "stiffness" (see text); *c*, superfusate changed to include 0.3 μM norepinephrine; *d*, norepinephrine, 3.0 μM. ΔL same in both stretches.

is exposed to an agonist in an organ bath depends on the rate of diffusion into the wall and the spread of excitation. The response usually reaches a peak and then declines to a steady level. The muscle becomes stiffer when cross-bridges are active (see below), a change that can be demonstrated by quickly stretching the tissue (Figure 9.5). Under isotonic conditions, where the muscle is required to maintain a constant force, length is the variable that changes and shortening occurs over roughly the same time course.

Some evidence suggests that the earliest response and peak originate from the release of intracellular Ca^{2+} stores, whereas the steady state is more dependent on an influx of Ca^{2+} from the extracellular fluid. In experiments where $[Ca^{2+}]_o$ is very low ($<1 \times 10^{-8}$ M), the peak is much lower and the plateau is greatly reduced compared to the response in millimolar Ca^{2+} solutions. On repeated stimulation, the rising phase becomes smaller and smaller, as if the internal sources were being exhausted. Nevertheless, a small, steady force persists, equal to approximately 5% of the response to the first stimulus, perhaps because binding of calcium to sites on the external membrane surface makes it impossible to reduce the extracellular concentration of that ion to zero.

In both the relaxed and activated states, muscle length, force, and velocity of shortening are interdependent, and the relationships are essentially the same as in cardiac muscle (Chapter 3). Active force increases along with length up to a peak (*optimum length*) and then declines at greater lengths, although the peak is often flatter and less well defined than in striated muscle. Velocity and force are inversely correlated in a curvilinear manner, with a finite intercept on the force axis, and estimates of maximum unloaded velocity can be made (v_{max}; Chapter 3).

Contractile machinery

In spite of marked differences in microscopic structure, the basic mechanism of contraction in vascular smooth muscle appears to be the same as in striated muscle, a cross-bridge–driven sliding of actin and myosin filaments.

Estimates of cycling time, the interval each bridge spends in attachment, force generation, detachment, and rest before the next attachment, range from 3 to 50 msec in striated muscle.

The cycling time for an active cross-bridge is not necessarily the same under all conditions. During sustained isometric contraction *in vitro,* for example, many bridges appear to be *latched,* cycling very slowly, if at all.[23] Under other experimental conditions, bridges cycle rapidly but generate little or no force (*weak bridges*).[10,32] Whether or not smooth muscle bridges can enter a noncycling state of *rigor,* where they are firmly attached but produce little force, is a matter of controversy. The physiological implications of all these states are under investigation.

Investigators of striated muscle have long attempted to correlate mechanical behavior with specific aspects of cross-bridge function, and some of the results are probably applicable to vascular smooth muscle. Active force, to cite an obvious example, is presumably an index of the number of force-generating bridges, if we assume that each normally functioning bridge generates a specific quantum of force. Other correlations have been derived from *quick-stretch* or *quick-release* experiments, in which muscle length is suddenly changed. This maneuver is intended to alter the length of elastic elements in the muscle instantaneously, before bridges can detach and reattach, which requires that the change be imposed in less than 1 msec. The ratio of change in force to change in length in a quick stretch ($\Delta F/\Delta L$) is called the *stiffness* of the muscle. Stiffness is thought to be indicative of the number of attached cross-bridges, and it is almost always proportional to active force.

Similar experiments can be used to measure unloaded shortening velocity (v_{max}), which is assumed to be directly correlated with the rate of cross-bridge cycling. This interpretation is based on the observation in a wide range of vertebrate and invertebrate species that actual shortening velocity is directly related to the level of actin-calcium–activated ATPase, which is essential for the cycling process.[12] The *load-bearing capacity,* or maximum load that the muscle will bear without yielding, is another experimental measure of muscle behavior.[23] The mechanical work done by muscle can also be calculated from measurements of force and length, a common practice in studies of myocardial function (Chapter 4), but that approach has been little explored in smooth muscle. Calculations of this kind on the oscillatory striated muscle of insects have shown that the work done by the muscle during sinusoidal stress is frequency dependent.[47]

Although the contractile machinery is currently assumed to be the same in smooth and striated muscles, some recent evidence casts doubt on that hypothesis. Most parts of a smooth muscle cell contain actin, but in some intracellular regions the actin is associated with myosin and in others with a different protein, filamin.[43] The chemical complex formed by actin and filamin may provide a physical mechanism for shortening in which cross-bridges play no part. Even in striated muscle, revolutionary changes in classical contraction theory may be on the horizon. Some recent investigations suggest that cross-bridges are synchronized in some way; others indicate that they may not rotate.[51]

Mechanical Experiments on Smooth Muscle

Vascular smooth muscle exhibits elasticity and viscosity in the relaxed state, and both properties are altered by excitation.[5] Arterial elasticity is evident in the distention that follows each heartbeat, normal pulse pressures producing a pulsatile enlargement that amounts to 10 to 16% of the average diameter in the pulmonary artery and 2 to 5% of that in the less distensible aorta. Distensibility is a major determinant of pulse wave velocity, which has been used as an index of the arterial state in cardiovascular disease (Chapter 2). Elasticity is also manifested in force–length diagrams of blood vessels, which are typically concave toward the force axis (Figure 6.6). Viscous behavior is evident in the phenomenon of *stress relaxation,* discussed in Chapter 6, and in the phase shifts observed during sinusoidal perturbations.

The mechanical properties of the blood vessel wall and of vascular smooth muscle are often studied by measuring force while controlled changes of length are imposed, or vice versa, as in the quick-stretch maneuver already described. The characteristics of actin–myosin binding, the rate of cross-bridge cycling, and other aspects of the contractile process can be examined in this way. Current theories of contraction in both smooth and striated muscles have been largely derived by correlating the results of such experiments with biochemical and x-ray diffraction studies.[1,32]

The procedures are usually carried out *in vitro* on strips of vascular wall suspended in an organ bath, where temperature and the fluid environment can be controlled, a vascular counterpart of the isolated papillary muscle preparation (Chapter 3). Alternatively, observations can be made on segments of vessels in their normal cylindrical configuration or on vessels *in situ* in intact animals. Very small perturbations, typically less than 1% of the initial muscle length, are employed to avoid nonlinearity and overt myogenic responses.

Two kinds of manipulation can be used: a quick stretch (or release), in which muscle length is abruptly increased (or decreased) from one isometric level to another,[29] or controlled sinusoidal oscillations of length at various frequencies.[16] The protocol can be reversed and the length measured as similar alterations of force are imposed, but we will confine ourselves here to examples in which length is the controlled variable, and also assume that myogenic responses do not occur in the vessels being studied.

Sudden, sustained stretching of a smooth muscle (i.e., a *step function* of length) causes force to rise abruptly to a peak and then fall relatively slowly to a new level (Figure 9.6B). The new steady-state force that is eventually reached is higher than that before the stretch by an amount that is directly (but nonlinearly) related to the increase in muscle length. The height of the peak depends on the velocity as well as the amplitude of the stretch. A similar response occurs when skeletal or cardiac muscle is stretched (Figure 9.6A), but the peak in heart muscle is followed almost immediately by a rapid return to the control level, after which it slowly rises again to a new state.[46] In skeletal muscle, several distinct variations in declining force have been identified in the first 100 msec after the peak; similar transients have not been observed in vascular smooth muscle.

The almost instantaneous rise in force that accompanies a quick stretch, even in relaxed, noncontracting vascular smooth muscle, suggests that purely elastic elements are being elongated. In the absence of muscle activation, assuming that no cross-bridges are attached, the elasticity presumably resides in nonmuscular components of the wall, including the muscle cell membrane and any structures associated with it. As mentioned earlier, this conclusion may not be entirely correct, because relaxed muscle may contain some bridges that are attached but not generating force,[32] but the greater part of the elasticity of

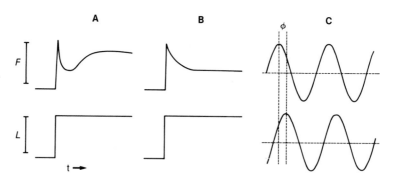

Figure 9.6. Force (*above*) and length (*below*) as functions of time (*abscissa*), when changes in muscle length are imposed experimentally. **A**, quick stretch, striated muscle. Note early decline of force after peak, followed by delayed redevelopment of force. In cardiac muscle, force falls quickly to almost the control level before rising again (not shown). **B**, quick stretch, smooth muscle. Force falls continuously after peak until a new equilibrium is reached. **C**, sinusoidal oscillations, smooth muscle. Force oscillates with the same frequency as the perturbations of length, but at low frequencies the peak force precedes peak length by a phase angle, φ. The phase difference shown here for purposes of illustration (55°) is much larger than that observed in muscle.

inactive blood vessels is almost certainly external to the muscle cells. This passive elasticity is much smaller in striated than in smooth muscle.

Quick stretching of a vessel wall in which the smooth muscle has been *stimulated* produces a greater force increment per unit stretch than is the case in the relaxed state (Figure 9.5). When graded isometric contraction of the smooth muscle is induced by adding successively higher concentrations of norepinephrine to the organ bath, for example, there is a similarly graded increase in stiffness. Quantitative studies of this phenomenon lead to the conclusion that the elastic elements in contracting muscle are largely in the cross-bridge structure itself,[29] although it is not clear whether they are located in the myosin head, tail, or attachment site. Whatever the location, they appear to be responsible for a large part of the stiffness of active skeletal muscle, and the same thing is probably true in smooth muscle.

Models

Interpretation of the results of such experiments is often based on mechanical models that consist of hypothetical elastic and viscous components arranged in various ways. Because smooth muscle exhibits viscoelastic behavior even when it is totally relaxed, it is customary for one part of the model to represent the passive elements of the wall and another the contractile apparatus. Such models can simulate the reactions of blood vessels, but it is important to remember that the apparently viscous behavior of active muscle owes at least as much to cross-bridge attachment and detachment as to classically viscous materials.

The standard unit used to account for a peak force followed by a decline is the *Maxwell element,* which consists of a spring and a dashpot in series (Figure 9.7A). The spring represents a *series elastic element* (*SE*) and the dashpot a purely viscous one. Quick stretch of a Maxwell element immediately lengthens the spring to an extent determined by its elasticity, which is often expressed as a spring constant, or stiffness, $\Delta F/\Delta L$. The dashpot, however, cannot be extended instantaneously, but elongates with a velocity that is inversely proportional to its viscosity and directly proportional to the applied force, a response analogous to that of a viscous fluid (equation 6.2). As the model is held at this new length, the viscous element slowly extends and the spring shortens, so that the force exerted by the SE declines and eventually reaches zero.

The simple Maxwell element is thus not an adequate model of muscle because it does not maintain a higher force when elongated, and a second spring, or *parallel elastic element* (*PE*), must be added to imitate the persistent elevation of steady-state force in the stretched muscle (Figure 9.7B). The initial stretch now extends both springs instantaneously, producing the peak force.

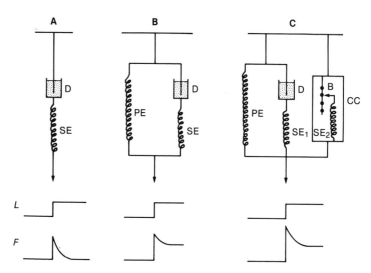

Figure 9.7. *Above*; mechanical models of muscle. *Below*; force response (*F*) to quick stretch (*L*) in each model. **A**, Maxwell model, consisting of elastic element (spring, *SE*) and viscous component (dashpot, *D*) in series. Quick stretch produces an instantaneous peak force, which is completely dissipated as viscous component slowly extends. **B**, Maxwell arrangement plus parallel elastic element (*PE*). Declining force after peak equilibrates at a higher level than before stretch. **C**, Model **B** plus contractile component (*CC*), including an attached cross-bridge (*B*) and bridge elasticity (*SE$_2$*). Force follows same time course as in model *B*, but is higher because of stretched bridge elastic elements, SE$_2$. Isometric force depends on total number of functioning contractile components and stretch of passive elastic elements *PE* and *SE$_1$*.

The viscous component yields slowly, as before, allowing the SE to shorten, which gradually reduces the total force. The PE remains stretched, however, and its elasticity determines the new equilibrium. This three-component array is the simplest model that approximates the passive responses of smooth muscle to externally applied force; the next step is to simulate the active elements.

Modeling of the myosin cross-bridge introduces a new kind of element, one that not only contributes additional elastic elements but also generates force. The contractile apparatus is represented in Figure 9.7C as a separate component (*CC*), containing a myosin cross-bridge (*B*) and an elastic element (*SE$_2$*) in the tail of the myosin molecule. (The component labeled *CC* represents just one of a large number of potentially active bridges in parallel). In an inactive muscle, the contractile component is assumed to be freely extensible, contributing nothing to the mechanical behavior. When the head binds to actin, the direction of the force it generates tends to shorten the whole array, but in an isometric preparation it elongates the myosin elastic element instead. This model is the basis for the idea that the stiffness measured on quick stretch is proportional to the number of attached cross-bridges.

In a steady state of isometric contraction, a vast number of bridges act asynchronously, cycling through attachment, force generation, and detachment, while the net effect averages out to a constant force. All of this force is exerted through the stretched cross-bridge elasticity in the model described here (SE_2), but experimental evidence suggests that part of it is stored in still other elastic elements not shown in the figure, which connect cells or muscle bundles in series.

The decline from peak force to a new equilibrium arises, according to one theory, from bridge detachment, recoil of SE_2 to its unstressed length, and reattachment at a new site farther down the actin filament. The overall length of the model remains constant by virtue of the isometric constraints of the experiment. The great number of bridges involved asynchronously conceals the stepwise nature of the process as one head after another "ratchets down" the filament. A new steady state develops when each head reaches a position where it can cycle repeatedly without seeking to shorten SE_2 further. Bridges continue to attach, generate force, and detach, but they have found a point of dynamic equilibrium. The constant overall force is now directly related to the number of functioning bridges, which depends on the intracellular concentration of Ca^{2+} and other messengers, which in turn depends on the strength of the stimulus (e.g., norepinephrine concentration). Equilibrium force is greater than before the stretch because the alignment of actin and myosin filaments provides more attachment sites and because of the effects of length on Ca^{2+} availability (Chapter 3), in addition to the passive contribution of the stretched PE.

Many other models of muscle contraction have been proposed,[1,12] and the one described above is no more than an introduction to the subject. One variant assumes that the act of stretching temporarily increases the number of participating cross-bridges, accounting for the fact that the muscle sustains a greater force during the declining phase than in the later steady state. This concept of *stretch activation* is reminiscent of the myogenic response, and the two phenomena may be related. Other models postulate a mixture of cross-bridge states, some units following the sequence just described and others varying in their cycling time and developed force.[23,32] Such models have been a fertile source of explicit, testable hypotheses about muscle function.

Sinusoidal perturbations

Sinusoidal changes of length in vascular smooth muscle[16] are accompanied by oscillations of force that have the same frequency but not the same timing (Figure 9.6C). In such experiments, the ratio of changes in wall force to those in diameter is a measure of viscoelasticity, analogous to that determined by quick stretch or release. The viscoelastic properties of blood vessels are fre-

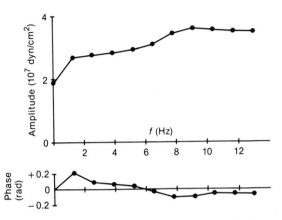

Figure 9.8. Spectrum of complex viscoelastic modules (E_c; Chapter 6) of canine femoral arterial wall with normal vascular tone, determined *in situ* by Fourier analysis of normal pulsations. *Abscissa*, frequency (Hz). *Ordinates: above,* E_c amplitude ($\times$ 10^{-7} dyn/cm²); *below,* E_c phase angle (radians). Positive phase angles indicate that force leads distension. Static elastic modulus is plotted at frequency of zero. (Reproduced from Milnor and Bertram,[37] with permission of the American Heart Association)

quency dependent. Typical measurements on a canine femoral artery are shown in Figure 9.8 in the form of a frequency spectrum of the complex viscoelastic modulus (E_c; Chapter 6). The physiological significance of arterial viscoelasticity lies in its influence on the work the heart must do to produce a pulsatile outflow and on the transformation of pulsatile waveforms as they travel through the arterial tree.[5] In the relaxed state at low frequencies, the amplitudes of the viscoelastic modulus in large systemic arteries are typically about 1.0×10^6 to 20×10^6 dyne/cm². Maximum stimulation can increase the amplitude about fivefold, increasing cardiac work (Chapter 4) and speeding the transmission of pulse waves.

Contractile activity also causes force to lead diameter oscillations by a larger time interval at low frequencies and to lag farther behind diameter oscillations at higher frequencies, time relationships that are expressed as phase angles. If a material is purely elastic, the change in length and the resulting force are exactly in phase (angle = 0°); if it is purely viscous, force leads length by 90°. In passive structures that exhibit both elastic and viscous behavior, force leads length by an angle smaller than 90°. This relationship obtains at low frequencies in blood vessels, where force *precedes* length below about 6 Hz, as shown in Figure 9.8.

The significance of the phase relationships in blood vessels at higher frequencies, where force *lags behind* length in most cases (Figure 9.8), is controversial. This phenomenon does not occur in conventional passive structures and is usually taken as a sign that the system is doing work as it is stretched and released. (In passive systems, all work is done by the instrument doing the stretching). One interpretation of the data in Figure 9.8 is, therefore, that sinusoidal stretch and release at frequencies above 6Hz stimulate contraction of vascular smooth muscle. A similar response has been found in the flight muscles of insects, the myocardium, and some skeletal muscles,[47] although the relation of work to frequency is not the same in all these tissues.

The results of sinusoidal oscillation, like those of quick stretch, thus support the notion that perturbations of muscle length can stimulate some degree of contraction. An alternative explanation of the negative phase angles of E_c, however, is that they arise from the nonlinearity of the relation between pressure and vessel diameter.[5] The physiological significance of these observations consequently remains debatable, but they raise the possibility that the pulsations to which the arterial tree is constantly subjected may have something to do with the autoregulation of blood flow (Chapter 12).

References

Reviews

1. Eisenberg, E., Greene, L.E. (1980). The relation of muscle biochemistry to muscle physiology. *Ann. Rev. Physiol.* 42:293–310.

2. Hirst, G.D.S., Edwards, F.R. (1989). Sympathetic neuroeffector transmission in arteries and arterioles. *Physiol. Rev.* 69:546–604.

3. Johansson, B., Somlyo, A.P. (1980). Electrophysiology and excitation–contraction coupling. In: *Handbook of Physiology, Section 2: The Cardiovascular System. Vol. II, Vascular Smooth Muscle,* D.F. Bohr, A.P. Somlyo, and H.V. Sparks, Jr., eds. Bethesda, Md., American Physiological Society, pp. 301–323.

4. Johnson, P.C. (1980). The myogenic response. In: *Handbook of Physiology, Section 2: The Cardiovascular System. Vol. II, Vascular Smooth Muscle,* D.F. Bohr, A.P. Somlyo, and H.V. Sparks, Jr., eds. Bethesda, Md., American Phsyiological Society, pp. 409–442.

5. Milnor, W.R. (1989). *Hemodynamics,* 2nd ed. Baltimore, Williams & Wilkins.

6. Pick, J. (1970). *The Autonomic Nervous System.* Philadelphia, J.B. Lippincott.

7. Ruegg, J.C. (1986). *Calcium in Muscle Activation. A Comparative Approach.* Berlin, Springer-Verlag.

8. Sparks, H.V., Jr. (1980). Effect of local metabolic factors on vascular smooth muscle. In: *Handbook of Physiology, Section 2: The Cardiovascular System. Vol. II, Vascular Smooth Muscle,* D.F. Bohr, A.P. Somlyo, and H.V. Sparks, Jr., eds. Bethesda, Md., American Physiological Society, pp. 475–513.

9. Speden, R.N. (1970). Excitation of vascular smooth muscle. In: *Smooth Muscle*, E. Bulbring et al., eds. London, Edward Arnold, pp. 558–588.

10. Stephens, N.L., ed. (1984). *Smooth Muscle Contraction*. New York, Marcel Dekker.

11. Szent-Gyorgyi, A. (1953). *Chemical Physiology of Contraction of Body and Heart Muscle*. New York, Academic Press.

12. Tregear, R.T., Marston, S.B. (1979). The crossbridge theory. *Ann. Rev. Physiol*. 41:723–736.

Research Reports

13. Apter, J.T., Rabinowitz, M., Cummings, D.H. (1966). Correlation of viscoelastic properties of large arteries with microscopic structure. I. Collagen, elastin and muscle determined chemically, histologically, and physiologically. *Circ. Res*. 19:104–121.

14. Barr, L., Berger, W., Dewey, M.M. (1968). Electrical transmission at the nexus between smooth muscle cells. *J. Gen. Physiol*. 51:347–368.

15. Benham, C.D., Tsien, R.W. (1987). A novel receptor-operated Ca^{2+}-permeable channel activated by ATP in smooth muscle. *Nature* 328:275–278.

16. Bergel, D.H. (1961). The dynamic elastic properties of the arterial wall. *J. Physiol*. 156:458–469.

17. Bozler, E. (1948). Conduction, automaticity and tonus of visceral smooth muscles. *Experientia* 4:213–218.

18. Brayden, J.E., Bevan, J.A. (1985). Neurogenic muscarinic vasodilatation in the cat: An example of endothelial-cell independent cholinergic relaxation. *Circ. Res*. 56:205–211.

19. Burnstock, G., Kennedy, C. (1986). A dual function for adenosine 5'-triphosphate in the regulation of vascular tone. *Circ. Res*. 58:319–330.

20. Casteels, R., Kitamura, R.K., Kuriyama, H., Suzuki, H. (1977). The membrane properties of the rabbit main pulmonary artery. *J. Physiol*. 271:63–79.

21. DeMey, J.G., Vanhoutte, P.M. (1982). Heterogeneous behavior of the canine arterial and venous wall. *Circ. Res*. 51:439–447.

22. Devine, C.E., Simpson, F.O., Bertrand, W.S. (1971). Freeze-etch studies on the innervation of mesenteric arteries and vas deferens. *J. Cell Sci*. 9:411–425.

23. Dillon, P.F., Murphy, R.A. (1982). Tonic force maintenance with reduced shortening velocity in arterial smooth muscle. *Am. J. Physiol*. 242 (*Cell* 11):C102–C108.

24. Duckles, S.P. (1983). Innervation of the cerebral vasculature. *Ann. Biomed. Eng*. 11:599–605.

25. Duling, B.R. (1972). Microvascular responses to alterations in oxygen tension. *Circ. Res*. 31:481–489.

26. Fabiato, A. (1985). Stimulated calcium current can both cause calcium loading in and trigger calcium release from the sarcoplasmic reticulum of a skinned canine cardiac Purkinje cell. *J. Gen. Physiol*. 85:291–320.

27. Fay, F.S. (1977). Isometric contractile properties of single isolated smooth muscle cells. *Nature* 265:553–556.

28. Filo, R.S., Bohr, D.F., Ruegg, J.C. (1965). Glycerinated skeletal and smooth muscle: Calcium and magnesium dependence. *Science* 147:1581–1583.

29. Ford, L.E., Huxley, A.F., Simmons, R.M. (1981). The relation between stiffness and filament overlap in stimulated frog muscle fibers. *J. Physiol.* 311:219–249.

30. Hendrickx, H., Casteels, R. (1974). Electrogenic sodium pump in arterial smooth muscle cells. *Pfluegers Arch.* 346:299–306.

31. Hirst, G.D.S., Neild, T.O. (1981). Localization of specialized noradrenaline receptors at neuromuscular junctions on arterioles of the guinea-pig. *J. Physiol.* 313:343–350.

32. Huxley, H.E., Kress, M. (1985). Cross-bridge behavior during muscle contraction. *J. Mus. Res. Cell Motility* 6:153–161.

33. Johansson, B., Mellander, S. (1975). Static and dynamic changes in the vascular myogenic response to passive changes in length as revealed by electrical and mechanical recordings from the rat portal vein. *Circ. Res.* 36:76–83.

34. Klockner, U., Isenberg, G. (1985). Calcium currents of cesium loaded isolated smooth muscle cells (urinary bladder of the guinea pig). *Pfluegers Arch.* 405:340–348.

35. Kukovetz, W.R., Holzmann, S., Wurm, A., Poch, G. (1979). Evidence for cyclic GMP–mediated relaxant effects of nitro-compounds in coronary smooth muscle. *Naunyn-Schmiedeberg's Arch. Pharmacol.* 310:129–138.

36. Marston, S.B., Lehman, W. (1985). Caldesmon is a Ca^{2+} regulatory component of native smooth-muscle thin filaments. *Biochem. J.* 231:517–522.

37. Milnor, W.R., Bertram, C.D. (1978). The relation between arterial viscoelasticity and wave propagation in the canine femoral artery in vivo. *Circ. Res.* 43:870–879.

38. Murphy, R.A., Herlihy, J.T., Megerman, J. (1974). Force-generating capacity and contractile protein content of arterial smooth muscle. *J. Gen. Physiol.* 64:691–705.

39. Palmer, R.M.J., Ferrige, A.G., Moncada, S. (1987). Nitric oxide release accounts for the biological activity of endothelium-derived relaxing factor. *Nature* 327:524–526.

40. Reuter, H. (1983). Calcium channel modulation by neurotransmitters, enzymes and drugs. *Nature* 301:569–574.

41. Roddie, I. (1967). Electrical and mechanical activity in turtle arteries and veins. *Bibl. Anat.* 8:1–4.

42. Siegel, G., Schneider, W. (1981). Anions, cations, membrane potential, and relaxation. In: *Vasodilatation,* P.M. Vanhoutte and I. Leusen, ed. New York, Raven Press, pp. 285–298.

43. Small, J.V., Furst, D.O., DeMey, J. (1986). Localization of filamin in smooth muscle. *J. Cell Biol.* 102:210–220.

44. Somlyo, A.V., Vinall, P., Somlyo, A.P. (1971). Excitation–contraction coupling and electrical events in two types of vascular smooth muscle. *Microvasc. Res.* 1:354–373.

45. Sparks, H.V., Jr. (1964). Effect of quick stretch on isolated vascular smooth muscle. *Circ. Res.* 15(Suppl. 1):254–260.

46. Steiger, G.J., Brady, A., Tan, S.T. (1978). Intrinsic regulatory properties of contractility in the myocardium. *Circ. Res.* 42:339–350.

47. Thorson, J., White, D.C.S. (1983). Role of cross-bridge distortion in the small-signal mechanical dynamics of insect and rabbit striated muscle. *J. Physiol.* 343:59–84.

48. Von Loh, D. (1971). The effect of adrenergic drugs on spontaneously active vascular smooth muscle studied by long-term intracellular recording of membrane potential. *Angiologica* 8:144–155.

49. Von Loh, D., Bohr, D.F. (1973). Membrane potentials of smooth muscle cells of isolated resistance vessels. *Proc. Soc. Exp. Biol. Med.* 144:513–516.

50. Warshaw, D.M., McBride, W.J., Work, S.S. (1987). Corkscrew-like shortening in single smooth muscle cells. *Science* 236:1457–1459.

51. Yangida, T. (1985). Angle of active site of myosin heads in contracting muscle during sudden length changes. *J. Muscle Res. Cell Motil.* 6:43–52.

10

CAPILLARY AND LYMPHATIC SYSTEMS

The capillaries are the site of communication between the circulatory system and the fluid that bathes all the cells of the body. Through the capillary walls pass nutrients, waste products, and regulatory substances that are absorbed into the bloodstream and delivered to appropriate tissues elsewhere. The capillaries are tubes of very small diameter, and their walls consist of a single layer of flattened endothelial cells, 0.1 to 0.3 μm in thickness, with nuclei that sometimes bulge into the lumen. Most of the movement of molecules between interstitial fluids and blood plasma takes place through the capillary wall, which thus controls the immediate environment of tissue cells. Some transfer of water, respiratory gases, and small molecules also takes place through the walls of terminal segments of arterioles and venules, but the potential total surface area of the capillaries is enormously greater. The lymphatic system also plays an important part in circulatory transport because it drains fluid from the interstitial space and empties into the great veins.

Capillary beds are interposed between the terminal branches of the arterial tree and the very smallest branches of the veins, and the anatomical arrangement of capillary beds is such that the distance for diffusion to and from local cells is relatively small. Arterioles and venules, unlike capillaries, are endowed with smooth muscle, and this muscle regulates capillary pressure and flow. Such regulation can increase capillary flow and exchange in one region while reducing them in another, to serve the needs of the moment. Because the arterioles, venules, and capillaries function as a physiological unit, they are often referred to inclusively as the *microcirculation*.

Architecture

The microscopic anatomy of the microcirculation varies from one organ to another, but the pattern is almost always some variant of that shown in Figure 10.1. From arterioles about 50 μm in diameter to venules of the same size, one or more direct paths can usually be traced through smaller vessels called *metarterioles,* which contain a small amount of smooth muscle. True capillaries branch from arterioles and metarterioles and form an irregular network in the space between the muscular vessels. In many cases, a few smooth muscle cells encircle the origin of a capillary where it leaves the arteriole, creating precapillary *sphincters* that can reduce or prevent flow through that particular channel. In addition, short, muscular *arteriovenous anastomoses* between an arteriole and a venule exist at a few locations.

In tissues that are essentially two-dimensional, like the mesentery and omentum, arterioles form arcades, with blood flowing up both sides of the arch and out into metarterioles or capillaries. The venules have a similar configuration. Each arcade supplies a discrete sector of tissue 2.5×10^{-4} to 8.1×10^{-4} μm^2 in area.[8] In tissues that extend in three dimensions, like skeletal muscle, the microcirculation follows a tree-like branching pattern and the capillaries form a complex meshwork, often supplied by several arterioles and drained by several venules. This architecture clearly provides for a great diversity of

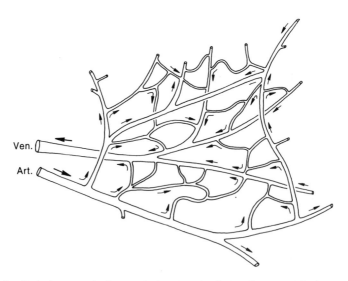

Figure 10.1. Typical segment of mesenteric microcirculation. One arteriole (approximately 30 μm in diameter) enters at lower left (*Art.*); another smaller one, at upper right. Venule exits at left (*Ven.*) *Arrows* indicate direction of flow through capillary paths between arterioles and venules. (Based on data reported by Zweifach et al.[8,39])

pathways through the microcirculation. The length of unbranched capillary segments varies widely, from 10 μm in some cases to more than 100 μm in others. The physiologically significant "length" is that of an average path through a capillary net, which is on the order of 400 to 1200 μm. The total path length from 50-μm arteriole to 80-μm venule is only slightly longer, perhaps 500 to 1500 μm.

Physiological responses make intensive use of the arteriolar-venular control system, adjusting the microcirculation to meet local needs. The smallest arterial terminations are called *arterioles,* but that designation includes vessels that range from 100 to 10 μm in diameter. For purposes of discussion, we will define the microcirculation as that portion of the vasculature that extends from 50-μm arterioles through the capillaries and on into the venules up to vessels about 80 μm in diameter. About 70% of the volume of blood in this region is in venules, and the remainder is in arterioles and capillaries.[8] The vessels in the system have been classified in various ways and given such names as *precapillary, terminal arteriole,* and so on, but we will designate precapillary and postcapillary vessels in the microcirculation as *arterioles* and *venules,* respectively, and identify segments by their diameter.

The total number of capillaries in the body can be estimated only by tedious microscopic counting in tissue samples, and the results are only rough approximations. In a classical work based on anatomical studies, Krogh[4] concluded that the total volume of capillaries in the human adult at rest is about 300 cm³, or 5% of the total blood volume. Only a small fraction of them are open at rest, when metabolic demand is relatively low. In the case of the capillaries of skeletal muscle, 1 or 2% are normally open, but during exercise the recruitment of channels previously closed increases that number 10- to 20-fold. The graded constriction or dilatation that occurs in arterioles is not possible in the capillaries because of their physical structure and lack of smooth muscle, so that these tiny vessels are usually either widely open or else completely closed. They are relatively indistensible, perhaps because of the gel-like character of their surroundings.[20] Increased tissue metabolism is served in part by more rapid flow through individual channels, in addition to the opening up of previously closed segments.

The details of the microcirculatory pattern are not exactly the same in all organ systems. The ratio of metarterioles to true capillaries, for example, is about 3:1 in the mesenteric bed and closer to 10:1 in skeletal muscle. This difference corresponds to the much greater physiological changes in metabolic demand that occur in skeletal muscle. In the human nail bed[39] and bat wing[30] capillaries branch directly from major arterioles through a sphincter, and metarterioles are virtually absent. In the liver, spleen, and bone marrow, capillaries widen out into broad sinusoidal spaces as great as 50 μm in width. Pulmonary capillaries have a unique configuration, forming a fine-meshed network around each alveolus (Chapter 11). Capillaries in the choroid plexuses of the brain and their special exchange characteristics (the *blood-brain barrier*) are considered in Chapter 12, as are the features of the renal and myocardial capillaries.

The number of capillaries also varies considerably from one organ to another. Total capillary surface in the canine myocardium is about four times that in the gastric mucosa, for example (Table 10.3). Histological counts in red skeletal muscle give values of about 1000 capillaries/mm² in the dog and in animals of similar size, but there are marked species differences and the density in white muscles is somewhat lower. The greatest distance from a tissue cell to the nearest capillary is about 9 to 17 μm in skeletal muscle, heart, and brain cortex of the dog and cat.

In spite of the variations that are characteristic of each organ system, some generalizations can be made about the dimensions of microcirculatory vessels. Most true capillaries are 4 to 8 μm in diameter, and the adjoining arteriolar and venular segments are not much larger than the capillaries that branch from them. Some idea of the relative numbers of vessels of different caliber can be gained from the estimate that in feline skeletal muscle one 50-μm arteriole supplies about 50 smaller arterioles 20 μm in diameter and 1500 capillaries.[8] The relation of pressure and flow in diameter in microcirculatory vessels is considered in a later section.

One of the most important regional differences in capillary structure is in the intercellular clefts, openings between endothelial cells that can be observed microscopically. Three kinds of capillaries have been distinguished by this criterion:

1. *Continuous*. In this type, narrow channels connecting the capillary lumen with the extravascular space lie between the endothelial cells (Figure 10.2A). The channels are 4 to 5 nm wide at the luminal opening and widen out to about 20 nm toward the abluminal side. This variety is widely distributed, occurring in skeletal and smooth muscle, connective tissue, fat, and the pulmonary circulation.

2. *Discontinuous*. The characteristic feature of this class is the presence of relatively large intercellular gaps a few hundred nanometers across (Figure 10.2C). Capillaries in the bone marrow, spleen, and liver sinusoids are of this type.

3. *Fenestrated*. Roughly circular openings or depressions called *fenestrae* (windows) are found in the endothelial cells of capillaries in the intestinal mucosa and renal glomeruli (Figures 10.2B, 10.3). These structures are sometimes as large as 100 nm in diameter, but many are

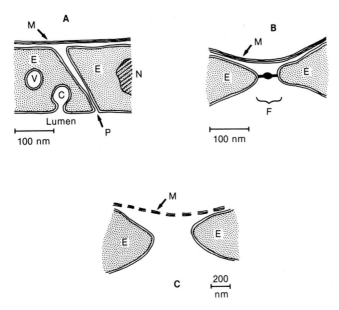

Figure 10.2.   Three types of capillaries, classified according to openings in their walls: **A**, continuous; **B**, fenestrated; **C**, discontinuous. *E*, endothelial cells; *N*, cell nucleus; *M*, basement membrane; *V*, vacuole; *C*, caveolus, or vacuole in communication with lumen; *P*, "pore" between endothelial cells; *F*, fenestration. (Reproduced with modifications from Renkin,[6] with permission of the American Heart Association)

smaller. Some of them are closed by a thin membrane with a central thickening, while others appear to be open and can pass particles at least as large as 20 nm in diameter.[35]. Even those that appear to be closed are capable of transmitting relatively large molecules. Fenestrations appear only in the thinner portions of endothelial cells.[6]

Functional studies of capillary permeability are more or less consistent with these morphological characteristics (see below). A thin *basement membrane* lies along the external surface of capillary endothelial cells, pierced by openings here and there in discontinuous capillaries but not in the other types.

   The cells of the endothelium are bounded by the usual lipid bilayer, which effectively blocks the passage of molecules that are not lipid soluble and tends to obstruct those that are polar. Nevertheless, it is possible for intracellular vesicles to transport such substances across endothelial cells. Vesicles up to 50 nm in diameter can be seen (Figure 10.2A); their action at the luminal cell boundaries is indicated by *caveoli* in the process of picking up or discharging contents.

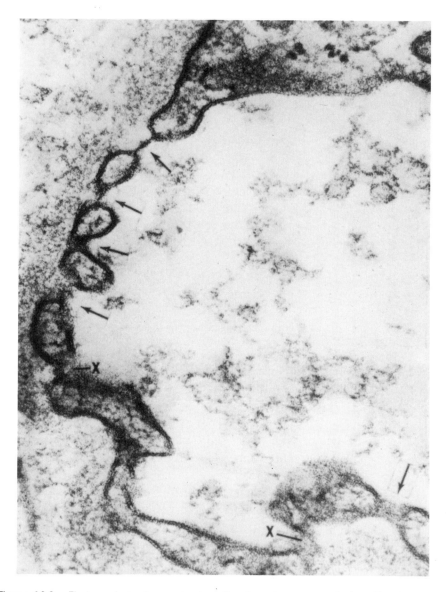

Figure 10.3.   Electron photomicrograph of section through venous end of capillary in mouse jejunum. Capillary lumen lies on right. *Arrows* indicate fenestrae in capillary wall. *X*, fenestrae lying partly out of section. (Reproduced from Casley-Smith,[13] with permission of *Microvasc. Res.*)

Hemodynamics

The flow of blood through channels that are often not as wide as a red cell cannot be expected to conform to the equations given in Chapter 6 for laminar fluid flow through cylindrical tubes. Erythrocytes must often be deformed to pass through capillaries, and plasma must flow around their edges, presenting problems that the most advanced engineering analyses have not yet completely solved. The variables involved include not only the deformability of red cells but also their tendency to aggregate; the latter affects pressure–flow relationships even in vessels two or three times larger than the red cell diameter (Chapter 13). The facts about capillary hemodynamics are thus largely empiric, but a large amount of such information is available.

Microscopic examination of capillary beds *in vivo* (the transilluminated mesentery, for example) shows that the pathways of flow vary from moment to moment. Under what seem to be constant conditions, capillaries that are closed at one instant open at another, diverting flow through a new series of segments. The resulting fluctuations appear to be random, but the capillaries lack any means of active vasomotion; thus, such changes must be due to local alterations of transmural pressure brought on by vasomotor activity of arterioles and venules. Arteriolar constriction tends to lower capillary pressure and venular constriction has the opposite effect, so that the balance between pre- and postcapillary action is the controlling factor.

Pressure

Accurate measurements of pressure can be made in microscopic vessels by a saline-filled micropipette inserted through the wall, combined with a servomechanism that senses the pressure required to prevent blood from moving into the pipette (Chapter 14). This technique gives continuous records of pulsatile pressure and has now been applied to the microcirculation in many different organs and species. Mean intracapillary pressure in most mammalian vascular beds in the systemic circulation is about 32 mm Hg, according to direct measurements in skeletal muscle, mesentery, omentum, and pia mater,[8] with a range under normal resting conditions of perhaps 26 to 38 mm Hg. These figures must be regarded as only illustrative, however, because local pressure and flow change in response to physiological stimuli. In capillaries of the human nail fold, for example, pressure rises appreciably when the environmental temperature is raised. The recurrent opening and closing of capillary segments impose additional changes. The drop in pressure in systemic capillaries typically ranges from 37 mm Hg at the arteriolar end to 27 mm Hg at the exit into a venule. This decrement is directly related to the length of the capillary pathway and averages 0.8 mm Hg/100-μm distance.

Some other vascular beds operate with quite different microcirculatory pressures. In the pulmonary capillaries, pressure is about 9 mm Hg at heart level, and varies from the top to the bottom of the lung in the erect posture in accordance with local hydrostatic effects (Chapter 11). Pressure within the capillary sinusoids of the liver is 2 to 6 mm Hg. In the capillaries of the renal glomeruli, pressure may be as high as 70 mm Hg, but it falls to about 12 mm Hg in the peritubular capillaries downstream (Chapter 12). The relation of pressure to filtration across the capillary wall will be discussed in a later section, but we may note here that capillary pressures measured by micropipettes have been found to be about 8 mm Hg higher than those estimated from transcapillary fluid flow in isogravimetric experiments (see below), perhaps because some water exchange takes place in the postcapillary venular segment, where pressure is lower than in the capillary segment.

A composite picture of the microcirculatory pressure gradients in organs similar to skeletal muscle is given by Table 10.1, where a mean pressure of 100 mm Hg in the major branches of the aorta has been assumed. The typical pressure drop across the microcirculation (as defined here) in a systemic bed is 50 to 60 mm Hg, the greatest part of it in the precapillary regions. In the absence of local physiological responses, the microcirculatory pressures rise and fall when major arterial pressures do, but this correlation is absent in regions where autoregulation keeps capillary pressures within a narrow range.

Table 10.1.   Typical Mean Blood Pressures and Velocities in Systemic Microcirculation[a]

VESSEL	DIAMETER (μM)	PRESSURE (MM HG)	VELOCITY (MM/SEC)
Arteriole, large	50	65	14.0
Arteriole, small	25	53	9.0
Capillary, entrance	8	37	
Capillary, midpoint	8	32	0.7
Capillary, exit	8	27	
Venule, small	25	20	3.0
Venule, large	70	15	9.0

[a]From data reported by Zweifach and Lipowski[8] for vessels of the cat mesentery, skeletal muscle, and omentum. Mean pressure of 100 mm Hg in main aortic branches is assumed.

Blood flow

The velocity with which blood moves through microscopic vessels can be measured by electronic, photometric, and laser techniques. Some methods operate by a correlation of signals from images of red cells moving single file through very small vessels. The result is a continuous display of velocity as a function of time, which can be converted into volumetric rate of flow when the diameter is known. In the case of the pulmonary circulation, pulsatile flow in the capillary bed as a whole can be measured by a body plethysmography technique (Chapter 11).

Mean velocities tend to fall in the arterial tree as the total cross section broadens out toward the periphery, and it is not surprising to find that they are only a few millimeters per second in the microcirculation, as contrasted with more than 10 cm/sec in the femoral and larger arteries. Typical values obtained from the cat mesentery are 9 mm/sec in 30-μm arterioles and 0.5 to 1.7 mm/sec in capillaries. Average velocities of 0.4 to 0.7 mm/sec have been reported in capillaries of the human nail fold. In vessels 20 to 100 μm in diameter, the velocity has been shown to be greatest in the axial portion of the stream, with a profile that is curved but more blunt than that of a parabola.[8,23]

The hematocrit within the microcirculation is distinctly lower than that of the body as a whole and ranges from 25 to 50% of the cell/whole blood ratio in large vessels. In 8-μm capillaries of the rabbit omentum, for example, the average hematocrit is about half that in systemic arteries.[8] This preponderance of plasma in microvessels is largely the result of *plasma skimming*. As blood in an arteriole moves past the entrance to a capillary, a disproportionate part of the flow entering the capillary comes from the cell-poor layer near the wall of the larger vessel. Red cells can be seen to be relatively scarce in the smallest microvessels, and some capillary segments contain only plasma for brief periods of time.

Blood flow through capillaries is pulsatile in most regions, with overall pulse amplitudes being 40 to 70% of the mean. The pulsations are damped out by the time blood has reached small veins 1 mm in diameter in the systemic circulation. The seemingly random variations in capillary flow mentioned earlier sometimes involve complete cessation of flow in selected channels for seconds or minutes. In other cases an irregular oscillation develops, with flow rising and falling from 1 to 15 times per minute. Some experiments suggest that the oscillations are associated with changes in capillary hematocrit, with flow decreasing as hematocrit rises, and vice versa.[19] The fluctuations are accompanied by swings in pressure above and below the osmotic pressure of plasma proteins, which must affect exchange through capillary walls. The passage of solutes into the interstitial space may be similarly intermittent, periods of efflux alternating with transfers into the capillary lumen.

Resistance

The complex pattern of the microcirculation and the squeezing of red cells through the smallest capillaries make it unreasonable to apply the Poiseuille equation (Chapter 6) in this region. The ratio of pressure to flow in any channel should still vary directly with length and blood viscosity, but there is no reason to expect that the flow for a given pressure gradient should be related to the fourth power of the radius. Nevertheless, the most detailed study of dimensions, pressure, and velocity in the microcirculation, carried out on unbranched segments in the cat mesentery by Lipowski and his associates,[29] shows that the relation between radius and resistance per unit length fits an inverse power function, with an exponent not significantly different from four! The relationship, in other words, is $(QL)/\Delta P = kr^4$, where k is a constant. The investigators attribute this fact to the opposing effects of low hematocrit and low velocity.

That explanation may be correct, but it is a little puzzling. The relation of vascular resistance to blood viscosity and vessel radius arises from the nature of viscous fluid flow. The viscosity of blood does, indeed, become greater at low rates of shear (i.e., low velocities) and smaller with low hematocrits (Chapter 13). The appearance of exactly the fourth power of the radius in the Poiseuille equation, however, is the result of assuming perfectly parabolic flow (Chapter 6), which is not present in the microcirculation. The friction between the wall and deformed red cells moving one by one through the smallest capillaries surely increases the pressure/flow ratio per unit length above that found in large vessels, while at the same time, the low hematocrit in the microcirculation must tend to diminish that ratio. The decreased resistance due to a scarcity of cells appears to be exactly counterbalanced by the increased resistance that comes from a low shear rate. It is difficult to believe that this balance is merely coincidence, but if the phenomenon has a physical origin, it remains obscure.

Flux Through the Capillary Wall

The transfer of materials across the endothelial wall is the central feature of capillary function, and an enormous amount of research has been devoted to that subject. Theoretic analyses and experimental strategies have become increasingly elaborate, and only a brief introduction to the relevant concepts will be presented here. A detailed summary of the field has recently been edited by Renkin and Michel.[7]

Three different paths exist between the capillary lumen and the interstitial space: (1) water-filled spaces, or *pores*, between endothelial cells; (2) direct routes through the lipid bilayer or plasma membrane of the cells, an alternative available only to the respiratory gases, O_2 and CO_2, and lipid-soluble sub-stances; and (3) intracellular vesicles that either shuttle from one side of the endothelial cell to the other or else form temporary chains across it. In the first two of these three processes, transport is passive in the sense that energy is not required. Although this discussion concerns the true capillaries, which are certainly the most important site of exchange with the interstitium, the arteri-olar and venular segments immediately adjacent to the capillary entrance and exit are also permeable to water, respiratory gases, and small molecules.

The principal mechanism for physiological regulation of capillary ex-change is the adjustment of intracapillary pressure. The physical properties of the capillary wall itself are usually assumed to be fixed and not under physio-logical control, except when permeability is altered by substances like hista-mine and bradykinin (Chapters 8 and 12). Arteriolar constriction tends to lower capillary pressure and thus reduce the number of open segments, decrease flow through the microcirculation, and lower the hydraulic pressure that moves fluid from capillary to interstitial space. Contraction of the precapillary sphincters has similar effects on capillaries immediately downstream. Evidence that such vasomotor activity alters the number of conducting capillaries, as well the rate of flow through the bed, comes from direct observation and experiments show-ing changes in total capillary surface area. Sympathetic stimulation in subcu-taneous adipose tissue, for example, causes a distinct decrease in capillary sur-face even when flow is held constant.[28] The conclusion that this change represents closure of many capillary channels is supported by the observation that the exchange of oxygen itself becomes limited, as if the average distance from cells to a patent capillary had been increased.

The arterioles are supplied with a sympathetic innervation that is more plentiful than in arteries, and it is mainly, although not exclusively, of the alpha-adrenergic constrictor type. Stimulation of sympathetic nerves in the mesen-tery, for example, constricts virtually all the local arterioles, particularly those 10 to 30 μm in diameter.[21] A sympathetic cholinergic vasodilator system exists in skeletal muscle (Chapter 12). The distribution of constrictor nerves within the microcirculation is both organ and species dependent, however, extending down to the smallest arteriolar branches in skeletal muscles of many species but not in the bat wing. Venular constriction *raises* capillary pressure and thus tends to promote fluid loss to the interstitial space, but at the same time it reduces the pressure head across the microcirculation (assuming constant ar-teriolar pressure) and consequently decreases flow, just as arteriolar constric-tion does. Fine tuning of local hemodynamics is accomplished by a combina-tion of precapillary and postcapillary vasomotion.

The ability of the capillary wall to transmit substances is studied by the classical physical approach of relating force to motion. First, information is required about the driving force, which consists of differences of hydraulic pressure (ΔP) and osmotic pressure ($\Delta \Pi$) across the capillary wall. Most experiments are designed so that one or the other of these pressures can be varied. Methods of measuring intracapillary pressure and the osmotic pressure of the plasma are available, but hydraulic and osmotic pressures outside the capillary are often assumed to be negligible. Tissue pressure is extremely difficult to measure without disturbing it, and whether it is normally a few millimeters of mercury above or below atmospheric pressure is a subject of debate. The osmotic pressure of interstitial fluid is also relatively low, and the normal interstitial concentration of some solutes (e.g., urea) is almost zero. When such substances are added experimentally to the bloodstream, their permeation through the capillary wall can be analyzed with measurements of only the intravascular concentration. The effect of concentration differences across a semipermeable membrane is quantitatively different from that of free diffusion in water, a topic that will be considered in a later section.

In measuring permeability, the volume of fluid and solute entering or leaving the capillary lumen per unit time must also be determined. These volumetric flow rates can be expressed in cubic centimeters per second, but they are often divided by the area through which the substances pass, to give flow per square centimeter. Depending on the application, the area involved may be the total capillary surface (A_m) or the total cross-sectional area of hypothetical channels between the endothelial cells (A_p). The relevant pressures are, by definition, forces per unit area.

Abundant morphological and functional evidence now leaves little doubt that channels between cells provide one important means of travel between the intravascular and interstitial spaces. The dimensions of these pores have been estimated by a variety of functional methods, and in general the results can be reconciled with physiological data on the capillary transfer of various substances. The stop-and-go nature of capillary flow presumably affects capillary filtration, and passage of solutes into the interstitial space may be similarly intermittent, but this aspect of the problem has been little studied. Some experimental data are inconsistent with a single class of pores of uniform size, and the existence of relatively large and small types has been postulated. In addition, the pores may not be wide-open pathways, but channels containing a sieve-like ultramicroscopic fiber matrix.[16]

Refinement of theoretic analysis has matched the ingenuity of experimental design that is characteristic of this field. Quantitative models are drawn from the principles of biophysics and physical chemistry, and it is generally agreed that two phenomena must be treated simultaneously: the bulk flow of fluid through the pores and the diffusion of solutes in that fluid. Molecular size is an important variable in both cases, and many experiments support the intuitive belief that it should be easier for small than for large molecules to traverse a given channel. Equations can be derived to describe the relationships, but certain simplifications are necessary. For example, most current theories assume regular geometric shapes for the channels and the molecules involved, although in reality both are irregular in form. The effects of electrical charge and viscosity are sometimes omitted from theoretic analyses, although they are as important as the driving force and physical dimensions of the pore.[2,11]

Physical principles

Exchange through capillary pores is viewed, then, as the net result of two processes: bulk flow and diffusion. *Bulk flow* consists of the simple movement of a fluid volume across the wall, carrying with it any dissolved molecules. The volumes of water and solute transported are considered separately. The net volume flow is the sum of the water and solute flows. *Diffusion,* on the other hand, is the movement of solute with respect to solvent. Some of the parameters used in describing capillary permeability are listed in Table 10.2.

The capillary wall can be regarded as a membrane separating two different concentrations of a solute, with a higher concentration and hydrostatic pressure on one side (representing the capillary lumen) than on the other. The net volumetric rate of flow across the membrane, J_v, is

$$J_v = L_p(\Delta P - [\sigma \Delta \Pi]) \qquad (10.1)$$

Table 10.2.   Terms Used to Express Capillary Permeability[a]

PARAMETER	SYMBOL	UNIT
Total capillary wall surface area	A_m	cm^2
Total pore area for water	A_p	cm^2
Total pore area for solutes	A_s	cm^2
Hydraulic conductivity, or filtration coefficient	L_p	cm^3/(sec mm Hg)[b]
Net volume flow (water + solute)	J_V	cm^3/sec
Mass flow rate of solute	J_S	moles/sec
Permeability to solute	M_s	cm^3/(sec cm^2) = cm/sec
Permeability–surface area product, or *transport capacity*	$M_s A_m$	cm^3/sec

[a]All terms are sometimes expressed in relation to tissue weight or capillary surface area.
[b]Units when driving pressure is expressed in millimeters of mercury.

where ΔP and $\Delta \Pi$ are the transmural gradients of hydrostatic pressure and osmotic pressure, respectively, and σ is a parameter called the *reflection coefficient*. L_p, which is referred to as the *hydraulic conductivity* of the membrane, is a proportionality constant that relates bulk flow of water to the driving force. The passage of fluid from the capillary lumen to the extravascular spaces is sometimes thought of as *filtration*, a term early physiologists used to describe the driving of a stream of liquid through the pores of a membrane. L_p is also called a *filtration coefficient*.[33] Typical L_p units are cubic centimeters per second per unit of driving pressure.

The concept of *reflection* is subtle but is widely used in descriptions of transcapillary exchange. It expresses the fact that the wall is selective in the sense that water passes through it with a higher velocity than solute molecules do. In the capillary, the osmotic gradient causes water to pass through the membrane toward the more concentrated solution, while solutes diffuse in the opposite direction, and these two processes interact within the membrane. Because the solute molecules are transmitted less readily than water, the net transfer of solute is less than would be the case in the absence of the membrane. Some of the solute is "held back," so to speak, and σ is the amount so "reflected" compared to the amount that would move during free diffusion in water. The reflection coefficient is thus a fraction, ranging in value from 0 to 1.

Diffusion can be expressed by assuming that when net volume flow is zero, solutes diffuse through the water-filled pores in the manner described by Fick's first law of diffusion, which states in effect that the rate of solute diffusion, J_s, is directly proportional to the area through which diffusion takes place and to the concentration gradient:

$$J_s = \frac{D_s A_s \, \Delta C_s}{\Delta x} \qquad (10.2)$$

where J_s is the mass rate of flow of solute (in moles per second, not volume) passing through an apparent pore cross-sectional area, A_s; $\Delta C_s / \Delta x$ is the concentration gradient of solute across the membrane; and D_s is the diffusion coefficient of the solute in water. D_s in this context is a proportionality coefficient that expresses (in square centimeters per second) the diffusion of the solute through water in the pores. The experimentally determined *free* diffusion coefficients of many substances are listed in reference books, but diffusion through a selectively permeable membrane is somewhat different because of the reflection phenomenon described above. Because of reflection, hydrostatic and osmotic forces affect both bulk flow and diffusion through membranes.

Equation 10.2 was used in the analysis of experimental results by early investigators, but a more complex expression that takes other relevant factors into account is now available.[2] The mass flow of solute can also be determined in a capillary bed by measuring blood flow (Q_b) and the arteriovenous concentration difference of the test substance ($C_a - C_v$), using an equation based on the conservation of mass:[32]

$$J_s = Q_b (C_a - C_v) \qquad (10.3)$$

The simplest and most general way to express the solute permeability, M_s, of a capillary bed of total wall area A_m is as a ratio of solute flux to concentration gradient:

$$M_s = \frac{J_s}{A_m \, \Delta C_s} \qquad (10.4)$$

By this definition, *permeability* is the volumetric flow of solute (cm^3/sec) moved through each cm^2 of capillary surface by a concentration gradient of one unit. Equation 10.4 gives M_s in cm/sec, but the significance of the term is more obvious when it is expressed in the expanded form cm^3/sec per cm^2 capillary surface. The permeability so defined is a measure of the *porosity* of the capillary wall, a variable that depends on both the number of pores per unit area and their radius. Because capillary surface can be estimated only approximately, the results of measurements of J_s and ΔC_s are often reported as the permeability–surface area product, $M_s A_m$ (sometimes represented by the alternative symbol *PS*) derived from equation 10.4. This product is a broad expression of the *transport capacity* of a vascular bed because it takes into account both the capillary density, or *vascularity,* of the tissue and the permeability per unit capillary surface.

Experimental observations

The earliest approach to quantitative analysis of fluid transfer in the microcirculation was made in 1896 by Starling,[36] who proposed that the net movement of water across the capillary membrane is the result of two opposing forces. The first, the transmural hydraulic pressure, tends to move water into the extravascular space, where pressure is lower than in the capillaries. The second, the osmotic pressure of plasma proteins, tends to move water back into the capillary lumen because the protein concentration is higher in plasma than in the interstitial space. Starling postulated that the rate of fluid transfer between plasma and tissue depended on the combination of hydrostatic pressure, osmotic pressure, and the physical properties of the capillary wall. His hypothesis was essentially the balance of forces stated by equation 10.1 (although the concept of the reflection coefficient had not yet been introduced and σ must be assumed to be unity). Starling's concept of an osmotic balance across the capillary wall was supported by his studies of blood proteins, which showed that their osmotic pressure was of the same order of magnitude as capillary pressure.

The passage of solutes between interstitial fluid and the capillary lumen had long been recognized, as had the intermittent drainage of the interstitial spaces by lymph flow, but the physiological role of this exchange was not clear. Starling suggested that the volume and low protein content of interstitial fluid were maintained by a small but finite net addition of fluid from capillaries, slowly returned to the vascular system by way of the lymphatics. The principle is illustrated diagrammatically in Figure 10.4, where a single channel between the arteriole and the venule represents the complex microcirculatory network in which fluid exchange takes place. In this hypothetical example, the hydraulic pressure supplied by the heart is assumed to be 34 mm Hg near the entrance to the capillary and 22 mm Hg at the exit. Tissue pressure is arbitrarily set at 2 mm Hg all along the exterior of the vessel. Colloid osmotic pressures of 26 mm Hg in the plasma and zero in the interstitial spaces are assumed, giving a net ΔΠ of 26 mm Hg. As a result, at the beginning of the capillary, the forces that tend to move fluid from the lumen to the interstitium outweigh those that tend to move it in the opposite direction. The two forces are about equal at the

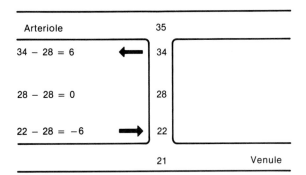

Figure 10.4. Starling hypothesis of fluid transfer in capillary between arteriole (*above*) and venule (*below*). *Numbers* within vessels indicate mean intravascular pressure in mm Hg. *Arrows* indicate direction of net fluid movement through capillary wall. Osmotic pressure of plasma assumed to be 26 mm Hg, and extravascular pressure 2 mm Hg, making a total of 28 mm Hg tending to move fluid into capillary from interstitial space. Intravascular pressure tends to move fluid in the opposite direction (i.e., out of capillary). Difference between these two opposing forces is shown in equations on the left, arbitrarily defining pressures that tend to move fluid into capillary as negative. There is a net loss of fluid from capillary at arteriolar end, approximate balance at the midpoint, and net influx into capillary at venular end.

capillary midpoint, and a net movement back into the lumen occurs beyond that point.

The net efflux at the arteriolar end of the capillary and the net influx in the prevenular segment indicated by the diagram doubtless occur under some conditions, but the figure represents only one of many possible states. Changes in precapillary or postcapillary resistance could produce reabsorption throughout the length of certain capillaries and outward filtration in others. A slightly lower than average intracapillary pressure has intentionally been adopted in this example, and the possibility of exchange through arteriolar and venular segments adjacent to the capillary has not been considered.

Starling put forth his ideas long before methods of measuring capillary pressure were available, but in 1927 Landis[26] published strong confirmatory evidence of the theory, based on his observations of single capillaries in the frog mesentery. Measuring pressure in capillaries cannulated by a micropipette and using microtools to occlude the vessels, he noted that red cells sometimes continued to move toward the occlusion, which he took to mean that fluid was being filtered out of the capillary between the red cell and the obstruction. Red cell motion in the opposite direction was interpreted as a sign of capillary reabsorption of fluid. The result of his experiments was the clear demonstration of a linear relation between capillary pressure and fluid exchange, with a balance point of neither gain nor loss at about 12 cm H_2O pressure (Figure 10.5). Subsequent work has in general supported this finding, although it is now known that permeability varies along the length of a capillary, being highest at the venous end. Landis also calculated the filtration coefficient for these vessels, arriving at a value of 0.0056 $\mu m^3/(sec\ cm\ H_2 0)$ per μm^2 of capillary surface, which is consistent with the results of more recent studies.[5,40]

The observations of Landis were an important advance, but even more information was forthcoming when Pappenheimer and Soto-Rivera[33] introduced an ingenious method of examining capillary hydraulic and osmotic pressures in a whole capillary bed rather than a single microvessel. They isolated, perfused, and weighed continuously on a recording balance the hind limb of a dog or cat, so that the rate of filtration of fluid between blood and tissues could be inferred from the gain or loss of limb weight. Perfusion pressures at the inflow and outflow of the system were adjusted until there was no net change in weight. When arterial pressure was lowered, not only did blood flow decrease but the limb began to lose weight; an upward adjustment of venous pressure could then reestablish an *isogravimetric* condition.

The investigators reasoned that with fluid neither entering nor leaving the capillaries, arterial inflow and venous outflow of blood would be equal. By the conventional definition of vascular resistance (Chapter 6), the relations among

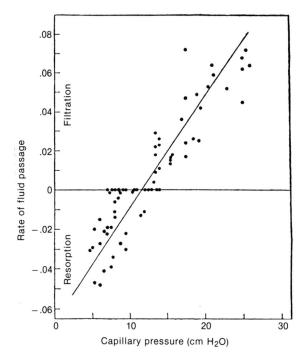

Figure 10.5. Relation between capillary pressure (*abscissa*, cm H_2O) and fluid movement across capillary wall (*ordinate*, $\mu m^3/\mu m^2$ sec) in single capillaries of frog mesentery. Negative flows denote movement into capillary from interstitium. (Reproduced from Landis,[26] with permission of the American Physiological Society)

venous pressure (P_v), pressure at the capillary midpoint (P_c), venous resistance (R_v), and blood flow (Q_b) would then be

$$P_v = P_c - (Q_bR_v)\Big|_{\Delta \text{weight}\ =\ 0} \qquad (10.5)$$

Constant weight could be maintained by an infinite number of pairs of arterial and venous pressures, each pair presumably yielding exactly the capillary pressure that prevented fluid exchange, although not necessarily the same blood flow. On trying many such combinations, the investigators found that isogravimetric venous pressure was related inversely to blood flow in a linear manner. Because plots of P_v versus Q_b followed a straight line, it seemed reasonable to extrapolate and assume that the P_c required for the isogravimetric state (P_{ci}) equaled P_v at the zero-flow intercept. Furthermore, the linearity implies that R_v does not vary with P_v or Q_b and equals the inverse slope of the plot (i.e.,

$\Delta Q_b/\Delta P_v$). This same equation can therefore be applied in nonisogravimetric situations, and P_c can be calculated if P_v and Q_b are known, as they usually are in such experiments.

These facts make it possible to determine hydraulic conductivity by altering P_v, measuring the change in weight as an estimate of J_v, and defining the driving pressure as $(P_c - P_{ci})$, thus providing the values needed to calculate L_p from equation 10.1. In the hind limbs of the cat and dog, the L_p so determined was 2.2×10^{-4} cm^3 fluid/sec mm Hg per 100 g tissue.[33] The same general principles can be applied by using a plethysmograph to measure the overall *volume* of an organ, rather than its weight, as an indication of changes in extravascular fluid, and that method has been applied to the human forearm. A modification of this procedure called the *osmotic transient* method[32] involves adding an osmotically active test substance to the perfusion inflow and measuring the resulting change in isogravimetric venous pressure. The alteration of capillary pressure required to prevent any change in weight is a measure of the osmotic pressure exerted by the added molecules.

The results achieved with these techniques strongly confirm the basic elements of the Starling hypothesis. Comparison with direct measurements of the osmotic pressure of plasma proteins *in vitro* shows that isogravimetric capillary pressure is opposite and almost equal to the osmotic pressure of plasma. The normal osmotic pressure of plasma is approximately 25 mm Hg, and the net gradient across the wall is only slightly less than that because the protein content of interstitial fluid is relatively low. The values for P_c obtained by micropuncture are usually 4 to 6 mm Hg *higher* than $\Delta\Pi$, whereas the isogravimetric P_c is 1 to 3 mm Hg *lower* than $\Delta\Pi$.[8,33] The results of these two methods are not really inconsistent, because the former measures hydraulic pressure at a single point, whereas the latter is a functional determination, averaged along the exchange path. The changing net gradient of transmural forces along the length of a capillary is difficult to measure precisely, but the important fact is that P_c and $\Delta\Pi$ differ by only a small amount, and the difference presumably shifts from positive to negative along the course of the channel. Interstitial pressure is an unknown element in this process, but it is very small, probably 1 to 2 mm Hg. Some investigators believe it to be slightly subatmospheric.

The repertoire of elegant techniques for studying capillary permeability was later enlarged by an application of the indicator-dilution method.[14,15] Two indicators are employed: one a substance to which the capillary wall is permeable, the other a solute that does not leave the vascular compartment. Radioisotopes of a freely diffusible ion like sodium are an example of the former, and isotopically tagged albumin or red cells are an example of the latter. The indicators are injected simultaneously into an artery, and venous blood is sampled rapidly to measure the resulting concentration curves. The difference between the curves is a measure of loss of the diffusible substance from the capillaries and gives an estimate of the number of moles lost per second (J_s). Data are usually taken from the early part of the curves, before much change in extravascular concentration can take place. More than one diffusible test indicator can be used to determine permeability to various materials.

To determine the permeability–surface area product (M_sA_m), the investigator must determine not only J_s but also the concentration gradient across the wall, ΔC_s (equation 10.4). If the interstitial concentration of the test substance is zero, the gradient can be approximated by the mean intracapillary concentration, C_m. Assuming that the concentration falls exponentially from the arterial to the venous end of the capillary, the mean can be calculated from the arterial and venous concentrations (C_a and C_v) derived from dilution curves:[15]

$$C_m = \frac{(C_a - C_v)}{\log_e(C_v/C_a)} \tag{10.6}$$

From equations 10.3, 10.4, and 10.6, it follows that the permeability–surface product is

$$M_sA_m = -Q_b(\log_e[C_v/C_a]) \tag{10.7}$$

Related expressions can be derived for situations in which the interstitial concentration of the test substance is not zero. The equations summarized above are obviously based on a number of simplifying assumptions, and other models that are more complex but more realistic have been described.[9]

All of the methods outlined above have been widely used, and the results for some lipid-insoluble molecules are listed in Table 10.3. As the data show, capillary permeability varies in different organs, Permeability for the solutes listed is roughly the same for cardiac as for skeletal muscle (as represented by limbs), but the myocardium is much more vascular than skeletal muscle, giving it a greater transport capacity (M_sA_m). Total capillary surface in a given organ cannot be determined with any precision, but the total area in canine myocardium has been estimated at 56,000 cm²/100 g tissue, as contrasted with 7,000 cm²/100 g tissue in skeletal muscle.[6] Tissue differences in permeability to water (not shown in the table) are similar to those for solutes; L_p (cm³/sec dyne) = 1.3×10^{-9} in mammalian intestinal mucosa, 2.5×10^{-11} in muscle of the feline hind leg, and 3.0×10^{-13} in rabbit brain.[6] The tabulated data for the capillaries of the brain show very low permeabilities, and the values may actually be overestimates. Transport of glucose and some amino acids in cerebral capillaries is not the result of simple diffusion but is carrier mediated.

Permeability in the wall of the stomach is relatively high, but this is the only organ considered in Table 10.3 in which the capillaries are fenestrated (see

Table 10.3. Capillary Permeability to Some Lipid-Insoluble Molecules[a]

	MOL. WT. (G/MOL)	D[b]	HIND LIMB (CAT)	FOREARM (MAN)	GASTRIC WALL (DOG)	HEART (DOG)	BRAIN (DOG)
			PERMEABILITY[c] (M_s, CM/SEC) $\times$ 10[6]				
Urea	60	1.90	26	28		27	4.6
Glucose	180	0.91	10.7	13.1	33	9.3	1.6[d]
Inulin	5,500	0.22	1.4	0.9		2.3	
Albumin	69,000	0.09	0.01			0.03	<0.001
Capillary surface (A_m, cm²/100 g) $\times$ 10⁻³			7.0	7.0	12.5	56	24
$M_s A_m$ (glucose) (cm³/sec)[e]			0.075	0.092	0.413	0.521	0.038[d]

[a]From various sources collected and cited by Renkin.[6]

[b]D = free diffusion coefficient in water at 37°C; (cm²/sec) $\times$ 10⁵.

[c]M_s as defined in equation 10.4.

[d]Fructose, not glucose. (Glucose transport in brain capillaries is carrier mediated.)

[e]Permeability $\times$ capillary surface for 100 g tissue.

below). Permeability and capillary type are not always closely correlated in other regions, however, as data on the pulmonary vasculature demonstrate. The capillaries of the canine lung are morphologically similar to those in skeletal and cardiac muscle, but the pulmonary M_s for urea is only 6×10^{-6} cm/ sec, less than one-fourth that in muscle.[6] Fenestrated capillaries like those of the gastrointestinal mucosa have a relatively high permeability to water and small molecules, and electron micrography shows that many of the fenestrae transmit particles 10 nm or more in radius.[35] One would expect such capillaries to be much more permeable than those of muscle to proteins, but that appears not to be the case. Values reported for M_s of macromolecular serum proteins with Stokes-Einstein radii ranging from 3.0 to 10.8 nm are approximately the same in the nonfenestrated capillaries of skeletal and cardiac muscle as in the intestine.[6] This anomaly may arise from a restriction of macromolecular diffusion by the basement membrane.

Pore dimensions

The analysis of flow through water-filled pores in the capillary wall was developed in part to learn the size of the pores.[32,33] As suggested earlier, two different phenomena are involved and must be described quantitatively. Pappenheimer's group began by assuming that the pores are cylindrical, and treated the bulk movement of water through such channels as a viscous flow in accordance with the Poiseuille equation (Chapter 6):

$$\frac{J_v}{\Delta P} = \frac{A_p r^2}{\Delta x 8 \eta} \tag{10.8}$$

The term J_v here represents the rate of flow of fluid through pores (volume per unit time), ΔP the driving force, η the viscosity of the fluid, Δx the thickness of the membrane (i.e., the length of the pores), r the pore radius, and A_p the total cross-sectional area of pores. (If n is the number of pores, then $A_p = n\pi r^2$). Analogous equations were derived for rectangular slits instead of cylindrical pores. The distinction between the pore area available for the passage of water, A_p, and that for solutes (A_s, equation 10.2) is an essential part of this version of pore theory. Because the diffusion of solute molecules is restricted by their size and other physical properties, A_s may be smaller than A_p.

An expression for the apparent pore size available to solutes can be derived[32] by combining equations 10.2 and 10.3 and applying van't Hoff's law ($\Delta C_s = \Delta\Pi/RT$) to eliminate ΔC_s:

$$\frac{A_s}{\Delta x} = \frac{Q_b(C_a - C_v)RT}{D_s\Delta\Pi} \tag{10.9}$$

where R is the universal gas constant, T the absolute temperature, and $\Delta\Pi$ the osmotic pressure difference across the wall.

All the terms on the right-hand side of equation 10.9 can be measured or are known constants, making it possible to determine experimentally the cross-sectional pore area available for diffusion of a given solute per unit pore length. Pappenheimer and his colleagues[32] used this equation in studying a variety of solutes ranging from NaCl to inulin and found, as expected, that the value of $A_s/\Delta x$ was inversely related to molecular weight (Figure 10.6). For example, the pore cross section available to inulin, a relatively large molecule, was only 17% of that for NaCl.

This same group of investigators[32] also invented a way of using their solute studies to estimate the unrestricted pore radius for water. Note that this radius could be calculated from equation 10.8 if the other variables in that expression were known. One of them, $J_v/\Delta P$, can be assessed in the isogravimetric type of experiment, taking the change in weight as J_v for an accompanying P_c. The viscosity of protein-free plasma, which is the appropriate η in this context, can be measured independently. Taking advantage of the relation between molecular weight and apparent pore dimensions (Figure 10.6), they estimated the remaining unknown, $A_s/\Delta x$ for water (mol. wt. = 18), by extrapolation from the solute data, arriving at a total pore area per unit path length of 1.3×10^5 cm in the capillaries of 100 g muscle.

This value, regarded as an estimate of $A_p/\Delta x$, completed the data needed to calculate unrestricted pore size from equation 10.8. The ratio $J_v/\Delta P$ had averaged 2.1×10^{-7} (cm³/sec)/(dyn/cm²) per 100 g hind limb by isogravimetric experiments, and measurements showed η to be 0.007 dyn sec/cm² at 37° C. Substituting these data in equation 10.8 gives a pore radius of 3.0 nm. Assuming[32] a pore length of 0.3 μm, this radius implies 1.4×10^{13} pores in 100 g muscle. If the total capillary surface is 7000 cm² (Table 10.3), there are 2×10^9 pores/cm² and the pore openings occupy only a tiny portion of the wall surface. This approach is incomplete to the extent that it does not include the reflection coefficient; that omission has since been remedied.[2]

Theoretic analysis along these lines has been carried further to incorporate steric factors that restrict entrance of the molecule into the pore, as well as the viscous drag that impedes its passage, defining a highly nonlinear relationship between the ratio A_s/A_p and the ratio of molecular to pore radius.[2,32] The early

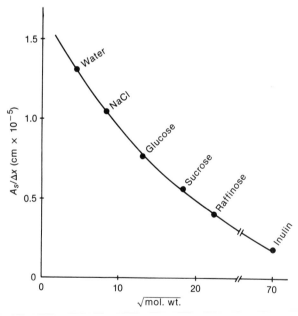

Figure 10.6.   Relation between molecular weight of solutes and area available for diffusion per unit pore length. *Abscissa*, square root of molecular weight. *Ordinate*, equivalent total pore area per unit pore length ($A_s/\Delta x$, equation 10.9), in cm × 10^{-5}. Value for water (mol. wt. = 18) obtained by extrapolation from other data. (Reproduced with modifications from Pappenheimer et al.,[32] with permission of the American Physiological Society)

data have also been adjusted to take into account the influence of a reflection coefficient on the van't Hoff relation between solute concentration and osmotic pressure.[2] Modern equations thus predict the experimental results to be expected for pores and molecules of any properties, allowing the formulation of testable hypotheses.

The intercellular pores are probably not immune to the stretching effects of vessel distention, and they may also be subject to the shearing forces at the capillary wall (Chapter 6). Investigation of this possibility has so far been limited to relatively large vessels, such as the aorta, where distention increases the passage of albumin into the vessel wall.[18] Some experiments show that shear stresses not much above the range *in vivo* increase the permeability of the wall to lipids as well as albumin, a fact that may be relevant to the development of atherosclerosis.[12] Another mechanism that may influence capillary permeability is motility of the endothelial cell itself. This possibility is no more than speculation at present, but the presence within the cell of actin and other contractile proteins suggests that its shape is not necessarily constant.

"Large" pores

Although capillary permeability is related inversely to the size of the solute molecule in almost all vascular beds, the relationship for large plasma proteins is much less steep than that for serum albumin and smaller molecules (Stokes-Einstein radius less than 3.5 nm). This fact, together with other evidence, is the basis for hypothesizing two classes of pores, small and large. The large channels, to judge from the relation of permeability to molecular size,[6,22,24] are 30 to 100 nm in radius, whereas the small ones are 3 to 4 nm. In some beds the large channels may be anatomical fenestrations, but similar functional behavior has been reported in capillaries where there is no electron microscopic evidence of fenestrae or other large pores.

A relatively new theory of selective capillary permeability suggests that the clefts between endothelial cells are not unobstructed watery channels, but a meshwork of fibrils, or *fiber matrix*.[16] The assumption that 5% of such a matrix consists of fibers 0.6 nm in radius would, in theory, account for many selective phenomena. The behavior of such a system would explain, for example, the observation that large molecules like albumin appear to be restricted by cylindrical pores 5.5 nm in radius in situations where water is passing through pores 8 nm in radius. The hypothesis further postulates that albumin adheres to or modifies the structure of the fiber network. This assumption is one way of accounting for the observation that hydraulic conductivity of the capillary wall is increased by removal of albumin from the perfusate. One provocative implication of the theory is that contractile elements in the endothelial cells might control the disposition of fibers in the matrix and thus contribute

.actively to regulation of permeability. Pappenheimer[31] has presented evidence for such activity in epithelial cells of the intestinal mucosa. Sodium-coupled transport in that tissue triggers contraction of an actomyosin ring around the junctions of such cells, thereby opening the junctions to increase mass transport of nutrients. The presence of glucose or amino acids in the intestinal lumen activates this process.

Transcellular exchange

The passage of substances across the capillary wall is not limited to pores but can also take place through the substance of endothelial cells. Although small, lipid-insoluble molecules are probably restricted to the intercellular channels, water can exchange across the endothelial cells by way of vesicles, and lipid-soluble materials can pass through the cell membrane. Pores are believed to provide the major pathway for water transport, but 2 to 30% of the hydraulic conductivity (L_p) appears to be transcellular.[6] Similar proportions of vesicular as contrasted with pore transport probably apply to urea (mol. wt. 60) and larger solutes that are not lipid soluble. The direction of current thinking is indicated by one estimate that transfer of water is 70% via small pores, 20% by way of large pores, and 10% through the cell.[6] In the case of macromolecules, the greater part of the exchange may be carried on by vesicles shuttling between the inner and outer surfaces of the cell, although just how this vesicular traffic is powered and regulated is not known. Intracellular vesicles up to 50 nm in diameter have been observed.

The distinction between vesicular and large-pore transport is difficult to make experimentally, although in theory, conduction by vesicles should not show the interaction between water and solute transport that is responsible for the reflection phenomenon (see above). Experimental attempts to exploit this difference have not been entirely satisfactory, but they do indicate that vesicular and large-pore transport both exist in capillaries.[6,34]

Lymphatic System

The lymphatic system, which drains the interstitial spaces, consists of a branching system of vessels with very thin walls. It parallels the blood vascular system and is filled with a colorless fluid of low protein content, the *lymph,* in which white cells often appear but erythrocytes are rare. The terminal lymphatic branches lie in the interstitial spaces and resemble the blood capillaries, except for being closed at one end. These *lymph capillaries* are fine tubes made up of a single layer of endothelial cells, which are the site for absorption of materials from the interstitium into the lymph. The microscopic channels join together to form larger and larger trunks, resembling the venous tree in this respect, and the larger lymphatics eventually enter lymph glands, where lymph flows through a rich plexus of small channels. The tissue of these glands acts as a kind of active filter for foreign particles, in addition to being an important part of the body's immune system. After passing through one or more glands, the lymph eventually enters the thoracic and right lymphatic ducts and thus empties into the innominate veins.

Lymphatics are found in virtually all tissues, and their smallest branches are almost as numerous as blood capillaries.[3] The lymphatic system functions as a homeostatic mechanism for the narrow but functionally important spaces that lie between the cells and the blood vascular system, maintaining the volume of the interstitial fluid and removing proteins, lipids, and foreign materials from it. The lymphatic capillaries are highly permeable to small molecules, but they can also admit particles 25 μm or more in diameter. The walls contain intercellular clefts similar to those in the blood vascular system, but there are also many quite large gaps, and they allow diffusion of substances with molecular weights of up to 6000 in whichever direction the concentration gradient favors. Transport by intracellular vesicles is prominent. Larger molecules and bacteria or other foreign particles can readily enter the lymphatics, and are either removed by the lymphatic glands or returned to the bloodstream via the thoracic duct. One striking example of physiological particle absorption can be seen in the intestinal lymphatics, where large numbers of lipid globules (*chylomicrons*) appear after a meal.

Exchange of water and solutes between interstitial fluid and the lumen of the smallest lymphatic vessels follows the general physical principles described earlier for capillaries of the blood vascular system. Ion concentrations in lymph are close to those in plasma, although lymph $[Ca^{2+}]$ is slightly lower and $[Cl^-]$ higher than the plasma concentrations. The protein content of lymph varies in different organs, the lymph/plasma ratio amounting to about 0.15 in skeletal muscle, 0.50 in the intestines and kidneys, and 0.67 in the heart and lungs. The highest lymphatic protein concentration is found in the liver, where it is almost as high as in blood plasma. Fibrinogen appears in lymph in a concentration approximately half that of plasma, and lymphatic fluid clots *in vitro,* although less rapidly than blood.

Although the permeability of the capillary wall to plasma proteins is relatively low, a slow net transfer into the interstitial spaces takes place normally. This movement is the origin of a kind of secondary "circulation" in which protein leaves the vascular system, enters the lymphatics, and eventually returns to the central veins. Between 80 and 200 g protein travels through this pathway daily, an amount approaching the total intravascular protein content. Most of the fluid transferred from capillaries to the extracellular compartment is promptly reabsorbed into the same microcirculatory vessels, but about 10% of it accompanies the extravascular recycling of protein through the lymphatics.

"Leakage" of protein from the capillaries at physiological rates is thus an entirely normal process. The return of this protein to the intravascular compartment cannot take place at the capillary level because of the adverse concentration gradient but is accomplished through the lymphatics. Inflammation and certain other pathological states, such as local hypoxia, can increase the permeability of the capillary walls to protein, as well as water and other solutes. Obstruction of the lymphatics by disease is one of the causes of *edema,* the accumulation of large volumes of fluid in tissue spaces. Although the interstitial space is often viewed as a fluid-filled compartment, it actually contains a gel-like substance, collagen fibers, and connective tissue, as well as aqueous spaces.[8,25] Several models for the transfer of proteins from interstitium to lymph have been proposed.[1,8]

Pressure in the lymphatic capillaries, like that in the interstitial space, is very low, from 0 to 2 mm Hg, and subatmospheric values of about -0.5 mm Hg have been reported.[38] Slightly higher pressures have been measured in the larger trunks when there is no lymph flow, but contraction of the surrounding skeletal muscles or external massage can raise the terminal pressures by 5 to 50 mm Hg and thus establish a strong centripetal gradient. The net flow of lymph toward the thoracic ducts depends mainly on such external compression, which causes lymph to move centrally because of the blind endings at the terminations and the existence of one-way valve leaflets in lymphatic vessels greater than about 200 μm in diameter.[3,25] Respiratory movements contribute to the extralymphatic forces in the lung, and peristalsis does so in the intestines. Smooth muscle cells are sparsely distributed in the walls of lymphatic vessels in some species, including man,[10] and their contraction may also contribute to the flow of lymph. Active constriction and relaxation in large segments of the lymphatic system have been observed in the bat wing and spontaneous contractions in lymphatics of the mammalian intestines.

Total lymphatic flow in human subjects is 2 to 4 liters/day, a volume roughly equivalent to that of plasma in the circulation, but flow varies widely in different regions and under different physiological conditions. Flow is minimal at rest but is rapidly increased by muscular activity, massage, increased venous pressure, or inflammatory reactions. The range of lymph flows observed experimentally is quite broad. In man and other mammalian species, the average total appears to be about 1.1 to 2.1 ml/hr per kilogram of body weight. A large part of this flow, some 25 to 50% of the total, comes from the lymphatics of the liver. Pulmonary, renal, and cardiac lymphatics each contribute approximately 3 to 10% of the total lymph duct drainage. A direct correlation between venous pressure and lymph flow has been observed in the lung, kidney, and other organs, and as the lymphatic flow increases, the protein concentration in the interstitial space falls. The heart is supplied with deep and superficial lymphatic plexuses, the former exposed to rhythmic external compression. The rate of flow in myocardial lymphatics increases when cardiac work is increased by pharmacological or other means.

Lymph flow is particularly important in maintaining fluid balance in the lung.[37] Capillary pressure is relatively low in that tissue, favoring the resorption of fluid from the very small space between capillary and alveolar wall. With high capillary pressures, however, excessive loss of fluid into the interstitial space can cause pulmonary edema as fluid moves from the interstitium into the alveoli. Lymphatic drainage tends to prevent such an event, and the flow of lymph from the lungs increases when left atrial and pulmonary venous pressure are raised experimentally. Interstitial protein concentration falls as lymph flow increases. These compensatory actions fail when capillary pressure reaches 20 to 25 mm Hg, and total lung water begins to increase.[17] Stretching of the capillary wall and enlargement of pore width have been suggested as the causes of fluid extravasation, but the conventional operation of filtration forces seems a more likely explanation.

An unusual example of the collaborative action of capillary and lymphatic transport is provided by synovial joints like the knee.[27] The synovial fluid is supplied through capillary walls and an overlying layer of synovial intima and drained by an extensive system of microscopic lymphatic vessels. Motion of the joint encourages lymph flow by external compression of the lymphatics. The synovial fluid is essentially an ultrafiltrate of plasma into which hyaluronate has been secreted. Pressure within the joint space is subatmospheric, averaging −5mm Hg and thus offering testimony to the "pumping" capacity of the local lymphatic system.

References

Reviews

1. Casley-Smith, J.R. (1977). Lymph and lymphatics. In: *Microcirculation, Vol. 2*, G. Kaley and B.M. Altura, eds. Baltimore, University Park Press, pp. 423–502.

2. Curry, F-R. E. (1984). Mechanics and thermodynamics of transcapillary exchange. In: *Handbook of Physiology, Section 2, The Cardiovascular System. Vol. IV, Microcirculation*. Bethesda, Md., American Physiological Society, pp. 309–374.

3. Drinker, C.K., Yoffey, J.M. (1941). *Lymphatics, Lymph, and Tissue Fluid.* Cambridge, Mass., Harvard University Press.

4. Krogh, A. (1929). *The Anatomy of Physiology of Capillaries.* New Haven, Conn., Yale University Press.

5. Michel, C. (1972). Flows across the capillary wall. In: *Cardiovascular Fluid Dynamics,* D.H. Bergel, ed. London, Academic Press, pp. 242–298.

6. Renkin, E.M. (1977). Multiple pathways of capillary permeability. *Circ. Res.* 41:735–743.

7. Renkin, E.M., Michel, C.C. (eds.) (1984). *Handbook of Physiology, Section 2, The Cardiovascular System. Vol. IV, The Microcirculation.* Bethesda, Md., American Physiological Society.

8. Zweifach, B.W., Lipowski, H.H. (1984). Pressure–flow relations in blood and lymph microcirculation. In: *Handbook of Physiology, Section 2, The Cardiovascular System, Vol. IV, Microcirculation.* Bethesda, Md., American Physiological Society, pp. 251–307.

Research Papers

9. Bassingthwaighte, J.B. (1974). A concurrent flow model for extraction during transcapillary passage. *Circ. Res.* 35:483–503.

10. Boggon, R.P., Palfrey, A.J. (1973). The microscopic anatomy of human lymphatic trunks. *J. Anat.* 114:398–405.

11. Brenner, B.M., Hostetter, T.H., Humes, H.D. (1978). Glomerular permselectivity: Barrier function based on discrimination of molecular size and charge. *Am. J. Physiol.* 234 (*Renal Fluid Electrolyte Physiol.* 3):F455–F460.

12. Caro, C.G. (1973). Transport of material between blood and wall in arteries. In: *Atherogenesis: Initiating Factors.* Ciba Foundation Symposium 12 (N.S.). Amsterdam, Associated Scientific Publishers, pp. 127–264.

13. Casley-Smith, J.R. (1971). Endothelial fenestrae in intestinal villi: Differences between the arterial and venous ends of the capillaries. *Microvasc. Res.* 3:49–68.

14. Chinard, F.P., Vosburgh, G.J., Enns, T. (1955). Transcapillary exchange of water and other substances in certain organs of the dog. *Am. J. Physiol.* 183:221–234.

15. Crone, C. (1963). The permeability of capillaries in various organs as determined by use of the 'indicator diffusion' method. *Acta Physiol. Scand.* 58:292–305.

16. Curry, F-R. E. (1986). Determinants of capillary permeability: A review of mechanisms based on single capillary studies in the frog. *Circ. Res.* 59:367–380.

17. Drake, R.E., Smith, J.H., Gabel, J.C. (1980). Estimation of the filtration coefficient in intact dog lungs. *Am. J. Physiol.* 238 (*Heart Circ. Physiol.* 7):H430–H438.

18. Duncan, L.E., Jr., Buck, K., Lynch, A. (1965). The effect of pressure and stretching on the passage of labelled albumin into canine aorta wall. *J. Atheroscler. Res.* 5:69–79.

19. Fagrell, B., Intaglietta, M., Ostergren, J. (1980). Relative hematocrit in human skin capillaries and its relation to capillary blood flow velocity. *Microvasc. Res.* 20:327–335.

20. Fung, Y.C., Zweifach, B.W., Intaglietta, M. (1966). Elastic environment of the capillary bed. *Circ. Res.* 19:441–461.

21. Furness, J.B., Marshall, J.M. (1974). Correlation of the directly observed re-

sponses of mesenteric vessels of the rat to nerve stimulation and noradrenalin with the distribution of adrenergic nerves. *J. Physiol.* 239:75–88.

22. Garlick, D.G., Renkin, E.M. (1970). Transport of large molecules from plasma to interstitial fluid and lymph in dogs. *Am. J. Physiol.* 219:1595–1605.

23. Goldsmith, H.L., Marlow, J.C. (1979). Flow behavior of erythrocytes. *J. Colloid Interface Sci.* 71:383–407.

24. Grotte, G. (1956). Passage of dextran molecules across the blood–lymph barrier. *Acta Chir. Scand.* 112(Suppl. 211):1–84.

25. Hargens, A.R., Zweifach, B.W. (1977). Transport between blood and peripheral lymph in intestine. *Microvasc. Res.* 11:89–101.

26. Landis, E.M. (1927). Microinjection studies of capillary permeability. II. The relation between capillary pressure and the rate at which fluid passes through the walls of single capillaries. *Am. J. Physiol.* 82:217–238.

27. Levick, J.R. (1980). Contributions of the lymphatic and microvascular systems to fluid absorption from the synovial cavity of the rabbit knee. *J. Physiol.* 306:445–461.

28. Linde, B., Gainer, J. (1974). Disappearance of [133]xenon and [125]iodide and extraction of [86]rubidium in subcutaneous adipose tissue during sympathetic nerve stimulation. *Acta Physiol. Scand.* 91:172–179.

29. Lipowski, H.H., Kovalcheck, S., Zweifach, B.W. (1978). The distribution of blood rheological parameters in the microcirculation of cat mesentery. *Circ. Res.* 43:738–729.

30. Nicoll, P.A., Webb, R.L. (1946). Blood circulation in the subcutaneous tissue of the living bat's wing. *Ann. N.Y. Acad. Sci.* 46:697–711.

31. Pappenheimer, J.R. (1987). Physiological regulation of transepithelial impedance in the intestinal mucosa of rats and hamsters. *J. Memb. Biol.* 100:137–148.

32. Pappenheimer, J.R., Renkin, E.M., Borrero, L.M. (1951). Filtration, diffusion, and molecular sieving through peripheral capillary membranes. *Am. J. Physiol.* 167:13–46.

33. Pappenheimer, J.R., Soto-Rivera, A. (1948). Effective osmotic pressure of the plasma proteins and other quantities associated with the capillary circulation in the hind limb of cats and dogs. *Am. J. Physiol.* 152:471–491.

34. Perl, W. (1975). Convection and permeation of albumin between plasma and interstitium. *Microvasc. Res.* 10:83–94.

35. Simionescu, N., Simionescu, M., Palade, G.E. (1972). Permeability of intestinal capillaries: Pathway followed by dextrans and glycogens. *J. Cell Biol.* 53:365–392.

36. Starling, E.H. (1896). On the absorption of fluids from the connective tissue spaces. *J. Physiol.* 19:312–326.

37. Staub, N.C. (1978). The forces regulating fluid filtration in the lung. *Microvasc. Res.* 15:45–56.

38. Wiederhielm, C.A., Weston, B.V. (1973). Microvascular, lymphatic, and tissue pressures in the unanesthetized mammal. *Am. J. Physiol.* 207:173–176.

39. Zweifach, B.W. (1950). Basic mechanisms in peripheral vascular homeostasis. In: *Third Conference on Factors Regulating Blood Pressure.* New York, J. Macy, Jr., Foundation.

40. Zweifach, B.W., Intaglietta, M. (1968). Mechanics of fluid movement across single capillaries in the rabbit. *Microvasc. Res.* 1:83–101.

11

PULMONARY CIRCULATION

Blood pressure and vascular resistance are much lower in the pulmonary than in the systemic circulation, and there are corresponding differences in vascular architecture. The large arteries and veins are shorter than their systemic counterparts, and the pulmonary vessels have thinner, more distensible walls containing less elastin and smooth muscle. The pulmonary artery and its main branches distend with each ejection of blood from the heart, just as the aorta does, and forward flow during diastole is maintained by recoil from this distended state. All the blood returning to the right atrium from the systemic circuit normally passes through the pulmonary bed, so that both ventricles must eject the same stroke volume except for brief periods of adjustment. Any temporary imbalance between right and left ventricular outputs[28] leads to an increase or decrease in the volume of blood contained in the pulmonary bed.

The external surface of pulmonary capillaries is exposed to the pressures within the alveoli, and the extravascular pressure of a large part of the pulmonary circulation is related to the subatmospheric pressure of the surrounding intrapleural space. Because these pressures change systematically with inspiration and expiration, there is an intimate relationship between pulmonary hemodynamics and ventilation of the lungs. In addition, the exchange of respiratory gases involves both ventilation and pulmonary blood flow, a collaboration illustrated most dramatically by the changes that take place at birth, when the lungs first inspire air.

Fetal and Neonatal Circulations

In the fetus the pulmonary alveoli are filled with amniotic fluid, and the respiratory exchange of O_2 and CO_2 is carried on entirely by the maternal lungs. Metabolism in the fetus thus depends critically on the umbilical artery and vein but requires little blood flow to the fetal lungs. Appropriate pathways for the distribution of flow are created by two sites of intervascular shunting, the ductus arteriosus between the aorta and pulmonary artery and the foramen ovale between the atria. The pattern of blood flow during intrauterine life is shown in Figure 11.1A. The relative amount of flow through the different paths is expressed in this figure as the percentage of combined ventricular outputs. Such figures offer a convenient comparison with the normal adult state, where each ventricle pumps half the combined output.

Studies of the fetal circulation in sheep[11] show that blood flow through the lungs during intrauterine life is much smaller than systemic blood flow. About three-quarters of the systemic flow returns to the right ventricle, the remainder being diverted into the left heart through an opening in the interatrial septum,

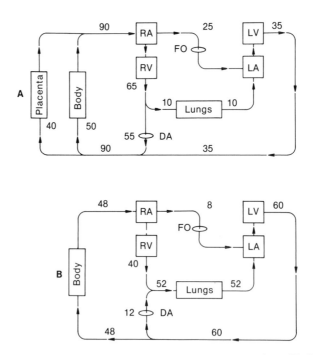

Figure 11.1.   Blood flow in the fetus (**A**) and transitional state in newborn (**B**). Numbers are an estimate of percentage of combined ventricular outputs (right plus left) flowing through each pathway. *RA*, right atrium; *LA*, left atrium; *RV*, right ventricle; *LV*, left ventricle; *FO*, foramen ovale; *DA*, ductus arteriosus. (After data published by Dawes[3] and Rudolph[11])

the *foramen ovale*. An even smaller amount flows through the lungs because about 85% of the right ventricular output goes from the pulmonary artery to the aorta through the ductus arteriosus. Pulmonary and systemic arterial pressures are approximately equal at this time,[3] 45 to 70 mm Hg, and pulmonary vascular resistance in the collapsed, fluid-filled fetal lung is higher than that of the systemic bed.

In the fetal lamb, umbilical venous blood is 85% saturated with O_2. A little more than half of the flow through the umbilical vein drains into the inferior vena cava near the atrium, while the remainder enters the liver and passes through the hepatic microcirculation before becoming part of the fetal systemic venous return.[11] Blood is not thoroughly mixed in the right atrium but streams along certain preferential paths. Most of the flow from the superior and distal inferior venae cavae crosses the tricuspid valve into the right ventricle, whereas blood delivered directly into the inferior vena cava from the umbilical vein tends to cross to the left heart by way of the foramen ovale. Because of the latter component, the O_2 concentration is higher in the left ventricle than in the right (65% as compared to 50%).

With the first breath after birth, pulmonary resistance falls precipitously and pulmonary blood flow increases, responses that are initiated by the mechanical expansion of the lungs and the change in alveolar tensions of O_2 and CO_2. Within a few hours after delivery the pulmonary resistance has decreased 10-fold, and blood flow in this neonatal period approximates that shown in Figure 11.1B. The ductus and foramen ovale are still open, but flow through the ductus has reversed, and part of the left as well as the right ventricular output travels to the lungs. This change in the direction of flow in the ductus occurs in a matter of minutes in the lamb but over a period of hours in human infants. The shunt through the foramen ovale is small and highly variable, depending as it does on the direction of the pressure difference between the atria.

The circulation of the newborn is in a transitional state, and it changes continually over the days and months that follow. The heavy elastic layers of the fetal pulmonary artery begin to disappear, and the arteriolar walls become thinner. In the pig, for example, the ratio of wall thickness to radius in vessels 200 μm in diameter decreases from 0.14 in the fetus to 0.06 after 1 wk.[30] The mean pulmonary arterial pressure of 45 to 70 mm Hg at birth falls to 20 to 40 mm Hg in 12 hours, and by 6 months of age the pulmonary arterial pressure and resistance are down to adult levels.[3,10]

The ductus arteriosus constricts rapidly in the first few hours after birth, primarily because of a direct constricting effect of O_2 on its smooth muscle. Complete closure does not occur immediately, but over the ensuing weeks the ductus becomes obliterated anatomically as its walls are gradually replaced by connective tissue. In most human infants 12 months of age, only slight fibrous traces of the ductus arteriosus can be found, although in rare instances a patent ductus persists into adult life. Shunting through the foramen ovale is greatly reduced after a few weeks because mean pressure becomes slightly higher in the left than in the right atrium, tending to hold shut the flap over the opening. In 50% of infants the flap seals to the septum within 1 yr.[3]

Cardiac output per unit body weight is relatively high in the fetus, the left ventricular output in the lamb averaging about 150 ml/min kg. It rises to as much as 400 ml/min kg at birth and then slowly falls to reach approximately 160 ml/min kg at 6 to 8 weeks.[11] This ability to sustain a high output cannot be attributed to neural stimulation because beta-adrenergic blockade reduces it only slightly, but it does require normal production of thyroid hormones during the late gestational period. The walls of the fetal right and left ventricles are approximately the same in thickness, but the muscle of the left ventricle increases rapidly after birth, while that of the right ventricle does not. Experimental manipulation of ventricular filling pressure shows that Starling's law (Chapter 4) operates in fetal and newborn lambs, but the increase in ventricular output caused by raising atrial pressure is relatively small, and the heart appears to be functioning near the top of the ventricular function curve. The values cited above for fetal and neonatal cardiac output probably also apply in humans, where a high output relative to body weight (though not surface area) persists throughout the first few years of life (Chapter 2).

Vascular Structure

In the pulmonary circulation, as in all vascular beds, the dimensions, numbers, viscoelasticity, and architectural pattern of the vessels determine hemodynamic conditions. Reasonably accurate information about these properties has been obtained in man and the dog, including detailed histological measurements throughout the bed.[14,45] Several quantitative models of the vasculature have been described.[9,49]

The main pulmonary artery has almost the same cross-sectional area as the ascending aorta but it is much shorter, extending only 3 or 4 cm in man before dividing into right and left main branches. This bifurcation is one of the rare points in the circulation where the total vascular cross section becomes smaller, the combined area of the two branches being about 80% that of the parent vessel. The main artery and the first few generations of branches are elliptical rather than circular in cross section (Chapter 2). The hemodynamic consequences of this departure from a cylindrical shape are of no great importance for practical purposes, although they are significant in exact analyses of pressure–flow relationships.

Branching in smaller vessels approximates a dichotomous pattern in which each vessel divides into two daughter branches of roughly equal cross section until the precapillary region is reached. The venous tree converges in a similar pattern, although there tends to be a larger number of veins than arteries at every level. The intravascular distance from pulmonic valve to capillaries ranges from 8 to 20 cm in man,[45] and the average vascular path from right ventricle to left atrium is about 30 cm.

The capillaries of the lung form a diffuse network around the pulmonary alveoli, presenting a very large capillary surface for gas exchange through the walls of the air spaces. The total area of the capillary membrane that serves this function in the human lung, according to careful histological measurements,[14] is 45 to 75 m^2. Pulmonary capillaries form an anastomosing network around each alveolus, as shown in Figure 11.2. Their diameter is 5 to 8 μm, and the overall pattern resembles a honeycomb, an arrangement of small capillary segments into roughly hexagonal units approximately 12 μm long on each side.[14] The time spent by a particle of blood in passing through the capillary bed under resting conditions is around 0.5 to 1 sec. Traditionally, the surface for pulmonary gas exchange has been considered to be limited to the capillaries, but it is now known that some diffusion also occurs in the terminal precapillary vessels.[22] About 1% of the cardiac output normally traverses the lung through unventilated regions or arteriovenous shunts and consequently takes no part in the exchange of respiratory gases.

Bronchial circulation

The bronchi, connective tissue, and other parenchymatous structures of the lung are supplied with blood by the bronchial arteries, which are part of the systemic circulation. Blood flow through the bronchial vessels is normally quite small, amounting to about 1% of the cardiac output.[19] The bronchial circulation has a complicated distribution.[2] It anastomoses with pulmonary vessels proximal to the capillaries, and there is free communication between the capillaries of the two systems along the bronchioles. A small part of the bronchial flow returns to the systemic circuit through the azygos vein, but the greater portion drains into the pulmonary veins. The highly oxygenated pulmonary venous blood is thereby contaminated by bronchial venous blood of lower O_2 content, but the bronchial flow is normally too small to have much effect on left atrial O_2 saturation. The influence of this anastomotic arrangement on pressures in the pulmonary microcirculation may well be significant, although it is difficult to evaluate beyond the general observation that pulmonary vasomotor responses to neural stimuli are altered by interruption of the

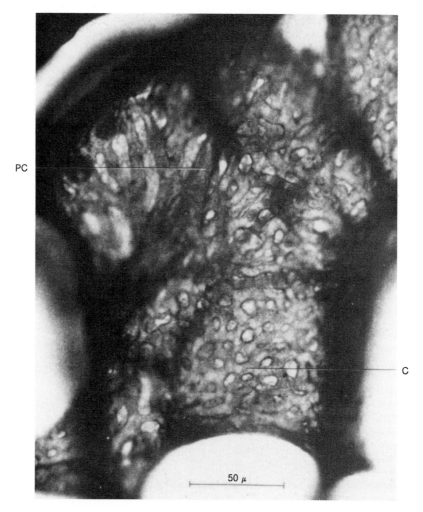

Figure 11.2.   Photomicrograph of capillary network (*C*) on one wall of a human pulmonary alveolus. *PC*, fan-shaped precapillary leading into network. (Reproduced from Weibel,[14] with permission of Springer-Verlag)

bronchial circulation.[2] The effects of vasomotor nerves and drugs on bronchial arteries are similar, in most respects, to those on other systemic arteries.

Pulmonary Hemodynamics

Pressures

The basal mean pulmonary arterial pressure has been found to lie between 10 and 20 mm Hg in a variety of mammals and is not related to body size. Representative values in man and the dog are given in Table 11.1, along with

Table 11.1. Typical Hemodynamic Conditions in Pulmonary Circulation

VARIABLE[a]	MAN (75 KG)		DOG (20 KG)	
	MEAN	PEAK/ MINIMUM	MEAN	PEAK/ MINIMUM
Heart rate (/sec)	1.20		1.50	
Radius, PA (cm)	1.40		0.75	
Pressure, PA (mm Hg)	15	24/10	17	26/11
Pressure, PC (mm Hg)	10	12/9	10	12/9
Pressure, PV (mm Hg)	8	9/6	7	8/6
Blood flow, PA (cm³/sec)	100	500/0	42	170/0
Blood flow, PC (cm³/sec)	100	280/40	42	95/15
Blood flow, PV (cm³/sec)	100	200/50	42	70/20
Blood velocity, PA (cm/sec)	16	80/0	24	96/0
Blood acceleration (max)(cm/sec²)	1,010		1,800	
PVR (dyn sec/cm⁵)	70		318	
Z_o (dyn sec/cm⁵)	22	(30/16)[b]	180	(245/130)[b]
Wave velocity (cm/sec)	180		270	
Pulse transmission time				
PA − PC (sec)	0.120		0.085	
PA − PV (sec)	0.180		0.110	
Blood volumes				
Arterial (cm³)	130		60	
Capillary (cm³)	150		68	
Venous (cm³)	160		72	
Total (cm³)	440		200	

[a]PA, main pulmonary artery; PC, pulmonary capillaries; PV, pulmonary veins at venoatrial junction.
[b]Maximum/minimum amplitude between 2 and 12 Hz.

other relevant hemodynamic variables. After the rapid fall from a relatively high level in the immediate postnatal period (see above), the mean pressure remains constant as the body grows to mature size and throughout adult life. The major increment in vascular length during the period of growth is in the large arteries, which contribute relatively little resistance,[27] and the expanding total vascular cross section is matched by the increase in cardiac output, so that mean pressure does not change. The pulsation amplitude in the main pulmonary artery is about as large as the mean value, and pressure may fall to only a few millimeters of mercury at the end of diastole, particularly if the heart rate is slow and the diastolic interval correspondingly long.

Since the magnitude of the pressure in the pulmonary artery is small compared with that in the aorta but the velocity of flow is approximately the same, the ratio of kinetic to pressure energy of blood flow is greater than in the aorta (equations 6.9 and 6.10). The relatively low pressures also make technical considerations in the measurement of pressure of greater importance; when the customary fluid-filled catheters are used, differences of a few centimeters in the selection of the *zero reference level* (the hydrostatic pressure on the gauge when determining the signal for atmospheric pressure) result in relatively large differences in the values recorded. As in other vascular beds, the drop in pressure along the arteries is greatest in the smallest branches. Although the pulsations of pressure are attenuated as they pass through the arterial bed, oscillations of some 3 to 5 mm Hg are transmitted into the capillaries. Blood flow in the pulmonary microcirculation is highly pulsatile but maintains some forward motion at virtually all times (see below).

Pulmonary capillaries

Pressure and flow in the pulmonary microcirculation are inevitably complex because the vessels are collapsible; the hydrodynamic, hydrostatic, and extravascular pressures are all of the same order of magnitude, and the interconversion of kinetic and potential energy can be significant. The pulmonary capillaries are particularly susceptible to the influence of extravascular and hydrostatic forces because of their low intraluminal pressure (see below). The extracapillary pressure in the sparse tissue separating the capillary from the adjacent air space is very close to the intraalveolar pressure, which ordinarily falls slightly with each inspiration. The influence of alveolar pressure on the diameter of capillaries is demonstrated by the great increase in resistance to flow through the pulmonary capillary bed when large positive pressures are applied to inflate the lung, as in some devices for artificial respiration.

The importance of hydrostatic pressure in the pulmonary vessels is evident from anatomical considerations; in the erect adult, vessels at the apex of the lung may be 15 cm above the pulmonary artery and those at the base an equal distance below it. Since the corresponding hydrostatic pressures are of the same order as the pulmonary arterial pressure, one might expect capillaries at the lung apices to be barely open (or perhaps entirely closed) in the erect position and those at the bases to be fully distended; measurements of regional pulmonary blood flow in human subjects show this to be the case.[15,48] This emphasizes once again the distinction between transmural pressures, which act on the walls of vessels, and the intravascular pressure gradients that produce blood flow (Chapter 6). Capillaries are not readily distensible, and the resistance of a capillary bed probably depends more on the relative numbers of vessels that are completely open or closed (as a result of transmural pressure) than on graded variations in individual diameter. The effects of gravity in the erect posture are discussed in more detail below.

Transmural pressure is also a factor in transcapillary exchange of water and solutes. Here the oncotic pressure of plasma (about 25 mm Hg) encourages the movement of fluid into the capillaries, whereas intracapillary pressure acts in the opposite direction (Chapter 10). Although microscopic examination reveals very little space between the alveolar walls and the capillaries, the total volume of interstitial fluid in the lungs is substantial, and there is continuous fluid exchange between the tissue spaces and the lumen of the capillaries.[20] The average volume of pericapillary fluid has been estimated as 220 ml in the lungs of adult human subjects and 4.2 ml/per kilogram of body weight in the dog,[41] quantities a bit larger than the intravascular blood volume of the capillaries (see Table 11.1).

The normal balance of forces across the capillary wall, together with effective drainage of the interstitial space by lymphatics, keeps the alveoli "dry" under physiological conditions. When capillary pressure is abnormally high or the endothelial wall is damaged, however, there is a net loss of fluid from the capillaries, which leads to an increased interstitial volume and eventually to the exudation of fluid into the air sacs. The presence of such fluid in the alveoli is called *pulmonary edema,* and it can interfere with gas exchange to a fatal degree. The most common clinical form of pulmonary edema is hemodynamic in origin, arising from excessive intracapillary pressure, but in some cases the fault lies in an elevation of capillary permeability caused by pulmonary or cerebral injury (see below).

Pulmonary veins

The drop in pressure from the venous end of the pulmonary capillaries to the entrance of the pulmonary veins into the left atrium is 3 to 4 mm Hg. The muscular coat of the venules is much less marked than that of the arterioles, and their resistance to flow is smaller. Nevertheless, the caliber of these small veins can be altered by vasomotor activity of their smooth muscle, and their resistance influences pressure in the capillaries upstream. In the larger pulmonary veins and across the venoatrial junction, the pressure gradients are so small that they are at the limits of resolution of present methods of measurement.

When a catheter is advanced out of the pulmonary artery until it "wedges" in a peripheral branch (a practice introduced in clinical investigation in an effort to estimate pulmonary capillary pressure), the pressure recorded probably approximates that in the small pulmonary veins. Under such conditions, blood stands stagnant in the vascular bed supplied by the occluded artery out to the point at which these vessels are joined by collaterals draining blood from unobstructed regions. Theoretically, what is recorded is the pressure at this junction—presumably somewhere in the microcirculation—but the significance of such measurements is limited because the site of the confluence is not known and the procedure may alter pressures in adjacent unobstructed areas.

Pulmonary blood flow

As the right ventricle ejects blood into the main pulmonary artery, the rate of flow rises to a peak and then falls, producing the contour shown in Figure 11.3. Peak flow is slightly lower and more rounded than in the aorta, although the areas under the pulmonic and aortic flow curves are equal, being proportional to stroke volume. Flow recorded from the midportion of the main pulmonary trunk shows a brief reversal at the end of systole, occasioned by a small backflow of blood that distends the root of the artery. The intermittent systolic ejections of the right ventricle are converted by the distention and recoil of the pulmonary artery and its major branches into a pulsatile flow that extends through diastole, as in the pulmonary venous flow record of Figure 11.3

Mean blood flow through the main pulmonary artery naturally equals the right ventricular output, about 6 liters/min in adult humans. The outputs of the

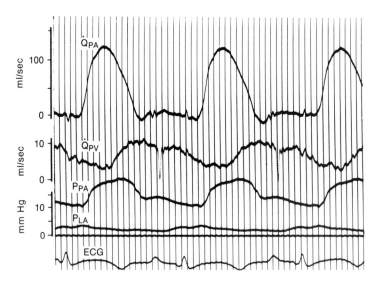

Figure 11.3. Records of pulmonary blood pressures and flows in a conscious, resting dog. *Q*, blood flow; *P*, pressure; *PA*, main pulmonary artery; *PV*, pulmonary vein within 2 cm of left atrium; *LA*, left atrium; *ECG*, electrocardiogram. Timing lines at intervals of 0.02 sec. Sharp spikes in the electromagnetic flowmeter record are electrocardiographic signals. (Reproduced from Milnor,[9] with permission of Academic Press)

right and left ventricle are identical, except for very small beat-to-beat differences that arise in part from respiratory effects on venous flow into the right atrium (see below). The average velocity of blood flow falls from about 16 cm/sec in the main pulmonary artery (the same as in the ascending aorta) to less than 0.1 cm/sec in the capillaries and back to almost its original speed in the large pulmonary veins.

In man, there is a small but consistent difference in blood flow to the two lungs, about 55% of the cardiac output flowing through the right lung and 45% through the left.[5] The distribution of flow within each lung varies in accordance with local hydrostatic pressures, and in the seated normal subject, the lower lobes are much better perfused than the upper lobes (see below). Flow is laminar in most pulmonary vessels because of the low velocities and small diameters. Although the Reynolds number is relatively high during peak flow in the main pulmonary artery, the flow profile appears to be relatively flat, with no gross evidence of turbulence. Severe congenital narrowing of the pulmonic valve orifice generates highly turbulent systolic flow, however, and an audible murmur (Chapter 6).

Pulmonary vascular resistance

Pulmonary vascular resistance is calculated from the standard resistance equation (6.5), which means that three variables must be measured: pulmonary arterial pressure, left atrial pressure, and pulmonary blood flow (cardiac output). Pulmonary arterial pressure alone is not sufficient, since that pressure may rise as a result of increased cardiac output or elevation of left atrial pressure. Studies of the approximate distribution of pulmonary vascular resistance within the bed show that the capillaries and venules contribute a larger share than is the case in the systemic circulation. The pressure drop across the microcirculation is difficult to measure and varies to some extent in different species.

Measurements by direct micropuncture in the cat show that the drop in pressure in vessels less than 40 μm in diameter is not quite one-half of the total gradient from pulmonary artery to left atrium. The remainder is about evenly divided between the arterial and venous beds.[39] Similar observations on the frog lung indicate that 15 to 30% of the total pulmonary resistance lies between precapillary and postcapillary vessels 80 μm in diameter.[35] In all species, total pulmonary vascular resistance can be altered significantly by events in any one of the three major divisions of the bed: arterial, capillary, or venous.

The diameter of each pulmonary vessel not only changes with active contraction or relaxation of the smooth muscle in its wall but also responds passively to changes in transmural pressure. This is true of all blood vessels, but in the thin-walled pulmonary vessels the effects are especially prominent, and the susceptibility of some pulmonary capillaries to partial or complete collapse makes the relation between blood flow and pressure particularly complex.[5] Three different factors affect the pulmonary vascular resistance:

1. The activity of vascular smooth muscle in various parts of the bed.
2. The intravascular component of transmural pressure, which depends on hemodynamic forces generated by the heart and the pressure gradients throughout the bed.
3. The extravascular component of transmural pressure, which is related to pressures in the intrapleural, interstitial, and alveolar spaces.

The effects of transmural pressure involve two phenomena. First, any increase in capillary transmural pressure tends to open up a greater number of capillaries and, to a lesser extent, distend those already open. This response depends on stress–strain relationships and critical closing pressures (Chapter 6). Second, and equally important, capillary patency depends on the relation between alveolar and venous pressures. If alveolar pressure is higher than intravascular pressure at the venous end of the pulmonary capillary, which is the normal condition in the upper parts of the human lung in the erect position, the capillary tends to collapse at its venous end. If pulmonary arterial and arteriolar pressures are higher than the intra-alveolar pressure, the collapse is not complete, and blood flow continues through the capillaries so affected. The capillary-to-venous pressure gradient is much higher per unit blood flow under these conditions than it is when the capillaries are widely open. In the lower parts of the lung, venous pressure is greater than alveolar pressure and most of the capillaries transmit flow freely. Total pulmonary blood flow is thus the sum of regional flows that differ considerably in different parts of the lung, a situation discussed in more detail below under "Gravitational Effects."

Because of the ample opportunities for passive responses to be superimposed on vasomotor activity, measurements of pulmonary vascular resistance have sometimes been regarded as of doubtful physiological significance. This view is unduly pessimistic if the principles governing the interpretation of resistance are strictly observed (Chapter 6). Indeed, measurements of pulmonary vascular resistance have found wide clinical and research application, being of particular importance in patients with congenital or valvular heart disease and in some general circulatory disorders. If a change in resistance is observed, the next question is whether the change is attributable to active vasomotion or to passive effects that do not involve activity of vascular smooth muscle, keeping in mind that the potential for passive alterations is greater in the pulmonic than in the systemic circulation. Active and passive vascular responses may both be present, of course. An agent that acts as a pulmonary vasoconstrictor in the isolated perfused lung, for example, may in the intact animal also raise right ventricular systolic pressure, increasing vascular transmural pressures and producing a net pulmonary vasodilatation.

Effects of exercise

One striking example of the modifications of pulmonary vascular resistance that occur *in vivo* is the characteristic response to exercise. As the cardiac output increases, mean pulmonary arterial pressure rises only moderately,[7] reaching 3 to 10 mm Hg above resting levels when the pulmonary blood flow has increased two- or threefold. The concomitant alterations in left atrial pressure have been measured rarely, but there appears to be little or no significant change. Pulmonary vascular resistance therefore falls during exercise, a response that develops within 2 min in dogs running on a treadmill[26] but may not appear in human subjects until the exertion has been maintained for more than 10 min.[7]

The decrease in resistance seems to be derived largely from *recruitment*, the opening up of capillaries that were closed before. Some of this recruitment may take place in the otherwise poorly perfused apical regions of the lungs. The increases in total capillary volume and diffusing capacity that occur with exercise[16,32] are so marked that they are unlikely to result solely from distention of already open capillaries to a larger cross section.

Diminished sympathetic constrictor discharge to pulmonary arterioles probably contributes to the lowering of resistance. No direct evidence for such an action has been presented, but the decrease in resting pulmonary resistance that follows thoracic sympathectomy shows that the potential for such a response exists. Whatever the mechanism, the net result is that pulmonary blood flow can be increased greatly without raising intravascular pressures to a degree that would encourage capillary transudation of fluid. The rapid blood flow keeps pace with the increased oxygen uptake required during exercise, and red cell velocity can increase to an extent that lowers their capillary transit time to half the resting value, but that speed does not prevent almost complete O_2 saturation of the pulmonary venous blood.[7]

Pulmonary vascular impedance

Resistance calculated from mean pressures and flows expresses only part of the opposition that must be overcome in moving blood through a vascular bed because it ignores the pulsatile waves, as discussed in Chapter 6. This omission can be corrected by determining pulmonary vascular impedance, the pulsatile analogue of resistance, from records of pulsatile flow and pressure.[17]

Impedance depends in part on vascular elasticity, and the main pulmonary artery has a thin, relatively distensible wall, its relative compliance $(dV/V_0 dP)$ being about 0.90%/mm Hg compared with 0.14%/mm Hg in the aorta (Chapter 2). The elastic modulus of the main pulmonary artery is much smaller than that of the aorta.

Because of this relatively high compliance, the characteristic impedance of the pulmonary arterial bed is much lower than that of the systemic circulation, approximating 20 dyne sec/cm^5 in the human pulmonary artery compared to 50 dyn sec/cm^5 in the ascending aorta. Pulse wave velocity, which is inversely related to compliance (Chapter 6), is 1 to 3 m/sec in the main pulmonary artery. The spectrum of pulmonary arterial input impedance is similar to that of the aorta, except that the amplitudes are smaller (Figure 11.4). The components of pulmonary arterial flow lead pressure slightly between 0 and 4 Hz; this relationship reverses at higher frequencies, as in the systemic circulation.

The physiological and pathological changes that can occur in pulmonary vascular impedance are under investigation in a number of laboratories, but their significance is not yet clear. During exercise the pulmonary vascular input impedance *rises,* an unexpected contrast with the fall in resistance; the mechanism of this response has not been identified.[26] Pulmonary impedance, like resistance, decreases immediately after birth, although only a few experimental

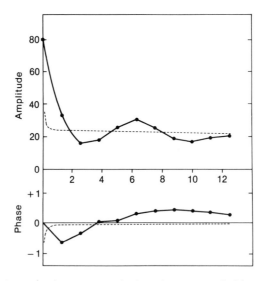

Figure 11.4. Spectrum of pulmonary vascular impedance computed from pressure and flow in main pulmonary artery of a human subject. *Ordinates,* impedance amplitude (*above,* dyn sec/cm^5), and phase angle (*below,* radians). *Abscissa,* frequency (Hz). Value plotted at $f = 0$ is input resistance (mean pulmonary arterial pressure/flow). Negative phase angles denote that flow leads pressure. (From Milnor and Nichols, unpublished data)

observations have been made in that period. Characteristic impedance in the pig is said to fall in the first 3 wk of extrauterine life to one-fifth of its value in the newborn.[29]

Transmission of pressure and flow pulsations

Pulsations of pressure and flow are transmitted through the pulmonary bed, and the shape of the waves changes because of viscous attenuation and reflections,[49] as in other parts of the circulation. Typical mean, systolic, and diastolic values from the mean pulmonary artery to the ends of the pulmonary veins are shown in Figure 11.5 The sharp drop in mean pressure in the microcirculation is evident in this figure, whereas mean flow is necessarily the same at all cross sections of the bed. The pulsations of pressure diminish in size as they travel; the pulse that reaches arterioles 100 μm in diameter is only 35 to 55% of the original wave in the main pulmonary artery.[35] Some 25 to 50% of the initial arterial pulse is transmitted to the capillaries of the lung, compared to 5% or less in the systemic bed.

Pressure waves are transmitted all the way to the ends of the pulmonary veins, where their amplitude is 10 to 30% of the main arterial pulsation.[9] Small retrograde waves of pressure and flow caused by the contractions of the left atrium appear in the distal veins, but most of the venous pulsation is transmitted from the right ventricle. The predominance of forward transmission is evident in experiments on isolated lungs in which a reservoir is substituted for the left atrium and the pulmonary artery is perfused by a pulsatile pump; pulmonary venous flow waves under such conditions are of the same shape and amplitude as those *in vivo*.[46]

Flow pulsations diminish in amplitude as they move through the pulmonary vascular tree, but not as much as the pressure pulses (Figure 11.5). This difference is characteristic of a system that contains reflected waves, which augment flow pulsations in regions where they attenuate pressures (Chapter 6). Damping of the flow waves is less marked in the pulmonary than in the systemic circuit. The pulse/mean ratio for flow in pulmonary capillaries is 2.0 to 2.5, for example, whereas it is close to 1.0 in the systemic microcirculation. Transmission ratios in different parts of the pulmonary vascular bed have been studied in detail in man and a number of experimental animals[9] (Chapter 6).

Because of the relatively high distensibility of pulmonary arteries, pulse wave velocity is slower than in the systemic arterial tree. The average value in the main pulmonary artery is 180 cm/sec in man, and somewhat higher in the dog (Table 11.1). The time required for waves to travel from the pulmonic valve to the end of the pulmonary veins[46] is 80 to 160 msec in canine lungs and 130 to 230 msec in human lungs (Table 11.1). As pointed out earlier, pulse waves

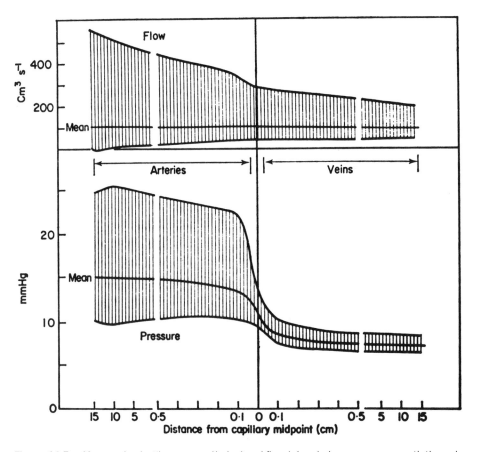

Figure 11.5. Mean and pulsatile pressure (*below*) and flow (*above*) along an average path through the human pulmonary vascular bed. Abscissa, distance from the capillary midpoint. Note changes of scale at 0.5 cm. Upper and lower boundaries of shaded area indicate systolic and diastolic values. (Reproduced from Milnor,[9] with permission of Academic Press)

move much more rapidly than the blood itself (Chapter 6). The average transit time for a drop of blood or injected dye through the human pulmonary circulation is 3 to 7 sec in normal adults at rest. The circulation time though the most rapid path in the pulmonary circuit, indicated by the earliest appearance in the left atrium of a substance injected into the pulmonary artery, averages 2 sec in man. The mean transit time through the pulmonary bed is slightly shorter for cells than for plasma, and the ratio of cell volume to plasma volume is somewhat less in the pulmonary vessels than in systemic venous blood. The source of such hematocrit variations is discussed in Chapter 13.

Pulsatile flow in the pulmonary capillaries was first demonstrated by direct microscopic observation in animals, but it can now be measured in human subjects by a technique that makes total capillary flow more accessible in the lungs than in any other organ.[34] The subject is enclosed in a body plethysmograph, and the rate of uptake of inhaled nitrous oxide is measured volumetrically. The pulsatile uptake of gas from the alveoli is taken as an indication of capillary flow at every instant, and a calibrated record of pulsatile flow can be derived (Figure 11.6). Peak flow varies directly with stroke volume, usually ranging between 130 and 300 ml/sec, and end-diastolic flow approaches zero when the heart rate is slow. The normal pattern indicates that about one-quarter of the total flow takes place during diastole. Red cells require about 0.75 sec to traverse the capillary bed.[7]

Pulmonary blood volume

The results of early animal experiments in which lungs were exsanguinated and more recent measurements using indicator-dilution methods[7,9,16] agree in showing that approximately 9% of the total blood volume is contained in the pulmonary vessels. This amounts to about half a liter in the average human adult, or 240 ml per square meter of body surface. A number of earlier reports in the literature that assigned more than twice this volume to the pulmonary bed were based on misinterpretations of the boundaries of the *central blood volume* determined by indicator-dilution, which includes the lungs, heart, and large central arteries and veins (Chapters 13 and 14).

The volume of pulmonary vessels is distributed almost equally among arteries, capillaries, and veins (Table 11.1). The capillary bed accounts for some 60 ml/m², or 34%, of total pulmonary blood volume,[16] while approximately 30% resides in the arteries and 36% in the veins. A large part of the total volume is thus in the capillary vessels, as might be expected in view of their respiratory function and the relatively short length of the arterial and venous trees. With exercise, the pulmonary capillary volume increases along with cardiac output,[16,32] and may reach twice its normal value (see below).

Changes in the distensibility of the pulmonary vessels or in their transmural pressures can raise or lower total pulmonary blood volume by 25 to 50%.[9] Examples of this expansion or contraction of the capacity of the pulmonary bed range from the decrease in pulmonary vascular volume on assuming the erect position to the accommodation of an increased volume[25] when vasoconstriction reduces the capacity of the systemic bed (Chapter 13). The lung vessels constitute a small blood reservoir in comparison with the systemic veins, however, since the total volume shifted into or out of the pulmonary bed in man probably rarely exceeds 200 ml. These alterations in pulmonary blood volume imply concomitant alterations in the caliber of some of the pulmonary vessels; as a rule, pulmonary vascular resistance rises when pulmonary blood

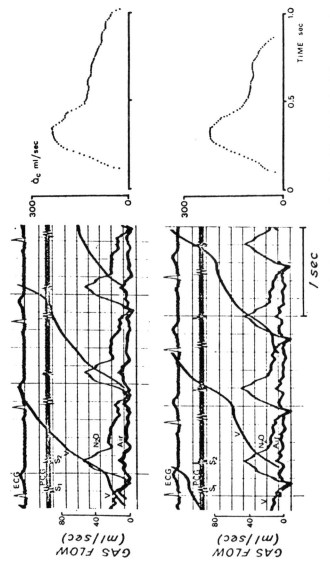

Figure 11.6. *Left*, data recorded in two measurements of pulmonary capillary blood flow by body plethysmograph in a normal human subject. *Right*, pulsatile flow calculated from records. *ECG*, electrocardiogram; *PCG*, phonocardiogram, showing first and second heart sounds (S_1, S_2); *V*, gas flow signal of the plethysmograph and its integral with time; Q_c, total pulmonary capillary flow. (Reproduced from Karatzas and Lee,[34] with permission of *Cardiovasc. Res.*)

volume falls, and vice versa. Regional blood volume and vascular resistance both depend on transmural pressure, smooth muscle tone, and all the other factors that affect vascular diameters.

Control and Regulation

Sensors

The baroreceptors in the walls of the largest pulmonary arteries were described earlier (Chapter 7), and the tissues of the lungs and pleura also contain stretch receptors of various kinds, which send afferent signals to the central nervous system by way of the vagus nerves.[1] One group, located in parenchymal, nonvascular tissue, is activated by expansion or inflation of the lungs. The *Hering-Breuer reflex* elicited by activation of these mechanoreceptors acts mainly on the mechanics of ventilation, but there are cardiovascular reactions as well. One component of the response is *sinus arrhythmia,* the waxing and waning of heart rate with inspiration and expiration. Lung inflation also causes reflex vasodilatation in skeletal muscle and, to a lesser extent, in the skin and splanchnic bed through a reduction of sympathetic constrictor impulses.[25] Although this response is insignificant during quiet inspiration and expiration, it presumably contributes to increased muscular blood flow when hyperventilation accompanies muscular exercise.

In addition to the inflation sensors, there is increasing evidence that some mechanically sensitive C-fiber endings in the pulmonary tissue (juxtacapillary or *J-receptors*) monitor the amount of fluid in the interstitial space. These nerve endings fire at a rapid rate whenever movement of fluid from pulmonary capillaries into the interstitium raises volume and pressure in that compartment. Reflex responses are thus generated by abnormal leakage from the pulmonary capillaries before exudation into the alveolar spaces develops, even though intravascular pressure may be normal.[1,42] Bronchoconstriction is part of the reflex, and rapid, shallow breathing is characteristic. One would expect reflex effects that would reduce pulmonary capillary pressure, but such responses have not been demonstrated, and in severe congestion of the lungs the picture is confused by the bradycardia and systemic hypotension that result from hypoxemia (Chapter 8).

Malfunction of the J-receptors may be involved in *neurogenic* pulmonary edema, an acute exudation of fluid into the alveoli that is often caused by severe head injuries and can be reproduced by experimental lesions of the medulla or hypothalamus. In some experiments a severe systemic hypertension, accompanied by a marked rise in left atrial, pulmonary capillary, and pulmonary arterial pressures, provides an adequate explanation for the net loss of fluid from the capillaries. In others, pulmonary edema develops in the absence of any rise in blood pressure, and an increase in capillary permeability is suspected. The mechanism by which permeability is altered has not been discovered, but the evidence strongly suggests a vasomotor origin. Beta-adrenergic agonists, for example, reduce permeability of the interendothelial junctions and tend to counteract stimuli that produce local edema in systemic organs.[8]

Autonomic vasomotor nerves

The existence of active vasomotion in pulmonary vessels was long regarded as doubtful because of varying interpretations of changes in pulmonary vascular resistance and the technical difficulty of measuring the small pressures in the pulmonary circulation. The discovery of a rich innervation in the vessels of the lung, together with the demonstration of a number of fairly unequivocal vasomotor responses under experimental conditions,[2,31] gradually removed this doubt, and the pulmonary vessels are now believed to be subject to autonomic controls like those of the systemic circulation. Under normal resting conditions, however, vasomotor tone is almost as low as it can get.

Pulmonary vessels are supplied with sympathetic vasoconstrictor and vasodilator fibers, both groups being atropine resistant.[2] Cholinergic parasympathetic fibers that cause pulmonary vasodilatation have also been identified in the vagus, but the possibility that these act on the bronchial rather than the pulmonary vessels has not been ruled out. The observation that stimulation of such fibers constricts or dilates the pulmonary vessels does not, of course, prove that they are part of the normal mechanism for circulatory control, but the evidence tends strongly in that direction. Additional clues that point to a constant active autonomic control of the pulmonary circulation are provided by the discovery of reflexes that originate in the systemic baroreceptors and moderate pulmonary vascular resistance. Stimulation of the carotid sinus baroreceptors leads to a reduction of pulmonary resistance, whereas stimulation of the carotid body chemoreceptors by hypoxic blood is followed by pulmonary vasoconstriction.

Cell receptors

Smooth muscle cells of the pulmonary vessels contain both alpha- and beta-adrenoceptors, which mediate constriction and dilatation, respectively. Norepinephrine, epinephrine, and other agonists that act on both types cause a net vasoconstriction. Alpha effects are predominantly those of the alpha$_1$ subtype, but the alpha$_2$ variety is also present. The action of antagonists identifies the beta adrenoceptors as the beta$_2$ subtype. The effects of all pulmonary vascular adrenoceptors are more prominent in arteries than in veins.

Muscarinic cholinergic receptors probably also function in pulmonary vascular smooth muscle, although that question is still under investigation. Acetylcholine or stimulation of vagus nerves induces pulmonary vasodilatation under carefully controlled experimental conditions, but the response is obvious only when definite constriction has been established in advance. The constrictor effects of serotonin, histamine, and some prostaglandins (PGE_1 and $PGF_{2\alpha}$) argue that receptors for those agents are also present. Some vagal terminals in the lung release vasoactive intestinal peptide, which relaxes smooth muscle in the airways and perhaps in some vessels (Chapter 8).

Local vasomotor responses

In addition to the responses elicited through vasomotor nerves and the central nervous system, the pulmonary vessels are capable of reacting directly to substances in contact with their walls. Like systemic vessels, they react to norepinephrine and other vasoactive materials that reach the vascular smooth muscle.

Hypoxia

One important local response is the pulmonary vasoconstriction brought on by low O_2 or high CO_2 tensions in the blood. This phenomenon was first described by von Euler and Liljestrand,[47] who postulated that the vasomotor response to respiratory gases is a mechanism for adjusting local alveolar perfusion to match ventilation. In this way, the local vascular resistance in different parts of the lung can be modified to favor perfusion of the best-ventilated alveoli. Further experiments have confirmed this hypothesis. General pulmonary vasoconstriction develops acutely in man when the O_2 saturation of systemic arterial blood falls below about 80%.[5] The effects of chronic hypoxia are similar, and residents at high altitudes may develop chronic pulmonary hypertension, along with enlargement of the right ventricle and an increase in the number of red cells. The pulmonary vascular effects of hypercapnia are more variable and depend on the production of acidosis, a decrease in blood pH acting as a stimulus to vasoconstriction (Chapter 9).

The pulmonary hypertension caused by hypoxia varies considerably in different species. Lowering arterial pO_2 acutely to 40 mm Hg causes mean pulmonary artery pressure to rise to about 60 mm Hg in the cow but to only 20 mm Hg in man. The effects of chronic hypoxia are also species dependent; cows, pigs, horses, and rats develop much greater pulmonary hypertension than sheep, dogs, llamas, and human beings do at high altitudes.[7] Some cattle are relatively resistant to this effect; the difference appears to be genetically determined.

Everything about the pulmonary vascular response to hypoxia has long been a subject for debate—the location of the O_2 sensor, the exact site of vasoconstriction, and the mechanism of the reaction. The first two of these questions can now be answered with some confidence, while the third is still the subject of various hypotheses. The present evidence suggests that the major constriction is in arterioles less than 50 μm in diameter and that the venules also constrict slightly.[7,39] Most observations support this conclusion in spite of wide variations in experimental technique. For example, the hypoxic increase in pulmonary vascular resistance is accompanied by a decrease in pulmonary arterial volume.[7] There is also an increase in the pressure gradient between the pulmonary artery and a wedged arterial catheter, but not in the gradient from the wedged position to the left atrium. Some investigators have found a small amount of postcapillary constriction as part of the pulmonary hypoxic response, although the precapillary change is far greater. In one study on the feline lung, the greatest hypoxic increase in resistance occurred between the pulmonary artery and arterioles 30 to 50 μm in diameter, but a small increment in resistance also appeared in the capillary and venous regions, demonstrating that constriction is not limited to the arterioles.[39]

The sensor as well as the major effector appears to have a precapillary location. Pulmonary resistance increases when hypoxic blood flows through the arteries, but not when flow is reversed and hypoxic blood is perfused by way of pulmonary veins.[18] With normally directed flow, low O_2 tensions in the alveoli are as effective as arterial hypoxemia in causing pulmonary vasoconstriction,[7] which is compatible with the theory that the arteriolar wall is the site of the O_2 sensor because gas diffusion takes place readily between alveoli and nearby terminal arterioles.[22]

If the pulmonary vascular response to hypoxia is triggered by low O_2 tensions in the walls of the terminal arterioles and brought about by active constriction in those same vessels, then the mechanism of constriction is probably the most obvious one, namely, that the contraction of arteriolar smooth muscle is a direct response to low O_2 tension. The mechanism of that response could be hypoxic depolarization and calcium flux into the muscle cells, a possibility supported by the finding that hypoxic pulmonary vasoconstriction is inhibited by calcium antagonists.[37] *In vitro* studies do not uniformly favor that hypothesis,[7] however, and the small but detectable venoconstricton cannot be explained in that way. No convincing evidence has been offered in favor of the standard alternative explanations, namely, a decrease in the concentration of some vasodilating substance or the release of a vasoconstrictor. Angiotensin-II is not a likely candidate for the latter role because hypoxia *reduces* the ability of the lungs to produce it.[12,13] The release of endothelial relaxing factor (Chapter 8) is depressed by hypoxia, but the removal of such a dilating stimulus is not enough to account for the marked pulmonary hypertension.

Vasoactive agents

Epinephrine, norepinephrine, angiotensin-II, and histamine act as pulmonary vasoconstrictors in the isolated lung, and serotonin is especially potent in this respect. In the intact animal, the effect of such drugs on vascular smooth muscle is sometimes outweighed by changes in transmural pressure secondary to their action on the heart and systemic circulation.[5] In the case of histamine, modifications of ventilation and intra-alveolar pressure resulting from the bronchoconstriction modify the vascular response. One form of pulmonary vasoconstriction that is still unexplained is the reaction to embolization of small pulmonary vessels, which causes intense constriction even in regions distant from the sites of obstruction. Tissues of the lung are also involved in hypersensitivity reactions, as all sufferers from asthma can testify. Immunological challenge causes release by the lung of substances that may be responsible for vasoconstriction and for some of the phenomena of anaphylactic reactions. Among these substances are leukotrienes, arachidonic acid derivatives that are potent constrictors of pulmonary vessels and bronchi.[33]

Extravascular Forces and the Pulmonary Circulation

The extravascular pressure applied to pulmonary capillaries is essentially that in the alveoli, whereas the pressure around the large pulmonary vessels not enclosed by lung tissue is determined by intrapleural pressure and its small respiratory excursions. Intrapulmonary vessels other than capillaries are exposed to a mixture of these forces and to the mechanical effects of stretching with inflation and deflation. Extravascular pressure is probably not the same near the pleural surface as in the deeper portions of the lung, and there is some evidence to suggest that interstitial pressure in some regions is more negative than the intrapleural pressure.[40]

Another external force on the pulmonary capillaries arises from the surface tension of the alveoli, which are not unlike microscopic bubbles. This surface tension is kept low by *surfactant*,[4] a substance that is secreted by the alveolar lining and contains dipalmitoyl phosphatidyl choline as one of its major constituents. The principal effect of surfactant is to stabilize the alveoli and prevent their collapse, but the low surface tension also tends to reduce the external force on the pulmonary capillaries.[15,21]

Effects of respiration

The dimensions of the pulmonary vessels vary with the degree of inflation of the lungs. Pulmonary vascular resistance is at a minimum when lung volume approximates the normal expiratory state *in vivo,* and it increases when the lungs are inflated or deflated beyond this range.[5,40] In the intact animal, respiratory variations in ventricular outputs, vena caval blood flow, and vascular transmural pressures are superimposed on these mechanical effects. The increased negativity of intrapleural pressure as it swings from the resting level of about −3 mm Hg down to −6 mm Hg on inspiration distends the intrathoracic portions of the venae cavae. Blood flow into these veins and the right atrium increases, and the right ventricle ejects a slightly larger stroke volume.[28] Elevation of intra-abdominal pressure by the respiratory movements of the diaphragm and abdominal muscles during inspiration may help to increase flow into the intrathoracic portion of the inferior vena cava. Extensive studies in the dog indicate that right ventricular stroke volume and peak flow in the pulmonary artery increase in the heartbeat immediately following the onset of inspiration, and that pulmonary venous and aortic flows then increase proportionately, usually in the next beat.[38]

Normal inspiration and expiration affect not only the venous inflow to the right atrium but also the pressures in the pulmonary vascular bed. The influence of inspiration on cardiovascular pressures is quite evident in experimental records, for pressures in the right atrium, ventricle, and pulmonary artery fall a few millimeters of mercury with each inspiration, just as intrathoracic pressure does. Motion of the chest wall and diaphragm bring about inflation and deflation of the lungs through changes in transpulmonary pressure, the difference between intra-alveolar and intrapleural pressure; it is difficult to distinguish between the direct mechanical effects of distending the lung and those of changes in transmural pressure. Mechanical stretching and compression appear to act mainly on the large vessels, whereas the changes in transmural pressure act predominantly on the microcirculation.

The net effect of these events on pulmonary vascular resistance is a subject on which investigators disagree, but it is certain that any respiratory change in pulmonary vascular resistance must be quite small. The resistance probably rises very slightly with inspiration, but not enough to prevent a simultaneous increase in pulmonary blood flow. The left ventricle initially increases its output to a slightly lesser extent than the right ventricle does, so that pulmonary blood volume enlarges with inspiration. During deep breathing or chronic pulmonary disease, these respiratory swings in flow, resistance, and volume are greatly exaggerated. The input impedance of the pulmonary circulation does not change during normal quiet inspiration and expiration.

Respiration and heart rate

Waxing and waning of the heart rate in phase with respiration is a common observation. It usually arises from variations in the firing rate of the normal pacemaker in the sinoatrial node and is therefore called *sinus arrhythmia*. The same phenomenon originates, in some instances, from a gradual wandering of the pacemaker from its normal site to fibers in the atrium or atrioventricular node and back again. Sinus arrhythmia is evoked through the vagus nerves and has its origin in at least two different sources: the stimulation of pulmonary stretch receptors by inflation of the lung and an interaction between the respiratory centers and the vagal nucleus. The physiological significance of this reflex is unknown, and perhaps none remains at this stage of evolution.

Increased intrathoracic pressure

When intra-alveolar and intrapleural pressures are raised by forced expiratory effort against a closed glottis or a column of water (the Valsalva maneuver), venous return to the right heart is impeded and the output of first the right and then the left ventricle declines gradually. The mean and pulse pressures fall in the brachial and other systemic arteries, but they return abruptly to levels above the control values when the increased pressure is released. Intrapleural pressures of more than +20 mm Hg can be developed, and prolonged maintenance of such high levels may be terminated by fainting. Coughing or straining also caused marked increase in intrathoracic pressure. Artificial respiration by mechanical devices affects the pulmonary circulation by altering the intra-alveolar and intrapleural pressures. Positive-pressure breathing, in which the lungs are inflated intermittently by applying positive pressure to the airway, can compress the pulmonary capillaries, so that pulmonary vascular resistance rises and right ventricular output falls with each inflation.

Gravitational effects

The physiological problems connected with pumping blood from the right ventricle up to the top of the lung in human subjects standing erect reveal the influence that hydrostatic and extravascular factors can have on the circulation. The pulmonary capillaries are not only devoid of smooth muscle and made up of a single layer of endothelial cells, but also possess relatively little external supporting structure. At zero transmural pressure, they collapse. Given the critical closing pressure exhibited by arterioles and venules (Chapter 6), it is to be expected that transmural pressures slightly above zero may not suffice to keep all segments of the pulmonary vascular bed open.

The external component of capillary transmural pressure is the pressure in the pericapillary tissue space, which is close to that in the alveolar air sacs. The internal component, the pressure generated by right ventricular contraction, is low, not only in comparison to systemic pressures but also in relation to hydrostatic pressures in the lung. In an adult human subject standing erect, a column of blood extending from the pulmonic valve up to the top of the lung is about 20 cm long, and it weight is equivalent to a pressure of about 15 mm

Hg. This weight exerts a downward force, a hydrostatic pressure amounting to -15 mm Hg, which tends to collapse microvessels at the apex of the lung. Net intravascular pressure in those vessels is the algebraic sum of the pressure generated by the ventricle and the hydrostatic force, but normal mean pressure in the main pulmonary artery can be less than 15 mm Hg, and the viscous attenuation of flow to arterioles reduces that amount by a few millimeters of mercury. As a result, transmural pressure in the microcirculation at the apex of the lung can be negative, that is, subatmospheric.

This line of reasoning suggests that the erect posture prevents perfusion of the uppermost part of the lungs, and that prediction has been fully confirmed experimentally.[48] The pulmonary microcirculation is like the collapsible vascular segments described in Chapter 6 and behaves like a Starling resistor (Figure 6.9). Intracapillary pressure is lower than the atmospheric pressure in adjacent alveoli in regions near the lung apex but is significantly higher at the bottom of the lung. Blood flow is consequently not the same in all parts of the lung; three hemodynamically different zones have been identified:[48]

Zone I: arterial < alveolar > venous pressure
Zone II: arterial > alveolar > venous pressure
Zone III: arterial > alveolar < venous pressure

The arterial and venous pressures referred to in this classification are those in the smallest vessels and include hydrostatic pressure. In the erect posture, the zones correspond approximately to the upper, middle, and lower parts of the lung, and blood flow is distributed accordingly. In Zone I, the capillaries are closed and there is no blood flow. In Zone II, the subalveolar pressure in the veins leads to partial collapse of the capillaries, as seen in Figure 6.9. Blood flow through this region is a function of the difference between arterial and alveolar pressures and is not influenced by pressure in the large pulmonary veins. This situation has been called a *vascular waterfall*[40] because flow is independent of downstream pressure; the mechanism is discussed in Chapter 6. Blood flow is greatest in Zone III, where intravascular pressure is sufficient to keep many capillaries widely open.

Vascular Endothelium

The endothelial cells lining pulmonary vessels, like those in other vascular beds, perform a number of physiological functions (Chapter 1), and the lung is the principal site of endothelial processing or degradation of certain hormones, peptides, and amines. Angiotensin-I is completely converted to angiotensin-II in a single passage through the bed by the action of *angiotensin-converting enzyme,* which is located near the surface of endothelial cells.[12] Bradykinin is removed from blood passing through the lungs, and the concentration of nor-epinephrine and serotonin is greatly reduced. Between 25 and 50% of circulat-ing norepinephrine is cleared by the lungs, as well as 80 to 95% of serotonin.[6] The pulmonary endothelium thus plays a part in regulating the levels of vaso-active agents in the systemic circulation, and current research suggests that a number of other substances may be removed from the blood in the same way. The potent vasoconstricting effect of angiotensin-II has led investigators to em-ploy drugs that inhibit angiotensin-converting enzyme in the treatment of sys-temic and pulmonary hypertension.[12]

Prostaglandins PGE_2, $PGF_{2\alpha}$, PGD_2, PGI_2, and thromboxanes (Chapter 8) are synthesized in pulmonary endothelial cells and by alveolar macrophages. These substances are not stored, and the amounts released depend on the rate of synthesis. The triggers for increased synthesis include (1) mechanical stimuli like hyperventilation; (2) biologically active materials such as bradykinin, angiotensin-II, and thrombin; and (3) pathological conditions such as anaphy-lactic reactions or hemorrhagic shock. Normal lung tissue also contains VIP and substance P, but these materials come from nerve endings, not the endo-thelium (Chapter 8).

The pulmonary vascular lining also possesses the antithrombogenic prop-erties common to all endothelia. Blood tends to clot in almost any container other than the vascular system, and the fact that it remains fluid in the circu-lation is largely due to the activity of endothelial cells. The mechanism involves prostacyclin (PGI_2) release[23] and ADPase activity at the endothelial surface. Under pathological conditions such as the presence of certain endotoxins, not only is the antithrombogenic activity diminished, but the endothelium may pro-duce substances that tend to promote coagulation.[44] Endothelial cells also ex-hibit a degree of adhesiveness for formed elements of the blood, and granulo-cytes tend to stick to small pulmonary vessels in a slowly exchanging pool.[36] The size of this pool varies inversely with the rate of pulmonary blood flow.

References

Reviews

1. Coleridge, H.M., Coleridge, J.C.G. (1986). Reflexes from the tracheobronchial tree and lungs. In: *The Handbook of Physiology; The Respiratory System, Vol. 2, Con-trol of Breathing, Part I*, N. Cherniak and J.G. Widdicombe, eds. Washington, D.C., American Physiological Society, pp. 395–429.

2. Daly, I. De B., Hebb, C. (1966). *Pulmonary and Bronchial vascular Systems.* Baltimore, Williams & Wilkins.

3. Dawes, G.S. (1968). *Foetal and Neonatal Physiology.* Chicago, Year Book Medical Publishers.

4. Dobbs, L.G. (1989). Pulmonary surfactant. *Ann. Rev. Med.* 40:431–446.

5. Fishman, A.P. (1963). Dynamics of the pulmonary circulation. In: *Handbook of Physiology, Section 2, Circulation. Vol. II,* W.F. Hamilton and P. Dow, ed. Washington, D.C., American Physiological Society, pp. 1667–1743.

6. Gillis, C.N., Pitt, B.R. (1982). The fate of circulating amines within the pulmonary circulation. *Annu. Rev. Physiol.* 44:269–281.

7. Grover, R.F., Wagner, W.W., Jr., McMurtry, I.F., Reeves, J.T. (1983). Pulmonary circulation. In: *Handbook of Physiology, Section 2: The Cardiovascular System. Vol. III, Peripheral Circulation and Organ Blood Flow,* J.T. Shepherd and F.M. Abboud, eds. Bethesda, Md., American Physiological Society, pp. 103–136.

8. Malik, A.B. (1985). Mechanisms of neurogenic pulmonary edema. *Circ. Res.* 57:1–18.

9. Milnor, W.R. (1972). Pulmonary hemodynamics. In: *Cardiovascular Fluid Dynamics, Vol. 2,* D.H. Bergel, ed. New York, Academic Press, pp. 299–340.

10. Nadas, A.S., Fyler, D.C. (1972). *Pediatric Cardiology.* 3rd ed. Philadelphia, W.B. Saunders, p. 672.

11. Rudolph, A.M. (1985). Distribution and regulation of blood flow in the fetal and neonatal lamb. *Circ. Res.* 57:811–821.

12. Ryan, J.W. (1982). Processing of endogenous polypeptides by the lungs. *Annu. Rev. Physiol.* 44:241–255.

13. Ryan, U. (1985). Processing of angiotensin and other peptides by the lungs. In: *Handbook of Physiology, The Respiratory System, Vol. 1,* A.P. Fishman and A.B. Fisher, eds. Bethesda, Md., American Physiological Society, pp. 351–364.

14. Weibel, E.R. (1963). *Morphometry of the Human Lung.* Berlin, Springer-Verlag.

15. West, J.B. (1987). *Pulmonary Pathophysiology.* Baltimore, Williams & Wilkins.

16. Yu, P.N. (1969). *Pulmonary Blood Volume in Health and Disease,* Philadelphia, Lea & Febiger.

Research Papers

17. Bergel, D.H., Milnor, W.R. (1965). Pulmonary vascular impedance in the dog. *Circ. Res.* 16:401–415.

18. Bergofsky, E.H., Haas, F., Porcelli, R. (1968). Determination of the sensitive vascular sites from which hypoxia and hypercapnia elicit rises in pulmonary arterial pressure. *Fed. Proc.* 27:1420–1425.

19. Bruner, H.D., Schmidt, C.F. (1947). Bloodflow in the bronchial artery of the anesthetized dog. *Am. J. Physiol.* 148:648–666.

20. Chinard, F.P., Enns, T. (1954). Transcapillary pulmonary exchange of water in the dog. *Am. J. Physiol.* 178:197–202.

21. Clements, J.A., Hustead, R.F., Johnson, R.P., Gribetz, I. (1961). Pulmonary surface tension and alveolar stability. *J. Appl. Physiol.* 16:444–450.

22. Conhaim, R.L., Staub, N.C. (1980). Reflection spectrophotometric measurement of O_2 uptake in pulmonary arterioles of cats. *J. Appl. Physiol.* 48:848–856.

23. Crutchley, D.J., Ryan, J.W., Ryan, U.S., Fisher, G.M. (1983). Bradykinin-induced release of prostacyclin and thromboxanes from bovine pulmonary artery endothelial cells. Studies with lower homologs and calcium antagonists. *Biochem. Biophys. Acta* 751:99–107.

24. Daly, I. de B., Daly, M. de B. (1959). The effects of stimulation of the carotid body chemoreceptors on the pulmonary vascular bed in the dog: The "vasosensory controlled perfused living animal" preparation. *J. Physiol.* 148:201–219.

25. Daly, M. de B., Hazzledine, J.L., Ungar, A. (1967). The reflex effects of alterations in lung volume on systemic vascular resistance in the dog. *J. Physiol.* 188:331–351.

26. Elkins, R.C., Milnor, W.R. (1971). Pulmonary vascular response to exercise in the dog. *Circ. Res.* 29:591–599.

27. Ferencz, C. (1969). Pulmonary arterial design in mammals. Morphologic variation and physiologic constancy. *Johns Hopkins Med. J.* 125:207–224.

28. Franklin, D.L., Van Citters, R.L., Rushmer, R.F. (1962) Balance between right and left ventricular output. *Circ. Res.* 10:17–26.

29. Greenwald, S.E., Johnson, R.J., Hawaorth, S.G. (1984). Pulmonary vascular input impedance in the newborn and infant pig. *Cardiovasc. Res.* 18:44–50.

30. Haworth, S., Hislop, A.A. (1981). Normal structural and functional adaptation to extrauterine life. *J. Pediatr.* 98:911–918.

31. Ingram, R.H., Jr., Szidon, J.P., Fishman, A.P. (1970). Response of the main pulmonary artery of dogs to neuronally released versus blood-borne norepinephrine. *Circ. Res.* 26:249–262.

32. Johnson, R.L., Jr., Spicer, W.S., Bishop, J.M., Forster, R.E. (1960). Pulmonary capillary blood flow, volume, and diffusing capacity during exercise. *J. Appl. Physiol.* 15:893–902.

33. Kadowitz, P.J., Hyman, A.L. (1984). Analysis of responses to leukotriene D4 in the pulmonary vascular bed. *Circ. Res.* 55:707–717.

34. Karatzas, N.B., Lee, G. de J. (1970). Instantaneous lung capillary blood flow in patients with heart disease. *Cardiovasc. Res.* 4:265–273.

35. Maloney, J.E., Castle, B.L. (1970). Dynamic intravascular pressures in the microvessels of the frog lung. *Respir. Physiol.* 10:51–63.

36. Martin, B.A., Wright, J.L., Thommasen, H., Hogg, J.C. (1982). The effect of pulmonary blood flow on the exchange between the circulating and marginating pool of polymorphonuclear leukocytes in dog lungs. *J. Clin. Invest.* 69:1277–1285.

37. McMurtry, I.F., Davidson, A.B., Reeves, J.T., Grover, R.F. (1976). Inhibition of hypoxic pulmonary vasoconstriction by calcium antagonists in isolated rat lungs. *Circ. Res.* 38:99–104.

38. Morgan, B.C., Abel, F.L., Mullins, G.L., Gunteroth, W.G. (1966). Flow patterns in cavae, pulmonary artery, pulmonary vein, and aorta in intact dogs. *Am. J. Physiol.* 210:903–909.

39. Nagasaka, Y., Bhattacharya, J., Nanjo, S., Gropper, M.A., Staub, N.C. (1984). Micropuncture measurement of lung microvascular pressure profile during hypoxia in cats. *Circ. Res.* 54:90–95.

40. Permutt, S., Riley, R.L. (1963). Hemodynamics of collapsible vessels with tone: The vascular waterfall. *J. Appl. Physiol.* 17:893–898.

41. Ramsey, L.H., Puckett, W., Jose, A., Lacy, W.W. (1964). Pericapillary gas and

water distribution volumes of the lung calculated from multiple indicator dilution nerves. *Circ. Res.* 15:275–286.

42. Roberts, A.M., Bhattacharya, J., Schultz, H.D., Coleridge, H.M., Coleridge, J.C.G. (1986). Stimulation of pulmonary vagal afferent C-fibers by lung edema in dogs. *Circ. Res.* 58:512–522.

43. Sancetta, S.M., Rakita, L. (1957). Response of pulmonary artery pressure and total pulmonary resistance of untrained, convalescent man to prolonged mild steady state exercise. *J. Clin. Invest.* 36:1138–1149.

44. Schorer, A.E., Rick, P.D., Swain, W.R., Moldow, C.F. (1985). Structural features of endotoxin required for stimulation of endothelial cell tissue factor production: Exposure of preformed tissue factor after oxidant-mediated endothelial injury. *J. Lab. Clin. Med.* 106:38–42.

45. Singhal, S., Henderson, R., Horsfield, K., Harding, K., Cumming, G. (1973). Morphometry of the human pulmonary arterial tree. *Circ. Res.* 33:190–197.

46. Szidon, J.P., Ingram, R.H., Fishman, A.P. (1968). Origin of the pulmonary venous flow pulse. *Am. J. Physiol.* 214:10–14.

47. Von Euler, U.S., Liljestrand, G. (1946). Observations on the pulmonary arterial blood pressure in the cat. *Acta Physiol. Scand.* 12:301–320.

48. West, J.B., Dollery, C.T., Naimark, A. (1964). Distribution of blood flow in isolated lung: Relation to vascular and alveolar pressures. *J. Appl. Physiol.* 19:713–724.

49. Wiener, F., Morkin, E., Skalak, R., Fishman, A.P. (1966). Wave propagation in the pulmonary circulation. *Circ. Res.* 19:834–850.

12

REGIONAL CIRCULATIONS

Each organ has a characteristic vascular pattern of its own.[1] The splanchnic system has two successive capillary beds connected by a portal vein, for example, and the coronary vasculature contains not only prominent superficial vessels but also small intramural branches that are unique in being compressed rhythmically by external pressure. The disposition of the pulmonary microcirculation around the alveoli of the lung is discussed in Chapter 11, and the special features of other major systems are considered in this chapter.

Many of the methods for measuring blood flow in these regional circulations have been applied in humans, and data from human subjects as well as experimental animals are available. Variants of the Fick principle were the basis for the earliest methods of measuring flow in almost all regions; modified by the more recent introduction of radioactive markers and external monitoring, they continue to be among the most effective techniques. Alternatively, catheter-mounted electromagnetic or ultrasonic flowmeters can be used to measure blood flow in the artery supplying a particular vascular bed, an approach especially suited to following rapid changes in flow.

The physiological demands of daily life, not to mention threats from the external environment, could not be met without mechanisms for regulating blood flow, keeping it constant in some regions, and modifying it in others as necessary. This regulation is carried on through signals from the autonomic nervous system, blood-borne hormones, and local reactions intrinsic to the region, as outlined in Chapter 8. The specific signals and their relative importance vary from one vascular bed to another, but the phenomenon known as *autoregulation* is found in almost all regional circulations.

Autoregulation

One of the most common—and most puzzling—characteristics of circulatory control is the maintenance of constant blood flow through certain regional vascular beds in spite of changes in the arterial pressure. This highly effective mode of regulation remains after denervation of the vessels, and indeed can be seen in isolated perfused organs, proving that it is a property of the vascular bed and the tissue it supplies, not something imposed by the nervous system or other extrinsic sources. The phenomenon is therefore called vascular *auto-regulation*; the mechanism by which is operates is unknown. This mode of blood flow regulation should not be confused with the autoregulatory mechanisms of myocardial function described in Chapter 4.

Autoregulation can be demonstrated experimentally by gradually raising the arterial perfusion pressure of an isolated kidney while keeping venous pressure constant (Figure 6.8). Blood flow begins when arterial pressure rises above the *critical closing* level (Chapter 6) and then increases as pressure is raised further. At some point, however, usually at arterial pressures between 60 and 80 mm Hg, flow levels out and then remains constant in spite of continued increases in pressure. This plateau may persist up to perfusing pressure of 180 mm Hg or more, after which further increments in pressure are accompanied by some increase in flow. The maintenance, within limits, of constant flow while driving pressure is rising implies that the vascular resistance is increasing. Vessels somewhere in the bed are reducing their diameter, in other words, and the puzzling element is the mechanism of this response. Autoregulation can thus be defined physiologically as the adjustment of vascular resistance in a direction that tends to maintain constant blood flow when there is an alteration of blood pressure, an adjustment brought on by mechanisms as yet unidentified. The effective range of autoregulation varies among different organ systems, but it has been observed in skeletal muscle, cardiac muscle, brain, liver, kidney, and the mesentery. The range available for autoregulation in each system depends in part on local vascular tone (Chapter 8).

The arterioles are the site of the resistance changes that are needed for autoregulation, and the appropriate responses have been directly observed in such vessels. An example is shown in Figure 12.1, which reproduces records from experiments on mesenteric arterioles of the cat *in vivo*.[41] The experimental procedure was a stepwise *decrease* in arterial pressure, just the opposite of the renal example described above. After a control period, the arterial pressure was lowered in three steps. In the control state, mean arterial pressure was in the neighborhood of 130 mm Hg, and arteriolar diameter was approximately 25 μm. The first step lowered pressure slightly, and arteriolar diameter increased by a small amount. The second step (1.8 min on the time scale) reduced mean

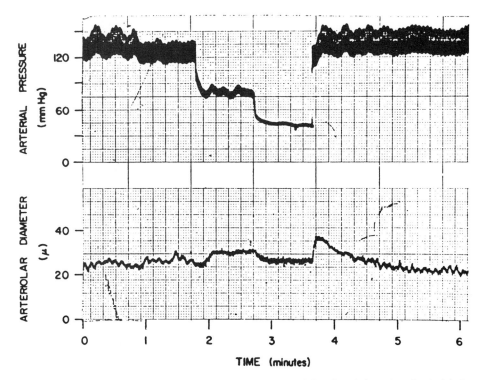

Figure 12.1. Records *in vivo* of systemic arterial pressure (*above*) and diameter of arteriole in feline mesentery (*below*), showing autoregulation. *Abscissa,* time in minutes. After a control period of approximately 1 min, the arterial pressure was lowered in three steps, each lasting slightly less than 1 min. First step lowered pressure by a small amount, and diameter increased slightly. Second step reduced mean arterial pressure to about 75 mm Hg, and the arteriole dilated to a diameter approximately 5 μm greater than in the control portion of the record. The third step lowered pressure to about 45 mm Hg; diameter decreased, but was still slightly greater than at the control pressure. When the clamp that had been used to lower arterial pressure was removed, the restoration of normal pressure was accompanied by a transient increase of diameter, showing that the vascular smooth muscle was more relaxed, and the vessel therefore more distensible, than had been the case in the earlier control state. Normal distensibility then returned slowly. (Reproduced from Johnson,[41] with permission of the American Heart Association)

arterial pressure to about 75 mm Hg, and the arteriole dilated to a diameter approximately 5 μm greater than in the control portion of the record. On the third step, mean pressure fell to about 45 mm Hg; the diameter decreased this time, but was still slightly greater than at the control pressure. In each case, the full response developed in approximately 10 sec. When the clamp that had been used to lower arterial pressure was removed, the restoration of normal pressure was accompanied by a transient increase in diameter, showing that the vascular smooth muscle was more relaxed, and the vessel therefore more

distensible, than had been the case in the earlier control state. Normal distensibility then returned slowly.

Experiments of this kind provide the most convincing evidence that autoregulation is an intrinsic response of some blood vessels. The arteriolar vasodilatation shown in Figure 12.1 when perfusing pressure falls is exactly opposite to the passive reduction in diameter that would ordinarily follow a lowering
of transmural pressure. On the other hand, the "overshoot" in diameter when
pressure was allowed to return to its normal high value is the response to be
expected when transmural pressure suddenly rises in a vessel that has become
more compliant during the preceding hypotensive periods. It must be added
that experimental results are not always as clear as those shown in the figure,
nor as consistent. Autoregulation is particularly sensitive to the experimental
arrangements and the condition of the preparation.

The three theories about the mechanism of autoregulation that have en-
joyed most popularity are referred to as the tissue pressure, metabolic, and
myogenic hypotheses. Attribution of the response to *tissue pressure* rests on
the assumption that extravascular forces pressing on the vessels are the controlling factor. It the tissue volume of an organ were constrained by a rigid
capsule, then an increase in pressure in the arteries contained therein would
tend to raise the extravascular pressure on all other vessels. The result, according to this argument, would be compression of the other vessels and an
increase in their resistance. The site of vascular compression could be arterioles and venules or, in another variant of the theory, an increase in extravascular fluid because of increased pressure in the capillaries.[12]

The structural arrangements essential to this explanation are present in
several organs. The kidney, with its relatively stiff capsule tightly packed with
tissue and fluid, seems to provide an ideal example of the architecture required,
and the decrease in renal blood flow observed when pressure is raised in the
renal vein or ureter is compatible with this theory. The brain has the most rigid
external constraint, of course, and most other organs are surrounded by limiting structures. Nevertheless, experimental support for the tissue pressure hypothesis has proved difficult to obtain, largely because of the artifacts and other
technical problems associated with measurements of tissue pressure. Although
this hypothesis still has its adherents, they are becoming fewer in number.

The *metabolic* theory attributes autoregulation to flow-dependent, local
concentrations of vasodilating metabolic products. The partial pressures of O_2
and CO_2 in the environment of the microcirculation, for example, are influenced by the rate at which blood flow delivers or removes them. This hypothesis asserts that flow is altered by metabolites in a way that keeps these tensions at a normal level. Whether the sensor is vascular smooth muscle or tissue
cells that respond to these respiratory gases by producing dilating metabolites

is not clear. The latter seems more likely because arterioles are apparently not affected by a simple change of pO_2 in their vicinity,[26] but the question remains open. Arterial hypoxia and hypercapnia certainly dilate a variety of systemic vascular beds and alter the contraction of large arteries *in vitro,* actions that may involve both direct smooth muscle stimulation and metabolic products. One variant of the metabolic theory postulates that pO_2 and pCO_2 *modulate* the strength of autoregulatory responses, which act through a separate, non-metabolic mechanism. Conflicting evidence for and against these hypotheses continues to appear, complicated by the fact that regional circulations vary considerably in their responsiveness to pO_2 and to various metabolites. The extreme sensitivity of the cerebral vasculature to CO_2, for instance, is not duplicated in other systemic vascular beds. The crucial experiment that would resolve the problem unequivocally has apparently not yet been conceived.

The *myogenic* hypothesis holds that vascular smooth muscle responds to stretching by increasing its contractile force, thus accounting for autoregulation. A quick stretch of any elastic structure to a new, constant length is necessarily accompanied by an equally rapid increment in force (Chapter 6); the *myogenic response* consists of a later, further development of force by the isometric muscle (Figure 9.3). This is in fact the oldest explanation for autoregulation, having been proposed by Bayliss in 1902 to explain his observations in the hind limbs of dogs and cats. The later discovery that smooth muscle in human umbilical arteries behaves this way[59] was followed by similar observations in smooth muscle of the intestine and bladder and in a few other blood vessels. The umbilical artery contains no neural elements, demonstrating that innervation is not required for the response.

In the umbilical artery, the initial peak force decays only slightly before the myogenic reaction intervenes. The details of the response vary in different vessels with respect to the speed and extent of stretch required and the duration of the myogenic contraction. In the umbilical artery, the phenomenon is elicited by a 25% stretch in 0.1 sec, occurs after a latency of 9 sec, and lasts for several minutes. Continuous autoregulation obviously requires more than a transient response, but normal arterial pulsations provide, after all, a repetitive mechanical stimulus. Some evidence suggests that periodic stretch by the pulse produces contraction in vascular smooth muscle, raising resistance.[50] The origin of the effect remains speculative, but stretching may stimulate the activity of pacemaker cells in the vascular smooth muscle. The existence of such pacemakers has been inferred from the spontaneous, rhythmic contractions seen frequently *in vitro* in portal, mesenteric, and other veins and occasionally in arteries. The portal vein responds to stretch with a burst of mechanical and electrical activity, although not with a clear, delayed myogenic force.[40]

One major obstacle stands in the way of the myogenic hypothesis as the explanation of autoregulation. If the myogenic activity that follows distention by an increased transmural pressure is to raise resistance and thus to autoregulate, it can do so only by constricting the vessel to less than its previous diameter, *removing* the stimulus. An increase in muscle length seems to be the change that evokes the myogenic reaction, but if the response is to maintain constancy of blood flow, then the muscle must shorten to less than its initial length. The stimulus for myogenic activity would then be gone, allowing the muscle to lengthen again, and it is difficult to see how a steady state could be established. Folkow suggested a way around this difficulty by assuming that an arteriole oscillates between relatively closed and open states, and that it becomes less open—on the average—during myogenic activity.[11] The distention needed as a stimulus still exists, the argument goes, but only in the brief open state. This idea is internally consistent, but one might expect the variations in caliber to be observable. Apart from oscillations in the venules of the bat wing *in vivo*, not associated with autoregulation, no such phenomena have been reported.

A more attractive solution is to postulate that the muscle senses *stress*, not length, as the stimulus for a myogenic response. This explanation recognizes that a rise in transmural pressure increases stress (force per unit area) in the wall as it distends the vessel, in accordance with the law of Laplace (Chapter 6), but it argues that transient, passive elastic stretching stimulates active shortening of the muscle. This myogenic shortening continues until a new balance is established between the vessel radius and the existing transmural pressure, in which the vessel has constricted but still has a higher wall stress than before it was stretched.

Cerebral Circulation

Anatomical considerations

Two anatomical features of the brain have particular relevance to the cerebral circulation: the rigidity of the skull and the complexity of the pathways for arterial inflow and venous outflow. The brain and spinal cord are enclosed in a bony compartment of constant volume, and the dura mater is almost indistensible. The intracranial tissues are virtually incompressible, and this arrangement makes it impossible for the total intravascular volume of the central nervous system to change significantly. Vasoconstriction or dilatation can occur in some regions of the brain, but they must be compensated for by opposite changes in some other part of the cerebral vasculature. Any increase in intracranial pressure affects the cerebral vessels, and the veins are particularly susceptible to such effects because their intravascular pressure is normally only slightly greater than that of the cerebrospinal fluid. The extravascular force exerted on microcirculatory vessels by elevated intracranial pressure can collapse them partially and bring into play the *waterfall* phenomenon (Chapters 6 and 11).

Arterial blood reaches the cerebral circulation in mammals through a number of different pathways, and venous outflow is even more complex. Four vessels, the paired carotid and vertebral arteries, supply the brain, and they interconnect through the circle of Willis. In man and the macaque, most of the arterial inflow travels through the internal carotids; occlusion of both common carotids in the neck causes unconsciousness in a few minutes. In the dog and cat, the vertebral and spinal arteries provide a larger proportion of total cerebral flow than they do in man. All of these arterial systems nourish various extracranial structures, as well as the brain. The vertebral arteries give off numerous branches, especially to the muscles of the neck, before entering the skull. The ophthalmic branch of the internal carotid supplies the orbit, ocular muscles, lacrimal gland, and part of the nasal mucosa. The external carotid communicates with cerebral arteries through a network of anastomoses in the cat and dog. The extensive plexuses of the vertebral veins can provide adequate venous flow even when the jugular veins are occluded.

This redundant system of multiple pathways provides a margin of safety in maintaining circulation to a crucial organ, but at the same time it makes difficult any experimental attempt to measure total blood flow through the brain. As in other organs, the behavior of large vessels, or superficial ones like the pial arteries, can be examined *in vitro* or *in vivo,* but the responses may differ from those in the microscopic vessels. Furthermore, measurements of total cerebral vascular resistance represent the net effect of changes that may not be similar in all parts of the brain.

Blood flow

Methods of measurement

Extensive measurements of cerebral blood flow in humans were first carried out by applying the Fick principle (Chapter 14). The subject inhales a low concentration of nitrous oxide (15%), and nitrous oxide concentrations are measured in a systemic artery and the jugular vein. Multiple blood samples are taken over a 10-min period, by which time equilibrium between brain tissue and venous blood has been reached. The arteriovenous nitrous oxide difference varies with time until equilibrium, and must therefore be integrated to determine the amount delivered to the brain during the collection period (equation 14.5). The coefficient defining the partition of nitrous oxide between blood and brain must be known from other experiments, so that the amount of gas taken up per gram of brain can be calculated from that coefficient and the venous concentration. The result is a measure of flow in milliliters of blood per unit tissue weight, usually expressed per 100 g of brain.[42]

Later investigators introduced the radioactive isotopes [85]Kr or ^{133}Xe as the inhaled gas, using the same basic principle. Breathed in very low concentrations through a closed circuit, these labels give blood flow measurements that do not differ significantly from those obtained with the nitrous oxide method. Whatever gas is used, the method assumes that the jugular venous bulb provides a representative sample of mixed cerebral venous blood, which is true in man for the cephalad portion of the vein.[42] The results are less accurate in species where a significant part of the jugular flow comes from extracranial tissues. Another technique of measuring cerebral blood flow, closely related in principle, is based on intra-arterial injection of ^{133}Xe dissolved in a small volume of saline. The washout of the isotope taken up by the brain is then followed for 10 to 15 min by an external array of radiation detectors.

In addition to these methods of measuring *total* cerebral blood flow, which continue to yield important information in research and clinical applications (especially when correlated with measurements of cerebral O_2 consumption), the recent addition of radiographic techniques for measuring *local* blood flow in small regions of the brain is an advance of major significance. Although the rigid enclosure of the brain limits changes in total cerebral blood volume, combinations of vasodilatation in one region and constriction in another are quite possible, and modern techniques show that they do occur. Maps of regional flow in the brain can be obtained by placing external detectors around the head before inhalation of ^{133}Xe, and a high degree of resolution has been achieved by arrangements containing as many as 250 detectors. Changes with time can be revealed by sequential images. The vast array of data is organized by a computer into a two-dimensional plot of a "slice" through the brain, making the procedure one form of *computer-assisted tomography* (Chapter 14). Local rates of blood flow can be identified by color coding in the final display.[60]

Normal values

The average cerebral blood flow in normal adult human subjects is 750 ml/min, or about 12% of the basal cardiac output. Brain weight is approximately 1400 g (roughly 2% of total body weight), and the normal range of flow per gram of brain tissue is about 46 to 62 ml/min 100 g (Figure 8.5). The brain thus resembles the myocardium and kidneys in having a relatively high flow per unit weight under basal conditions. Cerebral oxygen consumption in humans is normally 39 to 53 ml oxygen/min, averaging 3.3 ml oxygen/min per 100 g brain weight.

Brain function is sensitive to decreased cerebral blood flow, and the critical ischemia threshold is a flow of about 20 ml/min 100 g. At this rate, total extraction of the oxygen in arterial blood would just suffice to sustain normal cerebral metabolism.[12] Flow is not the only relevant factor, however, and unconsciousness can occur because of severe chemical disturbances even when flow is normal or increased, as in diabetic coma (Table 12.1). The mental state in clinical conditions correlates more closely with oxygen consumption than with blood flow. Confusion or other signs of mental impairment appear when cerebral oxygen consumption falls to 75% of normal,[42] and somatosensory afferent signals begin to fail below that level.[49] Complete cessation of blood flow during cardiac arrest or ventricular fibrillation precipitates immediate unconsciousness, and irreversible brain damage usually occurs within a matter of minutes. One of the primary objectives of cardiopulmonary resuscitation in those circumstances is to maintain some flow of oxygenated blood to the brain by cardiac "massage" and artificial respiration.

Localized responses

Local vasodilatation of specific parts of the brain during mental activity that involves those regions was reported long before the present sophisticated methods of measuring regional flow were available, and many examples of such *functional hyperemia* are now known. Shining a light on the retina causes a

Table 12.1.   Cerebral Blood Flow and O_2 Consumption in Human Subjects Under Various Conditions[a]

CONDITION	MEAN ARTERIAL PRESSURE (MM HG)	BLOOD FLOW (ML/MIN)	RESISTANCE (MM HG/ LITER MIN)	O_2 CONSUMPTION (ML/MIN)
Normal subjects (at rest)				
Breathing air	85	750	113	46
5–7% CO_2 in air	93	1293	72	46
Disease states				
Diabetic acidosis and coma	66	904	73	24
Hypertension (no cerebral complications)	155	778	199	47

[a]Breathing CO_2 causes cerebral vasodilatation. The vasomotor effect of hypercapnia is mediated by increased the hydrogen ion concentration, and other forms of acidosis cause similar vasodilatation. The change in cerebral blood flow depends on concomitant changes in arterial pressure. The high arterial pressure in essential hypertension is accompanied by cerebral vasoconstriction that keeps blood flow in the normal range, an example of autoregulation. (Calculated from data of Kety and Schmidt[42])

localized increase of blood flow in the visual area of the cerebral cortex; this response is not related to any change of blood pressure. The visual, sensorimotor, and auditory areas normally have greater blood flow than other regions, and the regional differences are abolished by anesthesia. In conscious subjects, localized vasomotor activity accompanies various emotional or mental stimuli.[42] Application of the ^{133}Xe method has shown that voluntary movement of the hand causes increased clearance of the isotope, implying increased flow, in the appropriate part of the motor cortex and premotor area, whereas merely *thinking* of moving the hand elevates flow in the premotor region only.[13] There is considerable evidence to indicate that local elevations of cerebral blood flow are closely tied to increased cell metabolism. Autoradiographic studies with a nonmetabolizable glucose analogue, for instance, show that it is taken up and phosphorylated more rapidly by active than by inactive brain cells.[58]

Control mechanisms

Changes in total cerebral blood flow associated with cognitive or motor functions of the brain are very small, and total flow remains almost constant in the face of physiological stresses that affect the rest of the circulation. Neural control is minor in comparison with responses to chemical stimuli and autoregulation.

Autoregulation

Cerebral blood flow is relatively independent of perfusing pressure over a range of about 60 to 150 mm Hg, although the regulation is not perfect and flow often rises slightly along with pressure.[10] Within the autoregulatory range, sudden changes in perfusion pressure are accompanied by transient changes of blood flow in the same direction, but the control state is reestablished in a few seconds. Below 60 mm Hg, flow falls along with pressure. Normal autoregulation can be impaired by brain injury or hypoxia. The mechanism of autoregulation is as debatable in this vascular bed as it is in others.

Metabolites

The cerebral circulation is extremely sensitive to the vasodilating effects of increased pCO_2 (Figure 12.2) and reacts in the opposite direction to hypocapnia. Such changes can be of considerable magnitude; inhalation of 5% CO_2 leads to a 50% increase in cerebral blood flow in humans. The influence of extracellular CO_2 tensions on vascular smooth muscle depends mainly on concomitant shifts of pH, however. Acidosis causes dilatation, and alkalosis the opposite, even in experiments where pCO_2 is kept constant.[43] The response to pH is rapid, developing fully in about 10 sec. O_2 tension also has an influence

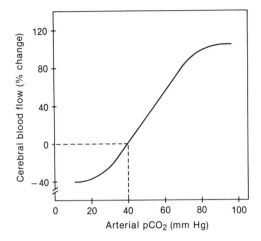

Figure 12.2. Relation between arterial pCO_2 (*abscissa*, mm Hg) and cerebral blood flow (*ordinate*, percent change from normal flow), measured in dogs. *Dashed lines* indicate average normal conditions. (After Harper[37] and Rowell[16])

on cerebrovascular resistance, and low partial pressures of O_2 in the arterial blood perfusing the brain increase cerebral blood flow by vasodilatation.

Once it was known that local vasodilatation and increased metabolism occur in regions of the brain that are being put to active use[38] (see above), the identity of the vasoactive agent was sought; the answer is still not certain. The usual suspects have been rounded up by analogy with the vasodilatation in exercising muscle: O_2, CO_2, pH, potassium, and adenosine. Metabolic changes in respiratory gas tensions and pH are rapid enough for the purpose, but are probably not large enough to be the full stimulus. Potassium dilates pial arteries, and the local concentration of this ion increases on electrical stimulation of the brain, but the rise is short-lived. Adenosine dilates superficial cerebral vessels when applied locally, and brain adenosine levels are greatly increased by ischemia, hypoxemia, or reduced perfusion pressure.[3] This purine nucleotide has the properties and effects required for the metabolic vasodilator, but unequivocal evidence that it is the agent responsible has yet to be found. It is entirely possible that all of these factors contribute to the response.

Neural control

Cerebral vessels are innervated by autonomic fibers, but their physiological functions are not clear and the neural supply is much less prominent than in extracranial vessels.[53] The response of cerebral vessels to stimulation of adrenergic nerves has been a matter of controversy for years, but the present consensus is that the sympathetic system sends no tonic sympathetic impulses to this vascular bed and has little or no part in its regulation. Sympathetic blockade does not alter cerebral blood flow, nor does baroreceptor[10] or chemoreceptor activity.

The evidence is mixed, however, and the older literature contains reports of localized, ipsilateral constriction of pial vessels upon stimulation of the cervical sympathetic ganglion in cats. This response is limited to a small region in the parietal cortex, and its significance remains obscure. In addition, some cerebral vessels, including the basilar artery, possess a small number of alpha-adrenergic receptors,[44] and catecholamine fluorescence has been demonstrated in pial arteries. Parts of the cerebral vasculature are thus capable of responding to adrenergic agonists, although they are less sensitive in this respect than other arteries. The existence in the basilar artery of an alpha-adrenoceptor with characteristics that differ from those of the alpha$_1$ and alpha$_2$ subtypes has been reported.[44]

Acetylcholine dilates the cerebrovascular bed, and there is morphological evidence of parasympathetic cholinergic innervation.[6] Specific histochemical markers of cholinergic terminals have been identified in the circle of Willis, as well as on the vertebral, internal carotid, and major spinal cord arteries, at least in the cat, rabbit, and dog.[28] Stimulation of the vagus nerve or local application of cholinergic agonists dilates pial arteries. Another source of cerebral vasodilatation is suggested by immunohistochemical studies showing the presence of VIP (Chapter 8) in some cerebral arteries,[45] where it appears to act by stimulating production of prostaglandins.

The blood-brain barrier

The function of capillaries in the brain differs in some respects from that in other organ systems. Substances can reach the extracellular environment by either of two routes. One is the capillary membrane exchange that exists in all tissues of the body, and the other is provided by the cerebrospinal fluid (CSF) that bathes the central nervous system. Both routes of access to brain tissue are restricted by mechanisms that are customarily referred to as the *blood-brain barrier*. As in other tissues, the cell membranes are relatively impermeable to lipid-insoluble substances in the extracellular fluid.

The principal source of CSF is secretion into the cerebral ventricles by the choroid plexuses, which are cauliflower-like projections containing arteriolar and capillary networks covered by a layer of epithelial cells. CSF is secreted continually, and it returns to the circulation from the subarachnoid space through villi that project into the venous sinuses. The CSF is generated from plasma by a selective mechanism, not simple diffusion; the concentration of Mg^{2+} is higher in CSF than in plasma, whereas that of K^+ and a number of other ions is lower. The choroid plexus epithelium where the cells bear some resemblance to those in renal tubules, is largely responsible for this selection.[5] This epithelial layer is tightly sealed and does not give passage to large molecules, even though the underlying capillaries are permeable to such substances as serum albumin. In contrast, the villi of the subarachnoid space allow egress of particles as large as 7 μm in diameter. The ependymal and pial linings of the ventricles are relatively permeable and could allow movement of solutes into the brain's extracellular fluid, but this transfer has been shown to be quantitatively of little significance. The function of the adrenergic and cholinergic nerves that innervate the choroid plexus is not known. CSF flow is augmented by agents that stimulate adenylcyclase, however, suggesting that it may be influenced by beta-adrenergic activity in the choroidal microcirculation. Capillaries in the brain substance also exhibit a selective permeability in the form of a carrier-mediated transfer of essential hexoses and amino acids from blood to brain, as well as from blood to CSF.[5] The exchange of glucose is described as *facilitated transfer* because plasma concentration influences the rate.

Intracranial pressure

Acute hypertension follows extreme elevation of intracranial pressure, an observation that has not diminished in importance since its description by Cushing[25] at the turn of the century. When CSF pressure is increased above its normal level of about 150 mm H_2O by a space-occupying brain tumor or an intracranial hemorrhage, one might expect that this extravascular force would compress intracranial vessels and increase the resistance of the cerebral vasculature. This does not happen with *moderate* increments of intracranial pressure, however. Neither cerebral blood flow nor arterial pressure changes, presumably an example of autoregulation, the arteriolar smooth muscle *relaxing* in response to *reduced* transmural pressure. Blood flow to the brain remains normal as transmural pressure falls, down to a point where the difference between intracranial and intra-arterial pressures is only 30 to 50 mm Hg.[35]

When intracranial pressure rises to extreme levels, a generalized, reflex vasoconstriction occurs by way of central nervous system centers, the *Cushing reflex,* and systemic arterial pressure rises. The critical CSF pressure has been estimated variously in different experiments, but it appears to lie between 50 and 80% of the systemic arterial pressure. The hypertensive response does not completely restore normal cerebral blood flow, but it makes the reduction less marked than would be the case without the reflex peripheral vasoconstriction. Human subjects with cerebral blood flows less than three-quarters of the normal value are usually confused or comatose, and death often follows.[35]

Coronary Circulation

Anatomy

Three major arteries supply blood to the heart in almost all mammals: the left anterior descending, left circumflex, and right coronary arteries. In most instances, the left coronary system supplies the left atrium and the anterior and lateral portion of the left ventricle; the right coronary artery delivers blood to the free wall of the right ventricle and to the right atrium. About 85% of total coronary blood flow is carried by the left coronary system in the dog and 15% in the right coronary system.[9,15] Anastomoses between the most distal parts of the two systems are abundant and range from 35 to 500 μm in diameter. The interventricular septum receives branches penetrating from the left anterior descending artery as it runs along the interventricular groove and from the posterior descending ramus. In the dog, rabbit, pig, and cow, but not in higher primates or man, a single septal artery directs 11 to 21% of left coronary flow to the septum. The sinoatrial and atrioventricular nodes in man are usually supplied by branches of the right coronary artery.

The posterior and inferior parts of the ventricles are regions where individual variations are common, and dominance of one of the major coronary branches depends on whether blood flow to this area comes from the left, right, or both arteries. The posterior descending branch, for example, may arise from the right or left circumflex arteries. *Left coronary dominance* is the rule in the dog, but that pattern appears in only about 20% of human subjects, the remainder showing either *right coronary dominance* or a balanced distribution.[9] The volume of the coronary vessels depends on arterial perfusion pressure; the capacity of the left coronary system is 11 ml blood per 100 left ventricle at a main coronary artery pressure of 70 mm Hg and almost twice that at 170 mm Hg.[15] As in other beds, the greatest part of this intravascular volume is in relatively large vessels.

The venous system of the heart consists of a superficial system of large veins, which drains most of the system, and a deep system of much smaller channels (Figure 12.3). The prominent coronary veins that parallel the arteries on the surface of the heart drain almost entirely into the coronary sinus and thence into the right atrium. Most of the flow through this sinus (about 90%) comes from the left coronary system. The anterior cardiac veins, which are visible on the epicardial surface of the right ventricle, empty directly into the right atrium. A large part of the right coronary flow drains through these veins and a smaller portion into the coronary sinus.

The deep venous system, which includes three classes of microvessels that empty into the cardiac chambers, carries only a small fraction of the total coronary blood flow,[51] perhaps 2%. *Thebesian veins* extend from some capillaries

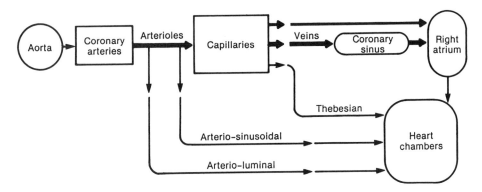

Figure 12.3. Pathways of blood flow through the vascular bed of the heart (see text).

or small vessels of the venous tree to the cavity of an atrium or ventricle. In a few branches of the left coronary system, including the septal and left atrial arteries, flow exits through Thebesian veins. *Arteriosinusoidal channels* consist of arterioles that lead into irregular, endothelial-lined spaces 50 to 200 μm in width. *Arterioluminal vessels* are communications between small coronary artery branches and one of the cardiac chambers. Capillary density in the myocardium is 3,000 to 4000/mm^2, much greater than in skeletal muscle. This concentration corresponds to an average of about one capillary for each muscle fiber,[4] and the capillary-to-cell diffusion distance is relatively small. Capillary density is some 15% lower in endocardial than in epicardial regions.

Blood flow

Methods

Coronary blood flow has been measured in many studies of unanesthetized animals and human subjects by the same nitrous oxide method[42] used for cerebral flow. The arteriovenous nitrous oxide difference is determined from samples taken through catheters placed in a systemic artery and in the coronary sinus. Care must be taken not to contaminate the venous sample with blood from the right atrium, where the nitrous oxide content may not be the same as in the myocardial venous drainage. As in the brain, flow is calculated from the blood gas concentrations and the partition coefficient, in this case the relative solubility of nitrous oxide in myocardium compared with blood. The blood flow measured is mainly that of the left ventricle, because the region drained by the coronary sinus is predominantly that supplied by the left coronary artery. Once coronary blood flow is known, myocardial O_2 uptake can be calculated from that value and the arteriovenous O_2 difference. Alternatively, blood flow through the heart can be determined by measuring the clearance of arterially injected isotopes with external detectors, using techniques similar to those already described for the cerebral circulation. The microsphere method (Chapter 14) has also been used to determine flow distribution in the ventricular wall. It shows that flow is slightly greater in subepicardial than in subendocardial layers.[15,20]

Normal values

Total coronary blood flow in resting adult human subjects averages 250 ml/min, or 4% of cardiac output. On the basis of heart weight, this is equivalent to about 0.6 ml blood/min/g. Total flow through the left ventricular myocardium averages 54 ml blood/min/100 g. These values represent the myocardial blood supply needed when the body is in a basal, resting state.

Under normal conditions, coronary blood flow and myocardial O_2 uptake are both closely correlated with heart rate and cardiac output (see below). O_2 consumption varies but ordinarily is 7 to 10 ml per 100 g heart muscle. The arteriovenous O_2 difference in the heart is normally higher than in other organs, 0.12 to 0.14 ml O_2/ml blood, giving blood from the coronary sinus a lower O_2 saturation than is found in most other veins. The minimal flow needed to sustain the metabolism of myocardial cells when they are *not* pumping blood has also been determined experimentally. When the ventricles are fibrillating or arrested by potassium solutions, and artificially perfused at the usual pressure by oxygenated blood, coronary oxygen uptake falls to 10 to 20% of its usual resting value.

Pulsatile flow

Flow in the main coronary arteries is pulsatile, as it is in all large arteries, and the pulsations have been recorded from vessels on the epicardial surface by electromagnetic and ultrasonic flowmeters. Surgically implanted miniature probes of such instruments can record coronary arterial flow from conscious, active animals.[15,24,34] The nature of the pulsations, shown in Figure 12.4, has been studied in detail in the dog, and the evidence indicates that the flow contours are similar in other mammals. The possibility that repeated pulsatile expansion has some myogenic effect on the vessels in this and other vascular beds[50] remains relatively unexplored.

Most of the flow in major coronary arteries occurs during diastole, differing in this respect from the flow to other organs. Diastolic flow normally amounts to about three-quarters of the total flow in each cardiac cycle, although this fraction is influenced to some extent by heart rate and force of ventricular contraction. Left coronary inflow reaches a peak early in diastole (Figure 12.4) and then falls gradually during the ventricular filling period. A

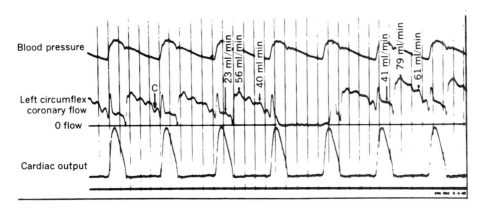

Figure 12.4. Aortic blood pressure, pulsatile blood flow in left circumflex coronary artery, and pulsatile flow in ascending aorta, in unanesthetized dog. Artery occluded temporarily in middle of record to determine zero flow signal. Numbers indicate flow rates at three instants in the cardiac cycle. Vertical time lines at intervals of 0.1 sec. Cardiac output = 4,116 ml/min; mean aortic pressure = 133 mm Hg; mean left circumflex coronary artery flow = 36 ml/min. (Reproduced from Gregg et al.,[34] with permission of the American Heart Association)

small, transient decrement in flow near the end of diastole has been observed in the left coronary arteries, apparently the effect of atrial systole. When ventricular contraction begins, flow drops abruptly, sometimes reversing direction briefly. Flow in a forward direction then rises to a peak and falls to a lower level throughout the remainder of systole.

This arterial flow pattern exists because the peripheral branches of the coronary tree lie within the ventricular walls, which compress the vessels as the cardiac muscle contracts. Pressure in the aortic root is the driving force for coronary flow, but the extravascular force exerted by myocardial contraction diminishes the caliber of intramural vessels during systole and raises coronary vascular resistance. The reduced flow during systole is related to the strength of ventricular contraction, as can be seen by the increased ratio of systolic to diastolic flow in animals with hemorrhagic shock and greatly reduced myocardial contractility. The suppression of systolic inflow is prominent in the left coronary bed, whereas right coronary flow is normally almost the same in systole as in early diastole,[48] a difference consistent with the magnitude of the pressures within the ventricular walls and chambers on the two sides of the heart. In abnormal states where right ventricular pressure is greatly elevated, the time course of right coronary flow begins to show the systolic reduction that is characteristic of the left side. The small arterial branches that supply the interventricular septum exhibit pulsations similar to those in the parent vessel, the left anterior descending artery, except that the transient retrograde flow is more marked and occurs slightly earlier in systole,[15] as might be expected from the early activation of septal muscle.

Venous blood flow in the left epicardial vessels is also pusatile, but flow is greatest during systole and drops to almost zero in diastole.[15] Inflow and outflow are thus exactly out of phase in the vascular bed of the left ventricle, and the volume of that bed must expand and contract appreciably with each heartbeat. The waveform of pulsatile flow in other veins has not been defined; venous branches over the anterior surface of the right ventricle are too small, and the Thebesian veins too deep, to be readily accessible for flow measurements.

Control mechanisms

The mechanisms for regulating the heart's blood supply are highly effective, for myocardial blood flow can increase greatly under the stresses of exercise. A fivefold increase in coronary blood flow has been reported in trained sled dogs during severe exercise.[62] Local metabolic products are the principal vasodilating agents involved. Neurogenic mechanisms also exist but appear to play a minor role. Myocardial metabolism is predominantly aerobic, no significant local O_2 debt can be incurred, and the high arteriovenous O_2 difference under basal conditions shows that the myocardium is already extracting some 70% of the O_2 delivered by the arterial blood. Increased coronary flow is thus the principal mechanism available for meeting the costs of any increase in cardiac work. A close matching of supply and demand is revealed by the direct correlation between coronary blood flow and myocardial O_2 consumption,[4,15] and much effort has been devoted to learning which hemodynamic variables influence the amount of O_2 required under various conditions. The specific factors that determine O_2 demand are still debatable.[4]

Myocardial oxygen requirements

The metabolic cost to the heart of exercise or other physiological stresses cannot be estimated reliably by a calculation of external cardiac work (Chapter 4). O_2 consumption is an index of metabolic rate, yet the highest rate of myocardial O_2 uptake occurs during isovolumic contraction, when *external* work is, by definition, zero. Two factors apparently determine the O_2 requirements of cardiac muscle, namely, the stress on ventricular walls (force per unit cross-sectional area) and the heart rate. This conclusion is supported by a variety of observations in dogs and man,[56] although it would be difficult to reach by exclusive concentration on the response to treadmill exercise, where rate, aortic pressure, cardiac output, work, coronary blood flow, and myocardial O_2 uptake all rise together.

A correlation between ventricular pressure and O_2 uptake was noted in early hemodynamic studies of exercise and led to the introduction of the *tension–time index*, an integral of pressure as a function of time. Later work confirmed the importance of the duration as well as the magnitude of pressure, but it became clear that wall *stress* is the critical variable,[56] meaning that wall thickness and chamber radius must be taken into account along with intraventricular pressure, applying Laplace's law (Chapter 6). Heart rate alone also correlates closely with myocardial O_2 consumption, presumably because a faster heart rate entails spending a greater part of each minute in contraction, in spite of the slight shortening of systole. A combined parameter called the *pressure–rate product* has been proposed as an empiric predictor of the metabolic needs of the myocardium.[54] The relevance of both variables has been demonstrated by studies of isometric, or static, exercise (e.g., supporting a weight of several kilograms), where blood pressure increases to a greater degree than heart rate, yet the correlation between pressure–rate product and myocardial O_2 consumption is the same as in bicycling or other dynamic exercise. The use of other experimental tools, including electrical pacing of the heart to vary the heart rate, suggests that cardiac output and external ventricular work themselves are not the crucial variables.[16]

Local mechanisms of control

The marked vasodilatation of the coronary bed that accompanies exercise is similar in many ways to that in contracting skeletal muscle, and speculation about the local stimulus has focused on the same list of metabolites: O_2, CO_2, pH, K^+, and the purine nucleotides.[7] The identity of the vasodilator substance remains unknown, but adenosine is the leading contender.

The question remains open because each of the metabolites satisfies the requirements in some respects and not in others, and the experimental data do not suffice to resolve the problem. Blood K^+ initially rises in tachycardia but does not maintain the elevated level needed to cause the sustained decrease of coronary resistance that is observed.[15] Experimental hypercapnia increases and hypocapnia decreases coronary flow,[7] but the role of endogenous CO_2 in coronary regulation has yet to be defined. Hypoxia elicits coronary vasodilatation, although the effect is not marked until arterial pO_2 falls below 50 mm Hg. It is difficult to know whether this response represents an action of pO_2 on vascular smooth muscle or on myocardial cells, considering the close tie between myocardial metabolic activity and coronary flow. A modest direct relaxation of coronary smooth muscle by low O_2 tensions appears to be the rule *in vitro*, some 5 to 20% reduction of force in experiments on drug-contracted coronary strips. Current evidence suggests that hypoxic vasodilatation is in general endothelium dependent and mediated by prostaglandins.[23]

Adenosine has for many years been suspected as the principal metabolic mediator of coronary vasodilatation, because its effects are potent and it is released into the myocardial circulation during ischemia and hypoxia of cardiac muscle.[3,4] The AMP and enzymes necessary for adenosine generation are present in the heart, and adenosine is normally found in myocardial cells and interstitium, but the site and mechanism of production are uncertain. Investigation of the process is hampered by the lack of consensus on methods of measuring intersitial adenosine and by the existence of a significant intracellular adenosine compartment. Adenylate cyclase is probably the adenosine receptor, suggesting a common final pathway with beta-adrenergic vasodilatation. The physiological mechanisms that control the level of adenosine in the interstitium have not been identified, but recently developed techniques show that it rises during systole and falls again in diastole.[15] Relaxation of strips in an organ bath by adenosine is inversely proportional to pO_2, suggesting an interaction between the effects of these two agents.[30]

Autoregulation

The coronary circulation exhibits an autoregulatory response, but the regulation is imperfect in the sense that coronary flow is not kept constant. Flow increases as perfusion pressure is raised, but in the range from 80 to 150 mm Hg the coronary resistance rises and makes the increase in flow smaller than would otherwise be expected.[4,15] Measurements of regional flows with radioactive microspheres indicate that the range of this regulation is not the same in all parts of the ventricular wall; it extends down to 40 mm Hg in epicardial regions but only to 70 mm Hg near the endocardium.[15]

Neural control

Coronary arteries are unquestionably well supplied with both sympathetic and parasympathetic nerve fibers, but the physiological significance of these fibers is difficult to assess.[7] Studies of neural control of the coronary circulation have been hampered by the virtual impossibility of stimulating coronary vasomotor fibers without activating at the same time the pathways that affect heart rate and myocardial contractility. The changes in coronary blood flow evoked by the latter, which have already been discussed, tend to obscure any evidence of purely neural responses in the smooth muscle of coronary vessels. For example, the coronary vasodilatation that follows stimulation of cardiac sympathetic nerves is not a direct neurogenic response of the vessels, but is largely the secondary effect of alterations in rate and myocardial performance. Myocardial blood flow actually *decreases* in the first few seconds of stellate ganglion stimulation before the cardiac effects develop and the aortic pressure, heart rate, and coronary flow begin to rise.

Nevertheless, in carefully designed experiments, it can be shown that sympathetic stimulation causes a nerve-mediated coronary vasoconstriction, and vagal stimulation causes a mild dilatation.[4,7,15] The relatively high degree of basal tone in coronary vessels is probably maintained in part by sympathetic constrictor impulses. Coronary vasoconstriction by sympathetic stimuli and catecholamine administration has been demonstrated in a variety of experiments. Coronary vascular resistance is increased by (1) concentrations of norepinephrine too low to affect pressure or rate; (2) sympathetic nerve stimulation after beta-adrenergic blockade; and (3) norepinephrine in potassium-arrested hearts. Alpha-adrenergic blockers prevent such constriction. Large doses of intravenous norepinephrine can produce coronary vasoconstriction even though myocardial activity and O_2 consumption are enhanced at the same time. The vasodilating action of parasympathetic nerves has been observed in similar experiments, although the responses are weak. Stimulation of the vagus nerve in perfused fibrillating hearts causes a small but distinct increase in coronary blood flow.[4]

The results of such functional studies show that coronary arterial smooth muscle possesses both alpha- and beta-adrenergic receptors. The enhancement of adrenergic constriction by beta-adrenergic blockade reveals the functioning of the alpha type, and dilatation of the coronary vascular bed by the beta-adrenergic agonist, isoproterenol, after potassium-induced arrest of the heart speaks for the presence of beta receptors. The use of selective drugs suggests that the latter are of the beta$_2$ subtype, in contrast to the mixed beta$_1$ and beta$_2$ population of myocardial cells. Whether these coronary beta$_2$ receptors, which generally mediate relaxation of vascular smooth muscle, are activated by stimulation of adrenergic nerves is a question that cannot be answered at present. Some evidence suggests that beta receptors dominate the response of very small coronary arterial branches to norepinephrine, whereas constriction by alpha-receptors is the rule in the larger vessels.

Circulation to the Skin

The skin is highly vascular and its vessels are richly innervated, appropriate characteristics in an organ that regulates body temperature and provides thermal insulation, not to mention protection against injury. Its arterial supply is through branches of deep vessels that penetrate layers of muscle before reaching the dermis. Arteriolar plexuses fed by a subdermal network of small arteries lie at a depth of about 1 mm in human skin and supply a profuse system of capillaries that loop up to the papillae of the corium. The capillaries drain into venules and a subpapillary layer of venous plexuses of relatively large capacity. Venous blood leaves the skin through one of the two sets of larger vessels: the superficial cutaneous veins or the deeper veins that in general parallel the arterial system. Arteriovenous anastomoses 20 to 40 μm in diameter are prominent in some parts of the circulation, especially in the nail beds and tips of fingers and toes.

The ability of the cutaneous bed to dilate and carry a large blood flow is a major element in thermoregulation of the body. Sweating is an additional human response to heat and shivering to cold, but the vasomotor reaction is the principal mechanism for adapting to high temperatures. The cutaneous vessels are capable of establishing marked gradients between the core temperature of the body and the environment.[16] Arterial blood cools relatively little in transit from the heart, and it reaches the hands and feet at 35° to 37° C under resting conditions in an environment that is not excessively hot or cold. The superficial veins are exposed and very effective at dissipating heat, whereas the deep veins are relatively insulated. Cutaneous veins and venous plexuses near the skin surface, with their large volume and slow velocity, are important sites of heat loss. Selective vasomotor activity in the cutaneous circulation can thus respond to hot environments by increasing blood flow near the body surface and decreasing it in deeper regions, a mechanism enhanced by the cooling effects of sweating. Exposure to cold elicits the opposite response. Because blood flow in the dermis is one means of thermoregulation, it is ordinarily far greater than would be required to satisfy the metabolic needs of the cutaneous tissue.

Blood flow

No completely satisfactory method of measuring total blood flow in the skin has been devised. Standard Fick procedures are impractical because it is virtually impossible to isolate an appropriate artery and vein, and heat is the only entity that can be said to be "cleared" more or less exclusively by the skin. Many studies have exploited the latter fact, using arteriovenous temperature difference and total heat exchange to calculate cutaneous flow.[16] Various other techniques for determining local flow have been described, none of them very accurate in absolute terms but some capable of detecting changes reliably. Determinations of thermal or electrical conductivity and clearance rates of dermally injected isotopes fall into this category. Venous occlusion plethysmography (Chapter 14) is probably the most useful method, although it cannot distinguish skin flow from that in muscle and bone. This limitation is minimal in the fingers, which contain relatively little muscle.

The rough estimates of total cutaneous blood flow obtained in spite of these problems range from 200 to 500 ml/min in normothermic human subjects. The *organ weight* involved is difficult to judge, but if we assume a skin thickness of 2.0 mm and a surface area of 1.8 m^2, the cutaneous volume[16] comes to 3600 cm^3. Blood flow is not uniform in all parts of the body, but these figures indicate an average total flow of around 10 ml/min per 100 g skin. Measurements of forearm blood flow suggest a lower value, approximately 2 ml/min/ 100 g to the skin and an equal amount to the forearm muscle.[16] External heating of the forearm raises cutaneous flow with little or no effect on the circulation to the underlying muscle. Maximum vasodilatation by heating can raise total cutaneous blood flow 10- to 20-fold, demonstrating the vast potential range of adjustment.[16] These extremes could not be reached without the increased cardiac output that is part of the physiological response to hot environments. Direct cooling of the skin to low temperatures can reduce local flow to virtually zero.

Investigation of constriction or dilatation in cutaneous vessels usually involves heating or cooling, and it is necessary to distinguish between direct and indirect ways of changing temperature. Local application of heat to the region being studied (*direct heating*) produces local vasodilatation in the skin by a direct effect on vascular smooth muscle. Cutaneous vessels are particularly sensitive to temperature, although vessels in other regions respond in this way to some extent. Direct heating of the body as a whole raises the temperature of most of the skin and eventually of the blood. The most common example of experimental *indirect heating* consists of placing one limb in hot water and observing the reflex vascular responses in the contralateral limb. In such experiments, the principal afferent arm of the reflex is the temperature of arterial blood perfusing the central nervous system.

The sensors responsible for reflex responses to thermal stress include those in the skin as well as those in the central nervous system, and the cutaneous elements quickly provide afferent signals when external temperature changes. Noncutaneous sensors for temperature regulation exist in the hypothalamus (Chapter 7), spinal cord, and probably skeletal muscle.[39] What they sense is referred to as the *core temperature,* which is not more than a few tenths of a degree Celsius different, in a steady state, from that conventionally measured in the sublingual space or rectum. When environmental and skin temperatures are raised, however, central venous blood temperatures may not approach skin temperature for 30 min or more.[16] Two sets of sensors are thus involved in thermoregulaton, a fast-acting system in the skin and a slower one in the hypothalamus and elsewhere.

Maximum cutaneous vasodilatation by direct whole-body heating causes a marked increase in heart rate and a modest enlargement of stroke volume, elevating cardiac output to perhaps twice its basal level. All of this increase in blood flow goes to the skin, and additional flow is diverted from the splanchnic and renal beds,[36] so that the end result can be delivery of 60% of the cardiac output to the skin. Cerebral blood flow changes little, if at all. Human thoracic and splanchnic blood volumes may fall as much as 600 ml with body heating; most of this blood is displaced to the venous system of the skin, with a corresponding increase in limb volume.[16] Arterial pressure tends to fall in the early stages of direct heating but then returns to its previous state.

Control mechanisms

Neural reflexes and local temperatures are the principal mechanisms of control for the cutaneous vascular bed. Autoregulation plays a relatively small part, but it does counteract the effects of hydrostatic pressure and maintain constant flow in the hand when the arm is raised or lowered vertically.[12] Sympathetic constrictor fibers innervate the cutaneous arterioles, and the smooth muscle of these vessels is plentifully supplied with alpha-, but not beta-adrenergic receptors. In neural environments the constrictor nerves maintain a high level of tone in what are called *apical* structures—the hands, feet, ears, and nose. Section or block of these nerves causes a marked increase in blood flow to the affected region, an observation that goes back to the beginnings of vasomotor physiology in 1852, when Claude Bernard noted such a response in the rabbit ear. A much lower degree of sympathetic tonic constriction exists in the skin of the trunk and limbs.

Vasomotor phenomena in the skin are for the most part related to the regulation of body temperature, but cutaneous arterioles are also involved in nonthermal reflexes like those generated by the arterial baroreceptors or changes in posture. The cutaneous bed is one of the efferent arms of such reflexes, and its resistance is altered by modulation of sympathetic constrictor tone. Cutaneous vasoconstriction in the cold is mediated by an increased frequency of sympathetic adrenergic impulses to the arterioles of the skin in virtually all parts of the body. The venous plexuses, unlike the arterioles, normally have little sympathetic tone but constrict at low temperatures. This response diverts blood flow to the deeper veins, which dilate with cold, shunting blood away from the surface when heat must be conserved.

Indirect heating reveals a difference in the vasomotor control of apical and nonapical parts of the body. Placing the legs in hot water, for example, rapidly leads to vasodilatation in both the hand (an apical region) and the forearm (nonapical), but the mechanisms are different. The response in the hand can be duplicated by sympathetic nerve block without heating, showing that it is caused by withdrawal of sympathetic constrictor tone. The reaction of the forearm differs in its time course and mechanism. In the absence of nerve block, blood flow in the skin of the forearm increases by 60% in the first few minutes of indirect heating. It remains constant for about 20 min and then begins to rise sharply, eventually reaching four times the control value. Blockade of the sympathetic innervation prevents this remarkable late increase in forearm flow,[16] indicating that nonapical structures like the forearm can call on some nerve-mediated mechanism of vasodilatation far more potent than suppression of constrictor impulses. Although this active dilatation is the principal means of human adaptation to hot environments, the nature of the process is not clear. It is less marked in other species.

Two possible sources of such dilatation have attracted particular attention: (1) activity of sympathetic dilator nerves and (2) a secretomotor process associated with sweat gland secretion. The results of interrupting sympathetic nerve pathways suggest that cholinergic sympathetic fibers may be the most important mechanism of cutaneous vasodilatation. In the skin of the forearm, sympathetic nerves must be intact for the maximum vasodilating response to indirect heat, yet the release of constrictor tone (presumably adrenergic) by nerve block alone causes a relatively small dilatation, as described above. These phenomena suggest an analogy with the sympathetic cholinergic vasodilatation of skeletal muscle in the defense reaction (Chapter 8). Nevertheless, vasodilatation in the skin, like that in exercising muscle, cannot be completely blocked by atropine. This makes it doubtful that the mechanism is entirely a direct cholinergic relaxation of vascular smooth muscle but raises the possibility of an indirect secretomotor reaction.

The phenomenon of vasodilatation in salivary glands (Chapter 8) is a reminder that cholinergic nerves can have indirect vascular effects through their action on secretory cells. The delayed, nerve-mediated rise in forearm flow described above begins at about the same time as sweating, which increases subsequently along with cutaneous blood flow. Microcirculatory vessels and sweat glands are in close proximity in the skin, and cholinergic stimulation of these glands causes them to release kallikrein, a precursor of bradykinin. The nerve-mediated event could, therefore, be activation of sweat glands, and the vasodilatation could be an effect of locally produced bradykinin. This attractive hypothesis does not quite fit the experimental findings, however. Most investigators have failed to find bradykinin in the venous effluent from limbs vasodilated by heat, but secretion of some unidentified vasoactive substance remains a strong possibility because active vasodilatation in the skin does not occur in subjects with congenital absence of sweat glands.[16] Adenosine, ATP, and prostaglandins are among the candidates being considered. Purinergic nerves have been proposed as the source of cutaneous vasodilatation in some species, but they have not been found in humans.

Splanchnic Circulation

The circulation of the gastrointestinal tract is, in effect, a single system in which the stomach, intestines, pancreas, spleen, and gallbladder receive arterial inflow from branches of the aorta and drain through the portal vein, liver, and hepatic veins.[14,17] The vasculature of these organs is referred to as the *splanch-nic* bed, from the Greek word for *viscera*. Blood flow through this system amounts to about one-quarter of the cardiac output at rest, and the splanchnic bed contains about one-fifth of the total blood volume. The urogenital organs, including the kidneys, are not considered to be parts of the splanchnic system.

Functional anatomy

Although various parts of the splanchnic circulation have their own large arteries and veins, all the venous blood normally flows into the portal vein and thus to the liver. The hepatic artery also supplies blood to the liver, and the total hepatic inflow—portal venous plus hepatic arterial—drains through the hepatic veins into the inferior vena cava (Figure 12.5). The portal vein subdivides into smaller branches in the liver, ending in venules that lead to the hepatic capillaries, which are actually large, irregularly shaped sinusoids. The hepatic arterial system terminates in arterioles that also enter the sinusoids, which consequently receive a mixture of arterial and venous blood. The sinusoids empty into efferent central venules of the liver lobules and thence into the hepatic venous system. Smooth muscle sphincters lie at the entrance of hepatic arterioles and portal venules into the sinusoids and at the sinusoidal exits.

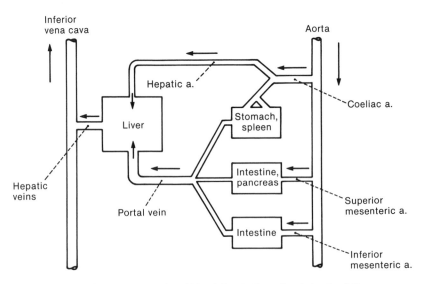

Figure 12.5.   Major paths of blood flow in the splanchnic circulation.

Hemodynamics

Splanchnic blood flow can be measured by application of the Fick principle, taking advantage of the fact that certain nontoxic dyes are extracted from the blood mainly by the liver. Perivascular flowmeters have also been used in experimental situations. Bromosulfophthalein and indocyanine green are commonly used as the dyes in man and other species. The dye is infused into a peripheral vein at a constant rate until equilibrium is established, at which time blood flow equals the amount infused per unit time divided by the arteriovenous concentration difference across the splanchnic bed (Chapter 14). A hepatic vein must be catheterized and a peripheral artery punctured to obtain the venous and arterial samples. Although the liver drains through several hepatic veins, there is no significant difference among them with respect to dye concentration.

Splanchnic blood flow averages 1500 ml/min in adult human subjects at rest. Maximum splanchnic vasoconstriction can reduce flow to 300 ml/min, and vasodilators can raise it to 2500 ml/min, indicating that considerable vascular tone exists in the basal state. A rough estimate of the subdivision of arterial inflow to the splanchnic organs is 60% to the intestines, 20% to the stomach, 10% to the pancreas, and 10% to the spleen, although those values are derived from the canine circulation, where splenic flow is larger than in man. The greater part of the blood supplied to the liver, 65 to 75%, comes from the portal vein and the remainder from the hepatic artery. Inasmuch as the venous blood leaving the liver has traversed two capillary beds in succession, one in the gastrointestinal tract and the other in the hepatic sinusoids, it cannot have exerted a pressure that completely balanced the colloid osmotic pressure of plasma in both of them. Intravascular pressures are about 26 mm Hg in the mesenteric capillaries, 6 to 12 mm Hg in the portal vein, and probably 2 to 6 mm Hg in the sinusoids. Lymphatic drainage from the liver is abundant, contributing one-fourth to one-half of the thoracic duct lymph flow.

The splanchnic vasculature, particularly the venous compartment, is a major blood reservoir that undergoes large changes in volume during reflex adjustments (Chapter 13). Human splanchnic blood volume is normally about 1 liter, 70% of it in the veins. As much as 40% of this volume can be displaced to other parts of the circulation by stimulation of splanchnic nerves, and similar shifts occur during exercise, heating, or hemorrhage. Blood redistribution of this kind has far-ranging effects elsewhere in the circulation, raising mean circulatory and ventricular filling pressures and furnishing a prime example of the importance of vascular capacitance in cardiovascular regulation. Changes in systemic venous pressure brought about by conditions external to the splanchnic bed can also influence its blood volume, which tends to rise passively when that pressure increases.

Control mechanisms

Liver

Autoregulation is the principal mode of control for blood flow through the liver. Even after hepatic denervation, total hepatic blood flow remains almost constant as arterial perfusion pressure is varied experimentally, and increased pressure in the hepatic or portal veins elicits hepatic arteriolar constriction. The portal venules do not share in this active constriction but are distended slightly by elevated hepatic venous pressure. This lack of active response is surprising because the portal and mesenteric veins are favorite vessels in the laboratory for demonstrating spontaneous contractions *in vitro*. The hepatic arterioles, representing a high-pressure source of sinusoidal inflow, must provide a relatively high resistance, and it is reasonable to assume that they are a major site of hepatic autoregulation. Nevertheless, considering the technical difficulty of measuring small pressure changes in the hepatic microcirculation, the possibility of regulation of hepatic venules cannot be ruled out at present.

The splanchnic arteries and veins are richly supplied with sympathetic adrenergic nerves, but these fibers are not tonically active. The basal tone is apparently the result of an autoregulatory process, which is probably myogenic. Nevertheless, the sympathetic pathways are capable of constricting splanchnic vessels. Stimulation of sympathetic nerves to the liver raises hepatic arterial resistance, but that response is transient, probably because autoregulation supervenes. Portal venous pressure is increased by sympathetic nerve stimulation, and here the response is maintained without "escape." Splanchnic veins in general have a heavy sympathetic innervation, and respond to reflex stimuli in the same way as the resistance vessels of skeletal muscle and kidney.[18]

Functional evidence indicates that both alpha- and beta-adrenergic receptors are plentiful in the smooth muscle of splanchnic vessels. Epinephrine in low concentrations vasodilates splanchnic arterioles, greatly increasing regional blood flow. If exogenous epinephrine is given in high doses, however, alpha-adrenergic effects predominate and splanchnic resistance is increased. Alpha-adrenergic venoconstriction has been thought to be the mediator of displacement of blood from the splanchnic region, but recent evidence raises doubts about that assumption. In some experiments on conscious dogs, beta-adrenergic receptor activation reduced the overall compliance of the systemic circulation to a greater extent than alpha-adrenergic stimulation did,[22] an unexpected result because beta-adrenergic agonists dilate vessels in many other regions. More information about this phenomenon is needed to clarify the role of adrenergic mechanisms in the regulation of venous blood volume.

In the realm of blood-borne agents, epinephrine is probably the only cir-

culating hormone that affects the splanchnic vascular bed, causing beta-adrenergic vasodilatation during severe stress. Angiotensin-II constricts the vessels,
as it does in other regions, but in man it does not normally appear in concentrations high enough to produce that effect. Vasodilating paracrine substances
are plentiful in the gastrointestinal tract, including substances released by the
mucosal glands and stimulated by the digestive process. Increased hepatic metabolism does not seem to be accompanied by local vasodilatation, as shown
by the absence of a significant change in hepatic blood flow when the liver is
stimulated by glucose, insulin, or glucagon. Cholinergic vasodilatation has not
been observed in hepatic vessels, but the release of cholinergic or peptidergic
neurotransmitters from sympathetic fibers that supply glands of the gastrointestinal mucosa initiates a secretomotor process in that region. Muscarinic cholinergic receptors have been demonstrated by radioisotope binding in the
canine portal vein, where they mediate contraction *in vitro,* but their function
in the intact animal is obscure.[52]

In some species, the splenic capsule and trabeculae contain smooth muscle, and stimulation of local sympathetic nerves expels blood from the spleen
into the general circulation. This phenomenon is prominent in the dog during
exercise or after hemorrhage, but it has not been demonstrated in humans.

Gastrointestinal tract

An overall picture of the intestinal vasculature is given by the estimated
dimensions of the canine mesenteric vascular tree listed in Table 1.1. The blood
supply of the stomach and intestines is distinguished by a great number of arterial arcades, an anastomotic system that protects the perfusion of each local
segment of the tract. Experimental ligation of more than 90% of the gastric
arteries, for example, has little effect on function.[12] The mucosal, submucosal,
and muscular layers of the gastrointestinal tract have more or less separate
systems of arterioles and venules, providing a mechanism for shunting and control of local capillary pressures. A dense capillary network lies beneath the
epithelium of the villi.

The stomach and intestines receive innervation from the sympathetic and
parasympathetic systems. Adrenergic terminals revealed by the fluorescence
technique show innervation of both precapillary and postcapillary vessels, with
the greatest density on the arteriolar side. Stimulation of regional sympathetic
nerves causes vasoconstriction, but after a few minutes flow returns almost to
the control level. This "escape" from neural control is probably the result of
autoregulation, as it is in the liver, although some investigators suspect that
beta-adrenergic receptor activation plays a part. The parasympathetic innervation affects secretion and motility, but the existence of true parasympathetic
dilator fibers to the blood vessels is uncertain. Stimulation of the vagus nerve

can increase blood flow in the gastric mucosa, but this response may be due to the secretion of kinins rather than to direct vasomotor activity.

The presence of food in the gastrointestinal tract induces regional vasodilatation, and splanchnic blood flow increases greatly after a meal. The mechanism for this response has not been precisely defined, but it is temporally related to gastrointestinal secretions. Production of gastrin by the stomach is accompanied by increased blood flow in the gastric wall. Secretin and cholecystokinin-pancreozymin, peptides released by the mucosa of the duodenum and upper intestine, induce hyperemia of small intestine. The question still to be answered is whether these substances act directly on vascular smooth muscle or indirectly by way of vasodilating metabolites. The analogous problem in the salivary glands and skin is discussed elsewhere in this chapter. The increased blood flow is almost entirely through the mucosa, not the muscular layers of the gut, which in a nondigestive state receive only about 20% of the gastrointestinal flow.[12,17]

Renal Circulation

A relatively large amount of blood flows to the kidneys in accordance with their function as regulators of the chemical composition of blood plasma, and the homestasis of body fluids is as important when the body is at rest as it is in the face of severe physiological demands. It is consequently appropriate that the renal vascular bed is unique in being almost fully vasodilated under normal resting conditions. Renal blood flow is usually kept constant by autoregulation, but during extreme bodily stress caused by severe exercise, heat, or hemorrhage, it may fall to less than half of its normal level.

Vascular patterns

The architecture of the renal bed conveys blood first to capillaries coiled within renal glomeruli and then to other capillary vessels that invest the tubules and collecting ducts.[21] Branches of the renal artery within the substance of the kidney lead to arcuate vessels at the corticomedullary border, which in turn give off branches that supply the afferent arterioles to glomeruli (Figure 12.6). The glomeruli, numbering about 1.6×10^6 in a human kidney, each receive flow from a single arteriole in most cases. The distal portion of the afferent arteriole lies near the juxtaglomerular apparatus, which was discussed in connection with the production of renin (Chapter 8), and close to distal tubules that loop back toward the cortex. The glomerular tuft itself is a web of capillaries of the fenestrated type, with pores some 0.1 μm in diameter (Figure 12.7).

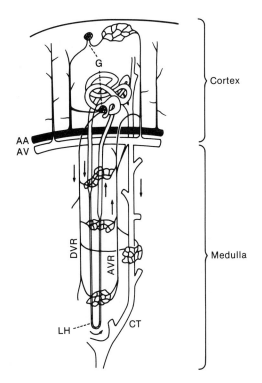

Figure 12.6. Schematic diagram of arrangement of intrarenal blood vessels, showing two glomerular capillary tufts (*G*) and the tubules associated with one of them. *AA*, arcuate artery; *AV*, arcuate vein; *DVR*, descending vasa recta; *AVR*, ascending vasa recta; *LH*, loop of Henle; *CT*, collecting tubule. See text for details. (Based on data published by Barger and Herd,[2] Johnson,[11] Beeuwkes,[21] and other sources)

The *lamina densa*, a basement membrane just external to the endothelial walls, is the site of ultrafiltration to the interstitial space and thence to the tubules. Studies of the permeability of this membrane show that it allows passage of molecules up to perhaps 9 nm in size.[32] Roughly 20% of the plasma in the glomerular capillaries filters through the membrane, and the remaining blood exits through efferent arterioles that eventually feed secondary capillary beds, some of them around proximal tubules and others investing distal tubules or collecting ducts in the renal medulla.

Efferent arterioles leaving glomeruli in the outer cortex ascend to lie near the renal surface before splitting into capillaries and creating a capillary plexus. Efferent arterioles from glomeruli near the corticomedullary boundary travel down through the medulla as *descending vasa recta*, which branch and turn at various levels into capillary plexuses and then *ascending vasa recta*. The de-

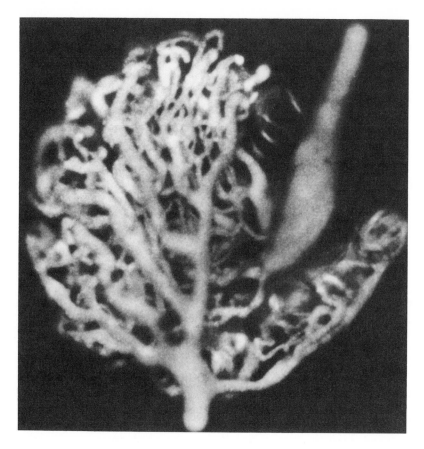

Figure 12.7. Renal glomerular capillary vessels after silicone rubber injection. (Reproduced from Barger and Herd,[2] with permission of the *N. Engl. J. Med.*)

scending vasa recta maintain the character of arterioles, having a layer of smooth muscle and a diameter of 10 to 20 μm. The ascending vessels are essentially a continuation of the peritubular capillaries and plexuses, with a fenestrated endothelium.[64] The two sets of vasa recta, descending and ascending, form bundles that are adjacent to collecting ducts and enveloped by the loops of Henle, providing the anatomical substrate for the countercurrent mechanism that regulates the exchange of water and solutes between the renal circulation and the tubules. In addition, the interconnecting capillaries and ascending vessels remove from the medulla substances that have been reabsorbed. Venous drainage is through interlobular and interlobar veins that parallel the arteries. Vasomotor nerve fibers are found throughout the renal vascular bed, but they are more prominent in the cortex than in the medulla.

Hemodynamics

Blood flow

Total blood flow to the kidney can be determined with modern perivascular flowmeters, but this vascular bed also provides ideal conditions for the Fick method because some solutes are almost completely removed from the blood as they pass through the renal circulation. The substance most often used in the measurement of renal blood flow is p-aminohippurate (PAH). Approximately 95% of the PAH that enters the renal artery leaves the plasma and appears in the urine, 20% being filtered through the glomerular membrane into the proximal tubules and 75% secreted from peritubular capillaries into the tubular lumen. The product of urinary PAH concentration (U) and the volume of urine formed per minute (V) form the numerator for the standard Fick equation, and the renal arteriovenous difference in PAH concentrations ($C_A - C_V$) is its denominator, so that renal blood flow (RBF) can be calculated by

$$RBF = \frac{UV}{k(C_A - C_V)} \tag{12.1}$$

where k is the fraction of PAH cleared by the kidneys (e.g., 0.95). Arterial and urinary PAH concentrations must be measured, but venous PAH concentration is usually very low and sometimes neglected. The PAH concentrations are measured in plasma but must be expressed as milligrams per milliliter of blood in equation 12.1, taking into account the hematocrit. Measurements obtained by this method agree closely with those from an electromagnetic flowmeter on the renal artery.[57]

Total renal blood flow through the two kidneys in adult humans at rest is typically 1200 ml/min, or about one-fifth of the cardiac output. The combined weight of both kidneys is approximately 300 g, making renal blood flow 400 ml blood/min per 100 g kidney on the average, greater than that for other major organs. The need for such a high flow arises from the kidney's excretory function and its regulation of water and electrolyte balance, not from the metabolic requirements of the renal cells alone. The amount of fluid filtered from the glomeruli into the urine, or *glomerular filtration rate,* is approximately 120 ml/min under normal conditions. Renal arterial flow is not distributed uniformly to all parts of the kidney. Regional flows within the organ have been determined by indicator dilution, microsphere distribution, and radioisotope techniques,[64] and the results uniformly show that the cortex receives the greater part of the renal blood flow. Typical figures for the distribution of renal arterial inflow are 75 to 85% to the cortex, 10 to 22% to the medulla, and 1 to 3% to the papilla.[61,64]

The renal arteriovenous O_2 difference is relatively small over a wide range of renal blood flows, about 1.3 ml/100 ml blood, and the O_2 uptake per unit weight is moderate, 5.3 ml/100 g kidney tissue. When blood flow is seriously reduced, as in shock, the organ does not extract more O_2 but curtails oxidative metabolism. The total volume of the renal vascular bed is not known with certainty because the results of various methods used to measure it do not agree. Some experiments based on mean transit time and renal blood flow (Chapter 14) and others using radioisotope-labeled red cells or plasma place the value in the neighborhood of 25 ml blood/100 g kidney, but higher and lower volumes have been reported.

Some feature of the postglomerular microcirculation produces a hematocrit in the vasa recta that is only half that found in the general systemic circulation.[63] That observation implies some degree of divergence in cell and plasma pathways and a relatively rapid transit of red cells. The video-microscopy techniques devised to measure flow in single vessels (Chapter 14) show average red cell velocities of 1.4 mm/sec in the descending vessels and 0.5 mm/sec in the ascending vessels.[64]

Pressures

The presence of two consecutive capillary beds, glomerular and peritubular, each preceded by arterioles, establishes a sequence of pressures that is a central factor in renal function. The formidable problems of measuring pressure in these minute vessels have gradually been overcome by applying micropuncture to the kidney of the rat.[31,33] Technical problems remain, however, and estimates of pressure at the afferent arteriolar entrance to the glomerular capillary range from 50 to 85 mm Hg at normal renal arterial pressures. All investigators agree that the subsequent pressure gradient across the glomerular tuft of capillaries is only a few millimeters of mercury. The resistance of the efferent arterioles appears to be fairly high, reducing pressure to about 12 mm Hg in the peritubular capillaries. Blood thus reaches glomeruli at a relatively high pressure for filtration, whereas the peritubular capillary bed, where reabsorption is a major function, is a low-pressure system. Many attempts have been made to compare intravascular pressures with those in the interstitium and in the tubules because of the importance of these variables to renal function, but the gradients are so small that it is difficult to place much confidence in the results.

Control mechanisms

Autoregulation of the renal circulation is the most frequently cited example of that mode of vascular control. It regulates renal blood flow effectively at arterial pressures from 80 to 150 mm Hg, although medullary blood flow tends to rise at pressures above 120 mm Hg. The relative indistensibility of the renal capsule was one of the arguments offered in support of the *tissue pressure* hypothesis of autoregulation, although that theory is not now widely accepted.

Sympathetic and endocrine mechanisms also have a part to play. Although the renal vascular bed is well dilated under normal conditions (Figure 8.5), a certain amount of nerve-mediated basal constrictor tone exists. This is shown by the increase in renal blood flow that follows denervation of the kidney, a response attributable to withdrawal of constrictor tone. The intact sympathetic pathways are, moreover, quite capable of bringing about renal vasoconstriction. Baroreceptor, thermoregulatory, and postural reflexes that call for increased systemic resistance impinge on the vessels of the kidney as well as other organs, although the renal constriction is much less marked than that of the splanchnic vasculature, and autoregulation tends to prevent much change in renal blood flow.

Afferent and efferent glomerular arterioles both receive sympathetic adrenergic constrictor fibers, but the innervation is dense in the afferent vessels and relatively sparse in the efferent vessels. The relative resistance in these two sets of arterioles is a major factor in the regulation of glomerular capillary pressure, which is jealously guarded to maintain a constant filtration rate. Afferent arteriolar dilatation combined with efferent constriction can compensate for a fall in arterial perfusing pressure, for example, maintaining constant pressure in the glomerular capillaries. The neural pathways that control vascular resistance at the entrance to the glomerulus are presumably separate from those at the exit.

Moderate stresses may reduce renal blood flow slightly but leave filtration rate unchanged. For example, passive tilting from the supine to an 80° head-up position can cause a detectable reduction of blood flow to the kidney, but the filtration fraction rises to maintain the filtration rate. Only in extreme emergencies like severe hemorrhage, strenuous exercise, or deep anesthesia are renal blood flow and filtration rate sacrificed in favor of preserving circulation to the brain and myocardium. When neural constriction occurs in the renal vascular bed, it is mediated by alpha-adrenergic receptors. Circulating epinephrine and norepinephrine both produce renal vasoconstriction, suggesting that very little of the adrenergic receptor population is of the beta type. Large doses of these catecholamines also constrict renal veins and raise the pressure in peritubular capillaries. Neither sympathetic nor parasympathetic cholinergic fibers are found in the kidney, and no direct neural mechanism of renal vasodilatation is known.

Stimulation of sympathetic nerves to the kidney or infusion of norepinephrine causes the release of renin along with constriction of glomerular arterioles, but whether this is a direct action on juxtaglomerular cells or a consequence of the vascular effect is uncertain. This response, together with the involvement of renin release in baroreceptor and other reflexes, demonstrates that the renin system is affected by sympathetic activity. Angiotensin-II, the vasoactive end product of renin release (Chapter 8), is a potent constrictor of the renal vascular bed, as it is throughout the systemic circulation. In adequate concentrations, it causes a distinct reduction of blood flow to the kidney. The same is true of ADH, which not only enhances the concentration of urine but also acts as a vasoconstrictor on the renal and other vascular beds. The relative effects of angiotensin-II and ADH on cortical as contrasted with medullary blood flow are controversial.

Extreme renal vasodilatation can be produced by only a few exogenous substances, notably pyrogens that cause hypertension, fever, and a marked increase in renal blood flow with no change in filtration rate. The same response can be observed in sympathectomized subjects, indicating that the pyrogens act directly on the smooth muscle of renal vessels. Infusions of acetylcholine or bradykinin also increase blood flow to the kidney. The possibility of vasodilatation by locally produced prostaglandins is under investigation, but the evidence for it is equivocal at present. The vasodilator prostaglandins PGE_2 and $PGF_{2\alpha}$ are synthesized by cells in the interstitium of the kidney, and their production is increased by angiotensin-II[64] suggesting that they may counteract local vasoconstriction under some physiological conditions. In addition, recent evidence indicates that renal prostaglandins act directly on juxtaglomerular cells, not as the primary stimulus for renin secretion but as a modulator of its rate.[29] To complicate the situation further, the beta-adrenergic agonist isoproterenol stimulates renin release, even when renal perfusion pressure is held constant, and some investigators believe that prostaglandins are involved in this response.

Skeletal Muscle

The most striking fact about the circulatory supply of blood to skeletal muscle is the enormous range over which it can be varied by physiological controls. In no other organ system can blood flow be increased to the extent that it is in exercising muscle. Local "metabolites" are the principal agents of dilatation in this vascular bed, but the vessels also respond to neural stimuli. The full explanation of muscle vasodilatation in exercise remains a subject of debate.

The pattern of the vascular tree is relatively simple. Branches of the large regional arteries pierce individual muscles and subdivide repeatedly to give small arteries that run parallel to the muscle fibers. Subsequent branching at oblique or right angles leads to a conventional arteriolar-capillary-venular microcirculation (Chapter 10). The capillary network is extensive, but the various types of muscle fibers that have been identified morphologically and histo-chemically (*red, white,* and *intermediate*) differ in diameter, so that capillary density is greater for some types than others (i.e., the number of capillaries per unit muscle cross section is greater in some muscles than others). Small, slow-acting muscle fibers have the highest capillary density and hence the shortest diffusion distance, as well as the greatest blood flow per unit. They also have a tortuous capillary mesh with many anastomoses surrounding each fiber. The soleus is an example of a tonic leg muscle made up predominantly of such fibers. Large fibers in which contraction is faster and shorter in duration have a less prominent capillary supply.[27]

Blood flow

Blood flow to skeletal muscles is difficult to measure *in vivo* with any accuracy. Most methods estimate flow to a limb or portion thereof, in which muscle is the dominant tissue mass but skin, bone, and connective tissue are included. Cooling the skin reduces the cutaneous component. Muscle alone is involved in techniques that measure the clearance of an intramuscularly in-jected isotope, but the results are influenced by a number of factors other than blood flow. The indicator-dilution method is the most satisfactory approach at present, using constant infusion of a dye or other indicator. This procedure can give fairly accurate estimates of flow during muscular exertion as long as skin flow is constant. Blood flow to the human leg, for example, has been measured during exercise by injecting cold saline continuously into the femoral vein and recording the temperature downstream with a thermistor.[19]

Blood flow to the approximately 30-kg mass of skeletal muscle in adult human subjects at rest is 800 to 1200 ml/min. This regional circulation therefore receives approximately one-fifth of the cardiac output when muscular exertion is at a minimum, but during heavy exercise 80 to 85% of the output goes to skeletal muscle.[16] Individuals differ greatly in the maximal cardiac output they can generate, the range in young adults being 20 to 40 liters/min (the latter only in highly trained athletes). Moreover, only about half of the total muscle mass is actively engaged during running, the form of exercise most frequently stud-ied. Blood flow to working muscle can thus rise from its basal level of about 33 ml/min per kilogram of muscle to at least 1000 ml/min kg. This value is much greater than early published estimates but is consistent with recent measure-ments by the microsphere method in exercising rats[46] and with observations based on thermodilution in man. Blood flow in the muscles that extend the knee was increased to 2500 ml/min kg muscle in one set of experiments on human subjects.[19]

The basal level of O_2 consumption by skeletal muscle in man is about 70 ml/min, or 2.3 ml/min per kilogram of muscle, and that value can increase well over 50-fold during severe exercise. Blood flow increases in the active muscles as a function of the intensity of exertion, and O_2 uptake of 350 ml/min per kilogram of exercising leg muscle have been reported.[19] Each kilogram of muscle uses only about 1% of the O_2 taken up by the lungs at rest but a vastly greater percentage during exercise. The blood volume of the muscle bed under basal conditions is 20 to 30 ml per kilogram of skeletal muscle in most experimental animals, about 70% of it in the veins.[47] The volume of this venous compartment changes only slightly with perfusion pressure, indicating that it plays little part as a blood reservoir.

Control mechanisms

Autoregulation operates effectively in resting skeletal muscle; as perfusion pressure is raised from 60 to 120 mm Hg, blood flow increases by only about 20%.[12] Mechanisms for neural control also exist in that the arterioles of skeletal muscle have a rich sympathetic innervation, although the venules have relatively little. Stimulating the sympathetic nerves can reduce muscle blood flow by 75%, confirming the presence of constrictor fibers, and interrupting them causes a twofold increase in flow, showing that some degree of tonic constrictor activity existed before the interruption. The constriction is mediated by alpha-adrenergic receptors, and when those receptors are blocked pharmacologically, sympathetic nerve stimulation *increases* muscle blood flow, although not nearly as much as exercise does. Infusion of acetylcholine has essentially the same effect, and atropine distinctly reduces the nerve-stimulated vasodilatation (although it does not completely prevent it), leading to the conclusion that sympathetic cholinergic dilator fibers supply vessels in the skeletal muscle bed. These dilator nerves play a part in the defense reaction (Chapter 8) but are probably of little importance during sustained exercise.

Although sympathetic adrenergic activity in the vascular bed of skeletal muscle is not an important element in the response to exercise, it plays a significant part in many reflex responses. Anything that elicits a general increase in systemic peripheral resistance calls forth a similar response in muscle. Even metabolic dilatation of the muscle bed can be reduced by sympathetic constrictor stimulation. The veins of skeletal muscle, on the other hand, apparently possess only a meager alpha-adrenergic receptor population, and stimulation of the sympathetic chains produces no more than mild venoconstriction, contrasting sharply with the marked reactivity of superficial cutaneous veins.[18]

One of the most curious vasomotor phenomena in the vascular bed of skeletal muscle is the effect of cholinergic stimulation on O_2 uptake by muscle. Blood flow increases, but venous O_2 saturation rises and O_2 uptake falls in spite of the greater amount being delivered per unit time, as if arteriovenous shunts had opened and bypassed the capillaries.[55] The response is quite different from that which accompanies exercise, and it constitutes one of the many arguments against a neural origin of exercise vasodilatation. One theory holds that neurogenic vasodilatation relaxes the arteriolar smooth muscle and lowers vascular resistance but does not affect the total number of capillaries open, perhaps because it fails to act on precapillary sphincters.[16] The metabolites of muscle activity presumably do both.

Abundant evidence supports the conclusion that products of local metabolism are responsible for most of the vasodilatation in active skeletal muscle, as they are in the myocardium. Just which products are the active ones remains a moot question, however. Blood osmolarity rises and muscle cells release potassium as soon as contraction begins, but neither of these factors follows a time course that would account for more than the first few minutes of vasodilatation. Adenosine and ATP are among the substances that could produce prolonged vasodilatation, as either nerve-released or paracrine agents. The possibility of secondary regional production of a vasodilating prostaglandin is being actively explored.

References

Reviews

1. Abramson, D.I., Dobrin, P.D. (eds.) (1984). *Blood Vessels and Lymphatics in Organ Systems*. London, Academic Press.

2. Barger, A.C., Herd, J.A. (1971). The renal circulation. *N. Engl. J. Med.* 284:482–490.

3. Berne, R.M., Rall, T.W., Rubio, R. (eds.) (1983). *Regulatory Function of Adenosine*. Boston, Martinus Nijhoff.

4. Berne, R.M., Rubio, R. (1979). Coronary circulation. In: *Handbook of Physiology, Section 2: The Cardiovascular System. Vol. I, The Heart*, R.M. Berne, and N. Sperelakis, eds. Bethesda, Md., American Physiological Society, pp. 873–952.

5. Davson, H. (1976). The blood-brain barier. *J. Physiol.* 255:1–28.

6. Edvinsson, L. (1975). Neurogenic mechanisms in the cerebrovascular bed. *Acta Physiol. Scand.* 427(Suppl):5–35.

7. Feigl, E.O. (1983). Coronary physiology. *Physiol. Rev.* 63:1–205.

8. Greenway, C.V., Stark, R.D. (1971). Hepatic vascular bed. *Physiol. Rev.* 51:23–65.

9. Gregg, D.E., Fisher, L.C. (1963). Blood supply to the heart. In: *Handbook of*

Physiology, Circulation, Vol. 2, W.R. Hamilton and P. Dow, eds. Baltimore, Williams & Wilkins, pp. 1517–1584.

10. Heistad, D.D., Kontos, H.A. (1983). Cerebral circulation. In: *Handbook of Physiology. The Cardiovascular System. Peripheral Circulation and Organ Blood Flow, Section 2, Vol. III, Part 1.* J.T. Shepherd and F.M. Abboud, eds. Bethesda, Md., American Physiological Society, pp. 137–182.

11. Johnson, P.C. (ed.) (1964). Autoregulation of blood flow. *Circ. Res.* 15(Suppl. 1):I1–I291.

12. Johnson, P.C. (1978). *Peripheral Circulation.* New York, Wiley.

13. Lassen, N.A., Ingvar, D.H., Skinhoj, E. (1978). Brain function and blood flow. *Sci. Am.* 239:62–71.

14. Lautt, W.W. (ed.) (1981). *Hepatic Circulation in Health and Disease.* New York, Raven Press.

15. Olsson, R.A., Bugni, W.J., (1986). Coronary circulation. In: *The Heart and Cardiovascular System,* H.A. Fozzard et al., eds. New York, Raven Press, pp. 987–1037.

16. Rowell, L.B. (1986). *Human Circulation: Regulation During Physical Stress.* New York, Oxford University Press.

17. Shepherd, A.P., Granger, D.N. (eds.) (1984). *Physiology of Intestinal Circulation.* New York, Raven Press.

18. Shepherd, J.T., Vanhoutte, P.M. (1975). *Veins and Their Control.* London, W.B. Saunders.

Research Reports

19. Andersen, P., Saltin, B. (1985). Maximal perfusion of skeletal muscle in man. *J. Physiol.* 366:233–249.

20. Bache, R.J., Ball, R.M., Cobb, F.R., Rembert, J.C., Greenfield, J.C. (1975). Effects of nitroglycerin on transmyocardial blood flow in the anesthetized dog. *J. Clin. Invest.* 55:1219–1228.

21. Beeuwkes, R. III, Bonventre, J.V. (1975). Tubular organization and vascular–tubular relations in the dog kidney. *Am. J. Physiol.* 229:695–713.

22. Bennett, T.D., Wyss, C.R., Scher, A.M. (1984). Changes in vascular capacity in awake dogs in response to carotid sinus occlusion and administration of catecholamines. *Circ. Res.* 55:440–453.

23. Busse, R., Forstermann, U., Matsuda, H., Pohl, U. (1984). The role of prostaglandins in the endothelium-mediated vasodilatory response to hypoxia. *Pfluegers Arch.* 401:77–83.

24. Chilian, W.M., Marcus, M.L. (1982). Phasic coronary blood flow velocity in intramural and epicardial coronary arteries. *Circ. Res.* 50:775–781.

25. Cushing, H. (1901). Concerning a definite regulatory mechanism of the vasomotor centre which controls blood pressure during cerebral compression. *Bull. Johns Hopkins Hosp.* 12:290–292.

26. Duling, B.R. (1974). Oxygen sensitivity of vascular smooth muscle. II. In vivo studies. *Am. J. Physiol.* 227:42–49.

27. Eriksson,, E., Myrhage, R. (1972). Microvascular dimensions and blood flow in skeletal muscle. *Acta Physiol. Scand.* 86:211–222.

28. Florence, V.M., Bevan, J.A. (1979). Biochemical determination of cholinergic innervation in cerebral arteries. *Circ. Res.* 45:212–218.

29. Freeman, R.H., Davis, J.O., Villarreal, D. (1984). Role of renal prostaglandins in the control of renin release. *Circ. Res.* 54:1–9.

30. Gelli, M., Norton, J.M., Detar, R. (1973). Evidence for direct control of coronary vascular tone by oxygen. *Circ. Res.* 32:279–289.

31. Gertz, K.H., Mangos, J.A., Braun, G., Pagel, H.D. (1966). Pressure in the glomerular capillaries of the rat kidney and its relation to arterial pressure. *Pfluegers Arch.* 288:369–374.

32. Giebisch, G., Lauson, H.D., Pitts, R.F. (1954). Renal excretion and volume of distribution of various dextrans. *Am. J. Physiol.* 178:168–176.

33. Gottschalk, C.W., Mylle, M. (1956). Micropuncture studies of pressures in proximal tubules and peritubular capillaries of the rat kidney and their relation to ureteral and renal venous pressures. *Am. J. Physiol.* 185:430–439.

34. Gregg, D.E., Khouri, E.M., Rayford, C.R. (1965). Systemic and coronary energetics in the resting unanesthetized dog. *Circ. Res.* 16:102–113.

35. Haggendal, E., Lofgren, J., Nilsson, N.J., Zwetnow, N.N. (1970). Effects of varied cerebrospinal fluid pressure on cerebral blood flow in dogs. *Acta Physiol. Scand.* 79:262–271.

36. Hales, J.R.S., Rowell, L.B., King, R.B. (1979). The redistribution of cardiac output in the dog during heat stress. *Am. J. Physiol.* 237 (*Heart Circ. Physiol.* 6):H705–H712.

37. Harper, A.M. (1965). The inter-relationship between P_{CO_2} and blood pressure in the regulation of blood flow through the cerebral cortex. *Acta Neurol. Scand.* 41(Suppl.14):94–103.

38. Ingvar, D.H., Lassen, N.A. (1962). Regional blood flow of the cerebral cortex determined by Krypton[85]. *Acta Physiol. Scand.* 54:325–338.

39. Jessen, C., Feistkorn, G., Nagel, A. (1983). Temperature sensitivity of skeletal muscle in the conscious goat. *J. Appl. Physiol.* (*Respir. Environ. Exercise*) 54:880–886.

40. Johansson, B., Mellander, S. (1975). Static and dynamic changes in the vascular myogenic response to passive changes in length as revealed by electrical and mechanical recordings from the rat portal vein. *Circ. Res.* 36:76–83.

41. Johnson, P.C. (1968). Autoregulatory responses of cat mesenteric arterioles measured in vivo. *Circ. Res.* 22:199–212.

42. Kety, S.S., Schmidt, C.F. (1948). The nitrous oxide method for the quantitative determination of cerebral blood flow in man: Theory, procedure, and normal values. *J. Clin. Invest.* 27:476–514. (First of five consecutive papers.)

43. Kontos, H.A., Raper, A.J., Paterson, J.L., Jr. (1977). Analysis of vasoactivity of local pH, P_{CO_2} and bicarbonate on pial vessels. *Stroke* 8:358–360.

44. Laher, I., Bevan, J.A. (1985). Alpha adrenoceptor number limits response of some rabbit arteries to norepinephrine. *J. Pharmacol. Exp. Ther.* 233:290–297.

45. Larsson, L.I., Edvinsson, L., Fahrenkrug, J., Hakanson, R., Owman, C., Schaffalitzky de Muckadell, O., Sundler, F. (1976). Immunohistochemical localization of a vasodilatory polypeptide (VIP) in cerebrovascular nerves. *Brain Res.* 113:400–404.

46. Laughlin, M.H., Armstrong, R.B. (1982). Muscular blood flow distribution patterns as a function of running speed in rats. *Am. J. Physiol.* 243 (*Heart Circ. Physiol.* 12):H296–H306.

47. Lesh, T.A., Rothe, C.F. (1969). Sympathetic and hemodynamic effects of capacitance vessels in dog skeletal muscle. *Am. J. Physiol.* 217:819–827.

48. Lowensohn, H.S., Khouri, E.M., Gregg, D.E., Pyle, R.L., Patterson, R.E. (1976). Phasic right coronary artery blood flow in conscious dogs with normal and elevated right ventricular pressures. *Circ. Res* 39:760–766.

49. McPherson, R.W., Zeger, S., Traystman, R.J. (1986). Relationship of somatosensory evoked potentials and cerebral oxygen consumption during hypoxic hypoxia in dogs. *Stroke* 17:30–36.

50. Mellander, S., Arvidsson, S. (1974). Possible "dynamic" component in the myogenic vascular response related to pulse pressure distention. *Acta Physiol. Scand.* 90:283–285.

51. Moir, T.W., Driscol, T.E., Eckstein, R.W. (1964). Thebesian drainage in the left heart of the dog. *Circ. Res.* 14:245–249.

52. Milnor, W.R., Sastre, A. (1988). Cholinergic receptors and contraction of smooth muscle in canine portal vein. *J. Pharmacol. Exp. Ther.* 245:244–249.

53. Nelson, E., Rennels, M. (1970). Innervation of intracranial arteries. *Brain* 93:475–490.

54. Nelson, R.R., Gobel, F.L., Jorgensen, C.R., Wang, K., Wang, Y., Taylor, H.L. (1974). Hemodynamic predictors of myocardial oxygen consumption during static and dynamic exercise. *Circulation* 50:1179–1189.

55. Renkin, E.M. (1971). The nutritive-shunt-flow hypothesis in skeletal muscle circulation. *Circ. Res.* 28(Suppl. 1):21–40.

56. Rooke, G.A., Feigl, E.O. (1982). Work as a correlate of canine left ventricular oxygen consumption, and the problem of catecholamine oxygen wasting. *Circ. Res.* 50:273–286.

57. Selkurt, E.E. (1974). Current status of renal circulation and related nephron function in hemorrhage and experimental shock. I Vascular mechanisms. *Circ. Shock* 1:3–15.

58. Sokoloff, L., Reivich, M., Kennedy, D., Des Rosiers, C.S., Patlak, K.D., Pettigrew, K.D., Sakurada, O., Shinohara, M. (1977). The [^{14}C]deoxyglucose method for the measurement of local cerebral glucose utilization: Theory, procedure, and normal values in the conscious and anesthetized albino rat. *J. Neurochem.* 28:897–916.

59. Sparks, H.V., Jr. (1964). Effect of quick stretch on isolated vascular smooth muscle. *Circ. Res.* 15(Suppl. 1):I254–I260.

60. Sugiyama, H., Christensen, J., Olsen, T.S., Lassen, N.A. (1986). Monitoring CBF in clinical routine by dynamic single photon emission tomography (SPECT) of inhaled Xenon-133. *Stroke* 7:1179–1182.

61. Thorburn, G.D., Kopald, H.H., Herd, J.A., Hollenberg, M., Barger, A.C. (1963). Intrarenal distribution of nutrient blood flow determined with ^{85}Kr in the unanesthetized dog. *Circ. Res.* 13:290–307.

62. Van Citters, R.L., Franklin, D.L. (1969). Cardiovascular performance of Alaska sled dogs during exercise. *Circ. Res.* 24:33–42.

63. Wolgast, M. (1973). Renal medullary red cell and plasma flow as studied with labeled indicators and internal detection. *Acta Physiol. Scand.* 88:215–225.

64. Zimmerhackl, B., Robertson, C.R., Jamison, R.L. (1985). The microcirculation of the renal medulla. *Circ. Res.* 57:657–667.

13

THE CIRCULATING FLUID: BLOOD

The blood that circulates through the cardiovascular system performs a multitude of functions. As a vehicle of transport, it carries nutrients and waste products, O_2 and CO_2, proteins, hormones and simple salts, as well as materials needed for hemostasis and immunity. O_2 is a special case, being transported predominantly by the hemoglobin in red cells, whereas the other essentials are carried as solutes. A continuous exchange between blood and the extracellular fluid, carried on through capillary walls, maintains an essentially constant internal environment for all the cells of the body.

The functions of this vital fluid are not limited to transport. The volume and viscosity of blood are critical variables in hemodynamic regulation, affecting blood pressure and cardiac performance (Chapter 6). The ability of blood to clot in damaged regions is an essential defense mechanism, although the formation of intravascular clots (*thrombi*) under pathological conditions can have harmful effects. The subject of blood coagulation is beyond the scope of this book but is covered in hematology textbooks.[10] Physically, blood is a suspension of cells in a viscous, yellowish fluid, the *plasma*, and the cells are kept in suspension by the motion of the blood. By far the greatest part of the formed elements consists of *erythrocytes*, or red cells, the remainder being *leukocytes*, or white cells, and blood *platelets*.

Plasma is about 90% water and contains a number of proteins that make up some 7% of its weight. Plasma albumin, which serves an important osmotic function in fluid balance across the capillary membranes (Chapter 10), makes up a large part of this protein content. Albumin also binds a number of biological substances reversibly (e.g., corticosteroids) and thus acts as a carrier in the blood stream. Other proteins include globulins involved in immune reactions, as well as fibrinogen and a host of other factors that provide the basis for coagulation of blood. Inorganic substances in plasma include the whole array of essential ions, the most important being sodium, potassium, calcium, magnesium, chloride, bicarbonate, and phosphate, all in strictly controlled concentrations. Glucose and amino acids are the principal nutrients. The solute content and volume of plasma are regulated primarily by the kidney.

Cellular Elements

Red cells, or *erythrocytes,* are biconcave discs about 8 μm in diameter and 2 μm in maximum thickness. They are readily deformable, a characteristic that allows them to pass through the smallest capillaries. The primary function of red cells is the transport of O_2, a specialization reflected in the fact that hemoglobin makes up 95% of their dry weight. The membrane of the erythrocyte contains phospholipids and cholesterol, along with glycoproteins and glycolipids responsible for blood group antigenicity. Erythrocytes swell up to become spherical when exposed to hypotonic solutions, and their membranes remain intact in 0.4% sodium chloride but rupture in salt-free water. Circulating red cells are metabolically active and maintain a high intracellular K^+, although they lack nuclei, mitochondria, or other organized structures. Some evidence suggests that the shape of the red cell and the stiffness of its membrane vary with ATP content, but not all investigators agree on that point.[3,27]

Erythrocytes are manufactured in the bone marrow, where the immature forms have nuclei and other intracellular organelles. The nuclei disappear as the cells develop, but mitochondria and ribosomes often remain when the red cell is first released into the bloodstream. A stainable reticulum can be demonstrated in such forms, hence the name *reticulocyte.* Such cells constitute fewer than 1% of circulating red cells under normal conditions, but they appear in greater numbers when blood production increases. Mature cells tend to agglutinate in stacks, or *rouleaux,* which can inhibit the flow of blood through narrow channels. The average life span of a red cell is 120 days, after which it degenerates and is removed from the circulation.[10] The net turnover rate of erythrocytes in a steady state is about 0.8% per day.

The rate of erythrocyte production is controlled by a hormone, *erythropoietin,* produced in the kidney and perhaps other tissues. Dietary iron, copper, and other substances are required for the synthesis of hemoglobin and the normal development of erythrocytes. Low arterial oxygen tensions are a potent stimulus to red cell production, increasing the number of erythrocytes in individuals who reside at high altitudes and in patients with certain congenital venous-arterial shunts. Androgenic hormones also promote production,[13] which may account for the observation that the normal average red cell concentration is slightly lower in females than in males.

Leukocytes are motile, nucleated cells. Three principal types are distinguished—granulocytes, lymphocytes, and monocytes—all much larger than red cells. They can pass through endothelial linings, and many more of them are found in extravascular spaces than in the circulating blood. Some leukocytes are carried freely in the bloodstream, whereas others hug the vessel wall and adhere to the endothelium. Such temporarily static cells, which are particularly prominent in the pulmonary vascular bed, form a pool that slowly exchanges with the overall population of white cells. Leukocytes function primarily as part of the body's defenses and are a central element in immunity and hypersensitivity reactions. Granulocytes and monocytes engulf bacteria and other foreign particles, degrading them by means of lytic enzymes.

Platelets are irregularly oval or spherical bodies in the circulating blood, derived from megakaryocytes in the bone marrow and usually 2 to 4 μm in their largest dimension. They have no nucleus but may contain a few reticulated intracellular fibers. Their average life in the bloodstream is about 10 days. One striking characteristic of platelets is their ability to agglutinate, or stick together, in clumps that help to seal an injured blood vessel. Normal endothelium presents a nonthrombogenic surface, but when the endothelium is damaged, platelets quickly adhere to the exposed subendothelial region, aggregating together and releasing substances that accelerate coagulation of blood, as well as potassium, ADP, and serotonin. Platelet aggregation is promoted by arachidonic acid, thromboxane A_2, and the enzyme thrombin. Platelets can also release a substance called *platelet-derived growth factor (PDGF)*, which stimulates mitosis in cultured fibroblasts and vascular smooth muscle cells,[15] suggesting that platelets are involved in the reparative processes that follow vascular damage. Platelets take up epinephrine, norepinephrine, histamine, and serotonin by active mechanisms. Human platelets contain alpha$_2$-adrenergic receptors, the function of which is not known.

Physical Properties of Blood

Red cells

The deformability of normal red cells is a useful property because some capillaries are less than 7 μm in diameter and erythrocytes must literally squeeze through, propelled by the driving pressure. Experiments *in vitro* have shown that erythrocytes can pass through channels as narrow as 2.5 μm in diameter.[3] The deformation is reversible, and red cells can resume their normal shape in about 60 msec. Part of the red cell membrane is in contact with the capillary wall, and the moving column of blood consists of a train of red cells separated at irregular intervals by plasma-filled segments. Typical capillary transit time for an erythrocyte is about 1 sec. The much larger white cells also pass through capillaries, changing their shape as necessary but temporarily obstructing the passage of red cells. Although they may take as long as 5 sec in transit, only a tiny fraction of the available capillaries is blocked in this way at any instant.

Obviously, the hemodynamic principles that govern blood flow in large vessels (Chapter 6) no longer apply under such conditions. Flow still depends in part on the pressure head, but it is also strongly influenced by the ability of the cells to assume appropriate shapes and by any tendency to adhere to the capillary wall. The red cell wall can be deformed into a variety of shapes, but the membrane area is not greatly altered in these changes. Stretching the total membrane area by more than a small percentage tears it, but that happens only with forces much greater than those required to deform the cell.[22] The erythrocyte as a whole is freely deformable because its internal contents are easily moved about, and the membrane is capable of sliding around the cell contents.

The tendency of red cells to aggregate is a potential source of microcirculatory blockage but presents no problems under normal conditions. Aggregation involves collision and rearrangement into rouleaux, which takes time and is not possible when the blood is moving rapidly. The critical parameter is the rate of shear in the blood (see below and Chapter 6), which is high enough throughout the arterial tree to discourage aggregation.[33] Even with the slower velocities on the venous side, aggregation into rouleaux is probably transient. Given the proper conditions, the half-time for aggregation is 3 to 5 sec, whereas disaggregation can occur in less than 0.1 sec. Rouleaux formation is thus a relatively slow process, but dispersion can occur very rapidly. Aggregation is also affected by plasma proteins, being directly correlated with the concentration of fibrinogen and, to a lesser extent, globulins. Albumin tends to decrease cell aggregation. Certain diseases, including diabetes mellitus, are accompanied by an increased tendency of erythrocytes to adhere to each other and to the endothelial wall.

Erythrocyte deformability and adhesiveness are critical in the function of the spleen as a kind of filter.[23] Red cells that are in any way abnormal adhere to the splenic pulp, which presents a large surface. Reticulocytes, which are "stickier" and less flexible than mature cells, are removed from the blood and held in the spleen for 1 or 2 days for further development. Red cells that have been made abnormal by experimental treatments such as stiffening by glutaraldehyde are trapped in the spleen in large numbers. Moreover, there appear to be two functional splenic compartments through which blood moves, one with a very slow transit time. About one-quarter of the cells in the spleen, many of them reticulocytes, are in the slow-moving region, and the cell concentration in the blood of the spleen is high, with an organ hematocrit of 0.70 to 0.80 (see below).

Sickle cell disease

Certain pathological states that affect the structure and conformation of the hemoglobin molecule restrict the deformation of the cell or cause it to assume abnormal shapes. The most striking example of this phenomenon is seen in a genetic disorder called *sickle cell anemia*.[10] A large proportion of the erythrocytes in sickle cell disease are bizarre in shape, sometimes taking on crescent-like forms that give the anomaly its name. Fewer cells of this kind appear in the heterozygous form of the disease than in the homozygous condition. The number of sickled erythrocytes is increased by low pO_2 or pH. The affected cells are relatively rigid, and whole blood viscosity is abnormally high.[2] The structure and conformation of an abnormal hemoglobin are responsible for the physical and morphological changes in this disorder, and serious disturbances follow from the obstructions that the relatively rigid cells can produce in the microcirculation. Some other diseases affect the flexibility of the red cell wall by altering the principal membrane proteins, showing that deformability may be altered by either membrane defects or hemoglobin abnormalities.

Cell/plasma ratios

The proportions of cells and fluid in the blood can be determined by centrifugation of a sample in a narrow, cylindrical, calibrated tube designed for the purpose. The red cells accumulate in a packed column at the bottom of the tube, with a thin layer of white cells on top of it and clear plasma above. The ratio of packed red cells to the total volume of the sample is called the *hematocrit*; the normal range is 0.47 ± 0.07 in adult human males and 0.42 ± 0.05 in adult females. When the blood has been drawn from a peripheral vein, the result is called the *venous hematocrit*. A small amount of plasma remains trapped among the red cells, and correction factors for this admixture have been determined experimentally.[10]

The ratio of cells to plasma in the vascular system as a whole can be measured by more elaborate procedures (see below), and the result, rather surprisingly, is not quite equal to the venous hematocrit. The ratio of total red cell to total blood volume, sometimes called the *body hematocrit,* amounts to only 91% of the value measured in venous blood on the average.[29] This difference arises in part from the relative scarcity of cells in small vessels and in part from differences in cell/plasma proportions in various organs. Within the kidney, for example, the local hematocrit may be only 0.20, whereas in the spleen it is at least 0.70. These fractions contrast sharply with the intermediate values found in the large veins, arteries, and heart, the *central* circulation. The body/venous hematocrit ratio is also highly species dependent.

The source of such differences is the dependence of local hematocrit on the relative velocities of red cells and plasma. If structural or other conditions in some region allow plasma to move more rapidly than red cells, then the cell/plasma ratio within that vascular bed at any instant will be greater than it is in the blood that enters the bed. This phenomenon is implicit in the equations that apply to the indicator-dilution method of measuring flow (Chapter 14); if Q denotes the volumetric rate of flow through a system, $\bar{t}$ the mean transit time, and V the volume of the system, then

$$V = Q\bar{t} \tag{13.1}$$

Assume, for purposes of illustration, that the hematocrit of arterial blood is 0.50 and that some organ receives an arterial inflow (Q) of 10 cm^3 whole blood per second, that is, 5 cm^3 of plasma and 5 cm^3 of cells per second. Suppose that the transit times through that organ's vascular bed are 4 sec for plasma and 16 sec for red cells. The volume of plasma in the organ at any instant will be 20 cm^3 ($= 5 \times 4$), and the volume of cells will be 80 cm^3 ($= 5 \times 16$).

Blood viscosity

The *viscosity* of blood (Chapter 6) determines to a large extent the amount of energy that must be supplied to move it through the vascular tree. Blood travels in most vessels with a parabolic velocity profile, the velocity ranging from a maximum in the axial stream to zero (theoretically) at the vessel wall. Because blood is viscous, this sliding of fluid laminae past each other at different velocities dissipates energy. Blood pressure and flow in the circulation consequently depend in part on blood viscosity. Even when the velocity profile is blunt, as it is in the ascending aorta, there is a sharp velocity gradient at the wall and energy is required to overcome the "friction," as it were, at that interface. Most of the work of the heart is employed in overcoming such viscous resistance to flow. Kinetic energy must also be supplied to put the blood in motion, but that component is very small compared to the cardiac work imposed by the viscous properties of blood (Chapter 4). The viscosity of human and canine blood at 37° C is normally 0.030 to 0.040 poise.[4] Larger and smaller estimates have been reported, but this range is the one generally accepted. The normal value for blood viscosity and hematocrit are not the same in all species.[10]

The particulate nature of blood as a suspension of cells has a great influ-

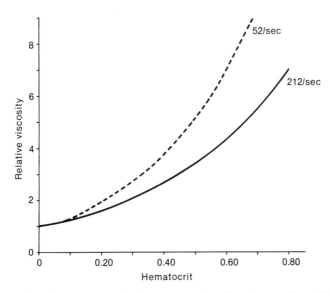

Figure 13.1. Effect of hematocrit and shear rate on viscosity of human blood. *Abscissa,* hematocrit. *Ordinate,* ratio of whole blood viscosity to plasma viscosity. *Solid line,* viscosities measured at shear rate of 212/sec. *Dashed line,* shear rate 52/sec. Blood viscosity varies directly with hematocrit and inversely with shear rate. (Redrawn from data collected by Whitmore[9])

ence on its flow properties, and blood viscosity is directly correlated with the hematocrit. Viscosity rises steadily as the proportion of cells increases,[39] although the relationship is nonlinear (Figure 13.1). High hematocrits thus place a burden on the heart by making it more difficult to move blood through the circulation. The plasma proteins, particularly fibrinogen, are another determinant of blood viscosity.

The behavior of blood places it in the class of non-Newtonian fluids, because its viscosity varies with the velocity of the blood and so fails to conform to the classical definition (equation 6.2). In Newtonian fluids, viscosity is entirely a property of the fluid and is unaffected by absolute velocity. The *anomalous viscosity* of blood is related to what is called the *shear rate* in the fluid, an expression of differences in velocity across the radius of the tube, and hence of internal friction. Rapid motion of the blood increases the shear rate. At high rates of shear (and constant hematocrit), the behavior of blood is close to that of a Newtonian fluid, but the apparent viscosity increases appreciably when the rate falls below about 60 sec^{-1}. Red cell aggregation is one factor that can increase whole blood viscosity at low shear rates.

Typical rates of shear in man and the dog are 40 to 70 sec^{-1} in the ascending aorta and 300 to 500 sec^{-1} in arterioles. Consequently, the increased apparent viscosity associated with a low shear rate becomes significant at relatively low rates of blood flow. It is difficult to be certain just how important this factor is *in vivo*. Some experiments have failed to show any rise in viscosity at low shear rates in tubes 30 to 60 μm in diameter, dimensions corresponding to a large part of the arteriolar and venular beds.[31]

The situation is further complicated by the influence of tube diameter per se. At high shear rates, the viscosity measured in a tube 20 μm in diameter is about half that in a 1-mm tube. The same phenomenon, called the *Fahraeus-Lindquist effect,* occurs in living vascular beds. Experiments in which a hind limb was perfused first with blood and then with physiological salt solution showed that the viscosity of blood relative to saline was 2.2 *in vivo,* compared with 4.0 when measured outside the animal in a viscometer.[39] The reason for the difference is the fall in local hematocrit in small tubes, the result of the axial concentration of red cells and the presence of a cell-poor region near the walls of the conduit. The physical explanation of this distribution is still debated, and the experimental evidence is conflicting.[9]

At the lowest shear rates, there is good evidence to suggest that some minimum force is required to keep blood in motion. The flow of blood through a narrow tube under a controlled head of pressure ceases when the pressure has been reduced to a very low but finite value, the *yield stress*. This phenomenon is similar to the critical closing pressure observed in living vascular beds (Chapter 6), but yield stresses are observed in rigid tubes and the cessation of flow arises from the properties of blood, not from closure of vessels. The same mechanism may operate *in vivo* at very low rates of flow in small vessels or during the lowest portion of pulsatile pressures. The absolute value of yield stress in normal human blood is quite small,[9] however, probably less than 0.1 dyn/cm^2, and its relevance to normal physiological functions has yet to be demonstrated.

A minimum yield stress is not found in saline suspensions of red cells at normal hematocrits, but only when fibrinogen is present.[17] This plasma protein is large in molecular weight, about 340,000, and the asymmetric, dumbbell shape of the molecule probably contributes to the effects on fluidity. In the absence of fibrinogen, the yield stress is less than half that measured in normal plasma. Plasma globulins also increase blood viscosity and promote aggregation, although not so strongly as fibrinogen. Albumin tends to decrease cell aggregation at low shear rates, and a negative correlation between plasma albumin and viscosity has been reported.

Blood Volume

The total amount of blood in the vascular system is about 6 liters in adult humans, varying with body size. Plasma volume averages 45 ml/per kilogram of body weight in normal adult males and cell volume 30 ml/kg, the normal range extending through ±20% of those values.[14] As might be expected from the low vascularity of fatty tissue, total blood volume correlates more closely with weight when body fat is excluded from the calculations (Figure 13.2), but elaborate procedures are required to measure lean body mass alone.[14] The total blood volume in other mammalian species ranges from 54 ml/kg in some varieties of rats to 92 ml/kg in the dog and possibly 110 ml/kg in race horses.[8]

Mechanisms of regulation

The total blood volume in any individual is kept relatively constant by a variety of mechanisms over periods of months or years. Neither cell nor plasma volumes vary much under ordinary conditions, but any pathological decrease in the cell fraction is followed by an increase in plasma that brings the total volume back to normal levels. As we have already seen, red cell volume is determined by a balance between the rate at which erythrocytes are produced and the rate at which they age and disintegrate. These rates are relatively fixed, whereas plasma volume can be altered fairly quickly by physiological mechanisms.

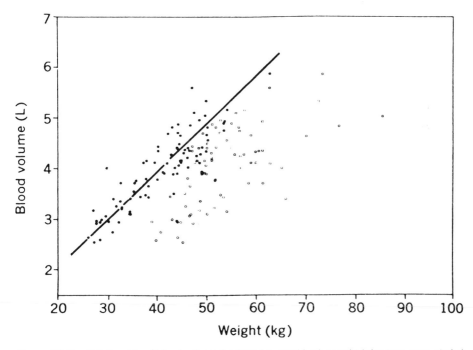

Figure 13.2. Relationship of blood volume (*ordinate*) to total body weight (*abscissa, open circles*) and lean body mass (total weight minus adipose tissue, *closed circles*) in adult human subjects. Blood volume is more closely correlated with lean body mass (*regression line*) than with total body weight. (From data published by Allen et al.[14])

Capillary transmural pressure and renal function are the two mechanisms that bring about gains or losses in the blood's fluid component. An increase in capillary pressure causes a net movement of fluid from vascular to extravascular space, thus tending to reduce plasma volume (Chapter 10). Increased pressure and low compliance of the interstitial space outside the capillaries act in the opposite direction, tending to prevent fluid loss from the vascular compartment. This system provides for physiological transfer between extracellular and intravascular fluid, one gaining at the expense of the other. Significant adjustments of plasma volume take place in this way, but the total volume of plasma and extracellular fluid together is not necessarily affected.

The second regulator of plasma volume is the kidney. The mechanisms here involve not only the pressure of glomerular, cortical, and medullary capillaries but also the reflexes generated by atrial and other mechanical receptors (Chapter 7). Both act to control renal excretion of salt and water, and so regulate extracellular as well as plasma volume. The reflex response to distention of the atria makes the atrial stretch receptors a sensing element in the plasma volume control system. An increase in blood volume, for example, raises atrial pressure, and the resulting reflex enhances renal excretion of sodium. The response is only in part a neural reflex and occurs even after the renal nerves have been cut.[20] The discovery that stretching of atrial walls also releases a *natriuretic factor* was discussed in Chapter 8, along with the part played by renin, angiotensin, aldosterone, and ADH.

Physiological variations in blood volume

Blood volume in relation to weight is higher in newborn infants, where it averages 100 ml/kg, than in adults. This value decreases over the first 3 yr of life, after which it maintains a more or less linear relationship to body weight. Although blood volume is carefully regulated by homeostatic mechanisms, physiological changes occur under a number of conditions. Blood volume in humans is higher in summer than in winter, for example, and moving from a cool to a warm environment raises it by 15 to 30% within a few days, almost all the change occurring in the volume of plasma.[19] Plasma volume also falls in patients restricted to a recumbent position in bed, and decreases of 10% of total blood volume over a period of 3 weeks have been observed.[35]

Posture

Plasma volume decreases slowly upon assuming the erect posture and may fall as much as 15%. The change is due to loss of fluid from the vascular compartment to interstitial spaces of the legs, which occurs because of the increased venous and capillary pressures in the lower extremities. Careful measurement of the circumference of the calf shows an increase of several millimeters after 15 min of standing quietly. A fall in blood volume also occurs in astronauts after periods of weightlessness. All of these adjustments to gravitational stress are considered more fully later in this chapter.

Exercise

Physical exertion is another cause of deceased plasma volume, although the extent of change varies with the degree and duration of activity. Running or bicycling can produce a reduction of several hundred milliliters in humans. The decrease occurs in the first 10 to 15 min and is related to the intensity of exertion.[25] On the other hand, some kinds of physical training tend to produce a distinct increase in resting blood volume, but others do not. Studies of individuals trained in gymnasia or on the track usually report blood volumes 10 to 20% greater than those in untrained controls. The rapidity with which blood volume can change has been demonstrated by increases of 10 to 19% over a 9-day period of ski training. In contrast, one study of men who had been training for 5 months as a rowing crew showed no significant change in blood volume.[32]

Nutrition

Malnutrition causes a decrease in red cells, and an increase in plasma, in proportions that lower total blood volume moderately. One well-controlled study was carried out on volunteers who remained in a state of semistarvation for 24 wk,[24] during which body weight decreased an average of 23%. Total blood volume decreased by 9%, but that net change was the result of a marked decrease in red cell volume and a modest increment in plasma, with a fall in hematocrit from 0.48 to 0.35. The red cell mass diminished by 33% and thus decreased in relation to body weight, as well as in absolute terms. Similar observations have been made in victims of famine. The anemia results from an inadequate supply of protein, iron, and other materials needed to produce normal red cells. The increase in plasma volume is a general response that moves to restore the total volume whenever the cellular component is reduced.

Pregnancy

Total blood volume rises gradually during pregnancy, increasing by 30 to 50% over the 9 mo of gestation. Plasma volume accounts for most of the rise in the first month or two. Cell volume may fall during the early stages, but then increases to well above control levels. The average blood loss at the time of delivery is about 250 ml; cell and plasma volumes usually return to normal in a few weeks.

Pathological changes

Hypovolemia, or abnormally low blood volume, is uncommon except in cases of hemorrhage, but it can occur with dehydration and disturbances that accelerate salt and water excretion. Reductions in red cell volume—chronic anemia, for example—interfere with optimum delivery of oxygen to the tissues but do not usually have much effect on hemodynamic conditions. Loss of as much as half of the normal red cell volume is compatible with life, although not with good health, if plasma increases so that total volume approaches normal and thus supports an adequate blood pressure. Some diseases reduce the amount of hemoglobin per red cell,[10] lowering the oxygen supply to the periphery even though the total red cell volume may be normal.

Hypervolemia, or excessive blood volume, can be caused by defects in the body's handling of salt and water, overproduction of red cells, or the injudicious infusion of blood or other solutions. It tends to raise pressures throughout the circulation, including veins and capillary beds, causing exudation of fluid into interstitial spaces (*edema*). Increased central venous pressure is sensed by receptors in the atria (Chapter 8), but the reflex response is not always successful in restoring normal blood volume. Congestive heart failure is one of the pathological states that lead to an increase in blood volume, the hypervolemia in that disorder arising from a failure of the kidney to balance intake and output of water and sodium. The overproduction of red cells caused by chronically low arterial oxygen tensions is an example of hypervolemia generated by an increase in red cell volume.

Measurement of blood volume

Blood volume is determined by the dilution of a nontoxic substance injected into the bloodstream, measuring the concentration of the marker after it has mixed thoroughly with the blood. Mixing is usually complete within 10 min. The ideal test material is one that *labels* either plasma or erythrocytes and thus stays in the vascular compartment for a reasonable length of time. Virtually all injected substances disappear from the blood sooner or later, but a label that binds to plasma proteins or some component of the red cells leaves the bloodstream very slowly.

Plasma volume is often measured by injection of radioisotope-labeled plasma albumin or by dyes like Evans blue (T-1824) that bind to albumin. Radioisotopes that *tag* hemoglobin or some other substance in the erythrocyte are employed to measure red cell volume. Incubation of a small amount of blood from the subject with ^{51}Cr for half an hour, for example, labels most of the red cells in the sample. After washing to remove unbound ^{51}Cr, a saline suspension of the cells is reinjected and the total red cell volume is calculated from the radioactivity of blood samples taken after a suitable mixing period. Radioactive compounds of ^{59}Fe, ^{32}P, and ^{42}K have also been used to tag red cells and ^{131}I to label plasma proteins.[29]

The basic procedures for measuring plasma volume and red cell volume are identical. A precisely measured amount of labeling material is injected into the bloodstream, usually by way of a vein, and blood samples are drawn from a contralateral vein at timed intervals. The concentration of label in these samples is then measured and plotted to allow extrapolation back to the time of injection. The concentration is high immediately after injection, falls as distribution throughout the system takes place, and then declines at a slow rate that reflects loss from the vascular compartment (Figure 13.3). Samples collected 10, 20, and 30 min after injection can be used to define the slope of concentration with time as the indicator slowly leaves the circulation; changes in the first 10 min are largely the result of mixing, not loss. Extrapolating back to the time of injection gives the concentration (C) of the label that would have existed after complete mixing if none had left the vascular compartment. If the marker

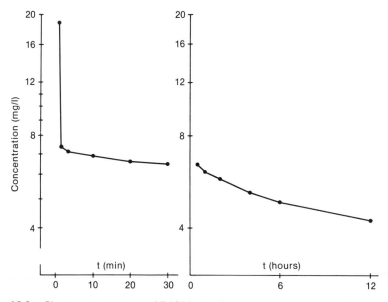

Figure 13.3. Plasma concentration of T-1824 dye after intravenous injection of 22.1 mg dye, in normal human subject. *Abscissa*, time; *ordinate*, plasma concentration of dye (logarithmic scale). Extrapolation from 10- to 30-min samples back to time zero indicates 7.16 mg/liter. Calculated plasma volume, 22.1/7.16 = 3.087 liters. (Milnor and Crary, unpublished data)

labels plasma, then plasma volume (V_{plasma}) can be calculated from C and the amount of dye injected (M):

$$V_{plasma} = \frac{M}{C} \qquad (13.2)$$

(A similar protocol can be employed to estimate total extracellular fluid volume by injecting a substance like sodium thiocyanate, which is distributed throughout the extracellular compartment, both intravascular and extravascular.)

Total blood volume (V_{blood}) can be calculated from measured plasma volume (V_{plasma}) and the hematocrit (h):

$$V_{blood} = \frac{V_{plasma}}{(1 - h)} \qquad (13.3)$$

Red cell volume can be estimated as

$$V_{cells} = V_{plasma} \times \frac{h}{(1 - h)} \qquad (13.4)$$

Analogous equations can be derived for calculating V_{blood} when V_{cells} has been measured by dilution. The hematocrit is usually measured on a venous blood sample, and the total blood volume calculated from these equations is consequently in error to the extent of the difference between venous and body hematocrits (see above). The difference was actually discovered by measuring total cell and plasma volumes simultaneously with two appropriate labels.

One weakness in the estimation of intravascular volumes by dilution methods is the somewhat arbitrary criterion for complete mixing. The label is certainly not evenly distributed in the first minute after injection; indeed, the earliest concentrations rise and fall in a reproduction of the indicator-dilution curves used to measure cardiac output. A slight, continuous fall in concentration begins after a few minutes and persists for hours due to loss from the vascular bed. The conventional compromise is to assume that mixing is complete when the label first achieves a slow, constant rate of disappearance, and this criterion is satisfied within 10 min in most cases. Even then, careful measurements show that the slope of concentration versus time cannot be considered constant for more than 10 or 20 min, whether treated as an exponential or a linear process. In spite of this theoretic problem, the method is useful and reasonably accurate.

Regional Volumes

The fraction of the total blood volume contained in each part of the vascular tree depends on the dimensions and compliance of the blood vessels. Considered from the point of view of the major organ systems, it is evident that organs differ widely in vascular volume, as can be seen from the data cited in Chapters 11 and 12. When arteries and veins are compared, it is clear that a disproportionate amount of blood, about two thirds of the total blood volume, is contained on the venous side of the circulation (Table 1.2). This preponderance arises not only from the dimensions of the veins, which are in general wider and more numerous than those of the parallel arteries, but also from their distensibility, which allows the relatively low pressures in veins to keep them distended. The relative distensibilities are reflected in the fact that an increment of 5 mm Hg in transmural pressure increases the vascular cross section by less than 1% in the canine ascending aorta but by 20 to 50% in the vena cava. The difference in compliance causes any increase in total blood volume to be accommodated largely in the venous system, with a relatively small increment on the arterial side.

The hemodynamic significance of veins thus lies in their capacity, contrasted with that of small arteries, which function primarily as a resistance. Arteries smaller than 1 mm in diameter create about 60% of the total systemic resistance but contain only 3% of the systemic blood volume. Veins of the same size hold roughly 50% of the systemic volume but are responsible for only 6% of the total resistance. Because of the contrasting properties of arterial and venous beds, the effects of vasomotor activity on the two sides are quite different. The principal effect of *arteriolar* constriction is to raise peripheral resistance, whereas active constriction of *veins* tends to alter local blood volumes, moving blood from one part of the circulation to another, with only minor changes in resistance. Arteriolar constriction can also affect venous volume indirectly if it lowers the pressure downstream, allowing a passive decrease in venous volume. Active constriction or relaxation of veins is a prominent element in many physiological responses. Venomotor activity affects the MCFP (Chapter 6), which rises with venoconstriction. The increase may amount to no more than few millimeters of mercury, but even that can have detectable effects on the circulation.

Regional compliances

Because shifts of blood from one part of the circulation to another are so important in physiological responses, many efforts have been made to describe specific intravascular compartments quantitatively. The goal is to define not only the normal blood volumes of the central, splanchnic, and other regions but also their compliance, or relation to transmural pressure.[5] In general, estimates of compliance form part of the reasoning about two circulatory phenomena: (1) the effect of changes in total blood volume on either central venous pressure or MCFP and (2) the characteristics of certain beds as *blood reservoirs*.

The problems encountered in making such estimates are related in part to the difficulty of measuring the volume of a specific segment of the vasculature without disturbing it, and in part to the theoretic limitations of the indicator-dilution principle (Chapter 14). In many cases, the volume determined by multiplying blood flow and mean transit time (equation 13.1) includes an indeterminate part of the arterial and venous trees adjacent to the organ under study. The pulmonary circulation is one of the few vascular beds where regional blood volume can be measured with some accuracy by dilution methods, because a single inflow vessel can be used for injection (the main pulmonary artery) and a single common terminus for collection (the left atrium). When the same method is applied to the splanchnic or central regions, the boundaries of the measured volume become less definite, extending into an ill-defined collection of parallel arteries and veins. External monitoring of radioisotope-labeled blood is an alternative approach that gives a fairly clear picture of shifts to or from a selected region, but it is not easy to make the measurements quantitative.

Attempts to measure regional compliance face even greater obstacles. Three major problems arise: (1) the ovrsimplification involved in describing one part of the circulation as a single compartment, when in fact its properties change continuously along the length of the vascular tree; (2) the nonlinearity of vascular pressure–volume relationships; and (3) the finite volume of most vessels at zero transmural pressure. Each of these problems has been recognized by investigators, but the experimental data remain no more than rough approximations.

To think of any large part of the vascular tree as having a certain volume and compliance is to adopt a *lumped-component* model of that region (Chapter 6), and this introduces another problem. If compliance is defined as $\Delta V/\Delta P$, what transmural pressure goes in the denominator? After all, pressure in any organ falls continuously from the principal arterial vessel to the major vein. Experimental procedures can be devised to stop flow, establish a uniform pressure, and measure the effect of adding to or decreasing the regional volume, but the results are not those that exist during normal blood flow. The compliance of a small vascular segment can be measured *in vitro,* but the compliance of a whole regional bed *in vivo* is some weighted average of many segments of different properties. It follows that estimates of regional compliances represent abstractions, but they are nevertheless an aid to physiological thinking.

Because of the large volume of blood in veins compared to arteries, investigators usually assume that venous pressure is the relevant one in measuring the pressure–volume relation in a lumped compartment. Accordingly, the compliance of the entire vascular system has been estimated by altering the total blood volume and measuring the effect on central venous pressure, with results in the range of 2.0 to 2.5 ml/mm Hg per kilogram of body weight in man and the dog.[5] (The values referred to here and in subsequent paragraphs are compliances defined as $\Delta V/\Delta P$ at the normal operating point on pressure–volume curves). Only 3 to 7% of this compliance is in the arterial bed, the remainder being venous.[34] Translated into absolute terms for a human subject weighing 75 kg, this corresponds to a value of about 170 ml/mm Hg. Transfusion of 500 ml of blood into such a subject would raise central venous pressure by about 3 mm Hg and MCFP by a similar amount, but *only* if there were no change in reflex activity or cardiac output. Physiological responses alter the effect in an intact animal, and this illustration merely suggests the magnitudes involved.

Regional compliances in the dog are approximately 0.68 ml/mm Hg per kilogram of body weight in the splanchnic circulation, the greatest part of it in the hepatic bed, and 0.30 ml/mm Hg per kilogram in the pulmonary vessels.[5] Extrapolated to human subjects, these values suggest splanchnic compliance of about 51 ml/mm Hg and pulmonary vascular compliance of 22 ml/mm Hg. No direct estimates of cutaneous vascular compliance have been possible, but indirect evidence indicates that the splanchnic and cutaneous circulations combined amount to approximately 80% of the 170 ml/mm Hg total vascular compliance already cited. These data convey the potential of the various regions as blood reservoirs that can be tapped when the blood volume is redistributed. Such reservoirs are part of the bloodstream, not isolated in any way from the rest of the circulation, and their function is based on the ability to change local volume with small changes in pressure.

Redistribution of Blood Volume

The distribution of blood between arteries and veins or between one region and another can be altered by physiological stresses even when the total blood volume remains unchanged. Such shifts have been studied in some detail in man as well as other species. In addition to the methods already described for measuring regional volumes, the relative amounts of blood in different parts of the body can be estimated by external detection of radiation from radioistopes injected into the bloodstream[6,18] (e.g., ^{99}Tc).

Central blood volume

One example of redistribution is the displacement from peripheral veins to a *central* region, namely, the chambers of the heart, the pulmonary vessels, and nearby segments of the aorta and vena cava. This central volume is for the most part a region of low pressure and relatively high distensibility, and it has a major conceptual and functional place in cardiovascular physiology. The pressure in the right atrium is often referred to as the *central venous pressure* for the systemic bed. Application of the indicator-dilution method to measure blood flow and transit times makes it possible to determine what is called the *central blood volume,* defined here as the volume between the right atrium and a systemic artery. (Some authors use the term to denote the region between the main pulmonary and systemic arteries.[11]) In adult supine human subjects, the central blood volume is about 1.2 liters, of which more than one-third is in the pulmonary vessels.[11] As pointed out above, the arterial boundaries of the compartment thus measured are ill-defined; the volume that dilutes the indicator includes arteries and veins that are temporally equidistant from the sites of injection and sampling.

One of the most important effects of peripheral venoconstriction is to raise central venous pressure and central blood volume. The significance of this change lies in its effect on cardiac function as expressed by Starling's law (Chapters 3, 4). Ventricular filling pressure rises, the ventricles deliver more energy, and in most circumstances stroke volume and cardiac output increase. A decrease in central blood volume and pressure has the opposite effect. As we have seen in previous chapters, the Starling mechanism is by no means the only one that governs ventricular function, but in this context it is particularly important.

A second effect of any adjustment that increases central blood volume is to engorge the pulmonary vasculature and enlarge the heart. Both changes are visible in x-ray or other images of the thorax. Pressure rises in the capillaries as well as in the other pulmonary vessels, with a predictable tendency toward loss of fluid into the interstitial spaces and alveoli. The pulmonary arteries and veins stiffen as they are distended, like other vessels, becoming a semirigid intrapulmonary framework that makes it more difficult to inflate and deflate the lungs.

These disturbances illustrate the most extreme effects that can be caused by displacement of blood from the periphery to central regions, but more often the same physiological mechanism operates with no harmful consequences. A considerable volume of blood can shift in either direction, as some examples will make clear. The general cardiovascular adjustments to various stresses have been considered elsewhere (Chapter 8); here we will concentrate on the direction and magnitude of redistributions of blood.

Postural changes

Gravity shifts blood from the upper to the lower parts of the body on changing from a supine to an erect position. Typically, about 250 ml moves from the central blood volume to the lower legs, decreasing vascular volume in the upper parts of the body and in all but the basal portions of the lungs. Central venous and mean systemic arterial pressures decrease slightly, and cardiac output falls 10 to 28% in spite of an increase in heart rate.[11] Venous blood volume in the legs rises,[1] sometimes by as much as 500 ml, due to the extra hydrostatic pressure imposed by the vertical distance between the legs and the heart. These responses are even more marked in experiments where the effects of gravity are simulated by sudden external application of suction to the lower part of the body (e.g., 50 mm Hg). Conversely, the "antigravity suit" developed for aviators and astronauts applies positive pressure on the lower extremities to prevent venous pooling during maneuvers that create strong footward g forces.

When an individual stands motionless, pooling of blood in the lower extremities is partially offset by sporadic, more or less voluntary contraction and relaxation of leg muscles (*muscle pumping*). Occasional small contractions suffice to restore normal central venous pressure and output.[1,37] To eliminate this variable in experimental studies of postural effects, the subject often lies on a motor-driven table that tilts the subject passively to a head-up position.

Compensatory reflexes are at work in the erect posture to make all of these effects less than they would otherwise be. Sympathetic vasoconstrictor activity, particularly in the upper arms and splanchnic bed, maintains arterial pressure at almost normal levels.[12] Venoconstriction is generally thought to be a part of the compensatory response, but experimental proof of such activity has been difficult to obtain.[6] Active venomotion could be detected only by demonstrating that venous compliance decreases to a level that is abnormal for the vessel diameter, and the evidence on this point is conflicting.

Some individuals suffer from a failure of reflex adjustment to the erect position. Their arterial pressure falls severely (*orthostatic hypotension*), often leading to dizziness or fainting.[1] Little is known about the cause of the disorder, except that is appears to arise from inadequacy of cardiovascular regulatory mechanisms. Chronic absence of gravitational stimuli, as in prolonged bed rest or space flight, produces similar intolerance to the upright posture in varying degrees, which gradually disappears when normal activity and gravitational conditions are restored. The total blood volume is decreased in such situations, which may account in part for the sensitivity to postural change. Red cell and plasma volumes both decrease about 12% in astronauts who remain under weightless conditions for long periods.[26] Patients on bed rest suffer a 5 to 15% loss of plasma volume in a few days, with no change in red cell mass.

Temperature

Hot environments bring about large changes in the distribution of the blood volume, and in doing so they place considerable stress on the cardiovascular system. The principal adjustments are a shift of blood from the splanchnic bed to the vessels of the skin (Chapter 12) and a smaller displacement into the central vascular compartment. Cutaneous blood flow increases to a marked degree. This response is an essential component of thermoregulation in man, placing a large volume of slow moving blood near the skin surface, where convection and sweating provide cooling. Other species in which panting is the major reaction to heat (the dog, for example) increase blood flow to the tongue, not to the skin. The description given here applies specifically to human subjects.

Although cutaneous blood volume cannot be measured with any accuracy at present it seems likely that body heating raises it at least fourfold, that is, by several hundred milliliters, and most of this blood is derived from the splanchnic compartment. Cardiac output increases, often leveling out at 12 to 13 liters/min after an hour of exposure to a temperature of 39° C. (The highest skin temperatures that can be tolerated[6] are 42° to 44° C.) The increased cardiac output is largely due to tachycardia, but there is also a moderate increase in stroke volume. Systemic arterial pressure falls at first but usually returns to the control level in a short time.

To cite a specific example reported by Rowell,[6] during whole-body heating at 40° C for 50 min, heart rate increased to 95 beats/min, stroke volume rose to 138 ml, central blood volume increased by 120 ml, and right atrial pressure fell to 1 mm Hg from a control value of 8 mm Hg. Splanchnic blood flow decreased by 40% and renal blood flow by 30%. The increase in stroke volume in spite of a fall in filling pressure demonstrates enhanced myocardial contractility, which, like the fast heart rate, is the result of reflex sympathetic stimulation. The enlargement of central blood volume is difficult to explain; although displacement of blood from the splanchnic bed often tends to increase the intrathoracic volume, most of the shift in this situation is into the cutaneous bed. Right atrial volume is presumably decreased, because pressure declines in that chamber and there is no reason to suppose that it becomes more compliant.

The sensors that provide information for these responses are temperature-sensitive regions of the skin, brain (Chapter 7), and possibly other internal locations; signals from these areas initiate selective reflex sympathetic vasoconstrictor impulses in response to heating of the body. The small, transient decrease in arterial pressure in the early phase of the response to heating is doubtless sensed by arterial barorecptors, but reflexes from that source probably have little to do with the redistribution of blood. The reflex response causes arteriolar constriction and reduced blood flow in the viscera, and would do so in the cutaneous circulation were it not for the powerful dilator mechanism that functions in the skin, plus the local effect of temperature on cutaneous veins (see below). As discussed in Chapter 12, active cutaneous vasodilatation is probably brought about by sympathetic cholinergic and secretmotor mechanisms. Much of the experimental evidence suggests that skin temperature controls the sympathetic constriction, whereas core temperature affects the active vasodilator components.[40] Although the skin detects changes in environmental temperature more quickly than the deeper core sensors do, the cutaneous and splanchnic circulations are more sensitive to changes in core temperature than to those in the skin.[28]

The efferent arms of the reflex responses to high temperatures are a sympathetic vasoconstriction of the splanchnic and renal beds, displacing blood from those organs, and dilatation in vessels of the skin, which favors redistribution of blood into that region. Arteriolar constriction in the splanchnic bed tends to lower venous pressure downstream, and a passive decrease in venous volume follows. Considering the approximately 700 ml of blood in the splanchnic veins, a large volume can be displaced. A similar but less marked reaction occurs in most abdominal viscera, including the kidneys, but they provide a smaller reservoir of blood. The vasoconstriction is largely neural in origin, but an increase in circulating epinephrine and norepinephrine is part of the sympathetic response. Plasma renin and angiotensin II also rise, and complete inhibition of angiotensin blocks about half of the renal vasoconstriction.[6] In contrast, the splanchnic constriction involves neither renin nor angiotensin II but is prevented by alpha-adrenergic blockade.[21]

Venomotor as well as arteriolar responses contribute to the redistribution of blood volume through splanchnic venoconstriction and cutaneous venodilatation. The arguments in favor of active splanchnic venoconstriction are rather indirect, but the veins of this bed are richly innervated, contain a large volume of blood, and can release at least half of their volume in reacting to exercise or stimulation of hepatic nerves.[16] It would consequently be surprising if that region did not furnish a large part of the blood translocated to the skin in hot environments. The veins of skeletal muscle are more sparsely innervated and are probably not involved.

The evidence for active relaxation of smooth muscle in veins of the skin is more specific. Relatively direct measurements can be made by occluding a segment of such vessels and measuring the intraluminal pressure; segmental volume being constant, any fall in pressure indicates relaxation of the venous wall. Active cutaneous venodilatation as a function of temperature comes about through two mechanisms. First, direct heating of superficial cutaneous veins reduces their responsiveness to incoming sympathetic constrictor impulses.[38]

This phenomenon is an inherent property of the local smooth muscle and can be demonstrated *in vitro*.[7] Second, the compliance of these veins is increased reflexly when core or skin temperature rises.[38] Deep cutaneous veins do not participate in this reaction, so that flow shifts away from the superficial vessels in the cold and toward them on exposure to heat.[7]

Heat and exercise

Exertion in a hot environment places a particularly heavy stress on the circulation, because the needs of contracting muscle compete with the requirements for cutaneous thermoregulation, and the metabolism of exercise adds an internal source of extra heat. The combined demands can exceed the ability of the cardiovascular system to meet them,[6] with severe and sometimes fatal results. The humidity of the environment and the subject's rate of sweating are important determinants of the stress that can be tolerated.

The problem that faces the regulatory system is to supply enough blood flow and oxygen to skeletal muscle while sustaining a high cutaneous flow and volume for heat exchange. Mean systemic arterial pressure is carefully protected, and falls little if at all. A tolerable physiological state can be established as long as the ambient temperature and the level of exercise permit physiological mechanisms to limit the increment in core temperature. With more severe stress some compromise must be reached, given the finite blood volume and the limited capacity of the heart to increase its output.

In general terms, the strategy the body adopts is to emphasize sympathetic vasoconstricton in the viscera so as to provide the necessary increase in flow to the skin and contracting muscle. Blood flow in the skin increases along with core temperature, as it does in nonexercising subjects, although at any given temperature cutaneous flow is lower during exercise than at rest. As discussed in the earlier section on the effects of heat per se, the splanchnic and renal blood flows in resting subjects are already lower than at neutral temperatures, while the heart rate, cardiac output, cutaneous flow, and blood volume of the skin are higher. Cardiac output increases further with the onset of exercise, but after prolonged exertion it tends to level off; stroke volume falls and the rate becomes faster. When the tachycardia reaches 200 beats/min and the core temperature approaches 40° C, exhaustion and collapse almost always occur. Cutaneous vasoconstriction occurs at the beginning of exercise but is soon replaced by vasodilatation, and blood flow to splanchnic and renal beds falls with exercise even more severely in hot environments than at normal temperatures.[6,18] Blood is thus transferred from visceral organs to skin regardless of temperature, but in a hot environment the visceral constriction is especially severe, leading in extreme cases to renal failure and gastrointestinal necrosis.

Individuals who reside and exercise moderately in hot, dry climates become physiologically adapted to these stresses in about 1 wk for reasons that are not clear. Such acclimatization reduces the tachycardia of exercise but does not affect cardiac output or peripheral resistance. An increase in plasma volume has been suspected of being one factor in the adaptation, but the experimental data do not uniformly support that hypothesis.[6]

References

Reviews

1. Blomqvist, C.G., Stone, H.L. (1983). Cardiovascular adjustments to gravitational stress. In: *Handbook of Physiology, Section 2: The Cardiovascular System, Vol. III, Peripheral Circulation and Organ Blood Flow, part 2,* J.T. Shepherd, F.M. Abboud, and S.R. Geiger, eds. Bethesda, Md., American Phsyiological Society, pp. 1025–1063.

2. Charm, S.E., Kurland, G.S. (1974). *Blood Flow and Microcirculaton.* New York, Wiley.

3. Cokelet, G.R., Meiselman, H.J., Brooks, D.E. (1980). *Erythrocyte Mechanics and Blood Flow.* New York, Alan R. Liss.

4. McDonald, D.A. (1974). *Blood Flow in Arteries.* London, Edward Arnold.

5. Rothe, C.F. (1983). Venous system: Physiology of the capacitative vessels. In: *Handbook of Physiology, Section 2: The Cardiovascular System, Vol. III, Part 1,* J.T. Shepherd, F.M. Abboud, and S.R. Geiger, eds. Bethesda, Md., Am. Physiological Society, pp. 397–452.

6. Rowell, L.B. (1986). *Human Circulation Regulation during Physical Stress.* New York, Oxford University Press.

7. Shepherd, J.T., Vanhoutte, P.M. (1975). *Veins and Their Control.* Philadelphia, W.B. Saunders.

8. Sjostrand, T. (1962). Blood volume. In: *Handbook of Physiology, Section 2, Vol. I,* W.F. Hamilton and P. Dow, eds. Washington, D.C., American Physiological Society, pp. 51–62.

9. Whitmore, R.L. (168). *Rheology of the Circulation.* Oxford, Pergamon Press.

10. Wintrobe, M.M. (1981). *Clinical Hematology,* 8th ed. Philadelphia, Lea & Febiger.

11. Yu, P. (1969). *Pulmonary Blood Volume in Health and Disease.* Philadelphia, Lea & Febiger.

Research Papers

12. Ahmad, M. Blomqvist, C.G., Mullins, C.B., Willerson, J.T. (1977). Left ventricular function during lower body negative pressure. *Aviat. Space Environ. Med.* 48:512–515.

13. Alexanian, R. (1969). Erythropoietin and erythropoiesis in anemic man following androgens. *Blood* 33:564–572.

14. Allen, T.H., Peng, M.T., Cheng, K.P., Huang, T.F., Change, C., Fang, H.L. (1956). Prediction of blood volume and adiposity in man from body weight and cube of height. *Metabolism* 5:328–345.

15. Antoniades, H.N., Scher, C.D., Stiles, C.D. (1979). Purification of platelet-derived growth factor. *Proc. Natl. Acad. Sci. U.S.A.* 76:1809–1813.

16. Brooksby, G.A., Donald, D.E. (1972). Release of blood from the splanchnic circulation in dogs. *Circ. Res.* 31:105–118.

17. Chien, S., Usami, S., Taylor, H., Liniberg, J.S., Gregerson, M. (1966). Effects of hematocrit and plasma protein on human blood rheology at low shear rates. *J. Appl. Physiol.* 21:81–87.

18. Clausen, J.P., Trap-Jensen, J. (1974). Arteriohepatic venous oxygen difference and heart rate during initial phases of exercise. *J. Appl. Physiol.* 37:716–719.

19. Conley, C.L., Nickerson, J.L. (1945). Effects of temperature change on the water balance in man. *Am. J. Physiol.* 143:373–384.

20. Davis, J.O., Holman, J.E. Carpenter, C.C.J., Urquhart, J., Higgins, J.T., Jr. (1964). An extra-adrenal factor essential for chronic renal sodium retention in presence of increased sodium-retaining hormone. *Circ. Res.* 14:17–31.

21. Escourrou, P., Freund, P.R., Rowell, L.B., Johnson, D.G. (1982). Splanchnic vasoconstriction in heat-stressed man: Role of renin-angiotensin system. *J. Appl. Physiol. (Respir. Environ. Exercise Physiol.)* 52:1438–1443.

22. Evans, E.A., Waugh, R., Melnik, L. 91976). Elastic area compressibility modulus of red cell membrane. *Biophys. J.* 16:585–595.

23. Groom, A.C. (1980). Microvascular transit of normal, immature, and altered red blood cells in spleen versus skeletal muscle. In: *Erythrocyte Mechanics and Blood Flow,* G.R. Cokelet et al., eds. New York, Alan R. Liss, pp. 229–259.

24. Henschel, A., Mickelsen, O., Taylor, H.L., Keys, A. (1947). Plasma volume and thiocyanate space in famine edema and recovery. *Am. J. Physiol.* 150:170–180.

25. Holmgren, A. (1956). Circulatory changes during muscular work in man. *Scand. J. Clin. Lab. Invest.* 8(Suppl. 24):1–97.

26. Johnson, P.C., Driscoll, R.B., LeBlance, A.D. (1977). Blood volume changes. In: *Biomedical Results from Skylab,* R.S. Johnston and L.F. Dietlin, eds. Washington, D.C., National Aeronautics and Space Administration, SP-377, pp. 235–241.

27. Nakao, M., Hoshino, K., Nakao, T. (1981). Constancy of cell volume during shape change of erythrocytes induced by increasing ATP content. *J. Bioenergetics Biomembranes* 13:5–6.

28. Proppe, D.W., Brengelmann, G.L., Rowell, L.B. (1976). Control of baboon limb blood flow and heart rate—role of skin vs. core temperature. *Am. J. Physiol.* 231:1457–1465.

29. Reeve, E.B. (1952). Use of radioactive phosphorus for the measurement of red-cell and blood volume *Br. Med. Bull.* 8:181–186.

30. Reeves, J.T., Grover, R.F., Blount, S.G., Jr., Filley, G.F. (1961). Cardiac output response to standing and treadmill walking. *J. Appl. Physiol.* 16:283–288.

31. Reinke, W., Johnson, P.C., Gaehtgens, P. (1986). Effect of shear rate variation on apparent viscosity of human blood in tubes of 29 to 94 μm diameter. *Circ. Res.* 59:124–132.

32. Reuschlein, P.S., Reddan, W.G., Burpee, J., Rankin, J. (1968). Effect of phys-

ical training on the pulmonary diffusing capacity during submaximal work. *J. Appl. Physiol.* 24:152–158.

33. Schmid-Schoenbein, H., Volger, E., Klose, H.J. (1972). Microrheology and light transmission of blood. II. The photometric quantification of red cell aggregation formation and dispersion in flow. *Pfluegers Arch.* 333:140–155.

34. Shoukas, A.A., Brunner, M.C. (1980). Epinephrine and the carotid sinus baroreceptor reflex: Influence on capacitative and resistive properties of the total systemic vascular bed of the dog. *Circ. Res.* 47:249–257.

35. Taylor, H.L., Erickson, L., Henschel, A., Keys, A. (1945). The effect of bed rest on the blood volume of normal young men. *Am. J. Physiol.* 144:227–232.

36. Trippodo, N.C., Cole, F.E., Frohlich, E.D., MacPhee, A.A. (1986). Atrial natriuretic peptide decreases circulatory capacitance in areflexic rats. *Circ. Res.* 59:291–296.

37. Wang, Y., Marshall, R.J., Shepherd, J.T. (1960). The effect of changes in posture and graded exercise on stroke volume in man. *J. Clin. Invest.* 39:1051–1061.

38. Webb-Peploe, M.M., Shepherd, J.T. (1968). Responses of dog's cutaneous veins to local and central temperature changes. *Circ. Res.* 23:693–699.

39. Whittaker, S.R.F., Winton, F.R. (1933). The apparent viscosity of blood flowing in the isolated hindlimb of the dog and its variation with corpuscular concentration. *J. Physiol.* 78:339–369.

40. Wyss, C.R., Brengelmann, G.L., Johnson, J.M., Rowell, L.B., Niederberger, M. (1974). Control of skin blood flow, sweating and heart rate: Role of skin vs. core temperature. *J. Appl. Physiol.* 36:726–733.

14

METHODS OF MEASUREMENT

Students of physiology rightly concentrate on the results of research as reported in textbooks and scientific papers, rather than on methodology, but they must also know something of the way those results have been obtained. Understanding a measurement technique not only reveals the accuracy and potential artifacts of the method but also conveys fundamental physiological principles. The relation between oxygen uptake and blood flow in the lungs, for example, is not merely the basis for a method of measuring cardiac output but a fact of functional significance. This chapter is a brief introduction to some of the methods by which important cardiovascular variables are measured. The detailed information needed to perform the procedures is given in specialized textbooks, which are cited in the appropriate sections.

Cardiovascular physiology is largely concerned with the measurement of physical dimensions like the force generated by heart muscle, the diameter of blood vessels, the area of capillary membranes, or the total volume of the blood. Other quantities, like rates of change with time or hydraulic energy, are derived from these variables. Chemical phenomena are no less important, as is evident in the binding properties of muscle receptors (Chapter 1) and the metabolism of cardiac muscle,[15] but we will concentrate here on the measurement of physical parameters.

The variables of interest are rarely measured directly. Instead, they are translated by instruments of varying degrees of complexity into other phenomena that can be manipulated and recorded. In modern laboratories, for example, the pressure within a blood vessel is usually evaluated by electrical currents in a transducer. The indirect nature of most experimental evidence should be kept in mind when results obtained with a new method of measurement seem to conflict with those given by earlier techniques. The conflict may lie in the interpretation of the results, not in the raw data produced by each method.

Instrumentation[4,12,21]

Physiological measurements are usually made by means of a *transducer,* a device that converts the entity being measured into another variable that can be displayed and recorded. The variable to which the transducer responds is called its *input,* and the signal produced by the transducing system is its *output.* In many transducers, the output is an electrical voltage or current, which may require amplification or other processing. The trend today is toward final conversion of data into digits that are stored in the memory of a computer or on a magnetic medium (see below).

Certain characteristics of performance are critical in virtually all instruments: sensitivity, method of calibration, stability, linearity, and frequency response. *Sensitivity* refers to the ratio of output to input; a transducer might convert a pressure of 100 mm Hg into an output of 5 V, for example, in which case the sensitivity, or *calibration factor,* would be $5/100 = 0.05$ V/mm Hg. If the data are handled by a digital computer, a pressure of 100 mm Hg at the transducer might produce a final output of 1,000 analogue-to-digital conversion units (ADU), corresponding to a sensitivity of $1,000/100 = 10$ ADU/mm Hg. Calibration in such terms is needed to express the final results in standard units. *Stability* refers to the constancy of calibration over periods of hours or days. Most instruments are designed to minimize drift of the zero baseline and calibration, but they should be checked frequently.

Instrumental sensitivity must be determined for two different kinds of inputs. The *static response* is the sensitivity measured when constant, time-invariant input signals are applied—for example, steady pressures at a number of different levels, or *steps*. The results are sometimes called the *DC response* by analogy with "direct" as opposed to "alternating" (sinusoidal) electrical signals. *Dynamic response* refers to the instrument's behavior when the input signal varies with time, and is usually tested by applying a series of sinusoidal waves of different frequencies. Dynamic performance can be displayed as a *frequency response* graph in which the outputs for constant-amplitude inputs are plotted against the frequency. The question of frequency response does not arise with all cardiovascular procedures, of course, being largely irrelevant with methods designed to determine an average value over a large number of cardiac cycles, as in the measurement of cardiac output. A *linear* static or dynamic response is one in which output is directly proportional to input regardless of input amplitude (within practical limits).

An ideal instrument would have the same sensitivity at all frequencies, including DC, so that the shape of the wave at the input would be precisely reproduced at the output, but such performance cannot be achieved in the real world. When the frequency of sinusoidal waves is steadily increased, sensitivity begins to fall at some point, as shown in Figure 14.1A. The essential requirement for a measuring instrument is that it have a uniform response up to frequencies higher than those contained in the physiological signal. The acceptable cutoff point is not the same for all variables. In human subjects, frequencies up to at least 20 Hz are contained in pulsations of blood pressure and flow, and up to 100 Hz in the electrocardiogram. The frequency content of cardiovascular signals depends in part on the heart rate (see below) and is consequently species dependent.

An exact description of instrumental behavior specifies just how uniform the frequency response is within a certain range—for example, "flat within ±5% from zero to 20 Hz." The response should extend evenly down to zero for most cardiovascular variables, including pressure and flow, but in electrocardiography the very lowest frequencies are often sacrificed, as in Figure 14.1C. Frequencies below 0.2 Hz in electrocardiographic records usually represent potentials that arise from the conjunction of skin, paste, and metal electrodes and are therefore of no physiological significance. Circuits can also be designed to filter out a specific band of frequencies, a modification sometimes used to eliminate 60-Hz interference from an electrical supply (Figure 14.1D).

The frequency response of an instrument depends on a host of factors, ranging from properties of the electronic circuitry to inertia of recording pens when they are employed. A complete specification of dynamic performance states the time delays between input and output (not shown in Figure 14.1), as well as the output/input amplitude ratios. Such delays are inescapable, although they may be very small. Perfect reproduction of the input signal requires preservation not only of the relative amplitudes of the various frequency components but also of their relative phase angles, or timing. Otherwise, the

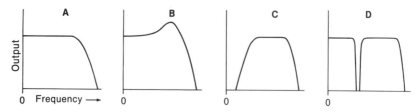

Figure 14.1. Typical instrumental outputs (*ordinate*) for sinusoidal input signals of constant amplitude, as a function of frequency (*abscissa*). **A**, overdamped system; **B**, underdamped system; **C**, cutoff at low as well as high frequency limit; **D**, "band-rejection" response. (Reproduced from Milnor,[12] with permission of Williams & Wilkins)

shape of the recorded wave will differ from that of the original. The response of an instrument to different frequencies is sometimes described in terms of the *damping* it imposes on inputs. A response that is uniform with respect to amplitudes up to some limiting frequency and falls off above that point is characteristic of an *overdamped* system. If, in addition, the device accurately reproduces the relative timing of the frequency components up to the cutoff point, it is said to be *critically damped*. An instrument that has an exaggerated response at some frequencies (Figure 14.1B) is referred to as *underdamped*.

The practical relevance of these considerations is that only a critically damped system can record pulsatile phenomena with perfect fidelity, and the frequency response of a measuring device is thus one of its most important characteristics. Most physiologists have no occasion to analyze the damping of their instruments, but they do learn to recognize the signs of a less than ideal frequency response. A system that does not transmit all the frequencies in the physiological signal not only fails to reproduce sharp details in the original waves but also records falsely low pulse amplitudes. In extreme cases, the pulsations virtually disappear, leaving only a tracing that indicates the time-averaged value of the variable. Underdamped systems can introduce *spikes* at their resonant frequency (the peak in Figure 14.1B); records of intraventricular pressure sometimes show an overshoot at the end of the rising phase for that reason. An electrocardiograph with an inadequate low-frequency response can produce records that resemble those in myocardial ischemia.

The best way to avoid distortion is to perform static and dynamic calibrations in the user's laboratory. Once the performance of an instrument is known, the data it delivers can be corrected for nonuniformities of response by electronic means or digital computation. Appropriate tests are relatively simple in the case of fluid-filled manometer systems, for example,[12] and more complicated but entirely feasible procedures can be devised to test most flowmeters. Creating testing conditions *in vitro* comparable to those in the intact animal is often the greatest problem. Transducer sensitivity to temperature and other environmental conditions is one of the factors to be taken into account.

Pressure and Force

Blood pressure can be measured directly by inserting a vertical tube into a vessel to discover how high blood will rise in it, as Stephen Hales did in 1733 to determine blood pressure in a horse.[3] As he discovered, pressure in a systemic artery will support the weight of a column of blood some 2 m in height. The idea that blood pressure can be expressed as the height of a column of fluid survives in our measurement of arterial pressure in millimeters of mercury or venous pressures in centimeters of saline. Pressure is by definition force per unit area, and the weight of a fluid column is a force proportional to its height. Lateral rather than end pressure (Chapter 6) is the variable of interest in most situations. Two different methods are commonly used to measure blood pressure: (1) direct sensing of intravascular pressure by the force it exerts on a pressure transducer, or manometer, and (2) external compression of an artery by the familiar blood pressure cuff around an arm or leg. The special problems that arise with direct measurements of pressure in microvessels require manometer systems designed for that purpose (see below).

The transducers in use today are designed so that the application of pressure modifies the electrical properties of some component by stretching or otherwise deforming it, the component usually being part of a resistor, capacitor, or inductor. Instruments specifically designed to measure force rather than pressure, which are used in studies of muscle contraction, for example, operate on similar principles. In the *strain gauge,* the most common type of pressure or force transducer, a strain-sensitive resistor serves as part of a Wheatstone bridge connected to a fixed external voltage. Stretching or compression of the sensing element changes its resistance and hence the electrical current flowing through the bridge. The structure is designed in a way that makes the change in current proportional to the applied stress, or pressure. The sensing element can be extremely small and mounted on the tip of a cardiovascular catheter. Most of the catheter-mounted sensors now available are accurate into the kilohertz range, eliminating any problems with frequency response.

Another type of manometry system employs an external transducer, mounted near the subject and connected to the lumen of a vessel through tubing and a saline-filled needle or catheter. The performance of such instruments depends on the characteristics of the connecting system as well as those of the transducer. Fluid-transmission systems are particularly prone to degradation of their frequency response, and they can produce distorted records unless strenuous efforts are made to eliminate gas bubbles. The length, diameter, and elasticity of the connecting tubing are also critical. The dynamic behavior of fluid-filled connections and transducers closely resembles that of second-order systems, and their behavior can be analyzed by appropriate equations.[5,12] The frequency response in a given arrangement can be tested in the laboratory by observing the response to an abrupt change in applied pressure, a waveform that can be created by bursting an inflated balloon (the "pop test"). The frequency response of the system can be calculated from the frequency and amplitude of the oscillations that follow such a *step function* of pressure.[12]

Most of the energy in pressure and blood flow pulsations lies in their first 10 harmonics, which means that they will be reproduced faithfully if the system responds uniformly at frequencies up to 10 times the fundamental, or heart rate—for example, 12 Hz when the heart rate is 72 beats/min. The fast heart rates in small animals require that the response be flat up to correspondingly higher frequencies. Moreover, the *10-harmonics* rule should be regarded as a minimum because spikes or notches in the pressure wave often come from frequencies above that range. In research using modern techniques, there is no reason to be satisfied with anything less than a response that extends up to at least 50 Hz in work on human subjects or dogs. A higher-frequency response equivalent to at least 20 harmonics is required for accurate measurement of differential pressures (dP/dt). In all cases, the low-frequency response should extend down to, and include, zero Hz (the DC response).

Cuff method

Clinical measurements of arterial pressure are usually carried out with a technique introduced by Riva-Rocci,[3] often referred to as the *cuff* method. This procedure depends on the *Korotkow sounds* that occur in a partially occluded artery. A specially designed cuff containing a rubber bladder is first wrapped around the arm and then inflated to a pressure above the arterial systolic pressure. Pressure is lowered gradually while the region just below the cuff is monitored with a stethoscope to detect sounds. At first, when the artery under the cuff is completely occluded, nothing is heard, but as soon as cuff pressure falls to the systolic level, a characteristic thudding sound occurs with each heartbeat. These sounds change abruptly in character when diastolic pressure is reached, becoming more distant and muffled. The technique is simple, easily learned, and surprisingly accurate, but not without its pitfalls.

Accuracy depends on attention to a number of details. The cuff should be wide enough to distribute pressure over a broad area, about 12 cm for the adult arm, smaller for children and larger for application to the thigh. The artery to be monitored should be located by palpation before inflating the cuff, so that the bell of the stethoscope can be positioned correctly; the bell should be applied firmly, but not with enough force to cause occlusion. Deflation should be carried out slowly, keeping in mind that the pressure drop between heartbeats determines the resolution of the readings. Various changes in the character of sounds occur during deflation, and it is important to distinguish them from the muffling that marks diastolic pressure. Sounds usually disappear entirely a few millimeters of mercury below the point of muffling, but in some pathological conditions they persist to levels well below the true diastolic pressure.

Pressure within the cuff should be completely released between tests, to avoid reflex responses as well as the discomfort that accompanies prolonged arterial occlusion. The psychological effect of having one's blood pressure measured should be taken into account, for the pressure measured is almost always higher on the first reading than it is on subsequent trials. For that reason, multiple determinations should be carried out until the subject is completely relaxed. With these precautions and a modicum of experience, the cuff method can give systolic pressures within ± 2 mm Hg of the values obtained by direct arterial puncture and diastolic pressure within ± 4 mm Hg. Pressure in the cuff is sometimes measured with a mercury manometer, eliminating the need for calibration. More often the dial of an aneroid gauge is employed; its accuracy should occasionally be verified.

Pressure in microvessels

Direct access to pressures in the microcirculation can be established through drawn glass micropipettes, but their small diameter (0.5 to 5.0 μm) would produce intolerable damping of pulsations if conventional fluid connections to a transducer were used. This obstacle has been circumvented by measuring not the blood pressure itself but the counterforce that must be applied to prevent blood from entering the tip of the micropipette.[48] The electrical resistance across the tip is measured continuously, and the resistance when pressure is just high enough to hold the saline–blood interface at the tip is taken as the null point for a servomechanism. If pressure in the pipette falls below pressure in the vessel, blood enters the tip, resistance increases, and a hydraulic system applies more pressure until balance is restored. Careful design of the servomechanism makes this response so efficient that the interface does not oscillate but remains very close to the tip. A standard transducer is employed to measure pressure in the pipette, and pressure pulsations can be recorded with a flat response from 0 to about 18 Hz in vessels smaller than 100 μm in diameter.

Cardiac Output

Fick method

Concept

A general principle applied in physiology by Adolph Fick more than century ago is the basis for a variety of methods of measuring blood flow.[9] The principle is, in effect, a restatement of the law of conservation of mass for some *indicator*, which may be an endogenous substance like oxygen or an exogenous one introduced by the investigator. One class of indicators is confined to the vascular system, examples being radioisotope-labeled red cells and dyes like T-1824 or indocyanine green that bind to plasma albumin. A second class consists of diffusible indicators such as ^{133}Xe, nitrous oxide, and hydrogen gas. Heat can also be used as an indicator by injecting saline that is warmer or colder than blood temperature. The indicator may gain access to the blood-stream by inhalation, as in the case of oxygen or inert gases, or injected.

There are two relevant variables:

$M(t)$, the amount of indicator taken up by the blood in a period of time t. This quantity may be expressed as grams or milliliters of indicator, depending on the indicator.

ΔC, the change in blood concentration of the indicator between the inlet and outlet of the system being examined, or in other words, the arteriovenous difference $(C_A - C_V)$, where C_A is the arterial and C_V the venous concentration. The units here may be grams of indicator per milliliter of blood or milliliters of indicator per milliliter of blood.

Both variables are measured over the same period of time. A general equation for blood flow through the system (Q) in situations where arterial and venous concentrations vary with time is

$$Q = \frac{M(t)}{\int_0^t (C_A - C_V)dt} \tag{14.1}$$

Modifications of this expression for diffusible indicators used in measuring regional blood flow are discussed in a later section.

Measurement of cardiac output

The Fick method is one of the oldest yet most accurate ways of measuring cardiac output, its only disadvantage in humans being the need to obtain samples of blood from the pulmonary artery by cardiac catheterization. The indicator is usually the O_2 taken up from inspired air, although the respiratory exchange of CO_2 can be used. The principle can be stated in a form that is equivalent to a rearrangement of equation 14.1: The O_2 taken up in the lungs in 1 min equals pulmonary blood flow per minute (the cardiac output) multiplied by the amount of O_2 that each milliliter of blood picks up in passing through the pulmonary bed.

O_2 uptake in the lung is easily measured by collecting inspired and expired air. The O_2 collected by the blood as it traverses the pulmonary capillaries is determined by subtracting pulmonary arterial from pulmonary venous O_2 concentration. A blood sample from a systemic artery provides an estimate of pulmonary venous O_2, because the concentration does not change as blood moves from pulmonary veins to peripheral arteries unless an abnormal shunt pathway exists. The O_2 concentration in blood entering the lungs must be determined by sampling from the pulmonary artery or right ventricle; more peripheral venous sites will not do because the sample must represent complete mixing of blood from the venae cavae and the coronary sinus, which differ in their O_2 concentrations.

Pulmonary arterial blood can be obtained readily in experimental animals by direct puncture, but in human subjects such sampling became feasible only with the introduction of right heart catheterization.[6,26] Cardiac catheterization is now performed daily in hundreds of hospital laboratories as a diagnostic procedure. A small, flexible catheter is introduced into a peripheral vein and advanced through the venous tree into the vena cava, from which site its tip can be guided under fluoroscopic observation into the right heart and pulmonary artery. Special catheters tipped with a tiny balloon that floats along in the bloodstream until it reaches the pulmonary artery can also be used.

A steady state is assumed, so that the denominator of equation 14.1 is simply the O_2 difference between arterial and venous samples rather than an integral:

$$\text{Cardiac output (ml/min)} = \frac{\text{oxygen uptake (ml } O_2/\text{min)}}{\text{AV } O_2 \text{ difference (ml } O_2/\text{ml blood)}} \quad (14.2)$$

Suppose, for example, that O_2 uptake by the lungs in a resting subject is found to be 250 ml/min and that simultaneous sampling from the femoral artery and the pulmonary artery shows their O_2 concentrations to be 0.190 and 0.150 ml per milliliter of blood, respectively. The arteriovenous O_2 difference is thus 0.040 ml per milliliter blood, and the cardiac output is 250/0.040, or 6,250 ml/min. The same principle can be applied to the transfer of CO_2 from pulmonary circulation to lung or to inhaled foreign gases.

The Fick method has been widely used. Its accuracy when carefully performed is probably about $\pm 5\%$, meaning that in 95% of cases it gives results that differ by no more than 5% from the actual cardiac output. The principal limitation is the need for a steady state; output and pulmonary gas exchange must remain constant while samples are collected, which in practice means a period of several minutes. For that reason, rapid changes in the circulation during the onset of exercise or other events cannot be studied by this technique.

The procedure described above is known as the *direct Fick method,* and before it was generally adopted, a variety of indirect applications of the same principle were devised. One approach was to infer the O_2 or CO_2 concentrations of pulmonary arterial and venous blood from measurements of gas tensions in the lung, assuming that alveolar air and capillary blood were in perfect equilibrium. Such methods have now generally been abandoned because they are more difficult in practice and less accurate in results than the direct Fick method and other techniques now available.

Exogenous indicators

The measurement of cardiac output from the dilution of exogenous indicators was introduced by Stewart in 1897 and has since been modified in many ways.[2,23] The basic principle is the same as that in the O_2 uptake method described above, but in this instance a certain volume of blood is labeled by intravascular injection of a measurable, nontoxic indicator, and the time-varying concentrations of the blood so marked are observed at the outlet of the system. For the measurement of cardiac output, the indicator must remain within the vascular compartment while changes in its concentration are measured. The indicator may be a dye like indocyanine green, radioisotope-labeled red cells or plasma albumin, or even cold saline (*thermodilution*), the "concentration" in the last case being blood temperature.

Indicator-dilution curves

In a typical protocol, the indicator is injected into a peripheral vein as a small bolus, and its subsequent concentration in a peripheral artery is recorded as it changes with time. The injectate, which should be no more than a few milliliters in volume, mixes with the bloodstream and is assumed to enter all subsequent vascular branches in proportion to their flow. The measurements of concentration may be made on a series of arterial blood samples collected in rapid succession or by a sensor mounted on an intravascular catheter. The thermodilution method has become particularly popular because the arterial dilution curve can be sensed by a small, catheter-mounted thermistor. Whatever the indicator, it reaches the arterial sampling site after an interval of a few seconds (the *appearance time*), and its concentration then rises to a peak and falls, as in Figure 14.2A. One advantage of the bolus-injection indicator-dilution method is that it requires constant conditions for only 15 to 60 sec, the time needed for the all of indicator to travel from the point of injection to the distal sampling site.

The falling portion of the curve is eventually interrupted by a secondary rise caused by indicator that has already traversed paths through arteries and veins once and is now making a second trip. The indicator concentration at the pulmonary arterial inlet is zero by the time the curve begins, so the integral with respect to time of the first-pass concentrations at the outlet (as represented by systemic arterial samples) is the denominator for equation 14.1. The infor-

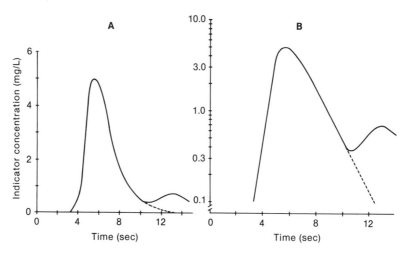

Figure 14.2.   Indicator-dilution curve in brachial artery after injection of 1.02 mg T-1824 dye into contralateral brachial vein. *Abscissa*, time after injection; *ordinate*, dye concentration in mg/liter blood. **A**, continuous record of arterial concentration by densitometer. Late secondary peak indicates recirculation of dye. **B**, curve in **A** replotted with logarithmic ordinate. *Dashed line*, extrapolation of downslope to separate the curve representing first circulation of the indicator ("primary curve") from recirculation. Area of primary curve = 15.57 mg sec/liter; therefore, cardiac output = 1.02/15.57 = 0.0655 liters/sec, or 3.93 liters/min.

mation relevant to cardiac output is thus contained in the *area* of the *primary* curve produced by the first circulation, and some way to exclude the recirculation part of the record must be found.

An empiric solution to that problem rests on the observation that the primary curve falls in an almost exponential manner, following a straight line when log concentration is plotted as a function of time (Figure 14.2B). Extrapolation of the downslope reveals the later portions of the initial passage of indicator, and the area of the primary curve can be determined by planimetry or other means. (The time at which the primary curve ends cannot be determined from a semilog plot, but it can be approximated by the time required to fall to 0.1% of the peak concentration.) Cardiac output can then be calculated from the amount of indicator injected (*I*, in milligrams) and the area of the primary curve (*A*, in milligram seconds per liter):

$$\text{Cardiac output (liters/sec)} = \frac{I}{A} \qquad (14.3)$$

A typical calculation accompanies Figure 14.2

This method is now more widely used than the O_2 uptake technique and has about the same accuracy. One advantage of the indicator-dilution technique

is that only a few seconds are required for each determination, so that measurements of output can be repeated rapidly. Instruments that carry out the
whole sequence of concentration measurement, extrapolation, and computation of output are available. The principal disadvantage of the indicator-dilution
method is its diminished accuracy when cardiac output is low; the curve then
becomes prolonged and reduced in height, making extrapolation of the downslope less reliable. An alternative technique is based on infusion of indicator at
a constant rate, rather than as a bolus; in this case the curve rises to a steady
plateau, and other methods of analysis must be applied.[2,9,23]

It is necessary to add that the accuracy *in vivo* of cardiac output methods
in general cannot be determined with any precision because no single standard
of proven reliability exists for comparison. Various lines of evidence suggest
that the error in the Fick and the indicator-dilution methods is probably about
±5%, and errors of this magnitude are usually unimportant. That figure may
overstate the accuracy of the dilution method, for its reproducibility in successive determinations can rarely be made better than ±7%, even with the most
careful attention to technique. Not the least of the potential sources of error is
the measurement of the exact amount of indicator injected. The reproducibility
of the O_2 uptake method can be brought to ±3% or ±4%. In any case, the O_2
uptake, indicator-dilution, electromagnetic, and ultrasonic methods (see below) all give essentially the same results, and the conclusion that they measure
cardiac output with a relatively small error is generally accepted.

Modifications of the indicator-dilution method serve a number of purposes, including measurement of regional blood flow in the forearm and other
systems[23] and studies of capillary permeability. The latter application employs
multiple indicators injected simultaneously. If one marker remains within the
vascular system and another is diffusible, two different curves are recorded,
and the rate at which the permeable substance passes through the capillary wall
can be determined by comparing them.[1]

Indicator transit times and regional blood volumes

The information contained in an indicator-dilution curve can be used to
measure not only the cardiac output but also the *mean transit time* and the
volume of distribution between the sites of injection and sampling. The reasoning behind such calculations becomes clearer when we realize that the area is
the product of the mean concentration, C_m, and the overall duration, t', of the
primary curve: $A = C_m t'$. If I represents the amount of indicator injected, then
the quantity I/C_m is the volume of blood labeled by indicator and t' is the length
of time required for its first passage. Just as the vertical dimensions of the curve
can be expressed as a mean concentration, so the sequence of values on the
abscissa during the primary curve can be expressed as a mean time for the first

passage of indicator. This mean depends on transit times through all the vascular pathways, long and short, traversed by some portion of the indicator. The procedures for calculating transit time appear in other textbooks.[2,9] Careful studies have shown that the distribution of transit times through any bed is a complicated function, and the so-called mean transit time is not a simple average.[1,23]

The product of blood flow and mean transit time is the volume of blood in all the pathways that contribute to dilution of the indicator. For example, when injection is into a peripheral vein and sampling is carried out at a peripheral artery, the product of cardiac output and mean transit time includes the blood volumes of the heart and the pulmonary vessels, as well as the venous path to the heart and the arterial conduit to the sampling site. The result of such a calculation is called the *central blood volume*, but its boundaries are not well defined because it includes all arterial and venous pathways that are *temporally* equidistant from the sites employed. The central volume has a physiological significance, however, because it increases when the heart enlarges or the pulmonary bed becomes distended (Chapter 13). In other situations, the boundaries of the volume determined by a dilution curve are more definite. The volume of the pulmonary vascular bed can be measured with some accuracy, for instance, by injecting into the pulmonary artery and sampling from the left atrium, or from the difference between volumes measured by injections at those two sites.[12,22]

The dilution principle has also been applied to measure ventricular volumes. When an indicator is injected into the left atrium or ventricle, the aortic concentration falls in a stepwise manner with subsequent heartbeats, and the decrement from each ejection to the next is a measure of the *ejection fraction* (the ratio of stroke to end-diastolic volume). If stroke volume is known from the heart rate and a determination of cardiac output by dilution (or an alternative method), ventricular volume at the end of diastole can be calculated.[2,32] Complete mixing of the indicator with blood in the ventricle is required, and samples must be taken from the ascending aorta to detect the sharp downsteps in concentration. For some reason, thermodilution measurements of this kind often give larger end-diastolic volumes and smaller ejection fractions than angiographic techniques do, and the latter are probably more accurate.

Estimates of blood flow by pressure analysis

Pulse pressure

The excursion of pressure from peak systole to end of diastole, or *pulse pressure,* is related to the amount of blood ejected and the physical properties of the outflow artery. This fact has led to various methods of estimating stroke volume from arterial pulse pressure, but all of them suffer from the need to assume values for arterial elasticity and viscosity. These properties vary from one subject to another, and quantitative estimates of stroke volume cannot be made from pulse pressure alone for that reason. In cases where the arterial properties can safely be assumed to be constant, however, abrupt changes in pulse pressure usually indicate an alteration of stroke volume in the same direction.

Pressure gradient

Equations given in Chapter 6 show that pulsatile flow in a blood vessel is at every instant a function of the longitudinal intravascular pressure gradient. This relationship is the source of methods that calculate instantaneous flow from simultaneous measurements of pressure at two sites.[12] The theory employed adopts a number of simplifying assumptions, not the least of which is the use of pressure differences over a distance of several centimeters to estimate dP/dx (x being an axial coordinate). The pressure differences observed are small, and the mean pressure gradient is at the limit of resolution for even the best manometric techniques. In spite of these limitations, approximate results can be obtained. Simple electrical analogue circuits can be designed to receive the two pressure signals as input and then deliver a voltage continually proportional to flow as their output. With the exception of a few specialized research problems, the advent of electromagnetic and ultrasonic flowmeters (see below) leaves little place for pressure gradient methods.

Regional Blood Flows

Constant-infusion methods

The ubiquitous Fick principle is the basis of a number of procedures for determining regional blood flow with inert, diffusible gases, notably the nitrous oxide method of measuring flow in the brian.[33] The subject inhales continuously a low concentration of nitrous oxide in air (15%), causing arterial and venous concentrations to rise steadily and become equal after about 10 min (Figure 14.3); during that period, the gas diffuses into the brain and other tissues. (Some investigators recommend a longer equilibration period.) Measurement of nitrous oxide in repeated samples from a peripheral artery and the internal jugular vein gives the time course of concentrations at the inlet and outlet of the system, and the area between those two curves (Figure 14.3) is the denominator for the calculation of cerebral blood flow from equation 14.1.

The numerator, the amount of nitrous oxide taken up by brain tissue during 10 min of inhalation, cannot be determined directly in humans, but it can be estimated with the aid of the *partition coefficient* (λ) that defines the relative

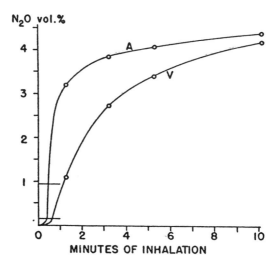

Figure 14.3.   Nitrous oxide concentrations (*ordinate*) in arterial (*A*) and jugular venous (*V*) blood as a function of time (*abscissa*) during a 10-min period of inhalation of N_2O. (Reproduced from Kety and Schmidt,[33] with permission of the American Society for Clinical Investigation)

distribution of nitrous oxide between blood and cerebral tissue. This parameter is the ratio, in a state of equilibrium, of tissue concentration ($C_{T\infty}$) to blood concentration ($C_{B\infty}$):

$$\lambda = \frac{C_{T\infty}}{C_{B\infty}} \tag{14.4}$$

The partition coefficient is relatively constant in man and the dog[33] (0.98 to 1.07). Tissue concentration is expressed in milliliters of nitrous oxide per gram of brain tissue and blood concentration in milliliters of nitrous oxide per milliliter of blood, giving λ in milliliters of blood per gram of tissue.

When equilibrium has been reached, $C_{B\infty}$ is equivalent to the venous concentration ($C_{V\infty}$), and the amount of nitrous oxide taken up by the brain during the equilibration period (*M* in equation 14.1) can be calculated as $M = \lambda\, C_{V\infty}$. The form of equation 14.1 for cerebral blood flow, *Q*, in milliliters of blood per minute per *gram of brain*, is

$$Q = \frac{\lambda C_{V\infty}}{\displaystyle\int_0^t (C_A - C_V)\,dt} \tag{14.5}$$

Nitrous oxide is not the only inert gas that can be employed; ^{85}Kr is often used to determine cerebral blood flow. The same principle can be used to measure myocardial blood flow, obtaining myocardial venous blood from the coronary sinus.

A variety of *washout* methods have also been devised.[9] The isotope ^{133}Xe has been used to measure local cutaneous flow, for example, by exposing a small area of epidermis to a chamber containing the gas for a time and then monitoring radioactivity in the area with an external detector. The activity declines with time as blood flow washes out the isotope, and a specific theoretic model must be assumed to calculate flow from the multiexponential curve that results. Analogous procedures have been adopted to measure local blood flows in the kidney and other organs.

Microsphere distribution

An approach widely used in experimental animals to compare blood flow in one part of the circulation with that in another is the injection of particulate matter that lodges in the capillaries.[30] If the particles mix thoroughly in the bloodstream so that they are distributed in proportion to flow in all branches of the system, and if they are completely trapped in the peripheral tissues so that no recirculation occurs, then the fraction of the injectate subsequently found in a given tissue region is the same as the fraction of blood flow that was delivered to it. The most common injectate is a suspension of plastic microsphere, typically 15 μm in diameter but commercially available in a range of sizes. The method can determine blood flow to a particular organ as a fraction of cardiac output, or flow to one segment of an organ as a fraction of flow to the whole organ.

For example, if one-tenth of the material injected into the left atrium is later found in the liver, then one-tenth of the cardiac output was distributed to that organ, and relative flow to different parts of the liver could be estimated from the local radioactivity. Absolute rather than relative regional blood flows can be calculated if cardiac output is measured simultaneously by another method or if the flow to another organ is known and used as a reference standard. The technique has been used in the kidney to determined the relative blood flows in the medullary, inner and outer cortical regions, and for analogous studies of skeletal muscle and the myocardium.

Flow in the microcirculation

In spite of the special problems presented by measurement of flow in the microcirculation, pulsatile records have been obtained by a number of different instruments, usually by photometric techniques for determining red cell velocity. The basic operation is electronic-optical detection of the edges of advancing erythrocytes and timing of the passage of cells between two points.[45] Refinements include the use of fluorescence, laser beams, and spectroscopic analysis.[38,44] Blood flow through the pulmonary capillary bed as a whole can be measured by inhalation of nitrous oxide while the subject is enclosed in a body plethysmograph (Chapter 11). The rate of uptake of nitrous oxide from the alveoli, measured volumetrically by the plethysmograph, is taken as an indication of capillary flow.

Pulsatile Blood Flow

The methods described for measuring cardiac output and regional blood flow average the outflow of blood from the heart over a period of time, and thus differ from techniques for recording the rapid changes of flow in a single cardiac cycle. The history of pulsatile flow measurement[12] is filled with devices now abandoned; the instruments in use today employ one of four fundamental techniques: electromagnetic fields, ultrasonic waves, radioisotope emissions, and nuclear magnetic resonance. The first two kinds are readily available and have been in use for some time; the last two are relatively new but in a rapidly advancing state. Most of the instruments sense blood velocity, not volumetric rate of flow, but they are nevertheless referred to by the generic name of *flowmeters*.

Electromagnetic flowmeters

This technique is based on an electromagnetic principle discovered by Michael Faraday early in the nineteenth century, namely, that the motion of a conductor in a magnetic field generates an electromotive force, or voltage, oriented at right angles to the motion. Blood is a conductor of electricity, so the imposition of a magnetic field on a blood vessel produces a difference of voltage across its diameter. Faraday himself attempted to apply this principle to measure flow in the river Thames as it moved through the earth's magnetic field, but the equipment available to him was inadequate to the task.

The voltages involved are extremely small in practice, frustrating many attempts over the years to measure the velocity of the bloodstream. The development of the modern electromagnetic flowmeter is largely the result of work by Kolin[34,35] and Wetterer.[47] The voltage generated by the movement of blood through a magnetic field can be sensed through electrodes on the walls of a blood vessel, and is directly proportional to the mean blood velocity and the strength of the field.[12] *Mean* velocity here refers to the average of the velocities in different lamina across the lumen (Chapter 6). The recorded pulsations thus represent the changing mean laminar velocity from instant to instant.

The pulsations can be averaged with respect to time by flowmeter circuits, and most instruments provide both pulsatile and nonpulsatile outputs, the latter being an indication of flow (or velocity) averaged over a great number of heartbeats. If the probe is on the ascending aorta or main pulmonary artery, this average is the cardiac output.

Electromagnetic transducers are of three types (Figure 14.4). The *cannulating* variety connects between two ends of a severed blood vessel; the cannula itself contains the voltage-detecting electrodes, and the block fitted around it contains the electromagnetic coils. The *perivascular* type is a cuff that slips around the vessel, fitted with sensing electrodes and coils for generating the field. The *catheter* type is mounted on the tip of a cardiovascular catheter, providing both electrodes and coils in a masterpiece of miniaturization. Typical records from perivascular probes appear in Figures 2.7 and 12.4

Perivascular and cannulating probes both require surgical exposure of the vessel and for that reason are used predominantly in animal experiments, although some studies of human arteries exposed during surgical procedures have been reported.[36] Perivascular probes must fit the vessel under examination closely but not constrict its lumen, which makes it necessary to have a selection of various sizes at hand. Cuffs with an internal diameter as small as 0.75 mm are commercially available. Too loose a fit fails to bring the electrodes in contact with the external surface of the vessel wall, resulting in a noisy or absent flow signal. Too tight a fit alters the pressure and flow in the vessel. Cuff-type probes can be used in acute studies or surgically implanted for conscious studies days or weeks later. In the latter case, a loose fit is desirable because a thin film of connective tissue and plasma clot soon anchors the cuff to the vessel wall. Catheter-mounted electromagnetic flowmeters have the obvious advantages of a less invasive procedure. Pressure sensors can be included on the same catheter, and cardiac catheterizations for diagnostic or investiga-

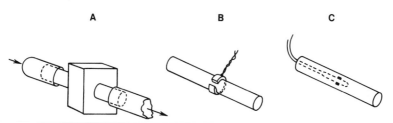

A   **B**   **C**

Figure 14.4.   Three types of electromagnetic flowmeter. **A**, cannulating type; vessel is cut transversely, and its ends are attached to the rigid inflow and outflow tubes of the probe. **B**, perivascular type, a rigid cuff that contains magnet and electrodes and can be slipped around the vessel. **C**, intravascular flowmeter; magnet coils and sensing electrodes are fitted to tip of catheter. (Reproduced from Milnor,[12] with permission of Williams & Wilkins)

tive purposes frequently make use of such instruments. The catheter should lie near the axis of the vessel for best results.

Static calibration of electromagnetic flowmeters can be carried out *in vitro* with ordinary laboratory equipment or determined *in vivo* by comparison of the mean signal from a flowmeter on the ascending aorta with cardiac output measured by some other method.[46] The latter procedure has the advantage of giving the calibration immediately in terms of volume flow (cubic centimeters per second); if the sensitivity is measured in terms of velocity (centimeters per second), the diameter of the lumen of the vessel must be known to convert to volume flow. Identification of the zero-flow signal, or baseline, is often the most difficult problem because it may be influenced by the electrical resistance of the probe's surroundings. Complete dynamic calibration is more complicated because it is difficult to construct a device that will generate sinusoidal flows at frequencies above 4 or 5 Hz. Fortunately, the high-frequency limits on response are not set by the electromagnetic principle but by the electronic circuits of the flowmeter, which can be tested.[12,28]

Ultrasonic flowmeters

Ultrasonic vibrations in the range 1 to 8 MHz can be applied to the measurement of blood flow in two different ways. One measures the *transit time* of the ultrasonic beam from one point to another in the bloodstream, and the other is based on the *Doppler effect*. In both cases, very short time intervals or small changes in frequency must be measured precisely,[8] placing stringent demands on the instrument designer. Much of the credit for early advances in this field belongs to Rushmer and his associates.[27] The later development of hand-held probes[25] enlarged the range of applications enormously (see below). Ultrasonic instruments now exist that can produce detailed images of blood flow in which the direction and velocity of motion are color coded.

Transit-time method

This technique makes use of the fact that ultrasonic vibrations are "carried along" with the flow of blood, so to speak, making their speed the algebraic sum of blood velocity and the inherent velocity of ultrasound. The vibrations move through blood and tissue with a speed close to that of sound in water, about 1,500 m/sec, whereas circulating blood velocities are much less than 1 m/sec, indicating the fine discrimination needed if a flowmeter is to separate them.

Ultrasonic flow probes, like the electromagnetic variety, often take the form of a perivascular cuff that fits around the vessel, but in this case precise fit is less important. Two crystals that can emit or receive ultrasonic signals are built into the cuff in positions that will transmit a beam through the bloodstream at a moderate angle to the vessel axis. Each crystal emits a brief pulse of ultrasound (hence the name, *pulsed transit-time flowmeter*) and then waits to receive the signal from its opposite number. The transit times are measured electronically, and the pulse is repeated at a rapid rate. The times occupied in transmission upstream and downstream differ because of the motion of the blood, and the difference is a function of blood velocity, the distance between the crystals, the angle of the beam, and the velocity of ultrasound. In practice, the difference is a matter of nanoseconds.[12] If the ultrasonic beam covers the full width of the vessel, the output of the instrument will be proportional to the average blood velocity in the vessel. Probes that cast a wider or narrower beam can introduce significant errors.

The accuracy of the ultrasonic transit-time method is approximately the same as that of the electromagnetic technique, and its uniform frequency response extends up to at least 50 Hz. The perivascular probe need not fit the vessel closely, because no electrodes in contact with the wall are involved. As with electromagnetic probes, static calibration can be performed *in vitro* with measured, steady flows. Catheter-mounted ultrasonic sensors that operate on the transit-time principle are also available.

Doppler method

Another application of ultrasound to the measurement of blood flow is founded on the Doppler effect, the phenomenon responsible for the abrupt change in tone of a train whistle as it speeds by. As the train approaches, the sound waves traveling toward the listener are compressed and hence higher in pitch than the one actually emitted. When the train passes and begins to move away, the frequency of the sound drops suddenly. The same principle applies to ultrasound reflected from a moving target when the emitter and detector are both stationary; the returning waves are not of the same frequency as those emitted, and the difference is a function of the target's velocity.

Doppler flowmeters use the moving red blood cells as reflectors and place the ultrasonic source and detector in a perivascular cuff or catheter.[31] The erythrocytes do not all move with exactly the same velocity, and a spectrum rather than a single frequency returns to the detector. Electronic circuitry processes this frequency spectrum to generate a final output signal. The results depend in part on the profile of velocities in the vessel being studied, and the analytic problems are complex, but in well-designed Doppler instruments the output is proportional to average cell velocity. Some amount of filtering at low frequencies is often imposed because motion of the vessel produces spurious signals in that range, with the result that velocities lower than 2 cm/sec are interpreted as zero in some instruments.

One type of Doppler meter[39] employs a single crystal for emission and detection, sending out repeated, brief pulses of ultrasound (the *pulsed Doppler* method, as contrasted with the *pulsed transit-time* technique described above). Detection of reflected waves occurs between these emissions but is restricted to a narrow time gate, and this gate can be adjusted so as to pick up only those reflections that occur at a selected distance from the crystal. In this way, the velocity of just one part of the stream can be measured with a spatial resolution reported to be 0.5 mm, making it possible to record velocity profiles in some vessels.

The simplest, yet most dramatic, application of the Doppler principle came with the introduction of transcutaneous recording of blood flow in peripheral arteries.[25,41] Transmitter and detector crystals are mounted side by side in a hand-held, pencil-like probe or in a block that can be strapped on a limb. An aqueous gel is used to eliminate any air space between the skin and the crystals, thus providing a continuous and effective medium for transmission of the ultrasonic waves. Records of pulsatile flow can be obtained from relatively superficial arteries like the carotid and femoral, but not from vessels that lie deep within layers of muscle or in the thorax. The potential usefulness of this instrument was quickly recognized, and many different applications have been reported.[7,42]

Ultrasound is employed to create images of cardiovascular structures, as well as to measure blood flow (see below). Like other imaging methods, it has been used to estimate stroke volume and thus cardiac output, but with less accuracy than the dilution and Fick procedures already described. In theory, end-diastolic, end-systolic, and stroke volumes could be measured from sequential three-dimensional pictures of the internal ventricular outlines, but volumes cannot be derived from the two-dimensional ultrasonic images that are usually recorded unless some assumptions are made about the geometric shape of the chamber. One could assume, for example, that the ventricles resemble a symmetric, longitudinally divided ellipsoid, but many other shapes have been tried and general agreement on the most appropriate model has yet to be reached. The goal is a clearly defined body with contours that are realistic and a volume that can be predicted from measurements of a limited number of linear dimensions. Much effort has been devoted to the task, testing various formulae and comparing the dimensions of radiological or ultrasonic images with postmortem casts of the ventricle, but the results thus far suggest an error of not less than $\pm 15\%$ in estimates of cardiac output by imaging techniques.

Thermal flow methods

The rate of flow of a liquid can be measured by its cooling effect on a heated body, and this principle is the basis for a technique that can determine profiles of blood velocity.[7,40] The instrumentation is similar to that of the *hot-*

wire anemometer, a device used by aeronautic engineers to measure air flow. The sensing element consists of a very thin, heated film of platinum or gold small enough to fit on an intravascular catheter or a needle that can be inserted through the vascular wall. The film is heated to a few degrees Celsius above the temperature of the blood, and a servomechanism maintains that thermal gradient. The higher the velocity of the blood, the greater its cooling effect; velocity is determined from the electrical power required to maintain the temperature of the metal strip. The probe is affected only by the motion of blood immediately adjacent to it, making it possible to explore local velocities at a number of points across the diameter of a vessel, with results like those shown in Figure 2.8. The response of such instruments extends up to at least 150 Hz, and they have been used to study the high frequencies that appear in turbulent flow.

Magnetic resonance flowmetry

The phenomenon of nuclear magnetic resonance not only provides a technique for creating images of cardiovascular structures (see below) but also promises to be a practical method of measuring flow velocity within blood vessels.[24] Protons moving in a magnetic field cause phase shifts in the magnetic gradient, and measurements of these shifts have been analyzed to produce velocity-coded images of the motion of blood.[43] This technique is still in its infancy, but it offers a noninvasive way of identifying separate lamina moving at different velocities in the bloodstream.

Imaging Methods

A host of new methods of creating images of the heart and blood vessels has been introduced in recent years, supplementing and for some purposes replacing the earlier x-ray techniques.[11] Standard radiological images of the heart and of radiopaque solutions in the bloodstream continue to be an important source of information, but newer approaches are based on the reflection of ultrasonic beams, the phenomena of nuclear magnetic resonance, and emissions from injected radionuclides.[13] These procedures not only reveal the size and shape of the cardiac chambers but also permit measurement of their changing blood volumes and the motion of the ventricular wall. Stroke volume can be estimated from the systolic and diastolic areas of the ventricular images, given certain assumptions about the shape of the chamber; a simple measurement of heart rate then permits calculation of cardiac output.

The modern proliferation of methods began when computer analysis was wedded to *tomography,* the radiographic picturing of "slices" through an organ, an alliance that has made *CAT scan* a household word.[17] The basic principle of tomography, namely, moving the source and detector through a series of angles to emphasize a single plane, has a long history in radiology, but the early pictures were far from perfect. Mathematical reconstruction of the image in one plane, a problem first encountered in electron microscopy and radioastronomy, is a task for which the digital computer is ideally suited, and the result was a vast improvement in clarity and resolution. This approach was first employed with x-rays, but it is now applied to a number of different imaging modes.

Ultrasonic imaging is at present the technique used most widely for examining details of cardiovascular structure and function.[16,18] It can produce pictures of the heart that rival or exceed in quality those obtained by x-ray angiography. The key operation is measurement of the time that elapses between emission of a pulse and reception of the "echo" from a distant site, an interval that is proportional to the distance because of the virtually constant velocity of the signal. A beam of ultrasound, usually in the 1- to 10-MHz range, is transmitted to the organ under investigation, and the waves reflected back from various structures are recorded. The distance from emitter to reflection site is calculated from the observed round-trip transit time and the wave velocity, which is of the same order as the speed of sound in water. The principle is similar to that involved in sonar or radar location of ships or aircraft. Application of the method to the heart is appropriately called *echocardiography*.

The use of ultrasonic imaging is simple in practice,[18] although a highly sophisticated instrument is required to measure the multiplicity of reflections and the very small transit times. A single transducer incorporating both emitter and detector is placed by hand on the thoracic wall at a position that sends the beam of ultrasound through the heart in the desired direction. Waves are reflected from interfaces between tissues of different acoustic impedance, so that signals return from the ventricular walls, septum, and valves; the result is displayed as an image on an oscilloscope or recording device. If a stationary beam is used, a narrow, cylindrical segment of the chest and heart is sampled (sometimes irreverently called an "icepick view"), revealing the position and motion of the reflecting structures. More often the beam is repeatedly swept through an angle, producing a two-dimensional view in which beat-to-beat changes can be observed. The detailed sequential images can be recorded on videotape and analyzed to give quantitative information about cardiovascular function. Multiple transducers and complex scanners can be designed to generate three-dimensional data. The diameter of blood vessels can also be monitored, and the resolution of the method is limited to one wave-length, about 0.3 mm for 5 MHz.

Radionuclides are a rapidly expanding technique of imaging. They use external detectors to record activity from short-lived, intravenously injected radiopharmaceuticals, a procedure that yields a high degree of contrast between the blood so labeled and the surrounding structures.[11,13] One method follows the first pass of tracer through the region of interest; another records events after an equilibrium has been established throughout the vascular compartment.

Two classes of radionuclides are of particular interest as tracers. *Positron emission tomography (PET)* uses substances that release a positron, which travels a short distance and then reacts with an electron to emit a pair of photons on paths 180° apart. The location of such events is determined by detectors placed diametrically opposite each other. Radionuclides of carbon (^{11}C), nitrogen (^{13}N), or oxygen (^{15}O) can be incorporated into amino acids or other substances and used in the PET method, so that metabolic data as well as images can be obtained. One disadvantage of this approach is the very short half-life of the compounds, which means that a cyclotron to produce them must be available nearby. An alternative technique is *single photon emission computerized tomography (SPECT)*, which is based on radionuclides like ^{99m}Tc that are now readily available at some distance from the production site and typically permit observations for longer than 24 hr. The imaging device in SPECT is usually a gamma-ray camera. Ventricular volume, stroke volume, ejection fraction, and wall thickness have been studied in man and other species by these methods.[11]

Nuclear magnetic resonance (NMR) operates on a quite different principle, but it is an equally versatile tool for studying blood flow and metabolism, in addition to the imaging of structures.[11,19] The technique is founded on the magnetic phenomena generated by the spinning of nuclei in certain atoms. When this magnetism is oriented uniformly by placing a tissue in a strong magnetic field, a probing radio-frequency beam will cause the sample to emit a signal. Each nuclear species is sensitive to a specific frequency, so that NMR can be adapted to measure the local concentrations of particular compounds, for example those containing phosphorus. In addition, the intensity of the signal emitted by stationary elements differs in strength and phase from that given by elements moving rapidly through the test region, making it possible to distinguish between blood in motion and surrounding structures. Techniques that can identify streams of different velocities within a blood vessel and display them as color-coded images are under development.

Computers

Digital computers have contributed to virtually every field of human endeavor, and research in cardiovascular physiology is no exception. Almost all cardiovascular laboratories make use of them to some extent, and everyone in the field should be familiar with their virtues and limitations. Among their most important characteristics are the ease of storing large quantities of data on magnetic tapes or disks and the rapid performance of complex calculations. Computer design and usage are advancing almost too rapidly to be caught in print, and only a few elementary comments will be attempted here.

Experimental data usually enter the computer by way of an analogue-to-digital (A/D) converter, which translates the electrical analogue signals from transducers into digits that are stored in the computer's memory. The overall frequency response of the measurement then depends not only on the transducer's characteristics but also on the A/D sampling rate and other properties of the converter. A rate of 10 samples/sec, for example, cannot describe accurately a signal that contains frequencies above 5 Hz, and that A/D rate is consequently not high enough for most physiological pulsations of blood pressure and flow. If signals from several different transducers are being recorded, it is important to know whether they are being converted simultaneously, or sequentially with a small but finite time interval between them.

Data received by the computer during the course of an experiment can be calibrated and printed out in appropriate units almost instantaneously. Moreover, the computer can be made to control the progress of an experiment, randomizing a series of tests or modifying a protocol in the light of current results. Measurements can also be displayed as time-based tracings on a monitor, thus taking the place of pen-writing oscillographs. There are advantages in having results continuously visible in such a graphic form because the human eye is remarkably efficient at recognizing artifacts and characterizing waveforms. The computer can be taught to do the same thing, identifying anomalies and measuring them precisely, but programming it to do so is an arduous task. Such programs already exist for some specific applications, however, the analysis of electrocardiograms and cardiac catheterization data being prominent examples.[29]

One application of computers is in the numerical analysis that follows experiments—statistical calculations, curve fitting and the like—operations that often cannot be planned until the results are all in. Automatic performance of this tedious number crunching is valuable but is probably the least of the computer's contributions. More important is the freedom it gives the investigator to frame hypotheses that would otherwise scarcely be considered. There need be no hesitation in exploring a nonlinear model, or seeking a multivariate solution, if the physiological circumstances suggest them and explicit equations can be written.

All of the above procedures require that the computer be directed by a program, and the writing of complex programs is a profession in itself. Nevertheless, the modern investigator is well advised to have at least an elementary knowledge of programming languages and to be able to call on specialized textbooks when necessary.[14,20] Repeated checking of the instructions that make up a program is essential; nothing is easier than to overlook some step or assumption that the researcher takes for granted but has forgotten to tell the computer.

References

Reviews

1. Bassingthwaighte, J.B., Sparks, H.V. (1986). Indicator dilution estimation of capillary endothelial transport. *Annu. Rev. Physiol.* 48:321–334.

2. Bloomfield, D.A. (1974). *Dye Curves: The Theory and Practice of Indicator Dilution*. Baltimore, University Park Press.

3. Geddes, L.A. (1970). *The Direct and Indirect Measurement of Blood Pressure*. Chicago, Year Book Medical Publishers.

4. Geddes, L.A. (1984). *Cardiovascular Devices and Their Applications*. New York, Wiley.

5. Grodins, F.S. (1963). *Control Theory and Biological Systems*. New York, Columbia University Press.

6. Grossman, W. (ed.) (1980). *Cardiac Catheterization and Angiography*. Philadelphia, Lea & Febiger.

7. Hwang, N.H.C., Normann, N.A. (1977). *Cardiovascular Flow Dynamics and Measurements*. Baltimore, University Park Press.

8. Hykes, D., Hendrick, W.R., Starchman, D.E. (1985). *Ultrasound Physics and Instrumentation*. New York, Churchill Livingstone.

9. Lassen, N.A., Henriksen, O., Sejrsen, P. (1983). Indicator methods for measurement of organ and tissue blood flow. In: *Handbook of Physiology, Section 2: The Cardiovascular System. Vol. III, Peripheral Circulation and Organ Blood Flow, Part I*, J.T. Shepherd and F.M. Abboud, eds. Bethesda, Md., American Physiological Society, pp. 21–63.

10. Levine, R.A., Gillam, L.D., Weyman, A.E. (1986). Echocardiography in cardiac research. In: *The Heart and Cardiovascular System*, H.A. Fozzard et al., eds. New York, Raven Press, pp. 369–452.

11. Miller, D.C. (ed.) (1988). *Clinical Cardiac Imaging*. New York, McGraw-Hill.

12. Milnor, W.R. (1989). *Hemodynamics*. 2nd ed. Baltimore, Williams & Wilkins.

13. Pohost, G.M., Okada, R., Boucher, C.A., Bourge, R.C. (1986). Radionuclide methods to assess cardiac function, perfusion, viability and necrosis. In: *The Heart and Cardiovascular System*, H.A. Fozzard, ed. New York, Raven Press, pp. 309–329.

14. Press, W.H., Flannery, B.P., Teukolsky, S.A., Vetterling, W.T. (1986). *Numerical Recipes. The Art of Scientific Computing*. Cambridge, Cambridge University Press.

15. Randle, P.J., Tubbs, P.K. (1979). Carbohydrate and fatty acid metabolism. In: *Handbook of Physiology, Section 2: The Cardiovascular System, Vol. I, The Heart*, R.M. Berne and N. Sperelakis, ed. Bethesda, Md., American Physiological Society, pp. 805–844.

16. Reneman, R.S. (ed.) (1974). *Cardiovascular Applications of Ultrasound.* Amsterdam, North Holland.

17. Robb, R.A. (1982). X-ray computed tomography: From basic principles to applications. *Ann. Rev. Biophys. Bioeng.* 11:177–201.

18. Schapira, J.N. (ed.) (1982). *Two-Dimensional Echocardiography.* Baltimore, Williams & Wilkins.

19. Schulman, R.G. (ed.) (1979). *Biological Applications of Magnetic Resonance.* New York, Academic Press.

20. Soucek, B. (1976). *Microprocessors and Microcomputers.* New York, Wiley.

21. Webster, J.G. (1978). *Medical Instrumentation. Application and Design.* Boston, Houghton Mifflin.

22. Yu, P.N. (1969). *Pulmonary Blood Volume in Health and Disease.* Philadelphia, Lea & Febiger.

23. Zierler, K.L. (1962). Circulation times and the theory of indicator-dilution methods for determining blood flow and volume. In: *Handbook of Physiology, Section 2: Circulation, Vol. 1,* W.F. Hamilton and P. Dow, eds. Washington, D.C., American Physiological Society, pp. 585–616.

Research Reports

24. Axel, L. (1984). Blood flow effects in magnetic resonance imaging. *Am. J. Roentgenol.* 143:1157–1166.

25. Baker, D.W., Stegall, F., Schlegel, W.A. (1964). A sonic transcutaneous blood flowmeter. In: *Proceeding of the 17th Annual Conference on Eng. Med. Biol.* 6:76.

26. Cournand, A., Ranges, H.A. (1941). Catheterization of right auricle in man. *Proc. Soc. Biol. Med.* 46:462–466.

27. Franklin, D.L., Schlegel, W., Rushmer, R.F. (1961). Blood flow measured by Doppler frequency shift back-scattered sound. *Science* 134:564–565.

28. Gessner, U., Bergel, D.H. (1964). Frequency response of electro-magnetic flowmeters. *J. Appl. Physiol.* 19:1209–1211.

29. Harrison, D.C., Ridges, J.D., Sanders, W.J., Alderman, E.L., Fanton, J.A. (1971). Real-time analysis of cardiac catheterization data using a computer system. *Circulation* 44:709–718.

30. Heymann, M.A., Payne, B.D., Hoffman, J.I.E., Rudolf, A. (1977). Blood flow measurements with radionuclide-labelled particles. *Prog. Cardiovasc. Dis.* 20:55–79.

31. Kalmanson, D., Toutan, G., Novokoff, N., Deral, C. (1972). Retrograde catheterization of left heart cavities in dogs by means of an orientable directional Doppler catheter-tip flowmeter: A preliminary report. *Cardiovasc. Res.* 6:309–318.

32. Keroes, J., Rapaport, E. (1972). Ventricular volume measurements in the awake dog using implanted thermistor beads. *J. Appl. Phsyiol.* 32:404–408.

33. Kety, S.S., Schmidt, C.F. (1948). The nitrous oxide method for the quantitative determination of cerebral blood flow in man: Theory, procedure and normal values. *J. Clin. Invest.* 27:476–514.

34. Kolin, A. (1936). An electromagnetic flowmeter. Principle of the method and its application to blood for measurements. *Proc. Soc. Exp. Biol. Med* 35:53–56.

35. Kolin, A. (1970). A new approach to electromagnetic blood flow determination

by means of a catheter in an external magnetic field. *Proc. Natl. Acad. Sci. U.S.A.* 65:521–527.

36. Lee, B.Y., Madden, H.L., McDonough, W.B. (1969). Use of square-wave electromagnetic flowmeter during direct arterial surgery. *Vasc. Surg.* 3:218–242.

37. Milnor, W.R., Jose, A.D., McGaff, C.J. (1960). Pulmonary vascular volume, resistance, and compliance in man. *Circ. Res.* 22:130–137.

38. Nilsson, G.E., Tenland, T., Obert, P.A. (1980). A new instrument for continuous measurement of tissue blood flow by light beating spectroscopy. *IEEE Trans. Biomed. Eng.* 27:12–19.

39. Peronneau, P.A., Hinglais, J., Pellet, M., Leger, F. (1970). Velocimetre sanguin par effet Doppler a emission ultra-sonore pulsee. A. Description de l'appareil. Resultats. *L'onde Electrique* 50:3–18.

40. Seed, W.A., Wood, N.B. (1970). Development and evaluation of a hot film velocity probe for cardiovascular studies. *Cardiovasc. Res.* 4:253–263.

41. Stegall, H.F., Rushmer, R.F., Baker, D.W. (1966). A transcutaneous ultrasonic blood-velocity meter. *J. Appl. Physiol.* 21:707–711.

42. Targett, R.C., Levy, B. Bardou, A., McIlroy, M.B. (1985). Simultaneous Doppler blood velocity measurements from aorta and radial artery in normal human subjects. *Cardiovasc. Res.* 19:394–399.

43. Van Dijk, P. (1984). Direct cardiac NMR imaging of heart wall and blood flow velocity. *J. Compt. Assist. Tomogr.* 8:429–436.

44. Wayland, H. (1982). A physicist looks at the microcirculation. *Microvasc. Res.* 23:139–170.

45. Wayland, H., Johnson, P.C. (1967). Erythrocyte velocity measurement in microvessels by a two-slit photometric method. *J. Appl. Physiol.* 22:333–337.

46. Weber, K.C., Engle, J.C., Lyons, G.W., Madsen, A.J., Fox, I.J. (1968). In vivo calibration of electromagnetic flowmeter probes on pulmonary artery and aorta. *J. Appl. Physiol.* 25:455–460.

47. Wetterer, E. (1937). Eine neue Methode zur Registrierung der Blutstromungsgeschwindigkeit am uneroffneten Gefass. *Z. Biol.* 98:26–36.

48. Wiederhielm, C.A., Woodbury, J.W., Kirk, S., Rushmer, R.F. (1964). Pulsatile pressures in the microcirculation of frog's mesentery. *Am. J. Physiol.* 207:173–176.

INDEX

Numbers in bold-face type indicate tables or figures.

Acceleration of blood, 125
Acetylcholine
  arrhythmias, effect on, 167
  cardiac effects, 70, 104
  endothelium and, 15, 260
  esterase, 260
  neurotransmitter, 25, 220, 223, 295
  presynaptic receptors, 70, 261, 263, 274
  receptors, 22, 295–296
  vascular effects, 260–263
Acidosis. See Hydrogen ions
Aconitine, 156
Actin, 66, 67, 91, 292
Action potentials. See Membrane potentials
Active state (muscle), 101
Adenosine, 266, 274, 301, 397, 406
  hypoxia and, 303
Adenosine triphosphate (ATP), 266, 273–274,
  307
  ATPase, 316
  co-release, 259, 301
  cross-bridges and, 130, 314
  endothelium and, 261, 296
  ischemia and, 273
  muscle-shortening velocity and, 130
  presynaptic receptors, 263, 274
  vasomotor effects, 273, 301
Adenylate cyclase, 15, 24, 70, 295, 406
ADH. See Antidiuretic hormone
Adrenal gland
  cortex, 280, 281, 429
  medulla, 220, 267, 278, 280, 298
Adrenoceptors. See Receptors, alpha-adrenergic;
  Receptors, beta-adrenergic
Adventitia, blood vessels, 6, 186
Afferent nerves. See Nerves
Afterload (muscle), 94, 118, 190
Afterpotentials, 157, 168
Aging, effects of, 52–54, 131
Agonists, 22
Airway irritation, 244
Aldosterone, 137, 238, 269, 270, 280
Allergic reactions, 274
All-or-none contraction, 98
Alpha-adrenergic receptors. See Receptors, alpha-
  adrenergic
Altitude, effects of, 377
Analogue-to-digital conversion, 205, 478
Anaphylaxis, 273, 379, 383
Anemometer, hot-wire, 474–475

Anesthetics, 31, 165, 166
Angina pectoris, 242
Angiotensin (I and II), 137, 269–270, 382
  clearance of, 269
  converting enzyme, 269, 382
  presynaptic receptors, 263, 270
  renin and, 269
  vasomotor effects, 269, 301, 378, 379, 422
Anoxia. See Hypoxia
ANP. See Atria: release of natriuretic peptide
Antagonists, 23
Anticoagulant actions, 16, 383
Antidiuretic hormone (ADH), 261, 270, 271,
  280, 301
Antidromic conduction, nerves, 266, 277
Antigravity suit, 447
Aorta. See Arteries
Aortic body, 239
Appearance time (indicators), 463
Arachidonic acid, 263, 272, 379
Arrhythmias, 155–169
  bigeminy, 160
  cardioversion, 163, 168–169
  catecholamines and, 164, 268
  drug actions on, 164–168
  ectopic foci, 154, 155, 156, 158
  extrasystoles, 155, 158–160
  fibrillation, 157, 161–163, 167, 168
  flutter, 161
  mechanisms of, 156–158
  myocardial injury and, 163–164
  parasympathetic stimuli and, 161, 167
  parasystole, 155
  reentrant, 155, 157–158, 162, 163
  sinus, 155, 375, 380
  tachycardias, 160–161, 167, 168
  triggered activity and, 156–157, 160, 168
Arterial hypoxia. See Hypoxia
Arteries, 6–10. See also Blood Vessels
  aorta, 39, 124, 304
  auricular, 296
  brachial, 44
  branches, area ratio of, 6, 360
  bronchial, 361
  carotid, 297, 303, 305, 393
  cerebral, 296
  coronary, 124, 303, 400
  cross section, 39–40, **41**
  distensibility, 125, 317
  ear, 297

Arteries (*continued*)
 elastic, 8, 187
 femoral, 304
 hepatic, 412
 muscular, 8, 187
 pial, 294, 393, 398
 pulmonary, 39, 297, 359, 360, 370,
   446
 pulsatile distention of, 50, 199
 receptors, smooth muscle, 294–295
 renal, clamping, 270
 spinal, 393
 stenosis of, 124, 131, 367
 umbilical, 307, 391
 vertebral, 393
 wall components, 6, 291
 Windkessel model, 202–203
Arterioles. *See* Microcirculation
Arteriovenous oxygen difference, **35,**
   285
Atherosclerosis, 54, 174
Athletic performance, 34, 37, 284
ATP. *See* Adenosine triphosphate
ATPase, 130, 168, 316. *See also* Adenosine
   triphosphate
Atria
 arrhythmias, 154, 160–161, 164, 238
 conduction in, 73
 contraction of, 51, 111, 237
 ectopic beats, 158–**159**
 pressure waves, 111, 114
 release of natriuretic peptide, 137, 238
 stretch receptors, 236–238, 279
Atrial natriuretic peptide, 137, 238, 270
Atrioventricular block, 153–154
Atrioventricular (AV) node
 block, 74, 106, 153–154
 blood supply, 400
 conduction in, 73–74, 147, 153, 154
 ectopic beats, 159
 innervation, 251, **252**
 membrane potentials, 151
 structure, **252**
Atropine, 260, 264
Attenuation, viscous, 212, **213**
Automaticity, 155, 156, 164
Autonomic nerves. *See* Nervous system, autonomic
Autoradiography, 22
Autoregulation, vascular, 191, 387–392
 arteriolar, **389**
 cerebral, 242, 395, 396
 coronary, 406
 renal, 420–421
 theories of mechanism, 303, 308, 323, 390–
   392
AV. *See* Atrioventricular node
Axial accumulation of red cells, 15
Axo-axonal signals, 261, 263
Axon reflex, 266, 274

Baroreceptive regions, distensibility of, 227
Baroreceptors, arterial, 226–236, 279, 376
 afferent signals, 227, **229,** 230–231
 central nervous system connections, 227, 230,
   233
 gain, 233
 histology, 227, **228**
 hypertension and, 234
 impairment of, 234
 norepinephrine and, 235–236
 pulmonary, 236
 reflex actions, 228, 231–232, 255
 resetting, 233, 234
 sensitivity, 235
 set point, 233
 as transducers, 230, 234–235
Basal state, 31
Bernard, Claude, 4, 264
Bernoulli principle, 182
Beta-adrenergic receptors. *See* Receptors, beta-
   adrenergic
Bezold-Jarisch reflex, 275
Bigeminal rhythm, 160
Biologic variation, 30
Block, conduction
 atrioventricular, 153–154
 bundle branch, 154
Blockers, calcium channel, 164, 166
Blood, 14, 428. *See also* Blood volume;
   Erythrocytes; Viscosity
 clots, 178, 429
 coagulation, 273, 383, 429
 density, 181
 erythrocytes, 429, 430, 431
 fibrinogen, 430, 435, 436
 hematocrit, 14, 433–434
 leukocytes, 431
 osmolarity, 306–307
 platelets, 273, 429, 431
 proteins, 342
 reservoirs, 280, 296, 444
 viscosity, 14, 118, 172, 336, 434, 435. *See*
   also Viscosity
 viscosity, normal, 434
 volume. *See* Blood volume
Blood-brain barrier, 330, 398–399
Blood flow, 17. *See also* Cardiac output;
   Hemodynamics; Regional circulations
 acceleration, 125
 aortic, 49
 capacitance and, **134**
 cerebral, 241, 393–395, 468
 in collapsible vessels, 194–198, 381–
   382
 critical closing pressure and, 193, 388
 cutaneous, 408–410, 450
 in distensible vessels, 191–192
 inertia, 113, 125
 laminar, 174, **175**
 mathematical analysis, 198, 204–209

methods of measurement, 49, 393–394, 401, 463–475
pressure gradient and, 171–172
pulmonary, 51, 366–367, 371–373
pulsatile, **50,** 51, 176, 198, **213,** 296, 335
regional, 393, 395, 401, 408, 413, 419, 423, 467–470
renal, 241, 419
resistance, **134,** 177–180
in rigid vessels, 191
skeletal muscle, 423
splanchnic, 241, 413
steady (nonpulsatile), 131, 172–176
turbulent, 175
velocity, **42,** 335, 367
velocity profile, 51, **52**
venous return, 132
Blood pressure, 9, 17. *See also* Pressure; Pressure, pulsations of
arterial, 44–49
in cattle, 43
central nervous control, 222–223, 225
"cuff" method of measuring, 459–460
diastolic, 44–45, 201–202
effects of age on, 45, 47
in giraffe, 43
hydrostatic, 182, 381–382
hypertension, 131, 179. *See also* Hypertension
hypotension. *See* Hypotension
mean, 200–201
normal, man, **44**-49
pulsatile, 198, 364
pulse contour, 46, **47**
pulse pressure, 45, 48, 200–201, 211, 466
sex differences, 45
sleep, 233
systolic, 44–45, 201
Blood vessels. *See also* Arteries; Microcirculation; Vasoconstriction; Vasodilation; Veins
adventitia, 186
branching of, 6, 40, 212
capacitance of, 258
changes with age, 52–53
circumferential stress, 185, **188**
collapsible, 194–198, 216, 381–382
compliance, 186, 443–445
conduit, 258
denervation, 259
diameter, 296
dimensions, **7,** 39–40
distensibility, 42, 184, 186–193, 296
elasticity, 42, 58
elliptical, 194
endothelium, 15–17, 186, 260, 275, 296
exchange, 258
functional classification, 257–258
genital, 260, 262
heterogeneity, 291, 297
injury to, 17
medial layer, 186

neural control, 253–257
receptors, smooth muscle, 23, 294–295
resistance, 177–180, 257
structure, 3–13
tone, 216, 290, 298, 306
viscoelasticity, 190–191
volume, 42
wall thickness, 6
wave velocity in. *See* Velocity
Blood volume, 274, 281
atrial stretch receptors and, 237, 438
blood "reservoirs," 280, 296, 444
capillary pressure, influence of, 438
central, 373, 446, 466
distribution of, **12,** 43
exercise and, 439
methods of measuring, 440–442
normal values, 436–437
nutrition and, 439
physiological variations, 438–440
plasma, 436–439, 442
posture, effect of, 438
in pregnancy, 439
pulmonary, 373–375
red cells, 436, 437
regional, 442–447
regulation, 437–438
shifts of, 191, 215, 373, 443, 445–451
transit time and, 444
Blushing, 225
Body plethysmograph, 51, 373
Body shape
and blood pressure, 43
and cardiac output, 57
Body size
and blood pressure, 43, 58
and cardiac output, 54–58, **56**
Body surface area, 34, 57
Bone marrow, 14, 329
Boundary layer, **176**
Bradycardia, 155, 241
Bradykinin, 241, 242, 261, 265, 296, 337, 382, 411
Brain. *See* Cerebral circulation; Nervous system, central
Branching coefficient, 40
Bromosulfophthalein, 413
Bronchial circulation, 361
Bundle branch block, 154
Bundle of His, 63, 73, 147, 153, 156
Bursts (action potentials), 297, **310,** 311, 391
Bypass, cardiopulmonary, 273

C fibers (nerve), 68, 225, 243
C filaments (muscle), 67
Cable theory, 90
Calcium "blockers," 164, 166
Calcium ions, 23, 315
calmodulin and, 313

Calcium (*continued*)
　cardiac effects, 107
　channels, 82, 300
　digitalis and, 168
　exchange for sodium, 82, 105, 168
　excitation–contraction and, 91, 313–314
　influx inhibitors ("blockers"), 164, 166
　intracellular concentration, 300, 306, 313
　membrane potentials and, 107, **305**
　muscle contraction and, 102, 103, 299, 313
　muscle length and, 93, 101, 309
　oscillatory release, 157
　sarcoplasmic reticulum and, 82, 103, 300
Caldesmon, 314
Calibration factor (instruments), 455
Calmodulin, 313, 314
cAMP. *See* Cyclic AMP
Capacitance
　cell membrane, 90
　vessels, 258
Capacitance vessels, 257–258, 443
Capillaries. *See also* Capillary wall, flux through;
　　Microcirculation; Regional circulations
　architecture, 327, 328–332
　basement membrane, 331
　blood flow in, 258, 333, 335
　blood volume, 369
　choroid plexus, 330
　classification, 330–331
　collapse, 382
　continuous, 330, **331**
　discontinuous, 330, **331**
　fenestrated, 330, 331, **332,** 346, 347
　fiber matrix in, 338, 350
　flux through wall, 258, 280, 331, 335, 336–
　　351
　glomerular, 334
　hematocrit in, 335
　hepatic, 329
　length, 329
　number of, 329, 330
　permeability, 274, 338, **339,** 465
　pores, 336, 338, 341, 347–351
　pressure, 49, 258, 333–334, 338, 342,
　　345
　protein leakage, 353
　pulmonary, 330, 334, 361, 373, 382
　pulsatile flow, pulmonary, 51, **372, 374**
　recruitment, 369
　resistance, 336
　skeletal muscle, 328
　splenic, 329
　structure, 330–331
　surface area, 11, 337, 338, 346
　transport capacity, 341
　vesicles in wall, 351
　volume
　　pulmonary, **12,** 372
　　total, **12,** 329
　wall, 330–331

Capillary wall, flux through, 336–351
　amino acids, 399
　bradykinin and, 337
　bulk flow, 339, 340
　carrier-mediated, 346
　by diffusion, 338, 339, 340
　filtration coefficient, 340
　glucose, 399
　histamine and, 337
　hydraulic conductivity, 340
　hydraulic force, 338, 341
　indicator-dilution measurement of, 345–346
　interstitial pressure and, 345
　isogravimetric studies, 343–345
　lipid-soluble substances, 337, 351
　molecular size and, 339, 348, **349,** 350
　osmotic pressure, 338, 342
　osmotic transients, 345
　permeability, 274, 338, **339,** 341, 346
　pores, 347–351
　pressure and, 337, 343, **344**
　principles, 337–341
　rate, 339
　reflection coefficient, 340, 350
　shear stress and, 350
　specific organs, 346, **347**
　surface area, 346
　vesicles, 337
Carbon dioxide. *See also* Hypercapnia
　cerebral vessels and, 304, 396
　chemoreceptor, 239
　pCO$_2$, 304, 396, **397**
　smooth muscle and, 304
　vascular effects, 304
Carbon monoxide, 277, 278
Cardiac cycle, events of, 5, 111, **112,** 113–
　116
Cardiac failure, 135–137, 238, 270, 281, 440
Cardiac glycosides. *See* Digitalis
Cardiac index, 34, 35, 56–57
Cardiac output, 17, 127, 255
　age, relation to, 32, 34
　in athletes, 34, 37
　body shape, relation to, 57
　body weight, relation to, 34, 54–58
　distribution of, 37, **39**
　with exercise, 282, **283,** 284, 450
　hypoxia and, 123, 241, 278
　measurement of, 32, 460–465
　normal, 31, **32, 33**
　after physical training, 284, 285
　posture and, 32
　sex differences, 32
　species differences, 35, **36**
　surface area, relation to, 34, **35,** 56–57
　temperature and, 448
Cardiac work. *See* Ventricles
Cardioversion, 168
Carotid artery. *See* Arteries
Carotid bodies, 239, 275

Carotid sinus
    afferent signals, 230–231
    arrhythmias and, 167
    baroreceptors, 227
    distensibility, 234
    external pressure on, 161, 167
    innervation, 227, **229**
    structure, 226–227
CAT scan. *See* Computer-assisted tomography
Catechol-O-methyl transferase, 299
Catecholamines. *see* Epinephrine; Norepinephrine
Catheter flowmeters, 471, 473, 475
Catheter manometers, 458, 471
Catheterization, cardiac, 462
Cell-to-cell conduction, 66, 297, 311
Central nervous system. *see* Nervous system,
        central
Cerebral circulation, 241, 242
    alpha-adrenergic receptors, 398
    anatomy, 392–393
    blood flow
        local, 394, 395–396
        total, **39,** 394, 395–396
    blood volume, 392
    cholinergic receptors, 398
    coma and, 395
    intracranial pressure and, 399
    ischemia, 281, 395
    metabolic effects, 396–397
    neural control, 397–398
    oxygen uptake, 394, **395**
    prostaglandins and, 398
Cerebrospinal fluid, 398
cGMP. *See* Cyclic GMP
Channels, cell membrane, 77–82, 298. *See also*
        specific ions
    conductance, 80
    gating, 77, 309
    inactivation, 78
    ionic currents, 79–82
    myocardial cells, **81**
    receptor-controlled, 300
    rectification, 81
    voltage-regulated, 300, 305
Chemoreceptors, 225, **226,** 281, 376
    aortic body, 239
    arterial, 226, 239
    blood flow and, 240
    bradykinin and, 241
    cardiac, 241
    carotid body, 239
    cerebral, 242
    lactic acid and, 241
    nerve-ending, 241, 275
    pCO_2, 239
    pH, 239
    pO_2, 239
    prostaglandins and, 241–242
    reflex responses, 341
    serotonin and, 275

Chloride ions, 81, 85
Cholecystokinin, 416
Cholinergic nerves. *see* Nerves
Cholinergic receptors. *See* Receptors
Cholinesterase. *See* Acetylcholine
Choroid plexus, 398–399
Chronotropic effects, 102, 252
Chylomicrons, 352
Circulation. *See also* Regional circulations
    dynamic equilibrium in, 131
    fetal, 48, 358–360
    lymph, 351–354
    pulmonary, 42, 48
    systemic, 4, 44
Circus movement. *See* Reentry
Cold. *See* Temperature
Cole, K. S., 71
Collagen, 6, 186, 292
Collapsible tubes, 194–198
Colloid osmotic pressure, 340, 342, 345
Coma, 395, 399
Compensatory pause, 99, 159
Complex numbers, 199
Complex viscoelastic modulus, 199
Compliance
    definition, 186.
    delayed, 190
    vascular, 187–190, 202, 443–445
    ventricular, 120, 124
Computer-assisted tomography, 394, 475–476
Computers, digital, 206, 477–479
Conductance, ion, 80, **83,** 89, 165
Conduction
    antidromic (nerves), 266
    atrial, 73
    atrioventricular, 73–74
    block, 74, 106, 153–154
    cable theory, 90
    cell-to-cell, 66, 297, 311
    disturbances of, 153–155
    electrotonic, 89, 297
    local circuits and, 88, 163
    mechanisms, 88–90
    membrane potential and, 89
    propagated, 89
    Purkinje fiber, 75
    sodium ions and, 89
    velocity, 73, 74, 88
    ventricular, 63–64, 74–75
Contractility, myocardial
    definition, 100–101, 124–125
    indices of, 125–127
    physical training and, 285
Control theory, 232
Co-release of neurotransmitters, 259, 301
    ATP and norepinephrine, 263, 301
    neuropeptide Y and norepinephrine, 301
    VIP and acetylcholine, 276
Coronary arteries. *See also* Coronary circulation
    blood flow, 402, **403**

Coronary arteries (*continued*)
  compression of, 194, 403
  pressures, 124
  receptors, 407
Coronary chemoreflex, 275
Coronary circulation
  adenosine effects, 405–406
  anatomy, 400–401
  autoregulation, 406
  blood flow, **39,** 400, 401–404, 469
  blood volume, 400
  capillary density, 401
  cardiac work and, 404
  chemoreflex, 275
  cholinergic vasodilatation, 262
  control mechanisms, 404–407
  coronary sinus, 400
  dominance, left or right coronary, 400
  hypoxic vasodilatation, 405
  metabolite effects, 404, 405–406
  neural control, 406–407
  oxygen uptake, 401, 402, 404–405
  pulsatile flow, 402, **403,** 404
  receptors, smooth muscle, 407
  venous system, 400–401
Corticosteroids, 429
Cortisol, 281
Coughing, 381
Coupling
  electromechanical, 298
  excitation–contraction, 312–314
  optimum, 134
  pharmacomechanical, 298
  ventriculo–arterial, 133–135
Creep, 190
Critical closing pressure, 193
Critical damping (instruments), 457
Cross-bridge (muscle), 130, 292, 299, 315, 317
  attachment, 313, 320
  cycling rate, 130, 316, 317, 321
  elasticity, 319, 320, 321
  latched, 316
  model, 320
  rigor, 314, 316
  weak, 316
Cushing reflex, 399
Cutaneous circulation
  axon reflex, 266
  blood flow, **39,** 408–410
  blood volume, 409
  neural control, 410
  sweat-gland secretion and, 411
  in thermoregulation, 408, 409, 410, 448, 449
  vascular bed, 407
  vasodilatation, 265–266, 410–411
  veins, 408, 410, 449
Cyanide, 240
Cyclic AMP, 23, 69, 103, 270, 313
Cyclic GMP, 24
Cyclic nucleotides, 23–24

Damping (instrumental), 457
Dashpot (in models), 96, 319, **320**
DC response (instruments), 455, 456
Defense reaction. *See* Reflexes
Defibrillation, 163
Denervation of blood vessels, 259
Dense bodies, 291
Depolarization, 77, 83, 142, 309–311. *See also*
    Membrane potentials
  conduction and, 88, 89
  graded, 297, 312
  by K^+, 304
  partial, 300, 312
  threshold, 83, 84
Desensitization (receptors), 69, 295
Desmin, 67
Diabetes mellitus, 395, 432
Diacyl glycerol, 24
Diastasis, 113
Diastole, 5, 113
Diffusion, 292, 326, 338, 339, 340, 378
Digitalis
  action in myocardial failure, 137
  arrhythmias and, 164, 167–168
  Na^+–K^+ pump and, 82, 107
  parasympathetic effects, 167
  toxic effects, 156, 167, 168
Dimensions of vascular system, **7,** 39–42
Dinitrophenol, 88
Dipoles, electrical, 141–143
Disc, intercalated, 64
Discontinuous capillaries, 330
Dissociation constant, 25
Distensibility, 186
Diuretics, 137
Diving reflex, 244
Dopamine
  cardiovascular effects, 276
  presynaptic receptors, 263, 274, 276
Doppler effect, 472, 473
Doppler flowmeter, 473, 474
Down regulation of receptors. *See* Receptors
Driving pressure, 172
Ductus arteriosus, 358, 359, 360
Dynamic modulus of elasticity, 199
Dynamic response (instruments), 455–457

ECG. *See* Electrocardiography
Echocardiography, 476
Ectopic pacemakers, 155, 158, 160
Edema, 353, 440, 274
  neurogenic, 375
  peripheral, 136
  pulmonary, 136, 279, 365, 375
Effectors, 20, 290
Eicosanoids, 271
Einthoven, W., 143
Ejection fraction. *See* Ventricles
EJP. *See* Excitatory junction potentials

Elastance, ventricular, 126
Elastic modulus, 185
    complex, 199, **322**
    dynamic, 199
    incremental, 188
    phase angle, pressure/distension, 199
    static, 188
    Young's, 43, 185
Elasticity, vascular, 42–43, 118, 186–190
    arterial, 52, 187–190
    compliance, 186
    effect on pulsatile pressure, 199, 201, 211
    nonlinearity, **188,** 189
    parallel elastic element, 319
    pulse wave velocity and, 193
    series elastic element, 319
    smooth muscle and, 189, 321–323
    stiffness, 199
    stroke volume and, 200, 201
    wall thickness and, 185
Elasticity of materials, 184–186
Elastin, 6, 186, 292
Electrical stimuli in treatment of arrhythmias,
        164, 168–169
Electrocardiography
    in arrhythmias, **159,** 160–162
    bundle of His, 151
    central terminal, 149
    Einthoven triangle, **145**
    frequency content, 148, 456
    leads
        bipolar, 144, **145**
        unipolar, 149–151
    principles, 140–143
    terminology, waves, 146–149
    vector analysis, **145**
Electromagnetic flowmeter, 470–472
Electromechanical coupling. See Coupling
Electrotonic conduction, 89, 297
Embolism, 379
Emotional stimuli, 225, 285
End-diastolic pressure, volume. See Ventricles
Endocrine mechanisms, 21, 249, 267–271, 301–
        302
Endoperoxide synthetase, 272
End-pressure, 182, 183
Endothelial cells, 15–17, 186
    actin filaments, 17, 351
    angiotensin and, 16, 382
    antithrombogenic properties, 16, 383
    beta-adrenergic receptors, 15
    cholinergic receptors, 15
    clearance of vasoactive agents by, 16
    endothelial relaxing factor, 15, 260, 275, 296,
        378
    histamine, effects of, 274
    injury, response to, 17, 431
    pores between, 336, 340, 347–351
    prostaglandins and, 16, 272, 383
    pulmonary, 382–383
    purinergic receptors, 261, 301
    serotonin and, 275
    stress and strain, 174, 350
    transport through, 351
    vesicles in, 331, 351
Endothelium-derived relaxing factor (EDRF). See
        Endothelial cells
End-systolic pressure, volume. See Ventricles
Energy, hydraulic, 180–184, 458
    Bernoulli principle and, 182
    cardiac, 127–131
    in collapsible vessels, 194, 195
    efficiency, 129
    gravitational, 181–182, 381–382
    impedance and, 209, 211
    kinetic, 128, 181, 434
    oscillatory, 131
    potential (pressure-flow), 129, 181
    pressure, 181
    pulmonary circulation, 364
    steady-flow, 131
Enkephalins, 277
Entrance effects, 175
Epinephrine
    adrenal medullary, 123, 267, 301
    cardiac response to, 103, 268
    neurotransmitter, 25, 26
    plasma levels, 268
    receptors, 268–269
    vascular responses to, 268, 301, 379
Equations
    cable, 90
    electrical field, 142
    Fick, 35, 461
    Fourier series, 207, 208
    impedance, vascular, 211
    Laplace's law, 185
    mass action, 25
    Navier-Stokes, 204
    Nernst, 79
    Poiseuille, 174
    Reynolds number, 176
    transmission line, 204
    van't Hoff, 348
    viscosity, fluid, 173
    Windkessel, 202–203, 204
Equilibrium potentials, 79–82
Erythrocytes, 14, 429, 430
    aggregation of, 430, 432, 435
    androgenic hormones and, 430
    deformation of, 15, 333, 430, 431–432
    immature forms, 430, 432
    life-span, 430
    membrane, 430
    rouleaux formation, 430, 432
    sickling, 433
    spleen and, 432
    total volume, 440–442
    velocity, 335, 432, 434
Erythropoietin, 430

Evans blue dye (T1824), 440, 460
Excitation. *See also* Muscle, cardiac; Muscle,
        smooth, vascular
    abnormal, 156–158
    ionic basis, 71, 79–82, 299–301
    membrane potentials and, 83, 297, 299
    myocardial, 70–76
    refractory periods, 75, **76**
    supernormal period, 75
    threshold, 83, 85
    vascular smooth muscle, 297, 299–301
    without action potential, 297, 312
Excitation–contraction coupling, 312–314
    calcium and, 91–92
    electromechanical, 298
    messengers, 23–25
    myocardial, 91–92
    pharmacomechanical, 298
Excitatory junction potentials (EJP), 297, 312
Exercise, **39**, 262, 282–285
    blood osmolarity, 307
    cardiovascular responses, 282–285, 307, 369,
        405
    with denervated heart, **283**, 284
    in heat, 282, 450
    at high temperatures, 450–451
    oxygen consumption, 283
    physical training, 284–285, 439
    plasma volume and, 439
    and pulmonary circulation, 369
    vascular impedance and, 211
    vascular resistance, 282, 369
    vasomotor effects, 243, 283
    ventricular volume, 282
Extensibility, 184
Extracellular fluid, 4, 306
Extrasystoles. *See* Arrhythmias

Facilitated transfer (capillary), 399
Fahraeus-Lindqvist effect, 436
Failure, cardiac, 135–137
Faraday, Michael, 470
Feedback, 231, 233, 263, 274, 294
Femoral artery. *See* Arteries
Fenestrated capillaries, 330–331
Fetal circulation, 357
    blood flow, 358–360
    cardiac output, 360
    pulmonary, vascular resistance, 359
    pulmonary arterial pressure, 359
    pulmonary arterial wall, 359
Fiber matrix, capillary pores, 338, 350
Fibrillation, 161–163, 168–169
    atrial, 157, 162
    mechanism, 161–162
    ventricular, **159**, 162–163, 395
Fibrinogen, 430, 435, 436
Fick, diffusion law, 340

Fick method
    cardiac output, 460–463
    principles, 393, 460–461
Filamin, 67, 292, 317
Flow waves, 49, **50**, **213**. *See also* Blood flow
Flowmeters
    electromagnetic, 470–472
    nuclear magnetic resonance, 475
    ultrasonic
        Doppler, 473–474
        transcutaneous, 474
        transit time, 472–473
Fluorescence, catecholamine, 254, **255**
Flutter
    atrial, 161
    ventricular, 161
Foramen ovale, 358, 359
Force, gravitational, 181–182, 381–382, 439,
        447
Force, muscular
    active, 95, 314, 316
    muscle length, relation to, 92–93, **97**, 117–
        118, 309, 315
    myogenic, 190–191, 307–309
    passive, 314
    velocity, relation to, 96, 97, 117–122
Force–length relationship. *See* Force, muscular
Force–velocity relationship. *See* Force, muscular
Fourier analysis, 205
Fourier series, **206**, 207–208
Frank, Otto, 96, 119
Free radicals, oxygen-derived, 279, 304
Frequency analysis, 205–209
Frequency content, pressure and flow waves,
        207, 456
Frequency response (instruments), 455, **456**
Functional hyperemia, 303, 395

Gain, 233
Galileo, 171
Galvanometer, 143
Gap junctions, 64, 88
Gastrin, 416
Gating of channels, 77–78, 309
Genitalia, vasomotor responses in, 260
Giraffe, 43
Glomerulus, renal, 416–417, **418**
Glycosides, cardiac. *See* Digitalis
Ground substance, vessel walls, 6, 187, 291
Guanine nucleotides, 295
Guyton, A. C., 132, 133

Hales, Stephen, 171, 202, 457
Harmonics, 207
Harvey, William, 4, 12, 171
Head injury, 375, 399

Heart, 4–5. *See also* Atria; Cardiac output;
  Coronary circulation; Muscle, cardiac;
  Ventricles
  afterload, 94, 95, 101, 118, 124
  aging, effects of, 131
  anatomy, 62–67
  atrioventricular node, 62, 73–74, 251, 252
  AV block, 153–154
  basal metabolism, 129
  bundle of His, 63, 73, 153, 156
  chronotropic effects, 102, 252
  conduction in, 63–64, 124, 153–155
  contractility, 100–102, 124–127, 239, 255,
    285
  contraction, sequence of, 124
  coronary vessels, 400, 401
  coupling to arterial system, 133–135
  development of, 5, 72
  efficiency, 129, 130
  electrical field of, 140–143
  embryology, 5, 72
  events of cardiac cycle, 111–116
  excitation, 70–71
  failure, 135–137, 238, 270, 281, 440
  innervation, 67–68
  inotropic effects, 102, 252
  massage, 395
  muscle. *See* Muscle, cardiac
  neural control, 123, 250–253
  pacemaker, 5, 62, 71
  power, mechanical. *See* Energy, hydraulic
  preload, 118, 124, 125
  Purkinje fibers, 75, 88, 154, 160
  rate, **33**, 34, 58, 155, 405
  sinoatrial node, 62, 73, 156, 251, 400
  sounds, 115–116
  Starling's law, 96, 119–121, 132, 446
  stimulation-response latency, 75
  stroke volume, **33**, 34, 171, 255
  valves, 5, 113–114
  ventricular volume, 36, **37**, 125, 126, 477
  work of, 120, 129, 130
Heat. *See also* Temperature
  direct heating, 409, 448
  indirect heating, 409, 410
Hematocrit
  arterial and venous, 433
  definition, 433
  plasma skimming and, 15
  regional, 14, 433–434
Hemodynamics, 17
  anomalous viscosity, 173
  boundary layer, 176
  in branching systems, 212–214
  in circular systems, 131, 214–215
  in collapsible vessels, 194–198, 216
  in distensible vessels, 191–193
  elastic modulus, 43, 185, 188, 199, **322**
  elasticity of vessels, 186–191
  energy, hydraulic, 180–182

  entrance length, 175
  fluid laminae, 172–175
  fluid viscosity, 173
  impedance. *See* Impedance, vascular
  laminar flow, 172–175
  Laplace's law, 185
  Newtonian flow, 174
  Newtonian fluids, 173
  parabolic flow, 174
  Poieuille equation, 174, 212
  pulsatile flow, 198
  pulse wave velocity, 193
  reflected waves, 212–214
  resistance, vascular, 177–180
  Reynolds number, 176
  in rigid tubes, 171–184
  shear rate, 173, 174
  turbulent flow, 175, 176
  vasomotion and, 215–216
  velocity profile, 175
  viscosity of fluids, 173
  wall stress, 173, 185
Hemoglobin, 430, 433
Hemorrhage, 270, 279–282, 383, 440
Hepatic circulation
  architecture, 412
  autoregulation, 414
  blood flow, 413, 414
  capillaries, 330, 334
  innervation, 414
  lymphatic, 353
  neural control, 414–415
  pressures, 413
  receptors, smooth muscle, 414–415
  resistance, 414
  sinusoids, 329, 412
  vasomotor activity, 414–415
Hering-Breuer reflex, 375
Heterometric regulation (heart), 122
High altitude, effects of, 377
Histamine, 261, 266, 274, 301, 377, 379
  blood pressure, effect on, 274, 301
  capillary permeability and, 274, 337
  endothelial cells and, 296
  receptors, 24, 263, 274
Hodgkin-Huxley theory, 77–78
Homeometric autoregulation (heart), 122
Hooke's law, 186
Hormones. *See also* Epinephrine; Norepinephrine
  androgenic, 430
  antidiuretic, 271, 301, 422
  oxytocin, 271
  posterior pituitary, 271
  thyroid, 253
Hyaluronate, 354
Hydraulic energy. *See* Energy, hydraulic
Hydrogen, as indicator, 460
Hydrogen ions
  acidosis, 281, 304, **395**
  and cerebral circulation, 304, 396, 397

and membrane potential, 304
and muscle relaxation, 304
vasomotor effects, 304, 305, 397, 405
(5-)hydroxytryptamine. *See* Serotonin
Hypercapnia, 123, 241, 242, 304, 377
Hyperpolarization, 104, 167, 305
Hypertension
    pulmonary, 179, 273, 377, 378, 383
    systemic, 54, 131, 179, 234, 253, 271, 375,
        383, **395,** 399, 422
Hypervolemia, 440
Hypotension, 274, 281, 375
    orthostatic, 447
Hypothalamus. *See* Nervous system, central
Hypovolemia, 440
Hypoxia, 277–279
    arterial, 277–278
    carbon monoxide and, 277–278
    cardiovascular effects, 123, 163, 241
    cerebral, 242, 396
    chronic, 377, 440
    high-altitude, 377
    myocardial, 405
    primary reflex effects, 241
    prostaglandins and, 303
    respiratory effects, 241
    species-dependent effects, 377
    tissue, 278–279
    vasomotor effects, 302, 376, 377–378, 405
Hysteresis, 190–191

Imaging methods, heart and blood vessels, 475–
        477
    nuclear magnetic resonance, 475, 477
    radionuclide, 476–477
    ultrasound, 474
    x-ray, 475, 476
Impedance, vascular
    as afterload, 118, 190, 209
    changes with age, 53
    characteristic, 211
    concept, 209–212
    elasticity and, 190, 211, 296
    input, 209
    of linear systems, 208
    normal values, **210,** 370
    phase angle, 209
    pulmonary, 211, 370, 380
    pulse pressure and, 211
    reflections and, 210–211
    spectra, 118, 209, 211
    systemic, **210**
    ventricule–arterial coupling, 135
Indicator-dilution measurements
    capillary permeability, 345–346
    cardiac output, 463–466
    ejection fraction, 466
    mean transit time, 465, 466
    regional blood volume, 465–466

thermodilution, 460, 463
time-concentration curve, 463, **464**
Indocyanine green dye, 460
Indomethacin, 168, 272
Inertia, 113, 125
Inflammation, 273
Inotropic effects, 102, 252
Input resistance, 179, 209
Internal environment, 4
Interstitial space, 306, 353, 375
Intestine. *See* Splanchnic circulation
Intima, blood vessels, 6, 186
Intracranial pressure, 242, 392, 399
Ion channels. *See* Channels, cell membrane
Ion pumps, 81, **82,** 309, 310
Ions. *See specific ions*
Isoelectric period (ECG), 147
Isoenzymes, renin, 269
Isogravimetric experiment, 334, 343–345
Isometric contraction, 94, **95**
Isomyosins, 67
Isoproterenol, 24, 103, 253, 407
Isotonic contraction, 94, **95**
Isovolumic contraction of ventricle, 113, 120

J receptors. *See* Juxtacapillary receptors
Joint capsules, 354
Joule (unit), 129
Juxtacapillary (J) receptors (pulmonary), 243, 375
Juxtaglomerular apparatus. *See* Kidney

Kallikrein, 265, 411
Kidney. *See also* Renal circulation
    aldosterone and, 137
    capillaries, 334
    filtration rate, 238
    glomerulus, **418,** 419, 421
    juxtaglomerular apparatus, 136, 269, 272
    macula densa, 269
    neural control, 137, 421
    prostaglandin synthesis, 272, 422
    regulation of plasma volume, 438
    renin production in, 136, 238, 269–271
    salt and water balance, 136, 438
    vascular resistance, 238, 421
Kinetic energy. *See* Energy, hydraulic
Korotkow sounds, 459

Lactate, 281, 283
Laminar flow, 172–175
Landis, E. M., 343
Laplace's law, 117, 185
Latched cross-bridge, 316
Latent period, 75, 300
Lateral pressure, 182, 183
Leucocytes, 429, 431
    adherence to endothelium, 383, 431

Leukotrienes, 271, 273, 275, 379
Lidocaine, 165
Linearity
    impedance and, 208, 211
    instrumental, 455
    pressure–diameter nonlinearity, 208
    of pressure–flow relations, 208
    principle, 208
Liver. *See* Hepatic circulation
Load-bearing capacity (muscle), 316
Lobeline, 240
Local circuits (in conduction), 88, 163
Lung. *See* Pulmonary circulation; Respiration
Lymphatic system, 15, 351–354
    glands, 352
    lymph capillaries, 351
    lymph flow, 342, 353
    lymph protein, 352
    pulmonary, 354, 364
    of synovial joints, 354
    valves, 353

Macula densa. *See* Kidney
Manometers, 457–459
Mass action, law of, 25
MCFP. *See* Mean circulatory filling pressure
Mean circulatory filling pressure (MCFP), 14,
    42, 132, 214, 279, 443, 445
Mechanoreceptors, 225, **226,** 236–238. *See also*
        Baroreceptors, arterial
    cardiovascular, 226, 236–238
    juxtacapillary (J), 375
    pulmonary, 243, 375, 381
    ventricular, 238
Media, blood vessels, 6, 186
Medulla. *See* Nervous system, central
Membrane potentials. *See also* Excitation
    action, 71, 83–86, 297
    afterpotentials, 157, 168
    contraction without action potentials, 312
    depolarization, 84, 165, 297, 308, 309–
        311
    effect of hypoxia, 378
    equilibrium, 79–82
    excitatory junctional, 297, 312
    hyperpolarization, 79, 104, 166, 305
    ionic basis, 84–87, 309
    myogenic response, 308
    nodal, **84,** 86
    pacemaker, 86–87, 107
    patch-clamping, 79
    phases 0–4, **83,** 84–86
    regenerative, 85
    resting, 71, 156, 310
    sinoatrial, 84, 86
    smooth muscle, 309–311
    threshold, 83, 85
    voltage-clamping, 79
Membrane-stabilizing agents, 164–165, 166

Messengers, intracellular
    adenylate cyclase, 15, 24, 70, 295, 406
    Ca^{2+}, 23, 91, 313–314
    cyclic AMP, 23, 69, 103, 270
    cyclic GMP, 24
    guanine nucleotide proteins, 24, 295
    guanylate cyclase, 24
    phosphoinositides, 23
Metabolic rate, 57
Metabolism, anaerobic, 244, 303
Metabolites, circulatory effects, 261, 283, 302–
        304, 390, 397, 405
Microcirculation. *See also* Capillaries; Regional
        circulations
    arcades, 328
    architecture, 328–332
    arterioles, 326, 333, 337
    arteriovenous anastomoses, 328
    blood flow, 335, 432, 469–470
    definition, 10, 327
    metarterioles, 328
    pressures, 333–334
    resistance, 336
    shunts in, 328
    sphincters, 328, 337
    venules, 274, 326, 333, 337
Microspheres, 469
Model, nerve, Hodgkin-Huxley, 71, 77
Models
    cross-bridge, 320
    Guyton, 132, **133**
    lumped-component, 204, 444
    Maxwell, 319, **320**
    muscle, 319–321
    RC networks, 202, 203
    transmission-line, 204, **205**
    T-tube, 53
    uses, 18–20
    ventricular, 117, 474
    Windkessel, 19, 202–203, 204
Monoamine oxidase, 299
Murmurs, cardiovascular, 176, 367
Muscarinic cholinergic receptors. *See* Receptors
Muscle, cardiac. *See also* Heart; Membrane
        potentials; Ventricles
    actin filaments, 66, 67, 91
    action potentials, 71, 83–86
    active force, 95
    afterload, 94, 95, 101, 118
    all-or-none response, 98
    cell receptors, 69–70, 253
    contractile element, 122
    contractility, 100–102, 120
    contraction, 90
    cross-bridges, 91, 93
    depolarization, 77, 80, 84, 86–87
    efficiency, 129, 130
    excitation, 70–71
    excitation–contraction coupling, 91–92
    force–length relation, 92, **93,** 117–122

Muscle, cardiac (*continued*)
  force–stimulus frequency relation, 98, 123
  force–velocity relation, 96, **97**, 117–122
  heterometric regulation, 122
  histology, **65**
  homeometric regulation, 122
  hyperemia, functional, 303
  hypertrophy, 253
  hypoxia, effects of, 163
  injury, 163, 164
  innervation, 67–69, 251
  ischemia, 72, 163, 242
  isometric contraction, 94
  isotonic contraction, 94
  latency after stimulation, 75
  myosin, 66, 67
  oxygen uptake, 130, 402
  papillary muscle preparations, 94–96, 118
  postextrasystolic potentiation, 99
  posttetanic potentiation, 99
  preload, 94, 118
  proteins, contractile, 67
  receptors, 69–70
  refractoriness, 88
  repolarization, 85
  sarcomere, **65**, 66–67, 90, 92–94
  sarcoplasmic reticulum, **65**, 91
  series elastic element, 93
  Starling's law, 96, 119
  striations, **65, 66**
  structure, 64–67
  troponin, 91, 93
  velocity of shortening, 98, 121, 125, 130
  viscous afterload, 96
Muscle, skeletal, 104, 318
  hyperemia, functional, 303
  oxygen uptake, 261
Muscle, smooth, vascular
  absent action potentials, 312
  calcium and, 313–314, 315
  contractile apparatus, 315–317
  contractile proteins, 292, 317
  contraction, 314–317
  dense bodies, 291
  electromechanical coupling, 298, 313
  endothelium and, 16
  excitation, 297–298, 299–301
  force–length relation, 315
  force–velocity relation, 315
  injury, 16
  innervation, 254, 292, **293**, 298
  latency, 300
  load-bearing capacity, 316
  mechanical action, 314–319
  membrane potentials, 300
  metabolites, responses to, 302–306
  models, 319–321
  multi-unit, 298
  myogenic contraction, 190–191, 307–309
  oxygen sensor, 303

  pacemakers, 256, 259, 297, 391
  pharmacomechanical coupling, 298, 313
  quick-release, 316, 317–319
  receptors, 254, 261, 291, 294–296
  rigor, 307, 314
  single-unit, 298
  sinusoidal oscillation, 317, 321–323
  structure, 291–292
  summation in, 311
  tone, 255–257, 290, 298
  v_{max}, 316
  vascular resistance and, 290
  viscoelasticity of, 317, 318, 319, 321, **322**
  work, 323
Muscle models, 319–321
Muscle pumping, 12, 283, 447
Myocardium. *See* Muscle, cardiac
Myogenic contraction, 190–**191**, 307–309, 317,
    321
  autoregulation and, 391
  membrane potentials, 308
  and wall stress, 392
Myosin
  cross-bridge, 313–314, 319
  filaments, 292
  light chains, 313
  phosphatase, 313
  polymorphism, 67

Navier-Stokes equation, 204
Nernst equation, 79
Nerves. *See also* Nervous system, autonomic
  afferent, 219, 243
  antidromic conduction in, 266, 277
  baroreceptor, 226–227, **229**
  cardiac, 67–69, 250–253
  chemoreceptor, 227, **229,** 239
  chorda tympani, 264
  conduction, relation to diameter, 89, 225
  co-release of transmitters, 259, 263
  cranial, 226, 239
  efferent, 219
    parasympathetic, 123, 220, 223
    sympathetic, 123, 220, 222, 223, 231
  endings
    chemosensitive, 241–242
    mechanosensitive, 236–238
  ganglia, 220, 250, 262
  hypogastric, 262
  inhibition of transmitter release, 260, 263
  nonadrenergic, noncholinergic, 250, 263, 266–
    267
  parasympathetic, 67–68, 254, 260, 262
  presynaptic receptors. *See* Receptors
  pulmonary, 376
  purinergic, 266, 267, 411
  secretomotor, 264–266
  sensory, as reflex input, 243, 244

serotoninergic, 266, 267, 275
signal frequency, 256, 258, 297, 300
sympathetic adrenergic, 254, 376
"sympathetic afferent," 226, 237, 238, 239, 241
sympathetic cholinergic, 254, 411
transmitters, 20, 249, 259
varicosities, **293**, 299
vasoconstrictor, 254, 258–260
vasodilator, 260–263
Nervous system, autonomic, 20, 249–250. *see also* Nerves; Nervous system, central
enteric, 250
ganglia, 250, 262
neurotransmitters, 20, 266, 267. *See also* Acetylcholine; Epinephrine; Norepinephrine
oscillators, 222, 230
parasympathetic division, 249, 250
"sympathetic afferents." *See* Nerves
sympathetic division, 249, 250
vasoconstriction and, 254, 258–259
vasodilatation and, 259–263
Nervous system, central, 219–225
afferent signals, 221, 243
blood flow
cerebral, 393–395
local, 394, 395, 396
choroid plexus, 398–399
circulation. *See* Cerebral circulation
cortex, cerebral, 225
depressor area, 223, 224
hypothalamus, 220, 224, 225, 284, 286, 375
ischemia, 242
medulla, 220, 222–224, 286, 375
nucleus ambiguus, 222, 224, 250
oscillators, 222, 230
pressor area, 223, 224
reflexes and, 21, 230
spinal cord, 220, 222
vagal nuclei, 223, 250, 381
vasomotor "centers," 220, **221**, 222–223
ventricles, cerebral, 398
ventrolateral portion, 223
Neuropeptide Y (NPY), 223, 259
Neurotransmitters. *See* Nerves
Newborn, circulation in, **358**, 371
Newton, Isaac, 171, 178
Newtonian fluids, 173, 174, 435
Nexus (cell), 64, 88
Nicotine, 240
Nitric oxide, 260, 296
Nitroglycerin, 24
Nitrous oxide, blood flow measurement with, 393–394, 401, 467–469
Nonlinear systems, 208
Norepinephrine
automaticity and, 156, 164
cardiac effects, 166, 268
neurotransmitter, 25, 27, 220, 299

optical isomers of, 22
plasma levels, 268
presynaptic receptors, 263
prostaglandins and, 272
receptors, 166, 253, 254, 268–269, 301
release from adrenal medulla, 102, 267, 301
shortening velocity and, **97, 98**
uptake mechanisms, 299, 383
vascular effects, 123, 268, 314, **315**, 379
Normal distribution curve, 30
Normal limits, definition of, 30
NPY. *See* Neuropeptide Y
Nuclear magnetic resonance, 475, 477
Nutrition and blood volume, 439

Ohm's law, 177
Open-loop conditions, 231, 232
Optimization, 211
Orthostatic hypotension, 447
Oscillatory power, ventricular, 131
Osmolarity, 269, 306–307, 425, 429
Osmotic pressure, 338
Overdamping (instruments), 457
Oxygen. *See also* Hypoxia
and autoregulation, 391
chemoreceptors and, 239
debt, 283, 284
fetal blood, 359
free radicals, 279, 304
pO_2, 278, 303
poisoning, 279
sensors, local, 378
superoxide, 279
transport by blood, 430
uptake, 35, 284. *See also* Regional circulations
vasomotor effects, 302
Oxytocin, 271

P wave of ECG, 146, 159
Pacemakers, cardiac
automatic, 156
development of, 71
ectopic, 72, 158
factors determining rate, 72
ionic currents, 86–87
potentials, 86–87, 311
smooth muscle, 256, 259, 297, 311
Pain
bradykinin and, 242
sensory fibers and, 243
serotonin and, 266
Parabolic flow, 174
Parabolic velocity profile, **175**
Paracrine mechanisms, 21, 249, 271–277
Parallel elastic element (muscle), 319
Parasympathetic nerves. *See* Nervous system, autonomic
Parasystole, 155

Partition coefficient, 393, 467, 468
Patch-clamping, 79, **80,** 165
pCO$_2$. *See* Carbon dioxide
Peptides, vasoactive, 276–277, 281
Pericardium, 124
Permeability of membranes, 338, 341, **347**
pH. *See* Hydrogen ions
Pharmcomechanical coupling. *See* Coupling
Phase angles, 207, 322
Phonocardiography, 116
Phosphocreatine, 314
Phosphoinositides, 23, 24, 272, 295, 300, 313
Physical training, effects of, 284–285, 439
Pituitary hormones, 271
Plasma, 429
    albumin, 350, 429
    globulins, 430
    gravitational effects, 447
    measurement of volume, 440–442
    proteins, 306, 341, 435
    skimming, 15, 335
    volume, 436–440, 442
Platelet-derived growth factor, 431
Platelets, 273, 429, 431
Plethysmography, 51, 408
pO$_2$. *See* Oxygen
Poise (unit), 173
Poiseuille, J. L. B.
    equation, 174, 177
    experiments by, 171
    law, 212
Polarization of cell membrane, 76
Polymorphism, molecular, 67
Postextrasystolic potentiation, 99
Posttetanic potentiation, 99
Posture, erect, effects of
    on blood-volume distribution, 447
    hydrostatic pressure, 381, 447
    pulmonary circulation, 381–382
    renal circulation, 421
Potassium ions
    channels, 87, 275, 311
    depolarization by, 106
    effects, 106
    membrane potentials and, 106, 305, 306, 309
    myocardial injury and, 163
    Na$^+$–K$^+$ pump, 82
    pacemaker potentials and, 87, 106
    vasomotor effects, 304–306, 397
Power, hydraulic. *See* Energy, hydraulic
P-QRS interval (ECG), 148, 153
Pregnancy, effect on plasma volume, 439
Preload (muscle), 94, 118
Premature beats, 158–159
Pressure. *See also* Blood pressure
    alveolar, 364, 368, 379, 380
    atrial, 113–114
    central venous, 440, 445, 446
    critical closing, 193, 388
    diastolic, **44**–45, 201–202

differential, 125, 459, 467
driving, 172
energy, 181
extravascular, 195, 390
gradient, and flow, 198, 467
harmonics, 207
hydrostatic, 182, 381–382, 447
interstitial, 353, 375
intracranial, 242, 392, 399
intrapleural, 380, 381
intrathoracic, 381
intravascular, 195
lateral vs. end, 182, 183, 184, 458
mean circulatory filling, 14, 42, 132, 214,
    279, 443, 445
measurement of. *See* Pressure manometers
microcirculation, 49, 333–334, 460
osmotic, 338
pressure–volume "loops," **119,** 120, **126**
profile, **9, 372**
pulmonary artery "wedge," 365, 378
pulsatile, 43, 198–204
pulse, 45, 200–202, 466
reflected waves, 212
sinusoidal, 208
stroke volume and, 200–201
systolic, **44**–45, 201
tissue, 390, 421
transmural, 49, 184, 192, 195, 296, 368
venous, **33, 363**
zero reference level, 181, 364
Pressure, pulsations of
    age effects, 47, 53
    amplification of, 212
    attenuation of, 214
    distortion of, 457
    reflection of, 212
    transmission, 198, **213,** 371
    types A, B, C, 47
    wavelength, 212
Pressure manometers, 457–458
    catheter-mounted, 458
    servo-controlled, 460
    strain gauge, 458
Presynaptic inhibition. *See* Receptors: presynaptic
Procaine, 165
Programs, computer, 478
Prostaglandins, 241, 242, 266, 274, 383
    and hypoxia, 303
    receptors, 263
    synthesis, 272, 383
    types, 271–272
    vasomotor effects, 272, 377
Protein kinase C, 25
Proteins
    guanine nucleotide, 295
    plasma, 306, 341, 350, 429, 430, 435
Pulmonary circulation, 273, 357
    alveolar pressure, 368, 379
    blood flow, **366,** 367

blood volume, 373–375, 446
bronchial circulation, 361
capillaries, 51, 334, 361, 364–365, 369, 371, 379, 382
  compliance, 370
  emboli in, 379
  endothelium, 382–383
  exercise and, 369, 370
  extravascular forces on, 379–382
  fetal, **358**, 359
  hemodynamics, **363**
  hydraulic energy, 364
  hydrostatic effects, 364, 381–382
  hypertension. *See* Hypertension: pulmonary
  hypoxia, effects, 377–378
  impedance, vascular, 369–371
  innervation, 376
  interstitial space, 243, 375
  intrathoracic pressure, influence of, 381
  mechanoreceptors
    inflation, 243
    interstitial, 243
  neural control, 376
  pericapillary space, 365, 381
  pO_2 effects, 377–378
  posture and, 373, 381–382
  pressures, 362–364, 368, 371
  pulsatile flow, 371–373, **374**
  pulse transmission, 371, **372**
  pulse wave velocity, 370
  receptors, smooth muscle, 376–377
  resistance, vascular, **179**, 359, 367–369, 378, 379–380
  respiration and, 364, 379–381
  transit time, 372
  vascular structure, 360–361
  vasoconstriction, 376, 377, 379
  vasodilatation, 263, 369, 377
Pulsatile flow. *See* Blood flow
Pulsatile flow measurements
  electromagnetic, 470–472
  magnetic resonance, 475
  microcirculation, 469–470
  plethysmograph, 51, 470
  thermal, 474–475
  transcutaneous, 474
  ultrasonic, 472–474
Pulse wave velocity, 193, 194
  cardiovascular disease and, 193
  effects of age, 54
  elasticity and, 193, 296, 370
  pulmonary artery, 370, 371
Purine nucleotides, 273–274
Purkinje fibers, 64, 75, 88, 154, 156, 160

QRS complex (ECG), 146–148, 154
QT interval (ECG), 149, 164
Quick-stretch or release, 316, 317, **318**
Quinidine, 164, 165

Radian (unit), 207
Radiography, 476
Radioisotopes, 345, 402, 444, 460, 476
  carbon (^{11}C), 477
  chromium (^{51}Cr), 440
  iodine (^{131}I), 441
  iron (^{59}Fe), 441
  krypton (^{85}Kr), 468
  nitrogen (^{13}N), 477
  oxygen (^{15}O), 477
  phosphorous (^{32}P), 441
  potassium (^{42}K), 441
  technetium (^{99}Tc), 445, 477
  xenon (^{133}Xe), 460, 469
Radionuclide imaging, 476–477
RC product, 202–203
Reactive hyperemia. *See* Functional hyperemia
Receptor–response coupling. *See* Messengers, intracellular
Receptors, 21–23. *See also* Receptors, alpha-adrenergic; Receptors, beta-adrenergic
  adenosine triphosphate, 274
  affinities, 25
  agonists, 22
  antagonists, 23
  binding, **26**
  blockade, 164
  cardiac, 24, 69–70, 166, 253
  cholinergic, 22, 24, 260, 295–296, 376, 398
  concentration, 27
  desensitization, 69, 295
  dissociation constants, 25
  down regulation, 69, 253, 259
  histaminergic, 24, 263, 274
  messengers, 23–25
  presynaptic, 70, 261, 263, 270, 274, 294
  purinergic, 301
  selectivity, 25–27
  serotoninergic, 275
  spare, 27
  total numbers, 27
  up regulation, 69, 253, 259
  vascular smooth muscle, 294–296
Receptors, alpha-adrenergic, 22, 294
  affinities, 166, 294
  cardiac, 166, 253
  cerebral vessels, 294, 398
  coronary vessels, 407
  pulmonary vessels, 376
  regulation, up or down, 23
  vascular, 268, 299, 300
Receptors, beta-adrenergic, 22, 69–70, 294–295
  affinities, 295
  arrhythmias and, 164, 166
  capillary permeability and, 376
  cardiac, 24, 69, 253
  catecholamines and, 268–269
  coronary vessels, 407
  cyclic AMP and, 23, 70
  desensitization of, 69

Receptors, beta-adrenergic (*continued*)
    endothelial, 15
    heart failure and, 69, 136
    pulmonary vessels, 376
    regulation, up or down, 69, 253
    regulatory proteins and, 295
    vascular, 24, 69, 268, 294
Recruitment (capillary), 369
Red cell. *See* Erythrocytes
Redistribution of blood volume, 445–451
    exercise and, 450
    postural, 447
    temperature-related, 448–450
Reentry, 157–158, 163, 164
Reflected waves
    effect on pressure waves, 212
    impedance, effect on, 210
    principles, 212, 296
    sources of, 212
Reflection coefficient, capillary flux, 340
Reflexes, 21
    atrial stretch, 238, 258
    axon, 266, 274
    Bainbridge, 238
    baroreceptor, 225, 232, 376
    Bezold-Jarisch, 275
    cerebral ischemia, 242
    chemoreceptor, 224, 376
    Cushing, 399
    defense reaction, 233, 261, 285–286
    diving, 244
    effectors, 255
    Hering-Breuer, 375
    hypoxia, 239–241. *See also* Hypoxia
    integrated reactions to stress, 277–286
    J (juxtaglomerular) receptor, 375
    postural, 447
    thermoregulatory, 448–451
Refractory periods, **76,** 88, 157, 161, 164
Regional blood flow, methods of measurement
    clearance, 419
    electromagnetic, 470–472
    Fick principle, 413, 467
    indicator-dilution, 423, 465
    microcirculation, 469–470
    microspheres, 402, 406, 423, 469
    nitrous oxide, 393–394, 401, 467–469
    nuclear magnetic resonance, 475
    radioisotope, 394, 401
    thermodilution, 423, 463
    ultrasonic, 472–474
    plethysmography, 51, 408
    washout, 469
Regional circulations. *See specific circulations*
Regulation, cardiovascular, 20, 116–123
Renal circulation, 241. *See also* Kidney
    anatomy, 416–418
    arterioles, 416, 417
    autoregulation, 420
    blood flow, **39,** 419

blood volume, 420
    glomeruli, **418,** 419, 421
    hematocrit, 419
    neural control, 137, 421
    oxygen uptake, 420
    pressures, 420
    prostaglandins and, 272, 422
    resistance, vascular, 238, 421
    vasa recta, **417,** 418
    vasomotor responses, 421–422
Renin, 238, 269–271
    prostaglandin stimulation, 272
Renin-angiotensin system, 136, 269–271, 280,
        421–422
Reperfusion syndrome, 279
Resistance, vascular, 9, 18, 37, 177. *See also*
        Regional circulations
    changes with age, 53
    in collapsible vessels, 194
    control of, 178, 257, 443
    input, 179, 209
    interpretation of, 178–180
    Poiseuille, 177–180
    relation to pressure and flow, 177
    in series vs. parallel, 180
    systemic, **179**
    ventricular–arterial coupling, 135
Resistance vessels, 257, 443
Resonant frequency (instrument), 457
Respiration
    chemoreceptors and, 275
    effect on cardiac output, 380
    effect on heart rate, 380–381
    hypoxia and, 241, 278
    and pulmonary stretch receptors, 375
    and pulmonary vascular resistance, 379, 380
Resuscitation, cardiopulmonary, 168, 395
Reticulocytes, 430
Retrograde P waves, 159
Reynolds number, 176
Rigor, 307, 314, 316
Riva-Rocci method (blood pressure), 459–460

Salivary glands, 263, 264–265
Salt and water balance, 136
Salt intake, 270
Sarcomere. *See* Muscle, cardiac
Sarcoplasmic reticulum (SR), **65,** 66, 300
Secretin, 416
Secretomotor vascular effects, 411, 264–265
Sensitivity (instrument), 455
Sensors. *See* Baroreceptors, arterial; Chemorecep-
        tors; Mechanoreceptors
Series elastic element (muscle), 319, **320**
Serotonin ([5-]hydroxytrypamine), 275–276,
        383,
    cardiovascular effects, 275, 301, 377, 379
    effect on chemoreceptors, 275
    in neurons, 223

pain and, 266
  receptors, 25, 241, 263
Servomechanisms
  hot-film anemomemeter, 474
  manometer, 460
Set point, 233
Shear rate, 173, 432, 435
Shear stress, 272
  in blood vessels, 173, 174
  permeability and, 350
Shock, circulatory, 281, 383, 420
Sickle cell anemia, 433
Side-struts (muscle), 67
Signal-averaging, 151
Similarity, principle of, 55
Sinoatrial (SA) node, **63**, 73
  blood supply, 400
  innervation, 251
  membrane potentials, 87, 156
  rate of firing, 156
Sinus arrhythmia, 155, 375, 380
Sinus venosus, 5, 72
Sinusoidal stress, 317, 321–323
Sinusoidal waves, 205–208, 317
Sinusoids (capillary)
  bone marrow, 329
  hepatic, 329, 412
  splenic, 329
Skeletal-muscle circulation
  architecture, 422–423
  arteriovenous shunting, 425
  autoregulation, 424
  blood flow, 423
  blood volume, 424
  exercise, effects of, 423
  metabolites and, 422, 425
  neural control, 424
  oxygen consumption, 423–424
  receptors, blood vessels, 424
  vasomotor responses, 424, 425
Skin. *See* Cutaneous circulation
Skinned muscle fibers, 306
Sleep, 233
Smooth muscle, vascular. *See* Muscle, smooth,
    vascular
Sodium–calcium exchange, 82, 105, 106, 168
Sodium ions, 269
  action potential and, 80–81, 84–85, 310
  cardiovascular effects, 105, 236
  channel conductance, 89, 165
  channels, 87
  conduction and, 89
  excretion, 136
  $Na^+ - K^+$ pump, 82, 236, 310
  pacemaker potential and, 87
Sodium–potassium pump, 82, 236
Somatostatin, 277
Spare receptors, 27
Spectral analysis, 206
Spinal cord. *See* Nervous system, central

Spinal shock, 222
Splanchnic circulation, 411, **412**
  anatomy, 412
  blood flow, **39,** 413
  blood reservoir, 413
  blood volume, 413, 448
  intestines, 241, 415
  liver. *See* Hepatic circulation
  pressures, 413
  resistance, 278
  spleen, 415, 432
  stomach, 415
  vasoconstriction, 279, 285, 449, 450
  vasodilatation, 263, 268, 416
Spleen. *See* Splanchnic circulation
SR. *See* Sarcoplasmic reticulum
ST segment (ECG), 148
Staircase phenomenon (muscle). *See* Treppe
Standard deviation, 30
Starling, E.
  on capillary exchange, 341, **342**
  law of the heart, 96, 119
  resistor, 195
Steady-flow power, ventricular, 131
Step-function, 318
Stiffness (smooth muscle), 315, 316, 319
Stomach. *See* Splanchnic circulation
Strain, physical definition, 184
Strain-gauge, 458
Stress relaxation, 190, 308, 317
Stretch activation (smooth muscle), 321. *See also*
    Myogenic contraction
Stretch receptors. *See* Baroreceptors, arterial;
    Mechanoreceptors
Stroke volume, 34, 171, 255. *See also* Ventricles
  measurement, imaging, 474, 475
  pulse pressure and, 200–201, 466–467
Submersion, effects of, 244
Substance P, 261, 277, 383
Summation, 311
Supernormal period, **76**
Superoxide
  dismutase, 279
  radicals, 279
Surface tension, alveolar, 379
Surfactant, 379
Sweating, 224, 265, 266, 411
Sympathectomy, 68, 259, 262, 278
Sympathetic nervous system. *See* Nerves; Ner-
    vous system, autonomic
Sympathoadrenal system, 267
Synovial joints, 354
Systole, 5, 113

T wave (ECG), 146, **147,** 148
Tachycardia, 155
  atrial, 154
  ventricular, 154
Temperature, 266. *See also* Heat
  acclimatization, 451

Temperature (*continued*)
  core, 409, 450
  cutaneous regulation of, 224, 265
  environmental, cardiovascular effects of, 448–451
  fever, effect of, 422
  hypothalamus and, 224
  pyrogens, effect of, 422
  sensors, 243, 409, 448
  skin, 448
Tension, 185. *See also* Force, muscular
Tension–time index, 130, 405
Thebesian veins, 400
Thermodilution, 460, 463
Thermoregulation, 408–410
Thompson, D'Arcy, 58
Thoracic duct, 352
Threshold. *See* Membrane potentials
Thrombi, 178, 429
Thrombin, 383
Thromboxanes, 271, 273
Thyroid hormone, 253
Tissue hypoxia, 278–279
Tomography, 475, 476, 477
Tone, vascular, 215, 255–257, 298, 306, 407
Transducers, 455
  baroreceptors as, 234–236
  blood flow, 470–475
  calibration, 455, 472
  catheter-mounted, 458, 471
  DC response, 455
  distortion by, 457
  dynamic response, 455
  electrical, 454
  force, 457
  frequency response, 455, **456,** 459
  pressure, 457–459
  sensitivity, 455
  stability, 455
  ultrasonic, 472–474, 476
Transmission line models, 204
Transverse tubules, 66
Treppe, 98, 123
Triggered activity, 156–157, 168
Triple response (skin), 266, 274
Tropomyosin, 314
Troponin, 91, 103, 313
Turbulent flow, 175, 176, 183

Ultrasound
  flowmeters, 472–474
  imaging, 474, 476
Umbilical vessels, 307, 359
Unconsciousness, 395
Underdamping (instruments), 457
Up regulation of receptors. *See* Receptors
Uterus, 263, 271

v_{max}. *See* Velocity
Valsalva maneuver, 381
Valves
  cardiac, 113, 114
  lymphatic, 353
  veins, 13
van't Hoff equation, 348
Vasa vasorum, 10
Vascular beds. *See* Regional circulations
Vascular smooth muscle. *See* Muscle, smooth, vascular
Vascularity of tissues, 257
Vasoactive intestinal peptide (VIP), 276, 296, 377, 383, 398
Vasoconstriction, 254, 258–259
  pulmonary, 376, 377
Vasodilatation
  cholinergic mechanisms, 260–261
  in functional hyperemia, 303, 395, 416
  maximum, 257
  metabolic, 261, 283, 302–304, 390, 425
  parasympathetic cholinergic, 262–263
  pulmonary, 369, 377
  purinergic, 273
  by reduced constriction, 259, 262, 263
  secretomotor, 264–266
  sympathetic cholinergic, 261–262
Vasomotion, 215–216, 253–256, 296
Vasopressin. *See* Antidiuretic hormone
Vectorcardiography, 146, 151–152
Veins, 11–13. *see also* Regional circulations
  as blood reservoir, 12, 257–258
  blood volume, **12,** 43, 215
  collapse of, 194
  coronary, 400
  distensibility, 215
  jugular, 194, 393
  mesenteric, 295, 297, 391
  portal, 295, 297, 304, 391, 412
  pulmonary, 365–366
  receptors, smooth muscle, 294, 295
  Thebesian, 400
  umbilical, 359
  valves in, **13**
  venae cavae, 295, 296, 412
  venomotor activity, 215, 258, 280, 373, 447, 449
  venous return, 132, **133**
  vertebral, 393
Velocity
  of blood, 41, **42,** 335
  kinetic energy and, 181
  of muscle shortening, 98, 121, 125, 130, 316
  pulse wave. *See* Pulse wave velocity
  Reynolds number, relation to, 176
  turbulence and, 175
  v_{max} (maximum unloaded shortening velocity), 98, **99,** 125, 316
Velocity profiles
  aortic arch, 51, **52**

blunt, 175
boundary layer and, **176**
entrance effects, 175, **176**
parabolic, **175,** 434
pulsatile, 198
Venomotor tone. *See* Veins: venomotor activity
Venous return, 132, **133**
Ventricles. *See also* Heart; Muscle, cardiac
    afterload, 124, 130
    compliance of, 120, 124
    conduction in, 63–64, 74–75
    contractility, 100–102, 120, **121,** 124–127
    coupling to arteries, 133–135
    diastole, 5
    ejection fraction, 36, 113, 125, 466
    elastance, 126
    end-diastolic volume, 36, **37,** 477
    end-systolic volume, 36, **37,** 125, **126,** 477
    extrasystoles, **159,** 160, 168
    failure. *See* Heart: failure
    fibrillation, 157, **159,** 161, 162, 168
    filling pressure, 194
    filling time, 123
    flutter, 161, 168
    force–length–velocity relations, 117–122
    function curves, 120, **121,** 125
    geometric shape of, 117
    heterometric regulation, 122
    homeometric regulation, 122
    interaction, 124
    isovolumic periods, 113, 120
    mechanoreceptors, 236, 238
    models of, 117
    pericardium, 124
    preload, 124
    pressure–volume relations, 119–120, **126,** 128
    Purkinje system. *See* Purkinje fibers
    residual volume, 36, 113
    Starling's law, 119–121
    stroke volume, **33,** 36, 474
    systole, 5
    tachycardia, 154, 161
    volume load, 130
    work of, 120, 127–131
Ventricular–arterial coupling, 133–135
    optimum, 211

reflected waves and, 135
Venules. *See* Microcirculation
Verapamil, 166
VIP. *See* Vasoactive intestinal peptide
Viscoelasticity, 184
Viscoelasticity of blood vessels, 190–191, **200**
Viscosity
    anomalous, 435
    blood, 14, 434–436
    definition, 173
    fluids, **173**
    solids, 184
    tube-diameter effect, 436
    yield stress, 436
Voltage-clamping, 79
Volume (blood, plasma, red cells). *See* Blood
        volume
Volume conductor, 141
Vortex
    in circus movement, 158
    in turbulent flow, 175
Vulnerable period, 75

Wall, vascular
    components, 186, **187**
    tension, 185
Water balance, 136
Waterfall, vascular, 198, 382, 393
Wave length, aorta, 58
Wave reflection, 46, 47, 53–54, 296
Wave velocity. *See* Pulse wave velocity
Weightlessness, 439, 447
Wenckebach phenomenon, 154
Wheatstone bridge, 458
Windkessel, 19, 202–203, 204
Work, cardiac. *See* Ventricles

X-ray diffraction, 317
X-rays, 475, 476

Yield stress, 436
Young's modulus of elasticity, 185